D0805433

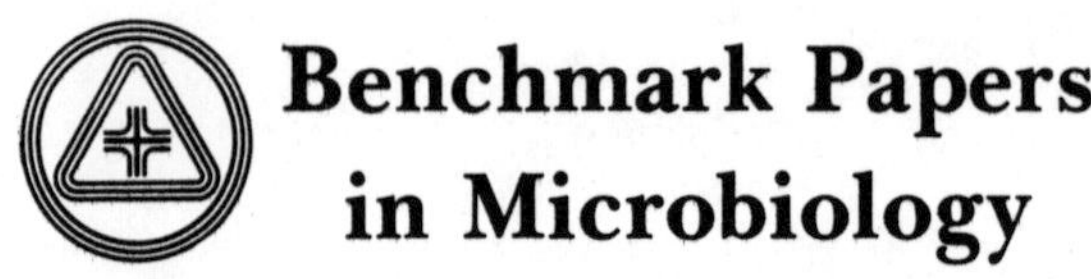

Series Editor: Wayne W. Umbreit
Rutgers University

Published Volumes and Volumes in Preparation

MICROBIAL PERMEABILITY
John P. Reeves
CHEMICAL STERILIZATION
Paul M. Borick
INFLUENCE OF TEMPERATURE ON MICROORGANISMS
J. L. Stokes
MICROBIAL GENETICS
Morad Abou-Sabé
MOLECULAR BIOLOGY AND PROTEIN SYNTHESIS
Robert Niederman
MICROBIAL GROWTH
P. S. S. Dawson
MICROBIAL METABOLISM
M. W. Doelle
ANTIBIOTICS AND CHEMOTHERAPY
M. Solotorovsky
MICROBIAL PHOTOSYNTHESIS
June Lascelles
INDUSTRIAL MICROBIOLOGY
Richard W. Thoma
MICROBIAL VIRUSES
S. P. Champe
TISSUE CULTURE AND BASIC VIROLOGY
R. J. Kuchler
MARINE MICROBIOLOGY
C. D. Litchfield

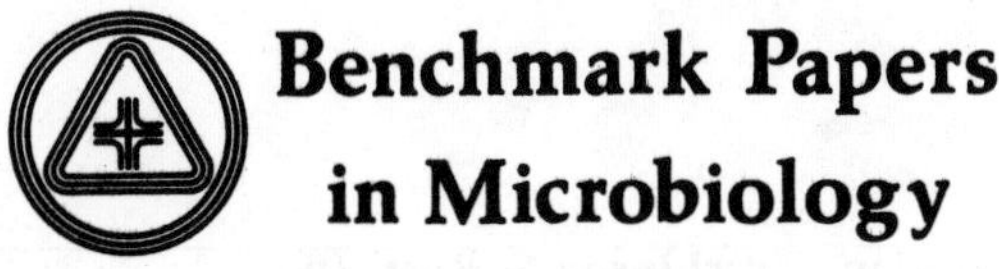

A *BENCHMARK*™ Books Series

CHEMICAL STERILIZATION

Edited by
PAUL M. BORICK
Ethicon, Inc.

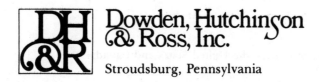

Dowden, Hutchinson & Ross, Inc.
Stroudsburg, Pennsylvania

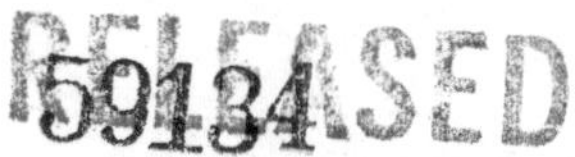

Library of Congress Catalog Card Number: 73-4967
ISBN: 0-87933-036-8

Library of Congress Cataloging in Publication Data

Borick, Paul M 1924- comp.
Chemical sterilization.

(Benchmark papers in microbiology)
1. Sterilization--Addresses, essays, lectures.
2. Anti-infective agents--Addresses, essays, lectures.
I. Title. [DNLM: 1. Sterilization. WA 240 C517 1973]
QR69.B67 614.4'8 73-4967
ISBN 0-87933-036-8

Manufactured in the United States of America.

Exclusive distributor outside the United States and Canada:
John Wiley & Sons, Inc.

Acknowledgments and Permissions

The following papers have been reprinted with the permission of the authors and copyright owners.

Academic Press, Inc.—*Advances in Applied Microbiology*
"Chemical Sterilizers"
"Cold Sterilization Techniques"

Academic Press, London—*Journal of Applied Bacteriology*
"The Mode of Action of Antibacterial Agents"
"The Sporicidal Properties of Chemical Disinfectants"

American Pharmaceutical Association—*Journal of Pharmaceutical Sciences*
"Interaction of Quaternary Ammonium Bactericides with Biological Materials. I: Conductometric Studies with Cephalin"
"Interaction of Quaternary Ammonium Bactericides with Biological Materials. II: Insoluble Monolayer Studies"
"Antibacterial Activity of Mixtures of Quaternary Ammonium Compounds and Hexachlorophene"

American Society of Hospital Pharmacists—*American Journal of Hospital Pharmacy*
"Buffered Glutaraldehyde: A New Chemical Sterilizing Solution"
"Classical and Modern Methods of Antimicrobial Treatment"

American Society for Microbiology
Applied Microbiology
"Limitations of Thioglycolate Broth as a Sterility Test Medium for Materials Exposed to Gaseous Ethylene Oxide"
"Sporicidal Effect of Peracetic Acid Vapor"
"Sporostatic and Sporocidal Properties of Aqueous Formaldehyde"
"Resistance of *Pseudomonas* to Quaternary Ammonium Compounds"

Journal of Bacteriology
"Effect of Inorganic Cations on Bacterial Activity of Anionic Surfactants"

American Sterilizer Company—*The Journal of Hospital Research*
"Chemical Disinfection and Antisepsis in the Hospital"

Annual Reviews, Inc.—*Annual Review of Microbiology*
"Gaseous Sterilization"

Association of Official Analytical Chemists, Inc.—*Journal of the Association of Official Analytical Chemists*
"Turbidimetric Evaluation of Bacterial Culture Resistance in Disinfectant Testing"

British Medical Association—*British Medical Journal*
"Contamination of Hospital Disinfectants with *Pseudomonas* Species"
"Cleaning and Disinfection of Hospital Floors"
"Methods for Disinfection of Hands and Operation Sites"

International Association of Milk, Food and Environmental Sanitarians, Inc.—*Journal of Milk and Food Technology*
"The Use of Antimicrobial Soaps and Detergents for Hand Washing in Food Service Establishments"

MacNair-Dorland Company—*Soap and Chemical Specialties*
"Detergent/Iodine Systems"
"Antiviral Action of Germicides"
"Evaluation of Disinfectants"
"Testing Sterilizers, Disinfectants, Sanitizers and Bacteriostats"
"Organotins: Biological Activity, Uses"
"Disinfectant Fogging Techniques"
"Antibacterial Residuals on Inanimate Surfaces"

Marcel Dekker, Inc., New York—*Disinfection*
"The Spore Problem"

Morgan-Grampian Publishers Ltd.—*Manufacturing Chemist and Aerosol News*
"Resistance of Bacterial Spores to Heat, Disinfectants, Gases and Radiation"

Society of Cosmetic Chemists of Great Britain—*Journal of the Society of Cosmetic Chemists*
"Fundamentals of Microbiology in Relation to Cleansing in the Cosmetics Industry"

John Wiley & Sons, Inc.—*Biotechnology and Bioengineering*
"Sterilization with Gaseous Ethylene Oxide: A Review of Chemical and Physical Factors"

Series Editor's Preface

Much of what man can do to prevent deterioration of his products or to ensure his safety from pathogens is dependent upon the control of microorganisms, and an important part of this control is dependent upon the use of chemical substances, usually agents having little specificity. Important as it is, this area tends to be neglected by the average microbiologist, in part because the information is scattered in journals not routinely used, in part because one is usually concerned with a specific organism rather than with sterilization in general. The complex technology, the variety of materials employed, the variation of conditions that must be met—even the methods that one can employ to select proper agents for the circumstances presented—are not as widely known as they should be. We are therefore delighted to have Dr. Borick, who has been instrumental in solving several of the problems of the field, select for us papers that summarize the nature of the problems, an approach to their solution, and some experience with a variety of agents. True, the effects obtained through sterilization depend on the nature of the organism, its physiological state, the agent employed, the conditions of application, and the method used to measure the effect. But what nature, what state, and what conditions are specifically indicated? It is to these questions that the articles selected address themselves. This collection adds to our readily available knowledge of an important area of microbiology.

Wayne W. Umbreit

Contents

Contents by Author

Introduction

Chemical sterilization is a complex technology that requires the expertise of the microbiologist experienced in the use of a wide variety of antimicrobial agents. A chemically prepared solution may be very effective in rendering a product or package sterile under a given set of circumstances, only to show sterility failure when the conditions are altered slightly. As an example, a wide range of antimicrobial agents may render a product sterile when vegetative bacterial cells of a gram-positive variety are present, but these may be ineffective when a wider spectrum of organisms, including gram-negatives, acid-fast types or spores, are to be destroyed.

Borick, in his work with chemosterilizers, showed that not only the intended use of the chemical agent, but also the conditions associated with its use, should be taken into consideration. More and more work is being done today on the microbial flora of numerous items in conjunction with good manufacturing practices. The reason is that, in defining the conditions required for sterilization, the process for achieving sterility is simultaneously defined. Obviously, one would not select an agent that failed to show antitubercular activity when tubercle bacilli were present in or on the product to be sterilized.

In this volume a series of papers were selected that will guide scientists or technical personnel in this task. The work by Hugo on the mode of action of antibacterial agents is useful in demonstrating the relative complexity of the action of disinfectants as a manifestation of their general nonspecificity. Some disinfectants have been used for years without an awareness of their "modus operandi." However, in studying the mechanism of their action, and knowing the site of attack (i.e., whether at the cellular level, through disruption of the cell, action through enzyme specificity, ultimate destruction of the plasma membrane, etc.) it has become possible for microbiologists to seek more effective agents to kill microbial cells, that is, more effective chemical sterilizing agents.

The use of ethylene oxide as a chemical sterilizing agent has gained wide acceptance because of its action where other methods could not be employed. The papers by Bruch and by Ernst and Doyle point out the pitfalls encountered if certain chemical or physical factors are overlooked in the use of this chemosterilizer. One must take into account whether or not stratification or diffusion barriers, as well as moisture-reducing or polymerization effects, are encountered. Because of its sporicidal nature, the use of ethylene oxide can be extremely effective, but it can also be detrimental, when various parameters are not defined. The aforementioned reports discuss the conditions to be considered in the use of this chemical agent.

The introduction of relatively new chemosterilizers requires a great deal of effort and cooperation on the part of many scientists, if we are to explore fully the factors involved in the destruction of microbes. Glutaraldehyde and peracetic acid were also shown to be sporicidal, and their use in chemical sterilization is well justified. Formaldehyde, which also shows sporicidal properties, has long been used in both the vapor and the liquid states. Russell discusses the resistance of bacterial spores to heat, disinfectants, and gases, and he concludes that spores which are highly resistant to one process are not necessarily insensitive to another process.

Steiger-Trippi, in discussing classical and modern methods of antimicrobial treatment, shows that beta-propiolactone, among other agents, is also an effective sporicide but emphasizes the appropriate precaution to be taken when applying it.

Klein and Deforest tested various classes of germicides and showed their effectiveness as viricidal agents as well as the differences in resistances among viruses. Laboratory data obtained from work with viruses must be extrapolated in terms of conditions during actual use. Claims for the ability of a given disinfectant to destroy influenza or other viruses, in addition to showing *in vitro* destruction of the virus, must show that spread of the disease can be prevented through use of the chemical agent. Indeed, reports by Burdon and Whitby and by Adair, Geftic, and Gelzer demonstrate that resistant bacteria such as *Pseudomonas* sp. can develop, even though the germicide had been shown previously to be effective in destruction of the same strain.

Various cleaning and disinfecting techniques are suggested that would help to eliminate microorganisms from the hospital or other working environments. Fogging techniques may be useful in cases in which the location is inaccessible to physical cleaning and where the area can be saturated with an effective antimicrobial agent. Fogging may act as an additional aid in a closed room or suite after the walls and floors have been thoroughly scrubbed and disinfected. Spaulding, in his treatise on chemical disinfection and antisepsis in hospitals, discusses not only the fogging and aerosolized techniques employed in hospitals but also the selection and use of chemical agents required for these applications.

Walter and Foris attempted to develop the relatively simple technique of obtaining uniformly contaminated surfaces to permit comparison of the efficacy of various antibacterial residuals. Other work shows the effectiveness of antimicrobial agents in a wide variety of applications, even at relatively low concentrations.

A great deal of controversy prevails in the use of antimicrobial agents in chemical sterilization, and Borick and Pepper discuss some of the problems encountered in working with microbial spores. Various factors that must be considered to improve the efficacy of chemical sterilizing agents are presented also.

It is the intent of this volume to present topics that will aid the scientist in selecting those antimicrobial agents and conditions that will achieve the desired end result—sterility. Although a great deal of work has been done in the past decade on new antimicrobial agents, as well as on the methodology for establishing their efficacy under varying circumstances, much still remains to be accomplished. Antiseptics and disinfectants may be active against vegetative microbial cells in minutes but may not have the strong penetrating power required to assure complete efficacy under trying circumstances.

Chemosterilizers, which are extremely potent because of their sporicidal properties, require long periods of time to accomplish the end result. The three to ten hours required to achieve sterility are often not available. Where spores are occluded or contained in a matrix, chemosterilizers do not have the penetrating power to attack the spore and destroy it. Wetting agents have been added to enhance their activity, but these can also increase the toxicity or impart sensitizing abilities, and so there may be some difficulty in working with them. Chemists, microbiologists, and other scientific personnel working together must set as their future objectives the discovery of antimicrobial agents that will rapidly destroy all microbial forms in the shortest possible time under varying circumstances.

Editor's Comments on Papers 1 through 6

1 **Borick:** *Chemical Sterilizers (Chemosterilizers)*

2 **Hugo:** *The Mode of Action of Antibacterial Agents*

3 **Opfell and Miller:** *Cold Sterilization Techniques*

4 **Bruch:** *Gaseous Sterilization*

5 **Ernst and Doyle:** *Sterilization with Gaseous Ethylene Oxide: A Review of Chemical and Physical Factors*

6 **Doyle, Mehrhof, and Ernst:** *Limitations of Thioglycolate Broth as a Sterility Test Medium for Materials Exposed to Gaseous Ethylene Oxide*

The first three articles were selected for their scientific merit, the practical uses of antimicrobial agents, and the theoretical aspects of their potential modes of action.

In the papers by Borick and by Opfell and Miller, those chemicals are shown which have sporicidal properties and may be considered to be chemosterilizers. It will be noted from these papers that the numbers of compounds contained in this category are extremely selective in spite of the fact that a wide variety of chemical agents show diversified antimicrobial properties. Hugo, in looking at the complexity of the action of disinfectants, ventures an opinion that it is not possible or even scientifically valid to try to determine the "mode of action" of a nonspecific drug by a study, however detailed, of a single changeable property.

In the final three papers of this group, work with gaseous sterilization is reviewed. In the publications by Bruch and by Ernst and Doyle we are given the benefit of years of experience by these microbiologists with ethylene oxide as a chemical sterilizing agent. They have pioneered in this relatively new technology and have established some of the basic parameters necessary in coping with problems involved in gaseous sterilization. The paper by Doyle, Mehrhof, and Ernst discusses the limitations that can occur as a result of the diffusion of this gaseous sterilizer, as well as the limits of the medium employed in sterility testing.

Reprinted from *Advan. Appl. Microbiol.* **10**, 291–312 (1968)

1

Chemical Sterilizers (Chemosterilizers)

PAUL M. BORICK

Ethicon, Inc., Somerville, New Jersey

I. Introduction

The continuous introduction into world markets of new materials that cannot be heat sterilized necessitates the use or development of other means of sterilization. A major modern method for this purpose is based on the use of chemical agents. Selectivity must be exercised in the employment of chemical compounds, however, as only those which show sporicidal activity can be classified as chemical sterilizers. A wide variety of antimicrobial agents is available, but in most instances these do not kill resistant bacterial spores. Microbicides are specifically limited to the destruction of the type of organism prefixed to *cide*, e.g., bactericide refers to killing of bacteria, fungicide to fungi, viricide to viruses and sporicide to spores, both bacterial and fungal. Since bacterial spores are the most difficult to destroy, sporicides may be considered synonymous with chemosterilizers. These may be defined as chemical agents which, when utilized properly, can destroy all forms of microbiological life, including bacterial and fungal spores, tubercle bacilli, and viruses.

The term chemosterilizer should be distinguished from the term chemosterilant as reported in "Chemical Processing," (Anonymous, 1964). Chemosterilizers are chemical compounds which are used to destroy all forms of microbiological life whereas chemosterilants are chemical substances used to sterilize insects and render them incapable of reproduction on mating with nonsterile partners. The term chemosterilant is unfortunately sometimes employed in chemical sterilization literature; it is suggested that such misuse of the term be avoided, and the term chemosterilizer be substituted to prevent further confusion.

Although, by definition, disinfectants and antiseptics should be capable of destruction of pathogenic microorganisms, they do not destroy the spores of pathogenic clostridial or aerobic bacilli. Chemicals intended for this use then cannot be classified as chemosterilizers, and it should be realized that they find only limited application. The chemical sterilizer, in addition to destroying fungi and bacterial spores, must be effective in destroying all types of microorganisms, including *Mycobacterium tuberculosis* within the recommended time. It should also be effective in destroying viruses, thus preventing the occurrence of viral diseases such as hepatitis when used to sterilize contaminated instruments, needles, or other medical equipment. Since only man is known, at present, to be susceptible to hepatitis viruses A and B and no laboratory methods are available for the evaluation of chemical sterilizers, it must be assumed that if other resistant viruses are destroyed, the hepatitis virus will also be killed. In this country, commercial use of chemical sterilizers is governed by the Federal Insecticide and Rodenticide Act and its control falls within the jurisdiction of the U.S. Department of Agriculture (USDA). Since test methods are not available for hepatitis virus, the USDA is most interested in this problem to ensure that chemical sterilizer claims are justified.

In the evaluation of a chemosterilizer, one must take into account the intended use and the conditions associated with its use. These applications may include wide areas, e.g., medical, hospital, and pharmaceutical use, food technology or sterilization of interplanetary space objects. If proven processes such as heat sterilization or irradiation cannot be employed, the proper chemical sterilizer should be selected. One must consider, then, the circumstances under which the chemosterilizer is to be utilized. Time, concentration, numbers and types of microorganisms as well as the type of material to be sterilized are important factors. If ethylene oxide gas were to be used, the limitations associated with this sporicide must be borne in mind. For example, many hours may be required with proper conditions of humidity, temperature, pressure, and gas concentration at the site of the microorganism. If the material to be sterilized were wrapped in a gas-impermeable membrane, the sporicidal agent, no matter how effective, could not reach the site to be sterilized.

Although chlorine is recognized by microbiologists as being a highly active antimicrobial agent with sporicidal properties, caution must be exercised in the presence of organic matter since the chlorine concentration, with a concomitant loss in activity, rapidly diminishes upon interaction with any form of organic material. Hence, sufficient active chlorine may not actually be available for adequate sterilization.

The manufacturer most probably has had the greatest experience with his product; it is wise then to follow his recommendations and accept the limitations of that particular agent. The practical applications of the use of chemical sterilizers should also be considered. Harsh or difficult conditions may make it impossible to achieve chemical sterilization under any circumstances. It is necessary then to consider chemical, physical, and biological factors in effecting sterilization and achieving sterility. It is the intent of this paper to discuss some of these objectives and present available information on the use of chemicals which can be regarded as effective chemosterilizers. It is also the purpose of this publication to clarify those issues which are borderline and tend to be misleading. The popular use of alcohols, for example, as antimicrobial agents gives one the impression that they can be used effectively as chemosterilizers and are sporicidal in nature. This is not so; alcoholic suspensions of viable bacterial spores have been retained for long periods of time and grown readily after transfer to the appropriate growth media.

II. Methods for Evaluation of Chemosterilizers

A. Sporicidal Tests

Although the broth dilution or serial dilution method and the agar-cup plate technique are widely employed for the rapid screening and evaluation of antimicrobial agents, their use in the appraisal of sporicidal agents is not recommended. Time is not a factor in these techniques and bacterial or fungal spores can revert to the vegetative state. Thus, it would be doubtful whether the chemical compounds tested were effective against the spore or the vegetative cell.

Tests for determining the presence or absence of sporicidal activity and potential effectiveness against various spore-forming bacteria under different conditions are recommended by the AOAC (Official Methods of Analysis, 1960). Either suture loops or porcelain penny-cylinders are infected with spores of bacilli or clostridia under the recommended conditions and exposed to the test agent for prescribed periods of time. The spore inoculum is removed from the test reagent, added to tubes of growth culture media, and incubated. The lack of positive cultures is considered as satisfactory evidence of the desired response, and it is expected that the use of these materials may be extrapolated to products of a similar nature under practical "in use" situations.

Resistance of bacterial spores with this method is determined by exposure to 2.5 *N* HCl. The test spores are expected to resist the HCl for at least 2 minutes, although many will resist the HCl for 30 minutes and longer. Vegetative cells should not show any significant resistance against this concentration of strong acid. Ortenzio *et al.* (1953) used constant boiling hydrochloric acid for short periods to destroy bacterial spores. The procedure was developed to minimize the hazard in handling dried spores of *Bacillus anthracis* or *Clostridium tetani* and to provide the bacteriologist with a constant source of dried spores for sporicidal evaluations. These workers showed the high degree of resistance of bacterial spores, and confirmed the work of Curran (1952) which indicated that the capacity of bacterial spores to withstand destructive agents is not equaled by any other living thing.

The test method for determination of sporicidal activity with suture loops is difficult to evaluate since Spaulding (1964) has pointed out that the suture loop is extremely resistant to sterilization by germicides. When the severity of the test condition was increased by using a heavy inoculum, some bacteria still showed long survival times. Why contaminated silk sutures should be so resistant to sterilization is not known, but it should be borne in mind that this type of situation, perhaps, cannot be extrapolated in practical terms to an actual in-use condition.

Stuart (1966) has reported on the current status of AOAC sporicidal test and has recommended changes in the procedure which would make it more precise. Tests with spores showed a high degree of resistance to chemical sterilizers. Rehydration treatments of spores prior to chemosterilizer exposure showed less resistance. Studies in this area were also conducted by Gilbert *et al.* (1964). It was pointed out that these procedures were applicable in evaluating the sporicidal activity of both liquids and gases, and that there can be no double standard for liquids or gases as sterilizing agents. This test is considered as satisfactory evidence of the desired response when applied to the carrier giving the lowest result; however, for a confidence level of 95%, killing in 59 out of 60 replicates is expected.

B. Additional Test Methods

Although the AOAC sporicidal method can be used readily for laboratory evaluations of chemosterilizers, Opfel and Miller (1965) have stated that a valid demonstration must be based on results and experiments duplicating the anticipated environment for each cell in the contaminating population and using microorganisms whose resistance to the sterilizing agent resembles that of the species in the contaminating population. Hence, a chemical sterilizer employed for medical instruments must be capable of destroying those microorganisms considered part of the normal flora of a hospital environment and practical "in-use" test evaluations must be performed subsequent to any initial laboratory evaluations.

A chemosterilizer, in addition to destroying bacterial spores and vegetative cells, must also be effective in (a) destroying *Mycobacterium tuberculosis,* which is known to be more resistant than other commonly encountered vegetative pathogenic bacteria, and (b) in destroying viruses, including proper sterilization of instruments and needles, for the prevention of human hepatitis.

Moessel (1963) developed a method for determining the overall rapid evaluation of a microbicide by providing a mixed culture of bacteria, spores, and yeasts. The suspension is treated with the antimicrobial; thus, if the manufacturer claims his agent is sporicidal, a viable spore count is required to determine this activity.

Portner *et al.* (1954) reported on the efficacy of membrane filters for testing the microbiological activity of formaldehyde solutions. This method offers the advantage that bacteria entrapped on membrane filters can be washed free of bacteriostatic material prior to subculture. In the adaptation of this test to sporicidal evaluations, clostridia or other bacterial spores may be used with sporistasis determined by inoculating the medium with spores of the test strain. Growth of the bacterium indicated that the test solution was not sporicidal.

III. Gaseous Chemosterilizers

A. Ethylene Oxide

The literature on sterilization by ethylene oxide is voluminous and a review of the subject would include hundreds of papers. One of the earliest extensive reviews regarding the bactericidal effectiveness and physical properties of ethylene oxide gas was published by Phillips and Kaye (1949). Phillips (1949) and Kaye and Phillips (1949) presented data which showed the effects of temperature, concentration, exposure time, and moisture upon sterilization with ethylene oxide. Methodology and procedures used in handling ethylene oxide for sterilization purposes in the pharmaceutical industry, surgical dressings and appliances, research institutions and hospitals were explored by Perkins (1956). This work and the properties of gaseous ethylene oxide mixtures were further reviewed by Lloyd and Thompson (1958). One of the first detailed reports regarding the inactivation of viruses by ethylene oxide was published by Ginsberg and Wilson (1950). Various investigators have reported on the use of ethylene oxide for sterilization of a wide variety of objects, e.g., the sterilization of bacteriological media and other fluids by Wilson and Bruno (1950) and viruses suspended in protein solutions by Auerswald and Doleschel (1962). Polley (1952) used ethylene oxide in the preparation of stable noninfective influenza and mumps antigen and Perkins (1960) employed ethylene oxide on a broad spectrum of pharmaceutical products. Ethylene oxide has also been used extensively in the food industry, e.g., for spices; however, there are limitations to its use in this industry since it can react with vitamins and other amino acids. For more recent reviews on the subject, the reader is referred to the work of Bruch (1961), Mayr (1961), Phillips (1961), Stierli *et al.* (1962), and Lloyd (1963).

The above literature demonstrates that ethylene oxide is widely used commercially for sterilization. It is not the intent of this article to pursue this matter, but rather to point out some of the restrictions in its applications. Serious limitations to its widespread use in hospitals were reported by Spaulding *et al.* (1958). It was also shown by Spaulding (1964) that the portable type of ethylene oxide sterilizer was less rapidly cidal than the autoclave type. Ernst and Shull (1962) showed that the relationships of reaction temperatures and concentration of gaseous ethylene oxide to the time required for inactivation of air-dried spores were highly complex and that use conditions of ethylene oxide should be selected on the basis of experimental support. It was further reported by Opfell *et al.* (1959) that the absence of hygroscopic substances appeared to increase the resistance of *B. globigii* spores to gaseous ethylene oxide sterilization. *B. globigii* spores were also shown to be more resistant than other bacterial spores by Lloyd *et al.* (1967).

Although Walter and Kundsin (1959) reported on the faulty functioning of a table model ethylene oxide sterilizer, sterilization problems are also frequently encountered by users of large autoclaves. During these test periods, it may be necessary to explore the many parameters involved in ethylene oxide sterilization. These include temperature, pressure, relative humidity, gas concentration, numbers and kinds of microorganisms to be destroyed, nature and permeability of the material to be sterilized, and, finally, the process and equipment used. If the material to be sterilized is a solid, and the gaseous sterilizer cannot penetrate it, some other means must be employed to achieve sterility. Doyle and Ernst (1967) showed, for example, that occluded spores could not be inactivated with ethylene oxide when a crystalline matrix of calcium carbonate acted as a barrier. It was pointed out by these investigators that spores entrapped in insoluble materials are extremely resistant to ethylene oxide, as well as to moist or dry heat.

The package used for sterilization with ethylene oxide is also of major importance. Many materials are impermeable to ethylene oxide, and where this is a problem, a vent may be included in the package and aseptic sealing applied after sterilization. If this is not practical, some other means for achieving sterility must be employed. The use of ethylene oxide for the preparation of sterile products was recommended by Guthrey (1967), using a polyester bag as a portable sterile hood.

B. Gases and Vapors

1. *Proplylene Oxide* (C_3H_6O)

According to Bruch (1961), propylene oxide has weak penetrating ability but strong microbicidal properties, and is frequently used as a substitute for ethylene oxide in sterilization. Russell (1965) has shown that spores of *B. subtilis* and *B. stearothermophilus* were destroyed after exposure to gaseous propylene oxide, and that *B. subtilis* was the more resistant of the two. Although Bruch and

Koesterer (1961) reported that the activity of propylene oxide decreased with increasing relative humidity, Himmelfarb *et al.* (1962) found that the death rate of *Bacillus subtilis* spores substantially increased with this increase in relative humidity.

Propylene oxide can be used in conjunction with ethylene oxide for chemical sterilization and, like ethylene oxide, requires dilution with inert gases for safety. Carbon dioxide was previously combined with these chemosterilizers; more recently, mixtures with Freon gas have come into popular usage. Flammability limits in air were reported by Bruch (1961) to be 2.1% to 21.5% by volume. Use of the above-mentioned inert gaseous mixtures can help to eliminate the flammability hazard. The acceptable concentration recommended for sterilization is in excess of 800 mg. per liter.

2. *β-Propiolactone*

β-Propiolactone, a heterocyclic ring compound, is a colorless, pungent liquid, vapors of which have been used for sporicidal activity. Hoffman and Warshowsky (1958) showed that β-propiolactone was lethal for cells of *B. subtilis* var. *niger*. Sporicidal activity was dependent on the concentration of the vapor and relative humidity above 70%. Bruch (1961) recommended the use of this chemical for sterilization in various areas and reported that tests performed with spore samples on paper strips showed that this method was used as an indicator for sterilization.

Allen and Murphy (1960) showed that β-propiolactone has a broad field of application provided that its limitations are recognized and that it is handled like other bactericidal agents with due regard for its toxic properties. Lo Grippo (1961), however, was able to sterilize biological material without toxic or allergic manifestations, employing β-propiolactone in the liquid state. The use of a specially purified β-propiolactone without the usual impurities of acrylic acid, acetic anhydride, and polymers was stressed. Vischer *et al.* (1963), Fellowes (1965), Barbieto (1966), and Pritchard *et al.* (1966), among others, have reported on sterilization by β-propiolactone and the advantages and limitations in its use. One of the major factors in limiting its development as a sterilizing agent is attributed to its carcinogenic and other physiologically undesirable properties as reported by Wisely and Falk (1960). However, the hydrolysis product—β-hydroxy propionic acid—does not appear to have these disadvantages as it is lower in toxicity and is noncarcinogenic.

3. *Formaldehyde Vapor*

Formaldehyde, in the vapor phase, has long been recognized for its chemical sterilizing ability. Formaldehyde vapor cabinets have been used to sterilize lensed instruments which cannot be subjected to heat. Although they have been employed effectively, a high degree of humidity and a prolonged exposure time is required if the formaldehyde is to exert its effect. Nordgren (1939) has summarized much of the earlier work together with his own experimental data on the action of formaldehyde vapor.

Although formaldehyde vapors have a high degree of microbiological activity, their ability to penetrate is weak, with the result that their application should be limited to surface sterilization. This method of sterilization appears to be losing its popularity and is being rapidly replaced by ethylene oxide or other gaseous sterilizers. The use of formaldehyde solutions as chemosterilizers will be dealt with separately in this article and the use of formaldehyde vapor in combination with other sporicides is discussed in a later section.

C. Consideration of Other antimicrobials as Chemosterilizers

A number of other chemical compounds have been reported as chemosterilizers, but the reader is cautioned in their use. As was pointed out earlier, in order to be considered a chemosterilizer, the anti-microbial agent must be sporicidal. Unfortunately, in most instances the microbiological population is unknown. Since spores may be present, it becomes necessary to destroy them as well. Thus, an agent may very well induce sterile conditions where vegetative bacterial cells are present, but not so in the presence of spores. Methyl bromide and ozone, for example, have weak microbicidal properties and, therefore, find limited application. In comparing methyl bromide vapors with ethylene oxide, Opfel *et al.* (1967) showed significant differences in the susceptibility of microbial populations to these agents, but the mixed vapors sterilized both spores and desiccated cells of *S. epidermidis.*

Ethylene imine was reported by Phillips (1949) to have a higher degree of microbiological activity than ethylene oxide or its methyl, chloromethyl or bromomethyl derivatives. This compound has not gained the wide acceptance of ethylene oxide nor has it been completely explored despite the fact that the work was reported almost two decades ago. A possible reason for the lack of popularity may be the occurrence of corrosion with the use of this chemosterilizer.

IV. Liquid Chemosterilizers

A. Strong Acids and Alkalies

Because of their sporicidal nature, strong acids or alkalies may be used as chemosterilizers. However, the acidic or caustic nature of these solutions places a strong limitation on their use. Solutions of 2.5 *N* hydrochloric acid are employed in AOAC sporicidal tests to determine the resistance of spores to this solution. Bacterial spores are rapidly destroyed within minutes and do not normally withstand an exposure limit beyond 30 minutes, although our own experiments with pure cultures of spores at concentrations of 1×10^5 to 1×10^6 per milliliter showed survival times in excess of 1 hour. This high degree of resistance is indicative of the complex nature of this biological material and its ability to survive under extremely difficult circumstances.

Sodium hydroxide also may require long exposure times to destroy bacterial spores. Although spores of *Clostridium sporogenes* were destroyed within 3 hours when exposed to 2.5 *N* NaOH, spores of *Bacillus megaterium* survived a 3-hour exposure to this concentration of alkali. It would appear that while strong caustic solutions may be used for the destruction of spores, long exposure times may be necessary to achieve sterility.

B. Phenolics

Phenolics have been widely used for disinfection by microbiologists; if they are to be effective as sporicidal agents, however, they must be employed in conjunction with heat. Klarmann (1956) reported that destruction of resistant bacterial spores could be effected by boiling with dilute aqueous solutions of synthetic phenolics of low volatility. This procedure was recommended for the sterilization of surgical instruments and it was shown that spores of *Cl. sporogenes* were destroyed by this method without corroding the instruments. While this procedure may be applicable in certain areas, it obviously cannot be utilized for sterilization of delicate-lensed instruments, e.g., bronchoscopes or cystoscopes. The use of 2% phenol and cresol by this method was contraindicated because a pungent odor intensified by heating was found to be objectionable. In accordance with the above, it appears that heating of cultures of sporulating organisms to kill vegetative cells will weaken the spores so that they will be more easily killed. For a review of the microbiological activity of the phenolics, the reader is referred to the works of Klarmann (1957) and Sykes (1965).

C. Halogens

Chlorine has long been employed as a chemosterilizer. Weber and Levine (1944) were able to show that hypochlorous acid was sporicidal over a pH range of 6 to 9. In a study of the effect of *N*-chloro compounds on *Bacillus metiens* spores, Marks *et al.* (1945) also found that, at each pH value, the log of time required for kill plotted against the log concentration gave a straight line, and the rate of sterilization decreased rapidly as the pH increased. This author's experience with dichloro-*S*-triazinetrione, an *N*-chloro compound, has also shown it to possess sporicidal activity. Where a concentration in excess of 400–500 p.p.m. available chlorine was used at neutral pH, bacterial spore populations were destroyed in a few hours.

Engelhard *et al.* (1961) studied the effects of an organic hypochlorous acid in a phosphate buffer and found that it was able to destroy various microorganisms including *Bacillus stearothermophilus* and *Clostridium sporogenes.* Chandler *et al.* (1957) had reported earlier, however, that hypochlorous acid compounds were not sporicidal when tested by two different methods. The activity of chlorine was markedly reduced in the presence of protein matter and storage temperatures in excess of 70°F.

Discrepancies regarding the sporicidal action of iodine, as with chlorine, are reported. The use of iodine as a chemical sterilizing agent was recommended by Gershenfeld and Witlin (1952). These authors found that 2% iodine solutions destroyed spores of *Bacillus subtilis, Bacillus anthracis, Bacillus mesentericus* and *Clostridium tetani* when tested on both absorbent and nonabsorbent surfaces. The relatively greater resistance of *B. subtilis* spores to an iodophor as compared with NaOCl was unexpected by Cousins and Allen (1967) because of the generally accepted view that iodine has greater activity against vegetative bacterial cells.

Iodine is frequently used for the destruction of microorganisms on the skin. Although it is effective in destroying a major percentage of microbes, the nature of skin is such that complete destruction of microbes cannot be achieved, hence, these solutions cannot be considered as chemosterilizers. The use of chemical sterilization, for the present at least, is limited to inanimate objects.

D. Formaldehyde

Since alcohols are not sporicidal, they cannot be considered as chemosterilizers. However, they are frequently used as carriers for other chemicals such as formaldehyde. Spaulding (1963) recommended the use of 8% formaldehyde or 20% formalin for the destruction of bacterial spores. His findings showed that formaldehyde was superior to iodophors insofar as sporicidal activity was concerned. The higher concentration of formaldehyde was essential since 1% or 2% formaldehyde solutions are not good sporicides. A solution of 8% formaldehyde in 70% isopropyl alcohol was sporicidal, and sterility was achieved in 3 hours according to Spaulding (1963).

Willard and Alexander (1964) concluded from their studies of the sterilizing properties of formaldehyde in methanol and water solutions that formaldehyde in methanol effected sterilization in 24 hours; formaldehyde in water sterilized in shorter periods of time and has a longer shelf life than formaldehyde in methanol. The test inoculum used in these studies was a water suspension of spores of *Bacillus subtilis* var. *niger*. According to these authors, the most recent suggested application of this chemical is for the sterilization of space vehicles.

Sykes (1965) reported that a formaldehyde-alcohol mixture is a more effective sterilizing agent than an aqueous solution of formaldehyde and that a 5% solution of formalin in alcohol will effectively sterilize all spores in 24 hours at 25°C. A 1% solution was also reported to kill in 24 hours at the higher temperature of 37°C. The kind of alcohol used as solvent was not specified.

Although formaldehyde has been widely employed for many years for the destruction of microorganisms, and my own experience has shown it to be a good chemosterilizer, one of the chief objections to its use is the pungent odor of the vapors given off by the sterilizing solutions.

E. Glutaraldehyde

Glutaraldehyde, a saturated dialdehyde having the formula $CHO—CH_2CH_2CH_2—CHO$, has been known for many years, but it is only recently that it has been developed commercially as a chemosterilizer. Borick (1965) reported that acid solutions stored at room temperature in a closed system remain stable whereas alkalinized glutaraldehyde solutions show a drop in pH and a decrease in glutaraldehyde concentration after 2 weeks (see Fig. 1). The alkaline solutions show a higher degree of sporicidal activity, however, and for this reason are preferred for chemical sterilization (see Table I). A comparison of 1% and 2% glutaraldehyde solutions with 4% formaldehyde solutions by Rubbo and Gardner (1965) showed that

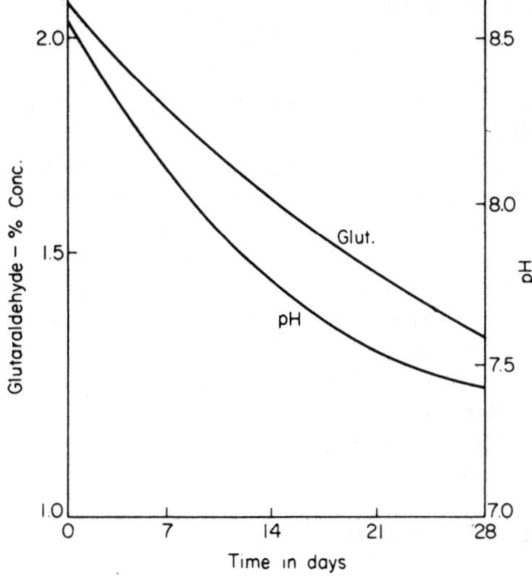

FIG. 1. Glutaraldehyde concentration and pH of alkalinized glutaraldehyde after standing 4 weeks. Reprinted from Borick (1965) courtesy John Wiley & Sons (Interscience).

TABLE I
ABILITY OF *Bacillus subtilis* SPORES TO SURVIVE 2% AQUEOUS GLUTARALDEHYDE SOLUTIONS AT DIFFERENT pH

	pH 5		pH 7		pH 9	
Exposure time (minutes)	Microbial count	Percent survivors	Microbial count	Percent survivors	Microbial count	Percent survivors
0	2.1×10^6	100	1.1×10^6	100	1.7×10^6	100
30	1.7×10^6	83	4.0×10^5	36	3.7×10^5	60
60	1.0×10^6	48	7.3×10^3	1	7.2×10^4	4
90	5.3×10^4	3	0	0	0	0
180	0	0	0	0	0	0

glutaraldehyde was able to destroy spores of *Bacillus anthracis* more rapidly than was formaldehyde. A comparison of the sporicidal activities of alcoholic glutaraldehyde and formaldehyde solutions (as seen in Table II) showed that a lower concentration of glutaraldehyde killed aerobic and anaerobic spores in a shorter period of time than a higher concentration of formaldehyde. The microbiological activity of saturated alcoholic dialdehyde solutions was reported by Pepper and Chandler (1963).

TABLE II
SPORICIDAL ACTIVITIES OF 1% ALKALINE ALCOHOLIC GLUTARALDEHYDE AND 8% FORMALDEHYDE SOLUTIONS USING PENICYLINDERS CONTAMINATED WITH A MIXED SUSPENSION OF VARYING NUMBERS OF SPORES[a]

			Exposure time[b]							
	Bacterial count[b]		0 hour		1 hour		3 hours		6 hours	
Test solutions	Aerobes	Anaerobes	Eug.[d]	Thio.[e]	Eug.[d]	Thio.[e]	Eug.[d]	Thio.[e]	Eug.[d]	Thio.[e]
1% Glutaraldehyde	380,000	210,000	+	+			−	−	+	−
1% Glutaraldehyde	2,100	3,000	+	+	+	+	+	+	−	−
1% Glutaraldehyde	100	100	+	+	−	+	−	−	−	−
8% Formaldehyde	380,000	210,000	+	+	+	+	+	+	+	+
8% Formaldehyde	2,100	3,000	+	+	+	+	+	+	+	+
8% Formaldehyde	100	100	+	+	+	+	+	+	−	−

[a] Reprinted from Pepper and Chandler (1963) courtesy of American Society of Microbiology.
[b] Key: + indicates growth and − indicates no growth.
[c] Spore counts were estimated from heat-shocked samples and shown as numbers of spores for cylinder.
[d] Eugon broth.
[e] Thioglycollate broth.
[d] Key: + indicates growth and − indicates no growth.

A wide spectrum of microorganisms was destroyed by aqueous glutaraldehyde solutions, according to various investigators: Borick (1964a, b, 1965), Klein and DeForest (1963), Spaulding (1963), Snyder and Cheatle (1965), and Stonehill *et al.* (1963). Since various test methods were employed by these investigators, details will not be reiterated here. The types of microorganisms destroyed can be seen from a perusal of Table III. A wide range of microorganisms, including vegetative bacterial and fungal cells, viruses, tubercle bacilli, and bacterial and fungal spores, were destroyed by 2% aqueous glutaraldehyde.

The ability of glutaraldehyde solutions to maintain their activity in the presence of organic matter was further reported by Borick (1964a,b).

Serum was neither precipitated nor coagulated in the presence of glutaraldehyde. When 2% glutaraldehyde was tested in the presence of 20% blood serum, its activity remained the same as that in the absence of organic matter.

TABLE III
EFFECTS OF AQUEOUS ALKALINE 2% GLUTARALDEHYDE SOLUTIONS ON VARIOUS MICROORGANISMS[a]

Microorganisms	Source	Killing time
Staphylococcus aureus	ATCC 6538	< 1 minute
Streptococcus pyogenes	ATCC 12384	< 1 minute
Diplococcus pneumoniae	U. of Michigan	< 1 minute
Escherichia coli	ATCC 6880	< 1 minute
Pseudomonas aeruginosa	ATCC 10145	< 1 minute
Serratia marcescens	Rutgers U.	< 1 minute
Proteus vulgaris	ATCC 6380	< 1 minute
Klebsiella pneumoniae	ATCC 132	< 1 minute
Trichophyton interdigitale	ATCC 640	< 1 minute
Micrococcus lysodeikticus	Ohio State U.	< 1 minute
Mycobacterium tuberculosis H37Rv	ATCC 7690	<10 minutes
Poliomyelitis types I & II	Temple U.	<10 minutes
Echo type 6	Temple U.	<10 minutes
Coxsackie B-1	Temple U.	<10 minutes
Herpes simplex	Temple U.	<10 minutes
Vaccinia	Temple U.	<10 minutes
Influenza A-2, Asian	Temple U.	<10 minutes
Adeno type 2	Temple U.	<10 minutes
Mouse hepatitis (MHV3)	Temple U.	<10 minutes
Bacillus subtilis spores	USDA	< 3 hours
Bacillus megaterium spores	U. of Texas	< 3 hours
B. globigii spores	USDA	< 3 hours
Cl. tetani spores	USDA	< 3 hours
Cl. perfringens spores	USDA	< 3 hours

[a] Reprinted from Borick (1965) courtesy John Wiley & Sons (Interscience).

The use of glutaraldehyde has gained wide acceptance in the medical field. Borick (1967a) advocated its use as an instrument germicide. It is especially useful in areas where heat cannot be employed, such as sterilization of lensed instruments, i.e., cystoscopes and bronchoscopes. Duquette and Snyder (1966) showed the superiority of glutaraldehyde over other antimicrobials for the control of hospital infection. The inactivation of biological activity of myxoviruses by glutaraldehyde was reported by Blough (1966). No incidence of irritation or sensitivity was reported by O'Brien *et al.* (1966) in over 4000 patients exposed to glutaraldehyde. Rittenbury and Hench (1965) used glutaraldehyde for sterilization of urological instruments and various anesthesia items, e.g., face masks, corrugated tubing, and endotracheal tubes. Use of glutaraldehyde in anesthesia was also reported by Meeks *et al.* (1967) and by Haselhuhn *et al.* (1967). Other areas of use of glutaraldehyde included the fixation of tissues for electron microscopy, as reported by Fahimi and Drochmans (1965).

Some of the advantages of glutaraldehyde as a chemosterilizer include: (1) no deleterious effects on the cement of lensed instruments, e.g., bronchoscopes, etc.; (2) it does not interfere with the electrical conductivity of rubber anesthesia equipment; (3) its low surface tension permits easy penetration and rinsing; (4) it is noncorrosive; (5) it does not affect rubber and plastic articles; (6) it does not coagulate blood or other proteinaceous material; (7) it does not affect the sharpness of cutting instruments; (8) it has a low vapor pressure—22 mm of mercury, compared to 24 mm for water; (9) it does not affect the markings on objects such as clinical thermometers.

F. Other Chemosterilizers

Various chemicals have been reported which demonstrate sporicidal activity, but have not been exploited as chemosterilizers. Included in this category are glyoxal, succinaldehyde, and other aldehydes. Pepper and Chandler (1963) showed that glyoxal-isopropanol solutions destroyed spores in a relatively short time. Work conducted by us also showed other aldehydes to have sporicidal activity. In this category, succinaldehyde solutions were intermediate between glyoxal and glutaraldehyde.

The peracids also have sporicidal activity and potential use as chemosterilizers. Peracetic acid is available commercially as a 40% solution and may be diluted with water to lower concentrations for use. A method for destroying thermophilic bacteria and spores in starch by the use of peracetic, perpropionic, and perbutyric acids was patented by Wurzburg and Kruger (1962). A 2% solution of *meta*-chloroperbenzoic acid in ethyl alcohol was tested by us and found to destroy both aerobic and anaerobic spores within 3 hours, using AOAC sporicidal test procedures. Both peracetic and perbenzoic acids showed sporicidal activity against spores of *B. subtilis* and *Cl. tetani.*

A patent covering the use of combinations of formic acid and epoxides for the sterilization of objects was issued to Kaye (1967). Both vaporized and liquid combinations of formic acid and epoxides were utilized; potentiation of activity of ethylene or propylene oxide was attributed to the combined use of formic acid and the epoxides.

V. Conditions for the Use of Chemosterilizers

In discussing the destruction of microorganisms by irradiation sterilization, Borick (1967b) reported that the many variables associated with destruction of microbial cells by physical means must be considered. This also holds true for chemical sterilization. Although a chemosterilizer may be sporicidal in its action, it cannot be effective unless it penetrates to the spore site. In our evaluation of chemicals to achieve sterility, laboratory experiments are too frequently planned without taking this factor into consideration. The microbiologist may make conditions so difficult that the chemosterilizer cannot perform its function under any circumstances. One of the methods employed here is to centrifuge a culture of microorganisms in order to obtain a high concentration of biological cells. Obviously a compact conglomeration of cells will not lend itself readily to penetration of the inner core, permitting destruction of those germs which are in the hard center. If these circumstances were extrapolated to practical everyday usage, there would indeed be few, if any, environmental conditions under which this phenomenon would occur.

The containment of the bacterial cell in a crystalline matrix would present a similar problem. A chemosterilizer which first acts as a solvent to dissolve the chemical and is still capable of destroying the bacterial cell would have to be employed. Another condition which may be applicable is the use of a chemical solution having a sufficiently low surface tension to permit penetration in narrow-bore instruments. Since air pockets can occur in these areas, it is necessary to ensure that the chemosterilizer will penetrate the narrowest crevice. According to Colbeck (1962), no method of chemical sterilization is reliable for the sterilization of uretheral catheters because it is difficult to ensure that the chemical will come into contact with the entire inner area. The positioning of long, narrow instruments in an upright position with slow immersion of the solution into the channel would prove more advantageous rather than placing them in a horizontal position.

Too often microbiologists feel that large concentrations of microorganisms are in themselves of paramount importance in the evaluation of chemosterilizers. Although numbers and types of microorganisms must be taken into consideration in the use of chemosterilizers, it should be remembered that environmental characteristics are also to be considered and that a high incidence of contamination may not necessarily be present in any given practical case. The types of microorganisms, too, may be such that they are readily destroyed or are nonpathogenic, so that their presence would be inconsequential. Van Winkle *et al.* (1967) pointed out that a most important factor in sterilization is a thorough understanding of the physical and biological nature of the product to be sterilized and the nature and level of organisms that must be destroyed. This is a practical approach to the problem and must be solved in each individual case in a rational way.

Granted that the chemosterilizer is unable to perform its sterility function under difficult, adverse circumstances, however, the use of heat, too, can result in sterility failure if improperly applied. Overloading of autoclaves and hot air sterilizers, inadequate time and temperature cycles, improper operation and undetected defects are not uncommon in heat sterilization. Some of these problems were extensively discussed by Shotten (1961) and Bowie (1961). In the use of chemosterilizers, time, temperature, pH, concentration, surface tension, the nature and types of chemicals employed, and the proper use of these chemicals are also all important factors. Let us consider each of these separately.

As most microbiologists are aware, time is a critical factor in the use of chemicals for microbiological activity. It is generally recognized that the longer the material is exposed to the microbicide, the better the chances are to achieve sterility. It is also known that present-day chemosterilizers do not act in minutes, but rather hours are required to achieve the desired effect. Here again, the individual must realize that some spores are readily destroyed whereas others are extremely difficult to kill and will, in fact, resist destruction. The simple analogy to a nut or a seed may be drawn. The brazil nut has a hard outer coat and it is only through a severe physical impact that we are able to shatter the tough outer coat to get at the meat. On the other hand, the almond or walnut has a softer shell and can be penetrated more readily. So, too, spores coats vary with different microbial cultures.

Temperature also plays an important role in the use of chemosterilizers as it is generally accepted that the killing efficiency of the chemical increases with increasing temperature. Since exceptions to this rule are possible, the temperature effects on each individual antimicrobial agent must be determined.

The pH at which the chemosterilizer exerts its optimum action must also be determined. According to Frobisher (1953), the lethal or toxic action of both chemical and physical harmful agents is affected by (H^+) or (OH^-). Cationic agents, for example, may be interferred with by an increased hydrogen ion concentration whereas increases in the hydroxyl ion will favor many of them.

As a general rule, the more concentrated the chemosterilizer, the more effective will be the action of the solution. This is applicable to a limited degree only, however, as once the maximum killing power of the chemical solution is obtained, additional increases in concentration may show little, if any, significant difference in killing power.

The addition of wetting agents to antimicrobial agents appears to enhance their activity. The lowering of the surface tension may impart greater penetrating ability to them and, hence, make them more readily able to reach the site to be acted upon. It is expected, then, that the time required to achieve kill would also be lowered.

The final criteria in an evaluation of chemosterilizers are the nature and types of chemicals and their proper use. The final choice of a chemosterilizer in any given situation will be determined by its intended use. Where facilities are available, it may be possible to test these solutions to determine which will be the most effective for that particular purpose. One should bear in mind that here, too, pitfalls can occur. Methyl-2-cyanoacrylate, an adhesive, was reported to be self-sterilizing. Page and Borick (1967) showed, however, that spores could be recovered from the entrapped chemical by breaking up the adhesive with glass beads.

TABLE IV
CHEMICALS WHICH EXHIBIT SPORICIDAL ACTIVITY AND ARE USED AS CHEMOSTERILIZERS

β-Propiolactone	Chlorine iodine
Ethylene oxide	Formaldehyde-formalin
Ethylene imine	Glyoxal
Propylene oxide	Glutaraldehyde
Strong acids and alkalies	Succinaldehyde
Phenolics (heat)	Per acids

All available antimicrobial agents which show activity have not been tested for their sporicidal action. Some years ago, Borick *et al.* (1959; Borick and Bratt, 1961) was instrumental in the discovery of a series of compounds of higher amine salts of carboxylic and saturated and unsaturated fatty acids. Although these show a high degree of microbiological activity against vegetative bacterial and fungal cells, to the best of the writers' knowledge, they have not been tested against bacterial spores. It is recommended that the individual chemical (Table IV) be tested before use to determine sporicidal activity and ensure its use as a chemosterilizer.

VI. Summary

Although large numbers of antimicrobial agents are available for use, only a limited number show sporicidal activity and can be classified as chemical sterilizers (chemosterilizers). As with other methods of sterilization, a number of factors must be considered when chemical sterilization is employed. These include time, temperature, concentration, pH, numbers, and types of microorganisms to be destroyed, surface tension, the nature and kind of chemical agent employed, and the proper use of the chemosterilizer.

Various chemicals employed for this purpose are discussed and their nature and properties presented. Both gaseous and liquid chemosterilizers are available. Included here are β-propiolactone, ethylene oxide, ethylene imine, proxylene oxide, strong acids, alkalies, phenolics accompanied by heat, chlorine and iodine, formaldehyde, formalin, glyoxal, glutaraldehyde, succinaldehyde, and the per acids.

References

Allen, H. F., and Murphy, J. T. (1960). *J. Am. Med. Assoc.* **172,** 1759–1763.

Anonymous (1964). *Chem. Process. (Chicago)* **27,** 13.

Auerswald, W., and Doleschel, W. (1962). *Med. Exptl.* **6,** 193–199.

Barbieto, M. S. (1966). J.A.H.A. **40,** 100–106.

Blough, H. A. (1966). *J. Bacteriol.* **92,** 266–268.

Borick, P. M. (1964a). *J. Pharm. Sci.* **10,** 1273–1275.

Borick, P. M. (1964b). Paper presented at the 148th Meeting of the Amer. Chem. Soc., Chicago.

Borick, P. M. (1965). *Biotechnol. Bioeng.* **7,** 435–443.

Borick, P. M. (1967a). Paper presented at the meetings of the Theobald Smith Soc., Somerville, New Jersey.

Borick, P. M. (1967b). *Appl. Microbiol.* **15,** 785–789.

Borick, P. M., and Bratt, M. (1961). *Appl. Microbiol.* **9,** 475–477.

Borick, P. M., Bratt, M., Wilson, A. G., Weintraub, L., and Kuna, M. (1959). *Appl. Microbiol.* **7,** 248–251.

Bowie, J. H. (1961). *In* "Recent Developments in the Sterilization of Surgical Materials" (Dept. Pharm. Sci., Pharm. Soc. G. Brit. and Smith & Nephew Res., Ltd., eds.), pp. 109–142. Pharmaceutical Press, London.

Bruch, C. W. (1961). *Ann. Rev. Microbiol.* **15,** 245–262.

Bruch, C. W., and Koesterer, M. G. (1961). *J. Food Sci.* **26,** 428.
Chandler, V. L., Pepper, R. E., and Gordon, L. E. (1957). *J. Am. Pharm. Assoc., Sci. Ed.* **46,** 124–128.
Colbeck, J. C. (1962). In "Control of Infections in Hospitals," Am. Hosp. Association 12, 69.
Cousins, C. M., and Allen, C. D. (1967). *J. Appl. Bacteriol.* **30**(1), 168–174.
Curran, H. R. (1952). *Bacteriol. Rev.* **16,** 111–117.
Doyle, J. E., and Ernst, R. R. (1967). *Appl. Microbiol.* **15,** 726–730.
Duquette, E., and Snyder, R. (1966). *Bacteriol. Proc.* **12,** 52.
Engelhard, W. E., Wiedman, J. G., and Jolliff, C. R. (1961). *Surgery* **49,** 651–656.
Ernst, R. R., and Shull, J. J. (1962). *Appl. Microbiol.* **10,** 337–341.
Fahimi, H. D., and Drochmans, P. (1965). *J. Microscopie* **4,** 725–748.
Fellowes, O. N. (1965). *Appl. Microbiol.* **13,** 1038–1039.
Frobisher, M. (1953). "Fundamentals of Bacteriology," 5th Ed., p. 222. Saunders, Philadelphia, Pennsylvania.
Gershenfeld, L., and Witlin, B. (1952). *J. Am. Pharm. Assoc., Sci. Ed.* **41,** 451–452.
Gilbert, G. L., Gambill, V. M., Spiner, D. R., Hoffman, R. K., and Phillips, C. R. (1964). *J. Appl. Microbiol.* **12,** 496–503.
Ginsberg, H. S., and Wilson, A. T. (1950). *Proc. Soc. Exptl. Biol. Med.* **73,** 614.
Guthrey, W. L. (1967). *Am. J. Hosp. Pharm.* **24,** 371–373.
Haselhuhn, D. H., Brason, F. W., and Borick, P. M. (1967). *Anesthesia Analgesia, Current Res.* **46,** 468–474.
Himmelfarb, P., El Bisi, H. M., Reed, R. B., and Litsky, W. (1962). *Appl. Microbiol.* **10,** 431–435.
Hoffman, R. K., and Warshowsky, B. (1958). *Appl. Microbiol.* **6,** 358–362.
Kaye, S. (1967). Canadian Patent No. 757,308.
Kaye, S., and Phillips, C. R. (1949). *Am. J. Hyg.* **50,** 296–306.
Klarmann, E. G. (1956). *Am. J. Pharm.* **128,** 4–18.
Klarmann, E. G. (1957). *In* "Antiseptics, Disinfectants, Fungicides, and Chemical and Physical Sterilization" (G. F. Reddish, ed.), pp. 506–557. Lea & Febiger, Philadelphia, Pennsylvania.
Klein, M., and DeForest, A. (1963). *Soap Chem. Specialties* **39,** 70–72.
Lloyd, R. S. (1963). *J. Hosp. Res.* **1,** 5–27.
Lloyd, R. S., and Thompson, E. L. (1958). "Gaseous Sterilization with Ethylene Oxide." Am. Sterilizer Co., Erie, Pennsylvania.
Lloyd, R. S.., Kereluk, K., and Gammon, R. (1967). Paper presented at the Soc. Ind. Microbiol., London, Ontario, Canada. Plenum Press, New York.
Lo Grippo, G. A. (1951). *Angiology* **12,** 80–83.
Marks, H. C., Wyss, O., and Strandskov, F. B. (1945). *J. Bacteriol.* **49,** 299–305.
Mayr, G. (1961). *In* "Recent Developments in the Sterilization of Surgical Materials" (Dept. Pharm. Sci., Pharm. Soc. G. Brit. and Smith & Nephew Res., Ltd., eds.), pp. 90–97. Pharmaceutical Press, London.
Meeks, C. H., Pembleton, W. E., and Hench, M. E. (1967). *J. Am. Med. Assoc.* **199,** 124–126.
Moessel, D. A. (1963). *Lab. Pract.* **12,** 898.
Nordgren, G. (1939). *Acta Pathol. Microbiol. Scand. Suppl.* **40,** 1–115.
O'Brien, H. A., Mitchell, J. D., Haberman, S., Rowan, D. F., Winford, T. E., and Pellet, J. (1966). *J. Urol.* **95,** 429–435.
"Official Methods of Analysis of the Association of Official Agricultural Chemists" (1960). 9th Ed., pp. 67–69. Assoc. Offic. Agr. Chemists, Washington, D.C.

Opfell, J. B., and Miller, C. E. (1965). *Advan. Appl. Microbiol.* **7,** 81–102.

Opfell, J. B., Hohmann, J. P., and Latham, A. B. (1959). *J. Am. Pharm. Assoc., Sci. Ed.* **48,** 617–619.

Opfell, J. B., Shannon, J. L., and Chan, H. (1967). *Bacteriol. Proc.* **13,** A77.

Ortenzio, L. F., Stuart, L. S., and Friedl, J. L. (1953). *J. Assoc. Offic. Agr. Chemists* **36,** 480–484.

Page, R. C., and Borick, P. M. (1967). Arch. Surg. **94,** 162.

Pepper, R. E., and Chandler, V. L. (1963). *Appl. Microbiol.* **11,** 384–388.

Perkins, J. J. (1956). "Principal Methods of Sterilization," Chapt. XXI. Thomas, Springfield, Illinois.

Perkins, J. J. (1960). *Drug Cosmetic Ind.* **87,** 178–179.

Phillips, C. R. (1949). *Am. J. Hyg.* **50,** 280–288.

Phillips, C. R. (1961). *In* "Recent Developments in the Sterilization of Surgical Materials" (Dept. Pharm. Sci., Pharm. Soc. G. Brit. and Smith & Nephew Res., Ltd., eds.), pp. 59–75. Pharmaceutical Press, London.

Phillips, C. R., and Kaye, S. (1949). *Am. J. Hyg.* **50,** 270–279.

Polley, J. R. (1952). *Proc. Soc. Exptl. Biol. Med.* **81,** 302.

Portner, D. M., Mayo, E. C., and Kaye, S. (1954). *Bacteriol. Proc.* p. 35.

Pritchard, G. R., Wright, J. S., and Johnston, M. S. (1966). *J. Thoracic Cardiovascular Surg.* **52,** 232–235.

Rittenbury, M. S., and Hench, M. E. (1965). *Ann. Surg.* **161,** 127–130.

Rubbo, S., and Gardner, J. S. (1965). "A Review of Sterilization and Disinfection," pp. 141–142, 224. Lloyd-Luke, London.

Russell, A. D. (1965). *Mfg. Chemist Aerosol News* **36,** 38–45.

Shotton, E. (1961). *In* "Recent Developments in the Sterilization of Surgical Materials" (Dept. Pharm. Sci., Pharm. Soc. G. Brit. and Smith & Nephew Res., Ltd., eds.), pp. 1–6. Pharmaceutical Press, London.

Snyder, R. W., and Cheatle, E. L. (1965). *Am. J. Hosp. Pharm.* **22,** 321–327.

Spaulding, E. H. (1963). A.O.R.N. J. **1,** 36–46.

Spaulding, E. H. (1964). *Soap Chem. Specialties* July, **40,** 71–74.

Spaulding, E. H., Emmons, E. K., and Guzara, M. L. (1958). *Am. J. Nursing* **58,** 1530–1531.

Stierli, H., Reed, L. L., and Billick, I. H. (1962). "Evaluation of Sterilization by Gaseous Ethylene Oxide," Public Health Monograph No. 68, Public Health Serv. Doc. No. 903. U.S. Govt. Printing Office, Washington, D.C.

Stonehill, A. A., Krop, S., and Borick, P. M. (1963). *Am. J. Hosp. Pharm.* **20,** 458–465.

Stuart, L. S. (1966). *J. Assoc. Off. Agr. Chemists* **49,** 34–36.

Sykes, G. (1965). "Disinfection and Sterilization," 2nd Ed., pp. 311–349. Spon, London.

Van Winkle, W., Borick, P. M., and Fogarty, M. G. (1967). Symp. on Radiation Sterilization of Medical Products, sponsored by the Intern. At. Energy Agency, Budapest, IAEA, Vienna.

Vischer, Von W. A., Buhlmann, X., and Bruhin, H. (1963). *Pathol. Microbiol.* **26,** 515–523.

Walter, C. W., and Kundsin, R. B. (1959). *J. Am. Med. Assoc.* **170,** 123–124.

Weber, G. R., and Levine, M. (1944). *Am. J. Public Health* **34,** 719–728.

Willard, M., and Alexander, A. (1964). *Appl. Microbiol.* **12,** 229–233.

Wilson, A., and Bruno, P. (1950). *J. Exptl. Med.* **296,** 91, 458.

Wisely, D. V., and Falk, H. L. (1960). *J. Am. Med. Assoc.* **173,** 1161.

Wurzburg, O. B., and Kruger, L. H. (1962). U.S. Patent No. 3,058,853.

Copyright © 1967 by Academic Press, London
Reprinted from *J. Appl. Bacteriol.* **30**, 17–50 (1967)

 PRINTED IN GREAT BRITAIN

(Symposium on Chemical Disinfection: Paper III)

2

The Mode of Action of Antibacterial Agents

W. B. HUGO
Department of Pharmacy, The University, Nottingham, England

CONTENTS

1. Introduction

AN OUTSTANDING FEATURE which is immediately noticed when surveying the literature on the mode of action of antibacterial compounds is not only the diversity of publications wherein data are found but also the diversity of experimental approaches used. It is interesting that this diversity often arises from the nature of the original discipline in which the research worker was trained.

Work in this field has been going on for nearly 60 years and it is now possible to see some semblance of a pattern in antibacterial mechanisms.

Since 1940 work on the mode of action of antibiotics has paralleled work on disinfectants and it is interesting to note that there are one or two substances classified as antibiotics, the mode of action of which closely parallels other substances classified as disinfectants or antiseptics, and it is hoped to draw attention to these similarities in the later discussion. Previous reviews on this subject include those made by Wyss

(1948), by Hugo (1957) and by Newton (1958). A review dealing with the action of cationic agents on microbial cells has also recently appeared (Hugo, 1965*a*).

It would be quite wrong to embark upon a discussion of weapons without knowing something about their ultimate target and in the case of chemotherapeutic agents something of the nature of the host. In this review, however, dealing as it does with disinfectants the prime target, the bacterial cell, is the one which must be considered.

2. Structure of the Bacterial Cell

The main structures in the bacterial cell which are relevant to this review are the cell wall, the cytoplasmic membrane within and the cytoplasm contained by this membrane. The internal osmotic pressure of this cytoplasm is quite high; in Gram positive bacteria it may be as high as 30 atmospheres, and for Gram negative bacteria the highest recorded internal osmotic pressure is 8 atmospheres, but even this exceeds the typical pressure in a motor car tyre by a factor of 4.

The cytoplasmic membrane has a very low mechanical strength, possesses special properties of permeability and regulates the passage of metabolites within the cell; it also contains certain essential enzymes. The cytoplasm, which is a semifluid material, contains all the remaining components necessary for the life of the cell, including enzymes not present in the membrane, reserves of food materials, structures involved in the synthesis of protein and the genetic material responsible for the inheritable character of the cell.

It is to be expected that the cell wall must be of considerable mechanical strength in order to protect the weak cytoplasmic membrane from rupture under the influence of cytoplasmic osmotic pressure and indeed this has been found to be so. The cell walls of bacteria contain a rigid macromolecular network comprising a polymer of *N*-acetylglucosamine and *N*-acetylmuramic acid peptide, called murein. This structure is the main component of the cell walls of Gram positive bacteria and may occur in these organisms as a macromolecule of three concentric shells. In Gram negative bacteria the rigid network is thought to be only one molecule thick but in addition their cell walls contain up to 25% of their weight of lipoprotein and lipopolysaccharide. This notion is entirely compatible with the known greater resistance of Gram positive organisms to a mechanical rupture and to the fact that their cytoplasm is maintained at a considerably higher osmotic pressure than that of the Gram negative cells. It is perhaps worth mentioning that in the mycoplasma or pleuropneumonia-like organisms which are devoid of the rigid cell wall component the internal osmotic pressure is only *c*. 3 atmospheres.

Bacterial membranes are characterized by a high lipid content. Detailed studies using special staining techniques and the examination of thin sections of bacteria in the electron microscope have suggested that the bacterial lipid is a multilayer structure consisting of up to three layers. Other membrane components include carbohydrates and proteins (Salton & Freer, 1965).

In addition to acting as an osmotic barrier controlling the passage of metabolites into and out of the cell, many enzymes have been shown to be located in the membrane. Thus, the cytochrome respiratory pigments are almost invariably found to exist in the membrane. Other membrane enzymes include succinic dehydrogenase, acid phosphatase, 2-keto-*d*-deoxy-6-phosphogluconate aldolase and reduced nicotinamide-adenine-dinucleotide oxidase (Hughes, 1962; Gray, Wimpenny, Hughes & Mossman, 1965). The group of enzymes implicated in the active transport of metabolites and known as permeases (Cohn & Monod, 1957) are also located in the membrane.

Clearly, therefore, damage to the membrane can result in both inhibition of key enzymes and/or changes in the essential permeability of the cell with consequent leakage of metabolites to an extent which may interfere with the integrated reaction sequences associated with the normal metabolic processes.

Many cells have, outside their true wall, additional so called extramural layers in the form of capsules or slime. These layers may be of significance in the resistance of bacterial to antiseptics. The possible role of surface lipid in this connection are considered in section 5(a).

3. The Interaction of Antiseptics with the Bacterial Cell

This may conveniently be considered as occuring in two phases:

(a) The primary reaction with the cell;
(b) Subsequent damage to a structure or structures in the cell.

(a) *Primary drug/cell interactions*

Using techniques which have been traditionally used by the physical chemist to study phenomena such as adsorption and electrophoretic mobility much has been discovered about the initial reaction of drugs and living cells.

(i) *Adsorption*

During the first decade of the present century Herzog & Betzel (1911) realized the importance of adsorption in the disinfection process in their studies with bakers yeast, and since then many others have measured the uptake of drugs by cells. These studies consist primarily of adding a suspension of the cells to a solution of the drug and at suitable time intervals removing a sample, centrifuging to remove the cells and determining the residue amount of drug in the cell free supernatant solution. Clearly if the cells are removing drug from solution the concentration of the drug in the supernatant fluid will diminish. From these data adsorption isotherms may be plotted and information concerning the rate of uptake and the total amount of uptake may be computed. Furthermore, by a consideration of the nature of the isotherm obtained some notion of the adsorptive mechanism may be inferred. This aspect of the work has been reviewed by Giles, MacEwan, Nakhura & Smith (1960).

In brief, these authors considered four patterns of adsorption which they called S, L, H and C. The "S (S-shaped) pattern" is found when the solute molecule (a) is monofunctional, (b) has moderate intermolecular attraction, causing it to pack vertically and (c) meets strong competition for substrate sites, from molecules of the solvent or by another adsorbed species. Monohydric phenols when adsorbed on a polar substrate from water usually give this pattern.

In the "L (Langmuir) pattern", the initial curvature implies that as more sites are filled it becomes increasingly difficult for a bombarding solute molecule to find a vacant site. It may be inferred further that the adsorbed solute molecule is not orientated vertically or that there is strong competition from the solvent, or if vertical orientation does occur there is strong intramolecular attraction between the adsorbed molecules. Amongst the phenols, resorcinol might be expected to show this type of behaviour. The "H (high affinity) pattern", as its name implies, is obtained when the solute is almost completely adsorbed. Sometimes the process is also accompanied by an ion exchange process as is found in many bacteriological staining procedures. It is also shown by the uptake of iodine from an iodophor by yeast (Hugo & Newton, 1964).

The "C (constant partition) pattern" is obtained when the solutes penetrate more readily into the adsorbate than does the solvent. It might be expected to occur in biological systems because it has been shown to occur, for example, when aqueous solutions of phenols are adsorbed by synthetic polypeptides. It might also be expected to occur when phenols are adsorbed from aqueous solution by bacteria containing a high proportion of lipid in their cell wall.

More recent studies on the adsorption of antibacterial substances by micro-organisms include the uptake of cetrimide (CTAB) by bacteria (Salton, 1951), the adsorption of hexylresorcinol by *Escherichia coli* (Beckett, Patki & Robinson, 1959) of iodine by *E. coli, Staphylococcus aureus* and *Saccharomyces cerevisiae* (Hugo & Newton, 1964), of chlorhexidine by *Staph. aureus* and *E. coli.* (Hugo & Longworth, 1964) of basic dyes by fixed yeast cells (Giles & McKay, 1965) and of phenols by *E. coli* (Bean & Das, 1966).

Further information on the site of adsorption may be obtained by studying the process at different pH values but it should be borne in mind that both the ionization of the disinfectant as well as receptor sites on the cell surface may be affected by changes in pH (Salton, 1957*a*; Hugo & Longworth, 1964).

(ii) *Changes in electrophoretic mobility*

Bacterial cells are normally negatively charged and, if suspended in water or a suitable electrolyte solution containing electrodes to which a potential has been applied, the cells will migrate to the positively charged electrode. This phenomenon may be placed on a quantitative basis by observing the rate of migration of a single cell to the electrode by timing over a measured distance using a microscope and calibrated eyepiece micrometer. Once the system has been standardized the effect of drugs on mobility may be studied and from the data so obtained some notion of the drug cell interaction and the effect of drugs on the charged bacterial cell surface may be deduced. The subject of bacterial cell electrophoresis has been reviewed in detail by Lerch (1953).

In addition, adjuncts to the electrophoresis of normal cells may be used to further elucidate the nature of the surface components and furnish information as to the nature of the active sites on the cell surface, and thereby possibly of drug/cell interaction.

de Jong (1949), in studies on the reversal of the charge on certain colloids by cations at varying concentrations, found that a characteristic pattern of behaviour was shown as between phosphate colloids, carboxyl colloids and sulphate colloids. Now if pretreatment of bacterial cells at the appropriate concentration with cations corresponding to one of the above colloidal types was found to protect these cells, if only in part, from the action of a cationic disinfectant (chlorhexidine, a quaternary ammonium compound (QAC) or a basic dye, for example) then it is presumptive evidence that the prime site of adsorption on the cationic binding site is of a similar chemical nature. Newton (1954) applied this technique in an investigation of the site of action of the polypeptide antibiotic, polymyxin.

Yet another technique which may throw light on the nature of the surface and, by suitably planned experiments, of the binding site of drugs is to study the effect of enzyme pretreatment on the electrophoretic mobility of cells (James, 1965) paralleled by experiments on mobility and drug uptake on the same cells. Studies of the effect of antiseptics on the electrophoretic mobility of bacterial cells have been extensive and the following are discussed by way of illustration.

One of the first papers describing the use of electrophoresis to study the interaction of an antibacterial compound with bacteria was that of Bradbury & Jordan (1942) who studied the action of sulphanilamide on *E. coli*. By comparing the behaviour of the bacterial cells when treated with the sulphonamide and by compounds with similar functional groupings such as aniline and *p*-aminobenzoic acid it was deduced that the association of the drug with the cell was *via* its free amino group.

The first agent to be investigated was cetylpyridinium chloride (CPC). Using 10 different organisms Dyar & Ordal (1946) found that in all instances as the concentration of the drug was raised the mobility of the cells towards the cathode gradually decreased, then became zero and eventually the charge was apparently reversed and the cells now moved towards the anode. The actual concentrations of the drug to produce this pattern varied from species to species, as might be expected, because it is unlikely that the number of charged groups or the composition of the surface layers of different bacterial species will be the same; clearly too, the presence of a capsule, microcapsule or slime might be expected to play some role in this phenomenon.

Again using CTAB the problem was further investigated by McQuillen (1950). With the Gram negative *E. coli* McQuillen confirmed the findings of Dyar & Ordal mainly with increasing concentration of CTAB, the surface negative changes as measured by electrophoretic mobility was gradually neutralized and reversed. However, with the Gram positive *Staph. aureus* and *Streptococcus faecalis* a difference in behaviour was found, for here the mobility, after a slight decrease with increasing concentration, thereafter remained steady until at a concentration of 50 μM it rose sharply to attain a maximum some $1\frac{3}{4}$ times that of the normal cells; it then fell back to zero and suffering eventual reversal. It will be recalled that Dyar & Ordal did not find any difference as between Gram positive and Gram negative species. McQuillen's explanation for the behaviour of the Gram positive cells was that the net negative charge, and hence the mobility to the anode, increased by the adsorption of negatively charged molecular released from the cell by the action of the drug on the permeability barrier of the cell. That such release occurs is undoubtedly true and is discussed in section 3(b), (i).

A direct correlation of mobility change and leakage would have been an interesting experiment in support of the above hypothesis. In addition, Gram negative cells, including *E. coli*, also lose cellular constituents of a similar nature to those lost by Gram positive cells on treatment with many types of antibacterial compound so that the situation is not necessarily yet fully explained.

Haydon (1956) calculated the zeta potentials (themselves a function of mobility) of *E. coli* from electrophoretic data and found that when the cells were suspended in a solution of phenol this potential decreased with contact time and fell to a steady minimum value after 15 min contact. Inorganic ions were found to retard the depressant effect of phenol on the zeta potential.

The problem was investigated again by James, Loveday & Plummer (1964), using *Aerobacter aerogenes* and phenol, *p*-alkylphenols and *p*-halogenophenols. These workers found that the electrophoretic mobility, i.e. the rate of migration to the positive electrode, increased with increasing concentration of all the phenols tested, the substituted phenols being more active than phenol itself. They compared the effects of their phenols on the mobilities and viabilities of the organisms and found parallelism between these two parameters. It existed in fact, not only between the maximum concentration required to produce minimum mobility but also between the minimum concentration required to produce maximum mobility, and if the logarithm of these values was plotted against the logarithm of the solubility of the phenols in water families of parallel regressions were produced.

The effect of cell age and the extent of capsulation was also examined. It was not possible from these results, however, to delineate the exact mechanism whereby the phenols kill bacteria but certainly supplied additional support for Ferguson's principle (Ferguson, 1939), which is discussed in section 4.

Hugo & Longworth (1966), in their studies on the mode of action of chlorhexidine, measured the electrophoretic mobility of *Staph. aureus* and *E. coli* in the presence of the drug and compared this value with the uptake of the drug by the cells as measured by adsorption: the mobilities of both organisms decreased with increase in drug concentration. They concluded that the failure of chlorhexidine to neutralize the charge on *E. coli* at concentrations several times greater than the amount required to form a monolayer around the cells suggested that the drug is not adsorbed in the form of a monolayer.

(b) *Secondary drug/cell interactions of a general nature*

It is unlikely that adsorption of antibacterial drugs by the cell is in itself a fatal event, however, after the adsorption process secondary processes can be shown to occur, and these contribute to a greater or less extent to the inhibition of the reproductive and metabolic processes of the cell (bacteriostatic effect) and even to a rapid loss of viability (bactericidal effect).

(i) *Modification of cell permeability and leakage of cell constituents*

The phenomenon of haemolysis is well known and has been extensively studied. It can be induced by surface active agents (Schulman & Rideal, 1937; Pethica & Schulman, 1953), and in 1940 Kuhn & Bielig made the suggestion that QAC, because of their ability to dissociate conjugated proteins, might act on the bacterial cell membrane, a lipoprotein conjugate, and in a manner analogous to haemolysis damage it to the extent that the death of the cell ensued. Four years later, Hotchkiss (1944) obtained proof at the biochemical level that membrane damage was in fact occurring, by demonstrating that nitrogen and phosphorus containing compounds leaked from staphylococci when treated with QAC and the polypeptide antibiotic, tyrocidin.

Gale & Taylor (1947) concluded that the lytic action of the antibacterial compounds they studied, which included CTAB and phenol, was sufficient to explain their disinfectant action.

Later, Salton (1950, 1951), amply confirmed these observations and demonstrated that the bactericidal activity of CTAB up to that required to effect a 99·99% kill was related to the amounts of purine or pyrimidine containing components (as measured by material absorbing in the UV region of the spectrum at 260 mμ) leaking from the cells in 5 min. Similar observations were made by Beckett, Patki & Robinson (1958, 1959) using hexylresorcinol; these workers found that with increasing concentration the amount of material absorbing at 250 mμ rose steadily and attained a maximum value which was short of the total pool of such material, i.e. the material releasable by mechanical disruption of the cell.

Hugo & Longworth (1964) studied the ability of chlorhexidine to promote leakage of intracellular material and found an interesting diphasic leakage concentration pattern. The authors deduced from colateral evidence that whereas the first part of the curve was due to the normal increase of leakage with concentration, at higher concentrations the protoplasmic contents or cytoplasmic membrane became gradually coagulated so that the leakage became progressively less. Certainly electron micrographs of thin sections of bacteria taken after suitable dose treatments provided evidence in support of this view (Hugo & Longworth, 1965).

Many solvents, including butanol (Pethica, 1958), ethanol (Salton, 1963) and toluene (Jackson & de Moss, 1965), will cause the release of intracellular constituents, while maintaining cells in the temperature of boiling water for 10 min will release far more of such material than does antiseptic or solvent treatment.

It is likely that solvents and antibacterial agents promote leakage of labile nucleic acids and their component purines, pyrimidines, pentoses and inorganic phosphorus, and in fact detection of all these substances is certainly used to determine membrane damage, but it is unlikely that this is a rapidly fatal process, and indeed there is evidence that this type of damage may sometimes be reparable (Pullman & Reynolds, 1965). However heat treatment probably releases ribosomal material, and Jackson & de Moss (1965) have produced evidence that toluene treatment of *E. coli* may release ribosomes.

Yet another aspect of cytolysis may be observed in studies on the time course of cytoplasmic leakage. Very often a rapid initial release is often followed after an additional time lapse which may be of the order of hours by a further release of material; this may be due to a breakdown by autolytic enzymes of large molecular weight, or to ribosomal bound compounds or to a further time dependent damage to a permeability barrier. The two phenomena may be distinguished by conducting the experiment at 2° and at 36–40°. Nonenzymic lysis will be little different at 2° from that observed at the higher temperature: lysis due to enzymic action (secondary lysis) will be much less at 2° than at 36–40°. Polyene antibiotics are thought to interfere with membrane integrity (Lampen, 1966).

(ii) *Lysis*

In the foregoing section the phenomenon of partial lysis resulting in loss of cytoplasmic constituents was described. Under certain conditions complete lysis may be observed as indicated by a total or partial clearing of a turbid bacterial suspension, a process which may be conveniently followed by observing optical density changes at a suitable wave length.

The phenomenon is well documented in the case of the enzyme lysozyme (Salton, 1957*b*; Gray & Wilkinson, 1965) and as a consequent of infection by bacteriophage, or of metabolic disturbance (McQuillen, 1950). In some instances it may be drug induced and may arise from (a) a secondary phenomenon due to the activation of autolytic enzymes, (b) a direct action on a component of the cell wall or (c) impairment of the biosynthesis of a rigid component of the cell wall.

(a) One of the earliest inferences regarding secondary lysis was made by Pulvertaft & Lumb (1948) who found that phenol, formalin, mercuric chloride, sodium hypochlorite and merthiolate at bacteriostatic concentrations caused the lysis of certain bacterial cultures. The organisms tested varied in the extent to which lysis occurred, advanced lysis being found with staphylococci, pneumococci. *B. subtilis* and several strains of *E. coli;* less marked lysis was found with *Shigella dysenteriae,* very little lysis was found with *Strep. haemolyticus* and a nonhaemolytic streptococcus. With some organisms. although lysis was encountered at a low concentration of the antiseptic, it did not occur at the higher concentration. For example, at a phenol concentration of 0·045% a culture of *E. coli* underwent complete lysis, whereas at 0·54% no lysis occurred. A suggested explanation of these facts was that at the lower concentration lytic enzymes present in the cell were acticated by phenol. At the higher concentration, the lytic enzymes were themselves inhibited and thus no lysis occurred. The lytic phenomenon was not seen in older cultures. Delpy & Chamsy (1949) found that thiomersalate increased the susceptibility of *B. anthracis* to lysis, and Norris (1957) confirmed this observation with *B. cereus.*

Schaechter & Santomassino (1962) noted that low concentrations of some mercurial compounds which included mercuric chloride, phenylmercuric acetate and merthiolate, caused lysis of growing cultures of *E. coli.* Isolated cell walls were not affected. They inferred interference with the formation of disulphide bonds in the cell wall but did not refer to earlier literature or suggest the activation of lytic enzymes.

(b) Bolle & Kellenberger (1958) found that sodium lauryl sulphate lysed non-respiring (cyanide treated) cells of *E. coli.* The rod shaped organisms enlarged into globular forms and then underwent rapid lysis. Actively metabolizing cells were not susceptible.

Working with walls isolated from 6 Gram negative bacteria Shafa & Salton (1960) found wall disagregation to occur and suggested that the breakdown was due to an action upon the lipid containing compounds of the wall. Lytic enzymes were not thought to be implicated in the observed effect.

(c) The original observation of Fleming (1929) on the action of penicillin was that it lysed bacterial cultures: 36 years of research has now proved almost unequivocally that penicillin interferes with the biosynthesis of the rigid mucopeptide component of the bacterial cell walls. It prevents the formation of a peptide bridge between layers of the acetylmuramic acid/*N*-acetylglucosamine polymer; lysis occurs by osmotic explosion (Wise & Park, 1965; Tipper & Strominger, 1965).

Although many antibiotics act by interference with cell wall biosynthesis only one other type of antiseptic, crystal violet, has been thought to possess this property, although the site of interference was thought to occur at a point earlier in cell wall synthesis than that at which the wall inhibiting antibiotics are known to act (Strominger, 1959). This experiment has not been repeated.

Clearly, therefore, if an antimicrobial drug can be demonstrated to possess a lytic action its final effect may be due to one of several modes of action and experiments must be devised to determine which may be the operative mode.

(iii) *Irreversible general coagulation of cytoplasmic constituents*

This drastic lesion is usually seen at drug concentrations far higher than those causing general lysis or leakage. Historically it was the first cytological effect to be reported and in fact most antiseptics were classified as general protoplasmic poisons or as protein precipitants. Indeed at concentrations used in many practical disinfection procedures this is undoubtedly the mechanism of rapid kill, the more subtle and more slowly fatal effects being completely masked.

The cytoplasmic components most likely to be coagulated or denatured are proteins and nucleic acids, most studies having been made on the former. Proteins are complex structures consisting of a linear polymer of amino acids (the primary structure) cross linked by hydrogen bonding (the secondary structure), by disulphide bonds and by bonds of weaker structure such as electrostatic forces to give the tertiary structure. Functionally, proteins are of two main kinds in living cells, structural and enzymic. The high specificity of enzymes is due to the unique surface contour they present in their tertiary structural form and to the distribution of charges on this contour. The charges arise from residual charges on the carboxylic acid or amino groups of the constituent amino acids uninvolved in peptide bond formation. It is not difficult to imagine therefore that a derangement of this uniquely contoured and electrically charged unit can easily upset its function.

As early as 1901, Meyer showed that the antibacterial action of phenols was proportionate to their distribution between water and protein thus suggesting that protein was a prime target. Cooper (1912) came to a similar conclusion working with bacteria and phenols and decided that phenols destroy the protein structure within the cell. Bancroft & Richter (1931) actually observed a coagulation of cell protein in *B. megaterium* and *A. aerogenes* using the light microscope.

Three main methods are available for studying protoplasmic coagulation—microscopy, light scattering and direct observation on cytoplasm obtained from crushed cells. Microscopic studies may include careful and skilful observation with the light microscope or by examination of treated cells, or thin sections of treated cells, in the electron microscope.

Example of studies by electron microscopy of whole cells treated with antibacterial compounds includes the work of Mitchell & Crowe (1947) (tyrocidin), Salton, Horne & Coslett (1951) and Dawson, Lominski & Stern (1953) (CTAB), and on thin sections, Chapman (1963) (colomycin) and Hugo & Longworth (1965) (chlorhexidine).

The last named authors found a correlation between the appearance of thin sections and inferential cytolytic damage obtained from measurement of cytoplasmic leakage. Thus at the concentration which caused maximum leakage, electron micrographs of thin section of cells treated at the same concentration showed a significant loss of electron dense material; at higher concentrations, which promoted no leakage due, it was thought to a general coagulation and sealing in of labile protoplasmic constituents, the electron micrographs showed a dense granular cytoplasm differing markedly in appearance from that seen in untreated cells.

An interesting technique for studying protoplasmic coagulation is based upon protoplast formation. It is well known that certain bacteria may be deprived of thin cell walls, and if this deprivation is carried out in a medium, the osmotic pressure of which balances the internal osmotic pressure of the cell, then globular protoplasts are formed; if the original cell was rod shaped, a change from a cylinder to a sphere also occurs. Now if the same operation is carried out on cells which have been treated with an agent which coagulates or fixes the protoplasm, then on dissolving the cell wall the expected globular form is not seen. Instead, a rod shaped protoplast is produced which, if coagulation is severe, does not undergo on subsequent dilution the expected general lysis due to osmotic explosion (see for example, Tomcsik, 1955; Hugo & Longworth, 1964). Coagulation of cellular protein may affect the light scattering properties of cells and is a sensitive method of assessing changes in the absorbing or reflecting properties of treated bacterial cells.

Yet another method consists of crushing the cells and investigating the action of the antiseptic directly on the cell free material so obtained. Although this system is in many ways an artificial one and the concentrations of the protoplasmic constituents may vary relatively and suffer enzymic degradation, it will give some indication of the order of concentration required to produce overt changes. Such experiments were made by Hugo & Longworth (1966) who, in their studies on chlorhexidine, found that protein and nucleic acid were precipitated from the cell-free juice of *E. coli* at concentrations of chlorhexidine far higher than those causing leakage.

(iv) *General effects on metabolism*

Early in the 1920's, at the beginnings of the era of studies on bacterial metabolism, a number of workers began investigating the effect of various antibacterial agents, including toluene, on metabolic processes. In general, experiments took the form of observations on bacterial respirations measured either directly by oxygen uptake or by recording the reduction of methylene blue in the classical Thunberg technique.

Quastel & Whetham (1925), during fundamental studies on the biological oxidation of alcohols by *E. coli*, noted that whereas at low concentrations ethyl and propyl alcohol were metabolized, methyl and the primary alcohols with chain lengths of C_4–C_8 were toxic to the cells; ethyl and propyl alcohols themselves were inhibitory at high concentrations and in order to function as a substrate had to be used at low concentrations. Another important observation was that the relative toxicity of the alcohols increased with increasing chain length. The studies were extended to phenol and to toluene, long used as a preservative in preparative and clinical biochemistry, and to other solvents such as benzene, cyclohexene, cyclohexane and acetone. All of these substances exercised a general inhibitory effect although some selectivity was observed. The cyclic hydrocarbons were much more toxic to succinic dehydrogenase (now known to be a membrane bound enzyme in many bacteria) than was phenol. Selectivity was also shown to be a function of the substrate being used. Thus sugar dehydrogenations were found to be much more susceptible than those involved in the dehydrogenation of lactate or formate. Acetone prevents reproduction of bacteria while leaving at least some dehydrogenases unscathed (Cathcart & Hahn, 1902).

Quastel continued in this field of study and in two papers (Quastel & Wooldridge, 1927*a*,*b*) produced evidence that the site of dehydrogenation reactions was the cell surface and that the reason for the selective action of toluene in inhibiting the dehydrogenations of the sugars was that the responsible enzymes were associated with lipid material. Although it was also considered that the permeability in the cell might be affected, the role of an altered permeability was not considered to be significant. Cook (1930) showed that the velocity of acetate oxidation by *E. coli*, as measured in the Barcroft respirometer, was slightly faster with the toluene treated cells than with untreated ones and suggested that this effect was due to an increase in cell permeability. He was also able to show that toluene treated cells still retained their ability to oxidize lactate, formate and succinate.

The next papers concerning the action of antiseptics on enzymes were published by Bach & Lambert (1937) who studied the effect of antiseptics and solvents on certain dehydrogenases of *Staph. aureus*. Their method was to expose the washed cells to the antiseptic for 30 min at 40° in both the presence and the absence of the substrate. Toluene, benzene and cyclohexanol were used in saturated aqueous solutions. The cells were than washed three times with water and their dehydrogenase activities measured by the Thunberg method. The lactic dehydrogenase was never totally destroyed by toluene, benzene, cyclohexanol, acetone or phenol and the presence of lactate reduced its apparent inhibition. In contrast iodine ($1/10^4$), mercuric cyanide ($1/10^6$), and copper sulphate ($1/10^2$) completely destroyed the enzyme and no protection was afforded by the substrate.

The work was extended to the glucose, succinate, formate, butanol, pyruvate, fumarate and glutamate dehydrogenases. The glucose, formate and butanol systems, like the lactate, were only partially inactivated by benzene, toulene, acetone or phenol, while systems activating succinate, fumarate, pyruvate and glutamate were completely destroyed.

Sykes (1939) also investigated the action of disinfectants on the succinate dehydrogenase of *E. coli*. His method differed from that of Quastel & Wooldridge and of Bach & Lambert in that the cells were treated at room temperature and after an interval substrate, buffer and methylene blue were added. The tubes were then evacuated and filled with nitrogen, placed in a water bath at 37° and the time taken to effect a 90% reduction of the dye measured. For phenol, viable counts were made on the suspensions after treatment; with other compounds subcultures were made to test for residual viability. Sykes concluded that the concentrations of *p*-chloro-*m*-cresol, hexylresorcinol, *p*-butylphenol, amyl-*m*-cresol, phenol and ethyl, *iso*propyl, *n*-butyl and *n*-amyl alcohols required to completely inhibit the succinate dehydrogenase were always slightly in excess of the minimum lethal concentrations.

Dagley, Dawes & Morrison (1950) grew cells of *A. aerogenes* in a synthetic medium containing glucose, potassium dihydrogen phosphate, ammonium sulphate and magnesium sulphate, and found that a progressively increasing lag phase was introduced by increasing the doses of phenol. This lag could be abolished or reduced by the addition of a culture filtrate of the synthetic medium in which the organisms had been growing, or by L-leucine, DL-methionine, or L-glutamic acid and also by α-oxoglutaric or succinic acids. On the other hand other amino and carboxylic acids were found to increase the lag period, DL-aspartic or fumaric acids being examples. The bacteriostatic effect of phenol was thought to be due to its inhibition of the synthesis of metabolites essential for rapid cell division.

Hugo & Street (1952) studied the effect of phenol and phenoxetol on the oxidation of certain substrates by washed suspensions of *E. coli*, and showed that 0·1–0·2% of either caused a stimulation (10–20%) of the rate of oxygen consumption when glucose, mannitol and lactose were used as substrate but a marked inhibition (10–15%) when lactate, pyruvate, acetate or succinate was the substrate. No changes in the viable population and no uncoupling effect could be demonstrated. It was thought that the enzymes mediating the stimulated reaction were situated within the cell and the first action of phenol and phenoxetol was to increase the permeability, thus facilitating the access of substrate to enzymes within the cell. The marked inhibition of lactate and succinate activity could be interpreted if the enzymes responsible for their oxidation were located at the surface of the cell. Partial confirmation was obtained (Hugo, 1956) by comparing the action of phenol and phenoxetol on a disrupted preparation of *E. coli* which was capable of oxidizing glucose and lactate. No stimulation of glucose oxidation was obtained with the disrupted preparation and the oxidation of lactate appeared less sensitive in the disrupted preparation than in the intact cell. Disruption of the cell would have the effect of destroying the *status quo* of enzyme location, thus the diffusion barrier represented by a cell wall or cell membrane would no longer function and a reaction stimulated by an increase in the permeability of the barrier would not be expected to undergo stimulation in a disrupted preparation. Similarly, enzymes located at a cell surface and therefore immediately exposed to the action of an adverse environment might appear less susceptible when the cells have been disrupted.

The action of 2:4-dinitrophenol (DNP) and certain other nitrated and halogenated phenols on the metabolic reactions of micro-organisms are of considerable interest. Shoup & Kimler (1934) found that DNP at first stimulated and then depressed the rate of respiration of certain luminous bacteria. Stimulation does not occur, however, with all substrates tested; Krahl & Clowes (1935) and Genevois & Creach (1935) detected no stimulation in the respiration of yeast with lactate, pyruvate or glycerol as substrates.

Simon (1953*a*, *b*) made a detailed study of the action of phenol and certain nitrated phenols on the respiration, assimilation and fermentation of glucose by a yeast isolated from a sample of commercial baker's yeast. 3:5-Dinitro-*o*-cresol in concentrations of 10^{-5} M stimulated the amount of oxygen used by as much as 1·7 times. At high concentrations the consumption of oxygen was inhibited and aerobic fermentation appeared, which reached a peak at about 10^{-4} M and then was progressively inhibited.

In the absence of inhibitors the uptake of oxygen by washed yeast suspensions with glucose is about only half that required for complete oxidation according to the equation $C_6H_{12}O_6+6O_2 = 6CO_2+6H_2O$. But in the presence of 2×10^{-5} M of the cresol, an oxygen consumption corresponding to 93% of the total requirement was obtained. It was assumed that the action of the cresol at concentrations rising to 10^{-5} M was to prevent assimilation of glucose, and this accounted for the increased use of oxygen, that proportion of glucose assimilated by normal cells being now oxidized by molecular oxygen. *o*- and *p*-Nitrophenol gave similar results. Phenol, although it did not stimulate respiration, did inhibit assimilation.

Simon (1953*c*) believed from an analysis of his result that dinitrocresol acts as an uncoupling agent and that both oxidative assimilation and the rate of glycolysis are controlled by the level of energy rich phosphate. He concluded that there was little doubt that both the stimulation of respiration and the inhibition of oxidative phosphorylation is profoundly influenced by nitrophenols. The results obtained with phenol provided no clear evidence of any effect on phosphorylation.

The general effect of nitration or chlorination of phenol is to increase its bactericidal properties but the additional uncoupling effect on metabolism should not be overlooked.

With the introduction of the QAC, detailed studies similar to the above were commenced with a view to investigating the mode of action of this class of compound. Thus Baker, Harrison & Miller (1941*a*, *b*) made a systematic investigation of the effects of anionic, cationic and nonionic synthetic detergents on the aerobic and anaerobic respiration of glucose by washed suspensions of *Staph. aureus*, *Staph. albus*, *Micrococcus tetragenus*, *E. coli*, *Proteus vulgaris*, *Salmonella paratyphi*, *Sarcina lutea*, *Pseudomonas aeroginosa* (*pyocyanea*), *A. aerogenes*, *Shig. dysenteriae* and a lactobacillus, and concluded that all the cationic detergents were effective inhibitors of respiration at concentrations of 333 μg/ml, that the Gram negative and Gram positive organisms were equally affected and that depression of metabolism and extent of kill were roughly parallel. The test of killing, however, was based on an end point method capable only of showing either a 0% or 100% kill. They also noted that certain detergents stimulated bacterial metabolism at subinhibitory concentrations, a phenomenon they found much more commonly amongst the anionic detergents.

Ordal & Borg (1942) studied the effect of CPC and sodium dioctylsulphosuccinate on the oxidation of lactate by *E. coli* and *Staph. aureus* using both molecular oxygen and methylene blue as hydrogen acceptors, and found that the lactate-methylene blue system of *Staph. aureus* was far more susceptible than was *E. coli*. When molecular oxygen was the final hydrogen acceptor, lactate oxidation by *Staph. aureus* was inhibited by both compounds, in contrast to *E. coli* in which only the cationic (pyridinium) compound was inhibitory. It was concluded that the terminal oxidative enzymes of lactate oxidation in *E. coli* are more susceptible than those responsible for the reaction when an artificial carrier is the final hydrogen acceptor, and it was suggested that the cytochrome system responsible in *E. coli*, for the mediation of the reduction of molecular oxygen was either more susceptible or more accessible to the action of the surface active agent.

Sevag & Ross (1944) made a systematic study of the action of the cationic compound Zephiran (an alkylmethylbenzylammonium chloride) on certain enzyme systems of baker's yeast. In the first place, at a concentration of 1000 μg/ml, the 545–565 and 605–625 mμ absorption bands of cytochrome c in yeast cells were reversibly diminished in intensity (quantitative measurements of the reduction in intensity of the bands were not made, their value being estimated by inspection with a hand spectroscope). The cytochrome-cytochrome oxidase system was investigated by following the oxidation of *p*-phenylenediamine colorimetrically and manometrically. Inhibition of this system was complete at a Zephiran concentration of 2·8 μg/ml, with a Zephiran-yeast ratio of 50–100 μg/mg dry wt of yeast. The oxidation of glucose by molecular oxygen was inhibited to the extent of 91% at Zephiran-yeast ratios of 33·3 μg/mg dry wt of yeast. When methylene blue replaced oxygen as the final oxygen acceptor, inhibition was 97% for Zephiran-yeast ratio of 25–33·3 μg/ml dry wt of yeast. Further experiments by the authors attempted to relate inhibition of growth with inhibition of respiration, using as substrate glucose in phosphate buffer. At Zephiran concentrations of 4·5–18·2 μg/ml, a stimulation of oxygen uptake of 54–60% was obtained whilst the inhibition of growth was 64–83%.

Knox, Auerbach, Zarudnaya & Spirtes (1949), studied the effect of 5 QAC and other detergents on the lactate oxidation and dehydrogenation, the glucose and hexose diphosphate oxidation and glycolysis, the oxidation of pyruvate, formate, alanine and succinate, arginine decarboxylation and the aldolase activity of *E. coli*. In the experiments on the inhibition of glucose oxidation, the percentage kill was determined at the end of the experiment by means of a viable count of the contents of the Warburg flask, and in certain cases cell free enzymes were prepared and the effect of the detergents on their activities compared with the effect on the intact cells. The concentration of each of the 5 compounds to produce 50% kill and 50% inhibition of glucose and lactate oxidation was determined and a correlation between killing and inhibition of glucose oxidation obtained. It is possible, however, that the figures for the viable counts reported in this work were low, as dilutions were plated out into Endo's agar and counts made after 24 h (it is customary to count after 48 or even 72 h), and no attempt was made to neutralize the cationic detergent or to overcome the clumping that occurs with this class of compound.

Some data on selective resistance of enzymes also emerged from this work. Thus the detergent/bacterial nitrogen or dry weight ratio for 50% inhibition of lactate oxidation of intact cells by Zephiran was 180 μg/mg of N (19·8 μg/mg dry wt of cells) a higher figure than the corresponding values for glucose (88–90 μg/mg of N, or 9·6–9·7 μg/mg dry wt of cells). A considerable stimulation of lactate oxidation by subbactericidal amounts of this detergent was reported. No actual figures were given for the extent of stimulation nor was further comment made on this observation. The arginine decarboxylase activity of intact cells was found to be remarkably resistant to Zephiran, and at certain concentrations marked stimulation of its activity noted. This stimulation was not shown to such a marked extent with a cell free arginine decarboxylase, and the authors interpreted it as being due to an increase in the permeability of the intact bacterial cell to the substrate.

A cell free preparation which catalysed the oxidation of lactic acid to pyruvic acid by molecular oxygen was prepared by grinding the cells for 3 h in a Booth-Green mill and centrifuging the resulting slurry after diluting with an equal volume of water.

The inhibition of this enzyme was of the same order as that of glucose oxidation by intact cells and the percentage killing of the cells. All these effects were proportional to the detergent/cell (or enzyme) N ratio rather than to the concentration of the detergent, and it was finally concluded that the specific inhibition of detergent sensitive enzymes can account for the metabolic inhibition, cell death and increased permeability observed in bacteria with bactericidal amounts of cationic detergents.

It is difficult to see how metabolic inhibition and cell death, which occur to the same extent, can be accounted for by the fact that a lactic oxidase, or for that matter any other enzyme, is inhibited by detergents, unless this reaction is shown to be essential for the metabolism of the cell. It is even more difficult to see how such enzyme sensitivity can account for the increased permeability shown. The stimulated lactate oxidation by intact cells in the presence of subinhibitory concentrations, however, may be attributable to a change in the permeability of the cell to substrate or co-enzyme, the reason given for stimulated arginine decarboxylase activity found.

More recently the problem has been re-investigated by Armstrong (1957). Using baker's yeast as the test organism, and with the aid of 6 cationic compounds, he examined the relationship between cytolytic damage, as measured by loss of total phosphorus from the cell, and metabolism, as measured by production of acid and carbon dioxide from glucose, and concluded that the initial toxic reaction was a disorganisation of the cell membrane and this was followed by inactivation of the cellular enzymes. He also noted that low concentrations ($0{\cdot}1 \times 10^{-3}$ M, equivalent to 0·8 μg/mg dry wt of yeast) of the QAC usually caused small and rather variable increases in acid production.

Scharff & Beck (1959) made a detailed investigation of the often reported stimulant effect on metabolic reactions caused by low doses of surface active agents. They studied the effect of benzalkonium chloride on the anaerobic and aerobic metabolism of glucose by baker's yeast and noted that glucose metabolism under anaerobic conditions underwent progressive inhibition at all concentrations of benzalkonium chloride tested, but that in the presence of air uptake of oxygen and output of carbon dioxide were stimulated, the former by 33% the latter by 50%, peak stimulation occurring at benzalkonium concentrations of 3·5 μg/mg dry wt of yeast. It was deduced in addition, both from measurements of CO_2 production and from glucose utilisation, that the Pasteur effect was inhibited. This work was extended by Scharff & Maupin (1960) who studied membrane damage as determined by the loss of potassium ion from the cell, and they distinguished two zones of activity depending on the concentration of benzalkonium chloride. In the first, the pre-lytic zone with concentrations of benzalkonium chloride of <4 μg/mg dry wt of yeast: (i) oxygen consumption was increased, (ii) the Pasteur effect was inhibited, (iii) membrane permeability was not appreciably altered and (iv) fermentation was not appreciably affected. In the second zone (>4–5 μg of benzalkonium chloride/mg dry wt of yeast): (i) cell permeability was affected as demonstrated by loss of K^+, (ii) fermentation was inhibited and (iii) decarboxylation of exogenous pyruvate was initiated.

Examining the carbohydrate metabolism more carefully they found that in zone 2, fermentation of glucose and decarboxylation of exogenous pyruvate were respectively, directly and inversely correlated. A close correlation between loss of potassium, inhibition of glucose fermentation and appearance of pyruvate decarboxylase activity over a range of QAC concentrations was observed. All experiments were performed at pH 5·5 on 'resting' cells of the yeast. The inhibition of fermentation was thought to be due either to the loss of essential cofactors or to an interference with glucose transport into the cell rather than to a direct action on the enzymes themselves, because the concentrations bringing about the inhibition did not inhibit the individual enzymes studied in isolation,

The conversion of pyruvic acid to acetaldehyde and ethanol at pH 5·5 only after treatment with the QAC was thought to be attributable directly to a change in membrane permeability to the substrate, thus allowing it to pass into the cell. In contrast, the metabolism of glucose-1- and -6-phosphate, fructose-6-phosphate, hexose diphosphate and 3-phosphoglycerate was not so facilitated. The enzymes responsible for the glycolysis cycle may not have been activated, either because the increased membrane permeability is not a factor in their activation or because the activity is impaired by loss of cofactors. This latter contention is certainly feasible as the potassium ion is an activator for ketohexokinase.

More recently the precise mechanism of the stimulation of oxygen uptake with glucose as substrate in baker's yeast by benzalkonium chloride has been elucidated by Bihler, Rothstein & Bihler (1961).

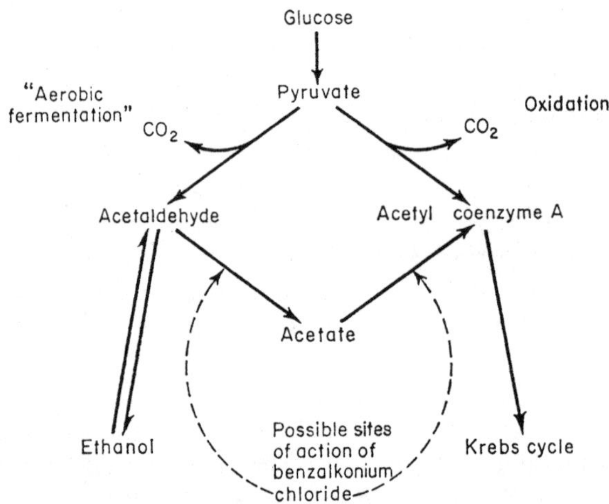

Fig. 1. Glucose metabolism by yeast, and possible sites of action of benzalkonium chloride.

The metabolic routes of glucose metabolism by yeast in the presence of air is shown in Fig. 1. Predisposition to the 'aerobic fermentative' pathway (so called because although taking place in air, the metabolic products are as found in glycolysis) is caused by a high initial glucose concentration in the medium. Thus with 0·11 M-glucose, the 'aerobic fermentation' was negligible but reaches a maximum with a ×100 increase in glucose concentration. The same result can also be obtained by adding excess of C_2 compounds (acetate or acetaldehyde) to the reaction mixture, and also with benzalkonium chloride at low (pre-lytic) concentrations. It is clear that the benzalkonium cannot increase the amount of glucose in the system but, by blocking the further oxidation of acetate in the Krebs cycle, it could cause an accumulation of acetate, thus producing the effect already noted when excess of the C_2 compounds are added. Hence it can be assumed that in yeast, the acetaldehyde⇋acetate, or the acetate⇋coenzyme A reaction must be unduly sensitive to benzalkonium chloride.

Stimulation and activation of enzymes may be due to the phenomenon of unmasking. Toluene, already aluded to, will activate β-galactosidase (Herzenberg, 1959), arabinose isomerase (Dobrogosz & de Moss, 1963) and alkaline phosphatase (Levinthal, Singer & Fetherhol, 1962) either by altering permeability by action on the cytoplasmic membrane or by removing a layer of lipid which is masking access to the active site.

In summary however, despite the large volume of work there is little evidence that the effect of antiseptics on bacterial metabolism is anything but the result of a number of secondary nonspecific effects, with the possible exception of the reaction described by Bihler *et al.* (1961) and the uncoupling effect noted with nitrated phenols.

(c) *Drug/cell interactions in which the nature of the interaction is known with some precision*

(i) *Interaction with thiol (sulphydryl) groups*

One of the constituent amino acids found in both structural and enzymic protein is cysteine, $SH.CH_2.CHNH_2.COOH$. The SH group derived from cysteine residues is essential for the activity of many enzymes, for example, coenzyme A and triosphosphate dehydrogenase (Barron, 1951). Undoubtedly, many disinfectants either react with or oxidize this essential group and, what is more interesting, this sulphydryl poisoning may be reversed in some cases by adding a sulphydryl compound to the environment in which the toxic action is taking place. Sulphydryl inactivation, as it is called, can be divided into two broad categories, one in which actual combination occurs and so gives rise to inactivation, and a second in which oxidation occurs again causing inactivation.

(a) *Combination with sulphydryl enzymes.* Many metals such as mercury, silver, copper and the element arsenic react with sulphydryl enzymes to form mercaptides. Thus with mercuric chloride the reaction may be envisaged:

$$\text{enzyme}\begin{matrix} \diagup \text{SH} \\ \diagdown \text{SH} \end{matrix} + HgCl_2 \rightarrow \text{enzyme}\begin{matrix} \diagup \text{S} \diagdown \\ \diagdown \text{S} \diagup \end{matrix}\text{Hg} + 2HCl.$$

The fact that this reaction occurred and can be reversed by a thiol compound was commented on as long ago as 1889 by Geppert, and it is interesting to note also that Robert Koch during his studies on the chemical disinfection of *B. anthracis* attributed a much greater value to the antibacterial activity of corrosive sublimate because combination of mercury with bacterial sulphydryl groups under some circumstances was reversible or was bacteriostatic only, and if the cells were placed in conditions where the mercurial salt could be removed from the SH groups the cells were capable of growth. Knowledge of the action of sulphydryl combinants and their reversants has been exploited in formulating inactivators for the sterility testing of solutions containing mercury or arsenic using thioglycollates (Sykes, Royce & Hugo, 1952; Cook & Steel, 1960) and in the formulation of dimercapt-*o*-propanol for the treatment of Lewisite (arsenic) poisoning, and in other metal intoxications which may occur during medication or accidental over dosage.

(b) *Oxidation of sulphydryl enzymes and the action of oxidizing agents.* Oxidizing agents may progressively oxidize sulphydryl groups to disulphides and even to sulphoxides or sulphones. Mild reducing conditions may be expected to reverse the reaction leading to disulphide formation, but if oxidation proceeds to the sulphoxide or sulphone stage this reaction is biologically at least, irreversible.

2 R-S-H- ⇆	R-S-S-R →	R-S-S-R ←	R-S-S-R
		↓	↓ ↓
(thiol		O	O O
compound)	(disulphide)	(sulphoxide)	(sulphone)

Examples of disinfectants which probably act in this way are the halogens (Knox *et al.*, 1949) and potassium permanganate, but the antibacterial activity of halogens may be due also to their ability to halogenate essential groups.

(ii) *The action of metal binding agents*

Another interesting facet of cellular oxidation is afforded by accummulated knowledge of the mode of action for 8-hydroxyquinoline (oxine). This mixed with potassium pyrosulphate was introduced as a disinfectant at the end of the last century under the trade name Chinosol. Because it is able to form co-ordination compounds with many metals it was thought that its action was due to the fact that it deprived the growing bacteria of metals essential for their metabolism (Zentmeyer, 1944). Detailed studies of Albert and his colleagues revealed that the compound was inactivated when iron or copper were absent from the culture medium and suggested that the lethal agent was the structure shown in formula I (Rubbo, Albert & Gibson, 1950).

N
↓
O—Fe^+

I

N
↓
O—Fe—O
↑
N

II

Even more interesting is the fact that if the concentration of oxine was increased its toxicity apparently decreased, the so-called concentration quenching (Albert, Gibson & Rubbo, 1953). This paradox was explained by the fact that at higher concentrations the mass action effect caused the formation of the structure shown in formula II.

This was relatively nontoxic, and it seemed therefore that the action of 8-hydroxyquinoline was to form structure I which then entered the cell and oxidized with sulphydryl groups. It has also been shown that in addition to iron and copper, nickel, zinc, cadmium, manganese and calcium were co-toxic with oxine. Cobalt, however, behaved in an interesting and anomalous way in that it protected bacterial and fungal cells from the toxic action of oxine and its chelate compounds with iron and copper.

It has been suggested that cobalt owes its unique property to its ability to destroy peroxide formed during the oxidation of cell constituents by metals or metal chelates in the presence of atmospheric oxygen. Hydrogen peroxide formation is considered a secondary cytotoxic reaction of certain metals or metal chelate but if this theory is correct then peroxide formation must be a major contribution to the toxicity of the metals. For a comprehensive review of the application of metal-binding agents in bacterial chemotherapy see Albert (1959).

It is interesting to note that many metals themselves exert a toxic action on bacteria and this action also may be reversed by thiol compounds. This effect was known although not understood by the Persians of antiquity who found that water stored in silver vessels did not develop an unpleasant taste; metals are not completely insoluble in water and sufficient will go into solution to exert a toxic effect. This phenomenon has been graced with the rather high sounding name of the oligodynamic action of metals.

(iii) *Interaction with amino groups*

Bacterial cells are known to contain amino groups, where they occur as residues in proteins and peptides and in the free amino acid pool. Formaldehyde, a potent and effective bactericide, is thought to act by combination with amino groups. Its action may be inhibited and sometimes reversed by the addition of ammonia or soluble amines.

Halogens, in addition to their oxidizing action, may also act by halogenating amino groups with the formation of chloramines.

(iv) *Interference with oxidation reduction systems*

Derivatives of nitrofuran are widely used as disinfectants, especially for the treatment of bladder infections. Cramer (1947) showed that these drugs are reduced by bacterial enzymes and postulated that their inhibitory action arises from their preferential reduction over the natural energy yielding substrates in the cell, thereby depriving the cell of the necessary energy for growth.

Nitrated phenols which although they are not used as bactericides are used extensively in agriculture, are able to interfere with oxidative phosphorylation (Hemker, 1964). Other manifestations of their action have been referred to under phenols (see section 3(b), (iv)).

(v) *The mode of action of triphenylmethane dyes*

Dyes, both natural and synthetic, were used in histology in the 1870's, and towards the end of the 19th century it was noted that certain of them inhibit bacterial growth. Systematic studies by Churchman and his colleagues (Churchman, 1912; Churchman &

Michael, 1912, 1913) elucidated the important generalization that basic dyes are more effective than acidic dyes, a generalization that was to be paralleled in later years by the finding that basic (cationic) surface active agents were more effective than acidic (anionic) ones.

Stearn & Stearn (1924*a*, *b*), in their studies on the mechanisms of bacterial staining and the effect of pH on the process, suggested that the cations of the triphenylmethane dyes combined with carboxyl residues in proteins and this reaction accounted for bacteriostasis. Quastel & Wheatley (1931), using the Thunberg technique, investigated the action of 29 dyes on the oxidation of glucose, lactate, succinate and formate by washed suspensions of *E. coli* and confirmed the findings of Churchman that the basic dyes were more toxic to the multi-enzyme systems necessarily studied by this technique than were the acid dyes.

In another significant experiment (Quastel, 1931), this time using fumarase from *M. lysodeikticus* and *E. coli*, it was noted from a comparison of the action of dyes on both intact cells and a cell-free enzyme that shows the pattern of differential action as between acid and basic dyes was repeated in experiments with whole cells, the toxicity of acid dyes was much greater, indeed approaching that of basic dyes in the cell free system. It was concluded that a cause of selectivity as between acid and basic dyes lies rather in their ability to penetrate the cell rather than in their intrinsic activity.

In further studies on the effect of dyes on metabolism, this time of baker's yeast, Armstrong (1958) again proved that in the case of whole cells, the basic dyes were far more inhibitory towards the production of acid and CO_2 from glucose than were acid dyes. Cell free preparations were not examined.

Much later Gale & Mitchell (1947) correlated the apparent lipid/water partition coefficient of a series of triphenylmethane (TPM) dyes with their bacteriostatic value towards *Strep. faecalis* and also with their ability to interfere with the intracellular metabolism of glutamic acid. It was inferred that the intensity of activity was dependent upon the ease in which the dyes could penetrate the cell, and lipid solubility was a property which assisted in this penetration because the cytoplasmic membrane was lipid in nature. These ideas are in accord with the findings of Quastel in his work on dyes and bacterial fumarase. On the other hand, Lowick & James (1957) showed that cells that had become resistant to crystal violet by training contained a lipid layer at their surface. It is clear from these experiments, and those of Hugo & Franklin (1966), that membrane lipid may behave quite differently to extramural lipid in its effect on drug penetration.

A further contribution to the understanding of the mode of action of TPM dyes followed from the observations by Gale & Mitchell (1947) and Elliot & Gale (1948) that crystal violet interfered with glutamic acid metabolism.

Fry (1957) later showed that glutamine synthesis in *Staph. aureus* was inhibited by several TPM dyes. The effect of pH and the magnitude of the basic dissociation constant of the 6 dyes examined was also investigated. It was thought likely that the dyes combined with the enzyme or enzymes concerned with glutamine formation, presumably a glutamic acid decarboxylase, and that the shape and charge on the dye cation—the active species—enabled it to occupy a site normally needed by the substrate for its activation and chemical reactivity.

Yet another interesting and specific metabolic lesion reported in the literature was that gentian violet was able to interfere and prevent the synthesis of the mucopeptide of the cell wall of *Staph. aureus* but at a point earlier in the sequence than that at which the wall inhibiting antibiotics are known to act (Strominger, 1959). However a repetition of this experiment with 6 different samples of crystal violet failed to demonstrate evidence of wall inhibition.

(vi) *Interference with the functioning of nucleic acids: the mode of action of acridine dyes*

Acridine dyes, first introduced into medicine as trypanicidal agents, have been extensively used as antibacterial agents, and a large amount of work has been carried out on their mode of action. As with the TPM dyes it was early realized that the cation was the active species. McIlwain (1941) showed that nucleic acids antagonised the antibacterial action of acridine dyes and Ferguson & Thorne (1946) after studying the effect of a series of acridine compounds on the growth and respiration of *E. coli* concluded that they inhibited reactions closely connected with synthetic processes.

In 1961, Lerman, in studies on the physical properties of acridine/DNA complexes, suggested that these dyes could fit or intercalate between adjacent base pairs in the double helix of the DNA molecule. Further experiments confirmed this fact, which is compatible with the observation of McIlwain (1941) that nucleic acids antagonize the action of acridines, with the observation of Albert (1966) that molecular size and shape are of importance in determining the relative potency of acridines and with Ferguson & Thorne's (1946) observation that acridines inhibit synthetic processes, for as a result of the intercalation the unique geometry of the DNA molecule is distorted with subsequent profound sequelae. This property of intercalation is shared by some antibiotics e.g. actinomycin.

For a detailed coverage of this facet of acridine action the review of Waring (1966) should be consulted.

4. Structure/Action Relationships

Since the introduction of phenol into medicine and its dramatic exploitation by Lister in the 1860's many derivatives have been used and tested. The accumulated data now available enables certain generalizations to be drawn and these will be considered briefly in relation to the effects of halogenation, nitration and alkylation. (For an extensive review on this topic the paper by Suter (1941) should be consulted).

Halogenation of the aromatic nucleus increases antibacterial activity, and so does alkyl substitution. Combinations of these two substituents also results in a compound with increased activity. With a single substituent group, be it halogeno or alkyl, *p* substituted products are more active than their *o* or *m* isomers.

With the alkyl substituent, a normal alkyl derivative is more active than the corresponding branch chained derivative of the same number of carbon atoms, and likewise multisubstituted alkylphenols are less active than the mono-alkyl substituent with the same number of carbon atoms, e.g. *sym*-trimethylbenzene (mesitylene) is very much less active than is *p*-*n*-propylphenol. On the other hand, activity in the normal alkyl series often reaches a maximum with the hexyl or heptyl compound. When substitution includes both an alkyl radical and a halogen, then in general (1) *o*-alkyl derivatives of *p*-halogenated phenol are more active than *p*-alkyl-*o*-halogenophenols.

Apart from the difference between phenol and any one alkylphenol, the behaviour of a regular series of phenols or alcohols has been undertaken into this extension of the structure action relationship. As early as 1926 Tilley & Shaffer compared the toxicity of a homologous series of primary alcohols (*n*-ethyl to *n*-hexyl) with their ability to kill *Salm. typhi* and their data showed a linear relationship between the logarithm of the lethal dose against the number of carbon atoms in the alcohol. This in turn is related to their relative solubility in water and in oil. Coulthard, Marshall & Pyman (1930) studied the relationship between the phenol coefficient and the degree of alkylation of the 4-(*p*-)alkylphenols. They found that peak activity was obtained with the *n*-pentyl (4-*n*-amyl) phenol. The solubility of these compounds in water decreased steadily and suggested that both surface activity and partition coefficients were of significance in determining the ultimate toxicity of the compound. Of equal interest too, was the finding that in studies on the *n*-l-alkyl derivatives of 4-chlorophenol maximum activity was not the same for all bacteria; thus for *Salm. paradysenteriae* the maximum activity was with the *n*-hexyl derivative, *Mycobacterium smegmatis* with the *n*-heptyl, and for *Staph. aureus* the *n*-octyl compound.

Richardson & Reid (1940) and Fogg & Lodge (1945) further demonstrated that the oil/water partition coefficients were significant in determining the relative potency of phenolic compounds towards bacteria.

At the beginning of this century Meyer (1901) had formulated a general theory to explain what they called narcotic action, or what may also be called general non-specific poisoning, and concluded that differing lipid solubility, or any differences in distribution between an oily phase and water, could account quantitatively for differences in observed effects; the above examples support it.

In 1939 a piece of research was published which rationalized the relationship between biological activity and water/oil solubility in a range of the so called nonspecific drugs (Ferguson, 1939). Ferguson realized that the intensity of biological action was a function of the equilibrium attained by the compound concerned as between the site in the cell at which it was exerting the measured effect and the external milieu. With the disinfection process in a liquid environment, the external phase is almost invariably water; in other instances—chemical fumigation, air disinfection, general anaesthesia with volatile anaesthetics—the external phase will be air.

Having realized this, it should follow that data could be treated by the application of thermodynamic principles and it would follow that at equilibrium the chemical potential of the drug *not* the concentration would be the same in all phases.

It should be borne in mind that the concept refers to an equilibrium state, and it is of course possible that true equilibrium in the theoretical sense is not achieved as between the cell and the drug containing environment. However, treatment of data using this principle does suggest that it is a reasonable explanation of the *status quo* at cell level.

The calculation of the chemical potential is yet another problem, for if it is to be applied using practical and available data again certain assumptions and approximations have to be made.

Chemical potential, like electrode potential, is defined in terms of a standard and is thus a difference between an observed value and that of the standard. Usually in considering solutions of electrolytes the activity is used as a measure of the chemical potential while the activity at infinite dilution is taken as the standard state. In the special case under consideration the chemicals are nonelectrolytes of low water solubility and it has been suggested that the standard state for measuring the chemical potential should be that of the saturated solution, so that instead of activity water solubility should be the physically measurable parameter of the chemical potential in any given circumstance. It follows from this that phenols in solution will exert the same degree of toxicity when the relative degree of saturation of the solutions is the same. Thus if several phenols are dissolved in water to the point of half saturation, their solutions should all exert the same biological effect.

Allawala & Riegelman (1954) extended the findings of Ferguson to other examples of antibacterial activity and verified the prediction that relative toxicity in a series could be related to their solubility which provided in the circumstances a measure of the chemical potential.

James *et al.* (1964) obtained further evidence in support of this interesting generalization; indeed their data, in showing the principle to hold for a series of *p*-halogenated phenols, suggested that it was applicable not only to homologous series but to series where the substituents are less closely related.

5. Resistance

It is often stated that micro-organisms do not develop resistance, at least to any significant extent, to drugs whose action is that of a general poison. On the other hand drugs the action of which is limited to interference with a single point in a biosynthetic pathway in a cell may be rendered ineffective if, by one or another of the processes of adaption, an alternative route for the formation of the otherwise inhibited end product can arise: in other words resistance to the drug develops. Equally, an organism may be able to develop enzymes capable of destroying the toxic agent. A classic example of this type of resistance is that shown towards the penicillins by penicillinase-producing organisms. Despite the above generalizations it is nevertheless true that reports occur in the literature of developed resistance to general toxic agents (Moyed, 1964).

To date there are two mechanisms of resistance definable with some precision: the first concerns the accumulation of lipid by the cell during its acquisition of resistance; the second, the ability of some strains of bacteria to actually decompose the antibacterial agent.

(a) *Lipid and bacterial resistance*

The first hint that bacterial lipid may be of significance in determining the relative resistance of bacteria to detergent was provided by an experiment of Dyar & Ordal (1946) with *M. aureus* (*Staph. aureus*) in which a strain containing more lipid than the parent showed a greater sensitivity to changes in electrophoretic mobility, as induced by cetylpridinium chloride, and acquired a greater apparent negative change in the presence of sodium dodecylsulphate. In one experiment no difference in susceptibility, as measured by viable counts, to this agent could be demonstrated.

By serial subculture Chaplin (1951) obtained a ×43 increase in the resistance of a strain of *E. coli* and a ×200 increase in the resistance of *Serratia marcescens* to a series of quaternary ammonium compounds. He was unable to demonstrate resistance with *Staph. aureus*.

The increase in resistance of *S. marcesens* was considerable and in a later paper (Chaplin, 1952) a possible mechanism was demonstrated. Staining with Sudan Black B and electrophoretic mobility studies pointed to an increase in the lipid content of the resistant cells. Strong support for the existance of this lipid and its involvement in resistance came when these cells on treatment with a lipase lost their resistant properties.

Fischer & Larose (1952) confirmed the bacteriological data of Chaplin and found the adaptive process to be dependent on pH. Thus resistance of a higher order per generation number was obtained if the experiment was performed at pH 6·8 than at pH 7·7. Chaplin's failure to induce resistance in *Staph. aureus* was thought to be due to the use of too high a concentration of the drug in the training experiments.

The effect of pH was thought to be on ionization of the QAC used and consequently on drug uptake. No reference was made to the involvement of lipid in the acquired resistance, or whether the different pH values used were effecting the biosynthesis of the lipid shown by Chaplin to be involved in the acquisition of resistance.

Lowick & James (1957) trained *A. aerogenes* to grow in the presence of crystal violet and demonstrated by electrophoretic techniques that the surface of the resistance cells was prédominantly lipid whereas in the case of untrained cells the surface was predominantly polysaccharide.

Work in support of the involvement of lipid in the acquisition of resistance to antibacterial drugs was published by Vaczi, Szita & Cieleszky (1957) who found that certain Gram negative bacteria, *E. coli*, *Salm. typhi*, *Salm. typhimurium*, *Salm. paratyphi* in the course of acquiring resistance to chloramphenicol suffered a change in their lipid composition; in fact an increase in the proportion of the ether soluble fraction of the cellular lipid closely paralleled the increase in resistance. Furthermore the cells resistant to chloramphenicol were also found to be more resistant to the quaternary, hexadecylpyridinium bromide, although resistance to phenol was less than the unadapted organisms, due, it was said, to the fact that phenols are soluble in lipid.

Later, Vaczi & Farkas (1961) found that a strain of *Staph. aureus* resistant to penicillin possessed a higher cellular lipid content than sensitive strains. Hill, James & Maxted (1963) in a detailed study of the cell wall lipid of *Strep. pyogenes* and the emergence of resistance concluded that changes in metabolism associated with resistance to tetracycline may also result in a stimulation in the production of lipid.

To investigate further the role of lipid in resistance Hugo & Stretton (1966*a,b*) by growing a selected group of micro-organisms in nutrient broth containing glycerol, achieved an enhancement of their cellular lipid. The organisms used were *Staph. aureus* (three strains), *B. subtilis* and *Strep. faecalis*. All the fattened organisms showed an increased resistance to quinacillin, methicillin, cloxacillin and benzylpenicillin.

Similarly, treating cells with pancreatic lipase so as to reduce their lipid content resulted in an increase in sensitivity.

Using the same model, Hugo & Franklin (1966) studied the effect of lipid enhancement in the Oxford strain of *Staph. aureus* on its resistance to phenols. They used a series of 4-*n*-alkylphenols from phenol itself (R = H) to hexylphenol (R = C_6H_{13}). Not until pentylphenol was reached did enhanced cellular lipid protect the cells from its inhibitory action, the protection was even greater with *n*-hexylphenol. The general conclusion from these experiments was that lipid protects the bacteria studied from the antibacterial drugs by a nonspecific blanketing mechanism and the amyl- and hexyl-phenols are probably locked at the interface between the cellular lipid and the liquid (aqueous) environment in which the cells are growing.

It was not found possible to enhance the lipid content of *E. coli* or *Ps. aeruginosa* by growth in glycerol but it should be borne in mind that these cells contain lipid in their own right (in the form of a lipoprotein and a lipopolysaccharide complex) as an integral part of the cell wall. The status of the lipid in the cell walls of fattened Gram positive cells has yet to be determined but electrophoretic data lend support to the fact that it is at or very near the cell surface.

Recent research on Gram negative bacteria however has added further weight to the thesis that cell wall lipid may play an important role in resistance.

It has been known for some time that ethylenediamine tetra-acetic acid (EDTA) renders the cell walls of certain bacterial species susceptible to digestion by lysozyme (Repaske, 1958). It has also been shown to enhance the activity of certain antibacterial agents (MacGregor & Elliker, 1958; Brown & Richards, 1965). A biochemical mechanism for this action has been revealed by the work of Eagon & Carson (1965) and Gray & Wilkinson (1965) in their studies on the action of EDTA on *Ps. aeruginosa*. The latter workers showed that EDTA at alkaline pH extracted a component from the cells for which there was strong chemical evidence that it was a lipopolysaccharide. Asbell & Eagon (1966) came to a similar conclusion.

Leive (1965) studied the effect of EDTA on *E. coli* and noted that this organism also became permeable to several unrelated molecules under such treatment.

Ivanov, Markov, Golovinskii & Kharisanova (1964) treated *Ps. aeruginosa* with light petroleum and found that 22% of the total cell lipid was extracted, that this extraction did not impair the viability of the cells and that the sensitivity of the cells towards streptomycin, chloramphenicol, phenol, acetone, alcohol, mercuric chloride, acids and alkalis was increased.

The possible involvement of cell wall lipid in the susceptibility of Gram negative cells to a variety of molecular species is certainly suggested by these experiments.

This survey of apparent lipid-dependent acquired resistance has highlighted several problems. Not the least of these is the need for an understanding of the biochemical mechanisms underlying lipid build up in cells. Growth in glycerol will enhance the lipid content of some Gram positive bacteria to the extent of 40% or more, other strains did not respond to growth in glycerol by building up cellular lipid.

What is the status of the built up lipid? Is it as a conjugate with cellular protein, or does it occur as an extramural coating? Growth in glycerol does not enhance the cellular lipid of Gram negative bacteria, yet reports show that both *S. marcescens*

Table 1

The utilization of aromatic compounds by bacteria as sole carbon sources for growth*

Test organism†	Test method‡	*p*-Cresol	*o*-Cresol	*m*-Cresol	Benzoic acid	Phenol	*p*-Hydroxybenzoic acid	Salicylic acid	*m*-Hydroxybenzoic acid	Hydroquinone	Resorcinol	Catechol	Phloroglucinol	3,4-Dihydroxy-benzoic acid	3,5-Dihydroxy-benzoic acid	Gallic acid	Methyl gallate	Ethyl gallate	Methyl *p*-hydroxy-benzoate
Pseudomonas convexa X.1	a	+	−	+	+	+	+	−	−	−	−	+	(+)	+	+	+	−	−	−
	b	+	−	+	+	+	+	−	−	−	−	+	(+)	+	+	+	−	−	−
Ps. fluorescens (NCIB 8248)	a	+	+	(+)	+	+	+	(+)	−	−	(+)	+	+	+	−	−	−	−	−
	b	+	+	+	+	+	+	−	−	−	(+)	+	+	+	N	−	−	−	−
Vibrio 01 (NCIB 8250)	a	(+)	−	−	+	+	+	−	−	−	−	+	−	+	−	?	?	?	−
	b	+	−	−	+	+	+	−	−	−	−	+	−	+	N	?	?	?	−
Pseudomonas sp. (NCIB 8858)	a	+	−	−	+	+	+	+	−	−	−	+	−	+	−	−	−	−	−
	b	+	−	−	+	+	+	+	−	−	−	+	−	+	−	−	−	−	−
Ps. fluorescens (NCIB 8249)	a	−	(+)	−	+	+	+	(+)	−	−	−	+	−	+	−	−	−	−	−
	b	−	−	−	+	+	+	−	−	−	−	+	−	+	−	−	−	−	−
p-Cresol organism (NCIB 8251)	a	+	+	−	+	(+)	+	−	+	−	−	+	−	+	−	−	−	−	−
	b	+	+	−	+	(+)	+	−	+	+	−	+	−	+	N	−	−	−	−
V. cyclosites (NCIB 2581)	a	+	−	−	+	+	−	−	−	−	−	+	−	−	−	?	−	−	−
	b	+	−	−	+	+	−	−	−	−	−	+	−	−	−	?	−	−	−
Ps. desmolyticum (NCIB 8859)	a	+	−	+	+	−	+	−	−	−	−	+	−	+	−	−	−	−	−
	b	+	−	+	+	−	+	−	−	+	−	+	−	+	−	−	−	−	−
Pseudomonas sp. (NCIB 8226)	a	+	−	−	+	−	(+)	−	−	−	−	+	−	+	−	−	−	−	−
	b	+	−	−	+	−	(+)	−	−	+	−	+	−	(+)	−	−	−	−	−

* Utilization: +, growth; (+), poor growth; −, no growth; ?, result uncertain. † NCIB, National Collection of Industrial Bacteria.
‡ Test method: a, results obtained from test tube experiment; b, results obtained from auxanographic experiment. N, Experiment not done.

and *A. aerogenes* when trained to grow in high concentrations of cationic detergents or crystal violet build up cellular lipid. Has this lipid the status of a component of the cell wall characteristic of the Gram negative bacteria, or is it located elsewhere—perhaps as an extramural layer?

Much more is now known about the lipids of bacterial cells and improved techniques now exist for lipid analysis. It should be possible therefore, to elucidate some of the interesting problems outlined above.

(b) *Resistance due to decomposition of the antiseptic*

Hugo (1965*b*) has already reviewed the available data on this topic and the main features are considered below. It has been known since the beginning of this century that substances added to soil as disinfectants (soil fumigants) disappeared from the soil with the passage of time. This phenomenon is due to the decomposition of the fumigant by micro-organisms and various workers have isolated from habitats such as gas works, bacteria able to decompose the components of some of the phenolic fractions of coal tar. Predominant amongst the bacteria were members of the sub-order Pseudomonadineae—the genera *Pseudomonas* and *Vibrio.* Beveridge & Hugo (1964) surveyed the ability of 9 micro-organisms to degrade 18 aromatic compounds, many of which are known antibacterial agents, and their findings are presented in Table 1.

In another investigation Hugo & Foster (1964) found a strain of *Ps. aeruginosa* able to utilize methyl and propyl *p*-hydroxybenzoates as the sole source of carbon. As these preservatives were at one time used in the preparation of eye drops, and because of the danger to the eye of infections by *Ps. aeruginosa*, it is clear that this pattern of resistance can be of extreme practical significance.

6. General Conclusions

The relative complexity of the action of disinfectants is in fact a manifestation of their general nonspecificity. Thus, whatever property of the cell is studied, whether it be its mobility in an electric field, its ability to dehydrogenate succinic acid, its ability to maintain its labile intracellular integrity, or simply to reproduce or even remain alive in the presence of the disinfectant a concentration dependent effect on this property will be obtained.

In the author's opinion it is no longer possible or even scientifically valid to try and determine 'the mode of action' of a nonspecific drug by a study, however detailed, of one changeable property. To do this it is essential to compare experimentally several facets of drug action, indeed the more the better, and always to relate them to the prime role of the drug, namely its ability to prevent multiplication or to kill.

To illustrate the theme of multiple attack and show its concentration dependence, the collected data of Hugo & Longworth (1964, 1965, 1966) obtained in their study of the actions of chlorhexidine on bacterial cells (Table 2) are interesting.

The large volume of work on the action of disinfectants on the metabolic processes of bacteria probably stem from the notion that a highly sensitive reaction might be found and hence reveal an intellectually satisfying mode of action. In most instances, in fact, differences in enzyme susceptibility which have been observed may be due

TABLE 2

Summary of results obtained for the action of chlorhexidine on E. coli

Reaction concentration µg/ml of chlorhexidine diacetate	Adsorption of chlorhexidine µg/mg dry wt *E. coli* cells (a)	Electro-phoretic mobility (µ/sec/v/cm)	Leakage µg/mg dry wt cells after 6 hr contact		Bactericidal activity mean single survivor time (min) (a)	Reduction of tetrazolium as % of reduction by untreated cells	Electron microscopic appearance after 6 h treatment (b)	% precipitation of cell free cytoplasmic constituents	
			E at 260 mµ (a)	pentoses (µg) (a)				protein	nucleic acid
0	0	4·62	0·04	0·8	—	100	"normal"	0	0
5	5	4·52	0·09	1·4	—	110	—	0	0
10	10	4·40	0·14	2·0	—	103	as control	0	0
90	72	3·40	0·53	9·2	3981	0	gross damage + leakage	0	0
200	160	2·50	0·175	3·6	417	0	coagulation of cytoplasm + surface	6	14
500	293	1·55	0·12	3·4	33	0	protuberances, no leakage	56	94

(a) Hugo & Longworth, 1964
(b) Hugo & Longworth, 1965

to the location rather than the intrinsic sensitivity of the enzymes; it could be expected that membrane-bound enzymes would appear more sensitive than those situated in the cytoplasm. Loss of co-factors essential for enzyme activity may also be occasioned by their leakage from the cells, again giving an impression of differences in susceptibility.

This is not to say, however, that no specific metabolic lesion will exist for drugs classified as disinfectants and usually expected to be nonspecific in their action The recently discovered subtle effect of acridine dyes is an example where the more recent techniques of molecular biology have revealed a very precise mode of action for a drug whose activities heretofore were cloaked in the broadest of generalities The interference of benzalkonium chloride with acetate metabolism, and of TPM dyes with glutamine synthesis, are also examples where more precise modes of action have been established from careful metabolic studies.

It is worth bearing in mind that if the drug under investigation produces a meaningful rate of kill of say 99·99% mortality in 20–30 min or is bacteriostatic at concentrations which appear to have no effect on the coagulation of protein, then a search for more precise modes of action might be worthwhile.

Finally, an underlying theme in all work in this field is to distinguish clearly cause and effect, a very difficult task with nonspecific drugs.

An interesting problem which remains after considering the survey of work in this review is to enquire what combination of properties in a molecule render it an efficient bactericide or bacteriostat; is it possible to see in the family of successful members of this class of compound any pattern common to all? If indeed such a spectrum of properties were to emerge clearly then could these be added to, included in, or serve as, screening characteristics?

Many of the newer successful bactericides have the property in common of causing membrane damage and a search for leakage of one of the relevant components might be a worthwhile routine. Examination of adsorption of drug uptake seems also to be important. Another thought which appears almost to give an *Alice through the Looking Glass* approach to the matter is to try and establish why certain chemicals are not, in the commonly accepted definition of the word, potential disinfectants (setting aside the obvious condemnatory properties of high chemical reactivity or gross systemic toxicity); again drug uptake and evidence of cytolytic damage might be properties which have to be shared by a compound destined to be useful as a disinfectant.

7. References

ALBERT, A. (1959). Metal-binding agents in chemotherapy: the activation of metals by deletion. In *The Strategy of Chemotherapy*, 8th Symposium of the Society for General Microbiology. Cambridge: University Press.

ALBERT, A. (1966). *The Acridines*, 2nd ed. London: Arnold.

ALBERT, A., GIBSON, M. I. & RUBBO, S. D. (1953). The influence of chemical constitution on antibacterial activity Part VI. The bactericidal action of 8-hydroxyquinoline (oxine). *Br. J. exp. Path.* **34**, 119.

ALLAWALA, N. A. & RIEGELMAN, S. (1954). Phenol coefficients and the Ferguson principle. *J. Am. pharm. Ass.* (*Sci. Ed.*) **43**, 93.

ARMSTRONG, W. McD. (1957). Surface active agents and cellular metabolism. I. The effect of cationic detergents on the production of acid and carbon dioxide by baker's yeast. *Arch. biochim. biophys.* **71**, 137.

ARMSTRONG, W. McD. (1958). The effect of some synthetic dyestuffs on the metabolism of baker's yeast. *Arch. biochem. biophys.* **73**, 153.

ASBELL, MARY A. & EAGON, R. G. (1966). Role of multivalent cations in the organisation structure and assembly of the cell wall of *Pseudomonas aeroginosa*. *J. Bact.* **92**, 380.

BACH, D. & LAMBERT, J. (1937). Action of some antiseptics on the dehydrogenases of *Staphylococcus aureus*. *C. Séane. Soc. Biol.* **126**, 300.

BAKER, Z., HARRISON, R. W. & MILLER, B. F. (1941*a*). Action of synthetic detergents on the metabolism of bacteria. *J. exp. Med.* **73**, 249.

BAKER, Z., HARRISON, R. W. & MILLER, B. F. (1941*b*). The bactericidal action of synthetic detergents. *J. exp. Med.* **74**, 661.

BANCROFT, W. D. & RICHTER, G. H. (1931). The chemistry of disinfection. *J. phys. Chem.* **35**, 511.

BARRON, E. S. G. (1951). Thiol groups of biological importance. *Adv. Enzymol.* **11**, 201.

BEAN, H. S. & DAS, A. (1966). The adsorption by *Escherichia coli* of phenols and their bactericidal activity. *J. Pharm. Pharmac.* **18**, 1075.

BECKETT, A. H., PATKI, S. J. & ROBINSON, A. (1958). Interaction of phenolic compounds with bacteria. *Nature, Lond.* **181**, 712.

BECKETT, A. N., PATKI, S. J. & ROBINSON, A. (1959). The Interaction of phenolic compounds with bacteria. I. Hexylrecorcinol and *Escherichia coli*. *J. Pharm. Pharmac.* **11**, 360.

BEVERIDGE, E. G. & HUGO, W. B. (1964). The resistance of gallic acid and its alkyl esters to attack by bacteria able to degrade aromatic ring structures. *J. appl. Bact.* **27**, 304.

BIHLER, I., ROTHSTEIN, A. & BIHLER, L. (1961). The mechanism of stimulation of aerobic fermentation in yeast by a quaternary ammonium detergent. *Biochem. Pharmac.* **8**, 289.

BOLLE, A. & KELLENBERGER, E. (1958). The action of sodium lauryl sulphate on *E. coli*. *Schweiz. Z. Path. Bakt.* **21**, 714.

BRADBURY, F. R. & JORDAN, D. O. (1942). The surface behaviour of antibacterial substances. I. Sulphanilamide and related substances. *Biochem. J.* **36**, 287.

BROWN, M. R. W. & RICHARDS, R. M. E. (1965). Effect of ethylenediamine tetracetate on the resistance of *Pseudomonas aeruginosa* to antibacterial agents. *Nature, Lond.* **207**, 1391.

CATHCART, E. & HAHN, M. (1902). Uber die Wirkungen der Bakterien. *Arch. Hyg.* **44**, 295.

CHAPLIN, C. E. (1951). Observations on quaternary ammonium disinfectants. *Can. J. Bot.* **29**, 373.

CHAPLIN, C. E. (1952). Bacterial resistance to quaternary ammonium disinfectants. *J. Bact.* **63**, 453.

CHAPMAN, G. B. (1963). Cytological aspects of antimicrobial antibiosis. III. Cytological distinguishable stages in antibiotic action of colistin sulphate on *Escherichia coli*. *J. Bact.* **86**, 536.

CHURCHMAN, J. W. (1912). The selective bactericidal action of gentian violet. *J. exp. Med.* **16**, 221.

CHURCHMAN, J. W. & MICHAEL, W. H. (1912). The selective action of gentian violet on closely related bacterial strains. *J. exp. Med.* **16**, 822.

CHURCHMAN, J. W. & MICHAEL, W. H. (1913). The selective bactericidal action of strains closely allied to gentian violet. *J. exp. Med.* **17**, 373.

COHN, G. H. & MONOD, J. (1957). Bacterial permeases. *Bact. Rev.* **21**, 169.

COOK, R. P. (1930). A comparison of the dehydrogenases produced by *E. coli communis* in the presence of oxygen and methylene blue. *Biochem. J.* **24**, 1538.

COOK, A. M. & STEEL, K. J. (1960). The antagonism of the antibacterial action of mercury compounds. IV. Quantitative aspects of the antagonism of the antibacterial action of mercuric chloride. *J. Pharm. Pharmac.* **11**, 162T.

COOPER, E. A. (1912). On the relationship of phenol and m-cresol to proteins; a contribution to our knowledge of the mechanism of disinfection. *Biochem. J.* **6**, 362.

COULTHARD, C. E., MARSHALL, J., & PYMAN, F. L. (1930). The variation of phenol coefficients in homologons series of phenols. *J. chem. Soc.* p. 280.

CRAMER, D. L. (1947). The mode of action of nitrofuran compounds. II. Application of physicochemical methods to the study of action against *Staphylococcus aureus*. *J. Bact.* **54**, 119.

DAGLEY, S., DAWES, E. A. & MORRISON, G. A. (1950). Inhibition of growth of *Aerobacter aerogenes*: the mode of action of phenols, alcohols, acetone and ethyl alcohol. *J. Bact.* **60**, 369.

DAWSON, I. A., LOMINSKI, I. & STERN, H. (1953). An electron microscope study of the action of cetyltrimethylammonium bromide (CTAB) on *Staph. aureus*. *J. Path. Bact.* **66**, 513.

Delpy, P. L. & Champsy, H. M. (1949). Sur la stabilisation des suspensions sporulèes de *B. anthracis* par l'action de certains antiseptiques. *C.r. hebd. Séanc. Acad. Sci., Paris* **228,** 1071.

Dobrogosz, W. J. & De Moss, R. D. (1963). Induction and repression of L-arabinose isomerase in *Pediococcus pentosaceus J. Bact.* **85,** 1350.

Dyar, M. T. & Ordal, E. J. (1946). Electrokinetic studies of bacterial surface. I. The effects of surface-active agents on the electrophoretic mobilities of bacteria *J. Bact.* **51,** 149.

Eagon, R. G. & Carson, K. J. (1965). Lysis of cell walls and intact cells of *Pseudomonas aeroginosa* by ethylenediamine tetra-acetic acid. and by lysozyme. *Can. J. Microbiol.* **11,** 193.

Elliot, W. H. & Gale, E. F. (1948). Glutamine-synthesising system of *Staphylococcus aureus;* its inhibition by crystal violet and methionine sulphoxide. *Nature, Lond.* **161,** 129.

Ferguson, J. (1939). The use of chemical potentials as indices of toxicity. *Proc. R. Soc.* **127B,** 387.

Ferguson, T. B. & Thorne, S. O. (1946). The effects of some acridine compounds on the growth and respiration of *Esch. coli. J. Pharmac. exp. Ther.* **86,** 258.

Fischer, R. & Larose, P. (1952). Factors governing the adaption of bacteria against quaternaries. *Nature. Lond.* **170,** 715.

Fleming, A., (1929). On the antibacterial action of cultures of a penicillium, with special reference to their use in the isolation of *B. influenzae. Br. J. exp. Path.* **10,** 226.

Fogg, A. H. & Lodge, R. M. (1945). The mode of antibacterial action of phenols in relation to drug-fastness. *Trans. Faraday Soc.* **41,** 359.

Fry, B. A. (1957). Basic triphenylmethane dyes and the inhibition of glutamine synthesis by *Staphylococcus aureus. J. gen. Microbiol.* **16,** 341.

Gale, E. F. & Mitchell, P. D. (1947). The assimilation of amino-acids by bacteria. 4. The action of triphenylmethane dyes on glutamic acid assimilation. *J. gen. Microbiol.* **1,** 299.

Gale, E. F. & Taylor, E. S. (1947). The action of tyrocidin and some detergent substances in releasing amino acids from the internal environment of *Streptococcus faecalis. J. gen. Microbiol.* **1,** 77.

Genevois, L. & Creach, P. (1935). Action du dinitrophenol (1,2,4) sur le levure de boulanger americaine. *C.r. Séance soc. biol.* **118,** 1357.

Giles, C. H., MacEwan, T. H., Nakhura, S. N. & Smith, D. (1960). Studies in adsorption. XI. A system of classification of solution adsorption isotherms and its use in the diagnosis of adsorption mechanisms and in measurements of specific surface areas of solids. *J. chem. Soc.* p. 3973.

Giles, C. H. & McKay, R. B. (1965). The adsorption of cationic (basic) dyes by fixed yeast cells. *J. Bact.* **89,** 390.

Gray, G. W. & Wilkinson, S. G. (1965). The effect of ethylenediamine tetraacetic acid on the cell walls of some Gram negative bacteria. *J. gen. Microbiol.* **39,** 385.

Gray, C. T., Wimpenny, J. W. T., Hughes, D. E. & Mossman, M. E. (1965). Regulation of metabolism in facultative bacteria. I. Structural and functional changes in *Escherichia coli* associated with shifts between the aerobic and anaerobic states. *Biochim. biophys. acta* **117,** 22.

Haydon, D. A. (1956). Surface behaviour of *Bacterium coli.* II The interaction with phenol. *Proc. R. Soc.* **145B,** 383.

Hemker, H. C. (1964). The mode of action of dinitrophenols on the different phosphoylating steps. *Biochim. biophys. acta* **81,** 9.

Herzenberg, L. A. (1959). Studies on the induction of β-galactosidase in a cryptic strain of *Escherichia coli. Biochim. biophys. acta* **31,** 525.

Herzog, R. A. & Betzel, R. (1911). Zur Theorie der Desinfektion. *Hoppe-Seyler Z.,* **74,** 221.

Hill, M. J., James, A. M. & Maxted, W. R. (1963). Some physical investigations of the behaviour of bacterial surfaces. X. The occurrence of lipid in the streptococcal cell wall. *Biochim. biophys. acta* **75,** 414.

Hotchkiss, R. D. (1944). Gramicidin, tyrocidine and tyrothricin. *Adv. Enzymol.* **4,** 153.

Hughes, D. E. (1962). The bacterial cytoplasmic membrane. *J. gen. Microbiol.* **29,** 39.

Hugo, W. B. (1956). The action of phenol and 2-phenoxyethanol on the oxidation of various substrates by *Escherichia coli* and by a disrupted cell preparation of the organisms. *J. gen. Microbiol.* **15,** 315.

Hugo, W. B. (1957). The mode of action of antiseptics. *J. Pharm. Pharmac.* **9,** 145.

Hugo, W. B. (1965*a*). Some aspects of the action of cationic surface active agents on microbial cells with special reference to their action on enzymes. In *Surface Activity and the Microbial Cell:* S.C.I. monograph no. 19. London: Society of Chemical Industry.

HUGO, W. B. (1965*b*). The degradation of preservatives by micro-organisms. Sci. and Tech. Symp. 122. *Ann. meeting Amer. pharm. Assoc.* C-111, p. 1.

HUGO, W. B. & FOSTER, J. H. S. (1964). Growth of *Pseudomonas aeruginosa* in solutions of esters of *p*-hydroxybenzoic acid. *J. Pharm. Pharmac.* **16**, 209.

HUGO, W. B. & FRANKLIN, I. (1966). The influence of cellular lipid on the resistance of micro-organisms to antibacterial agents. *IX Int. Cong. Microbiol. Abs.* p. 21.

HUGO, W. B. & LONGWORTH, A. R. (1964). Some aspects of the mode of action of chlorhexidine. *J. Pharm. Pharmac.* **16**, 655.

HUGO, W. B. & LONGWORTH, A. R. (1965). Cytological aspects of the mode of action of chlorhexidine diacetate. *J. Pharm. Pharmac.* **17**, 28.

HUGO, W. B. & LONGWORTH, A. R. (1966). The effect of chlorhexidine on the electrophorotic mobility cytoplasmic contents dehydrogenase activity and cell walls of *Escherichia coli* and *Staphylococcus aureus*. *J. Pharm. Pharmac.* **18**, 569.

HUGO, W. B. & NEWTON, J. M. (1964). The adsorption of iodine from solution by micro-organisms and serum. *J. Pharm. Pharmac.* **16**, 49.

HUGO, W. B. & STREET, M. E. (1952). The effect of phenol, 2-phenoxyethanol and cetyltrimethyl ammonium bromide on the oxidation of various substrates by *Escherichia coli*. *J. gen. Microbiol.* **6**, 90.

HUGO, W. B. & STRETTON, R. J. (1966*a*). Effect of cellular lipid on the sensitivity of some Gram positive bacteria to penicillins.. *Nature, Lond.* **209**, 940.

HUGO, W. B. & STRETON, R. J. (1966*b*). The role of cellular lipid in the resistance of Gram-positive bacteria to penicillins. *J. gen. Microbiol.* **42**, 133.

IVANOV, V., MARKOV, K. I., GOLOVINSKII, E. & KHARISANOVA, T. (1964). Importance of surface lipids for various biological properties of a *Pseudomonas aeruginosa* strain. *Z. Naturf.* **196**, 604.

JACKSON, R. W. & DE MOSS, J. A. (1965). Effects of toluene on *Escherichia coli*. *J. Bact.* **90**, 1420.

JAMES, A. M. (1965). The modification of bacterial surface structures by chemical and enzymic treatment. In *Cell Electrophoresis*, Ed. E. J. Ambrose, London: J. A. Churchill.

JAMES, A. M., LOVEDAY, D. E. E. & PLUMMER, D. T. (1964). Some physical investigations of bacterial surfaces. XI. The effect of phenol and substituted phenols on the electrophoretic mobility of *Aerobacter aerogenes*. *Biochim. biophys. acta* **79**, 351.

DE JONG, H. G. B. (1949). Reversal of charge phenomena. Equivalent weight and specific properties of the ionised groups. In *Colloid Science*, vol. 2. Ed. H. R. Kruyt. London: Elsevier.

KNOX, W. E., STUMPH, P. K., GREEN, D. E. & AUERBACH, V. H. (1948). The inhibition of sulphhydryl enzymes as the basis of the bactericidal action of chlorine. *J. Bact.* **55**, 451.

KNOX, W. E., AUERBACH, V. H., ZARUDNAYA, K. & SPIRTES, M. (1949). The action of cationic detergents on bacteria and bacterial enzymes. *J. Bact.* **58**, 443.

KRAHL, M. E. & CLOWES, G. H. A. (1935). Some effects of dinitrocresol on oxidation and fermentation. *J. biol. Chem.* **111**, 355.

KUHN, R. & BIELIG, H. J. (1940). Uber invertseifen. I; die Einwirkung von Invertseifen auf Eiweiss-Stoffe. *Ber. dt. chem. Ges.* **73**, 1080.

KUHN, R. & DAM, O. (1940). Uber Inverseifen II; Butyl-, Octyl-, Lauryl und Cetyldimethylsulphonium Jodid. *Ber. dt. chem. Ges.* **73**, 1099.

LAMPEN, J. O. (1966). Interference by polyenic antifungal antibiotics (especially nystatin and filipin) with specific membrane function. In 16th Symposium of the Society of General Microbiology. Cambridge: University Press.

LEIVE, LORETTA (1965). A non-specific increase in permeability of *Escherichia coli* produced by EDTA. *Proc. natn. Acad. Sci. U.S.A.* **53**, 745.

LERCH, C. (1953). Electrophoresis of *Micrococcus pyogenes* var *aureus*. *Acta. path. microbiol. scand.* **98**, 1.

LERMAN, L. S. (1961). Structural considerations in the interaction of DNA and acridines. *J. molec. Biol.* **3**, 18.

LEVINTHAL, C., SINGER, E. R. & FETHERHOL. K. (1962). Reactivation and hybridization of reduced alkaline phosphatase. *Proc. Natn. Acad. Sci. U.S.A.* **48**, 1230.

LOWICK, J. H. B. & JAMES, A. M. (1957). The electrokinetic properties of *Aerobacter aerogenes*. A comparison of the properties of normal and crystal violet-trained cells. *Biochem. J.* **65**, 431.

MACGREGOR, D. R. & ELLIKER, P. R. (1958). A comparison of some properties of strains of *Pseudomonas aeruginosa* sensitive and resistant to quaternary ammonium compounds. *Can. J. Microbiol.* **4**, 499.

McIlwain, H. (1941). A nutritional investigation of the antibacterial action of acriflavine. *Biochem. J.* **35**, 1311.

McQuillen, K. (1950). The bacterial surface. I. Effect of cetyltrimethylammonium bromide on the electrophoretic mobility of certain Gram positive bacteria. *Biochim. biophys. acta* **5**, 643.

Meyer, H. (1901). Zur Theorie der Alkoholnarkose. III. Mittheilung: Der Einfluss Wechselnder Temperatur auf Wirkungstarke und Narcotica. *Arch. exp. Path. Pharmak.* **46**, 338.

Mitchell, P. D. & Crowe, G. R. (1947). A note on electron micrographs of normal and tyrocidin lysed streptococci. *J. gen. Microbiol.* **1**, 85.

Moyed, H. F. (1964). Biochemical mechanisms of drug resistance. *Ann. Rev. Microbiol.* **18**, 347.

Newton, B. A. (1954). Site of action of polymyxin on *Pseudomonas aeruginosa:* antagonism by cations. *J. gen. Microbiol.* **10**, 491.

Newton, B. A. (1958). Surface active bactericides. *In The Strategy of Chemotherapy;* 8th Symposium of the Society for General Microbiology. Cambridge: University Press.

Norris, J. R. (1957). A bacteriolytic principle associated with cultures of *Bacillus cereus*. *J. gen. Microbiol.* **16**, 1.

Ordal, E. J. & Borg, A. F. (1942). Effect of surface active agents on the oxidation of lactate by bacteria. *Proc. Soc. exp. Biol. Med.* **50**, 332.

Pethica, B. A. (1958). Bacterial lysis. Lysis by physical and chemical methods. *J. gen. Microbiol.* **18**, 473.

Pethica, B. A. & Schulman, J. H. (1953). The physical chemistry of haemolysis by surface-active agents. *Biochem. J.* **53**, 177.

Pullman, J. E. & Reynolds, B. L. (1965). Some observations on the mode of action of phenol on *Escherichia coli*. *Austral. J. Pharm.* **46**, 580.

Pulvertaft, J. V. & Lumb, C. D. (1948). Bacterial lysis and antiseptics. *J. Hyg., Camb.* **46**, 62.

Quastel, J. H. (1931). The action of dyestuffs on enzymes: fumarase. *Biochem. J.* **25**, 898.

Quastel, J. H. & Wheatley, A. H. M. (1931). The action of dyestuffs on enzymes. I. Dyestuffs and oxidations. *Biochem. J.* **25**, 629.

Quastel, J. H. & Whetham, M. D. (1925). Dehydrogenations produced by resting bacteria. I. *Biochem. J.* **19**, 520.

Quastel, J. H. & Wooldridge, W. R. (1927*a*). The effects of chemical and physical changes in environment on resting bacteria. *Biochem. J.* **21**, 148.

Quastel, J. H. & Wooldridge, W. R. (1927*b*). Experiments on bacteria in relation to the mechanism of enzyme action. *Biochem. J.* **21**, 1224.

Repaske, R. (1958). Lysis of Gram-negative organisms and the role of versene, *Biochim. biophys. acta* **30**, 225.

Richardson, E. M. & Reid, E. E. (1940). a,ω,Di-p- hydroxyphenyl alkanes. *J. Am. chem. Soc.* **62**, 413.

Rubbo, S. D., Albert, A. & Gibson, M. I. (1950). The influence of chemical constitution on antibacterial activity. Part V. The antibacterial action of 8-hydroxyquinoline (oxine). *Br. J. exp. Path.* **31**, 425.

Salton, M. R. J. (1950). The bactericidal propeties of certain cationic detergents. *Aust. J. scient. Research* **B3**, 45.

Salton, M. R. J. (1951). The adsorption of cetyltrimethylammonium bromide by bacteria, its action in releasing cellular constituents and its bactericidal effects. *J. gen. Microbiol.* **5**, 391.

Salton, M. R. J. (1957*a*). The action of lytic agents on the surface structures of the bacterial cell. In *Proc. 2nd Int. Congr. Surface Activity*. London: Butterworth.

Salton, M. R. J. (1957*b*). The properties of lysozyme and its action on microorganisms. *Bact. Rev.* **21**, 28.

Salton, M. R. J. (1963). The relationship between the nature of the cell wall and the Gram-stain. *J. gen. Microbiol.* **30**, 223.

Salton, M. R. J. & Freer, J. H. (1965). Composition of the membranes isolated from several Gram-positive species. *Biochim. biophys. acta* **107**, 531.

Salton, M. R. J., Horne, R. W. & Coslett, V. E. (1951). Electron microscopy of bacteria treated with cetyltrimethylammonium bromide. *J. gen. Microbiol.* **5**, 405.

Schaechter, M. & Santomassino, K. A. (1962). The lysis of *Esch. coli* by sulphhydryl-binding agents. *J. Bact.* **84**, 318.

Scharff, T. G. & Beck, J. L. (1959). Effects of surface-active agents on carbohydrate metabolism in yeast. *Proc. Soc. exp. Biol. Med.* **100**, 307.

SCHARFF, T. G. & MAUPIN, W. C. (1960). Correlation of the metabolic effects of benzalkonium chloride with its membrane effects in yeast. *Biochem. Pharmac.* **5**, 79.

SCHULMAN, J. H. & RIDEAL, E. K. (1937). Molecular interaction in monolayers. I. Complexes between large molecules. *Proc. R. Soc.* **B122**, 29.

SEVAG, M. G. & ROSS, O. A. (1944). Studies on the mechanism of the inhibitory action of Zephiran on yeast cells. *J. Bact.* **48**, 677.

SHAFA, F. & SALTON, M. R. J. (1960). Disaggregation of bacterial cell walls by anionic detergents. *J. gen. Microbiol.* **23**, 137.

SHOUP, C. S. & KIMLER, A. (1934). The sensitivity of the respiration of luminous bacteria for 2,4-dinitrophenol. *J. cell. comp. Physiol.* **5**, 269.

SIMON, E. W. (1953*a*). The action of nitrophenols in respiration and glucose assimilation in yeast. *J. exp. Bot.* **4**, 377.

SIMON, E. W. (1953*b*). Dinitrocresol, cyanide and the Pasteur effect in yeast. *J. exp. Bot.* **4**, 393.

SIMON, E. W. (1953c). Mechanisms of dinitrophenol toxicity. *Biol. Rev.* **28**, **453**.

STEARN, E. W. & STEARN, A. E. (1924*a*). The chemical mechanism of bacterial behaviour. I. Behaviour towards dyes—factors controlling the Gram reaction. *J. Bact.* **9**, 463.

STEARN, E. W. & STEARN, A. E. (1924*b*). The chemical mechanism of bacterial behaviour. III. The problem of bacteriostasis. *J. Bact.* **9**, 491.

STROMINGER, J. L. (1959). Accumulation of uridine and cytidine nucleotides in *Staph. aureus* inhibited by gentian violet. *J. biol. Chem.*, **234**, 1520.

SUTER, C. M. (1941). Relationships between the structures and bactericidal properties of phenols. *Chem. Rev.* **28**, 269.

SYKES, G. (1939). The influence of germicides on the dehydrogenases of *Bact. coli*. *J. Hyg., Camb.* **39**, 463.

SYKES, G., ROYCE, A. R. & HUGO, W. B. (1952). A sterility test for Neoarsphenamine B.P. and Sulpharsphenamine B.P. for injection. *J. Pharm. Pharmac.* **4**, 366.

TILLEY, F. W. & SHAFFER, J. M. (1926). Relation between the chemical constitution and germicidal activity of the monohydric alcohols and phenols. *J. Bact.* **12**, 303.

TIPPER, D. J. & STROMINGER, J. L. (1965). Mechanism of action of penicillins: A proposal based on their structural similarity to Acyl-D-alanyl-D-alanine. *Proc. natn. Acad. Sci. U.S.A.* **54**, 1133.

TOMCSIK, J. (1955). Effects of disinfectants and of surface active agents on bacterial protoplasts. *Proc. Soc. exp. Biol. Med.* **89**, 459.

VACZI, L. & FARKAS, L. (1961). Association between lipid metabolism and antibiotic sensitivity. I. The lipid composition of antibiotic sensitive and resistant *Staphylococcus aureus* strains. *Acta microbiol. hung.* **8**, 205.

VACZI, L. SZITA, J. & CIELESZKY, V. (1957). The role of lipids in induced chloramphenicol resistance of bacteria. *Acta microbiol. hung.* **4**, 437.

WARING, M. J. (1966). Cross-linking and intercalation in nucleic acids. In *Biochemical Studies of Antimicrobial Drugs:* 16th Symposium of the Society of General Microbiology. Cambridge: University Press.

WISE, E. R. & PARK, J. T. (1965). Penicillin: Its basic site of action as an inhibitor of a peptide cross linking reaction in cell wall mucopeptide synthesis. *Proc. natn. Acad. Sci. U.S.A.* **54**, 75.

WYSS, O. (1948). Chemical disinfectants. *A. Rev. Microbiol.* **2**, 413.

ZENTMEYER, G. A. (1944). Inhibition of metal catalysis as a fungistatic mechanism. *Science* **100**, 294.

Reprinted from *Advan. Appl. Microbiol.* **7**, 81–102 (1965)

3

Cold Sterilization Techniques

JOHN B. OPFELL[1] AND CURTIS E. MILLER[2]

Dynamic Science Corporation, South Pasadena, California

I. Introduction

Cold sterilization processes are those effective below temperatures where heat alone can sterilize. For the most part, these processes are applied at temperatures below 50°C.

Cold sterilization processes are important because they can be applied to many materials or objects which are damaged or destroyed by heat sterilization processes. In many cases, however, cold sterilization processes are chosen for heat-sterilizable materials to gain savings in money, time, or effort. The degree to which these savings can be realized depends on the application intended for the sterilized object (whether it is a material or the interior surfaces and gas within an enclosed space). Usually, the very nature of the sterilization process is controlled by the sequence

[1] Present address: Aeronutronic Division of Philco Corporation, Newport Beach, California.

[2] Present address: Space-General Corporation, El Monte, California.

of operations which precede and which follow sterilization as well as by the nature of the constituent materials of the sterilized object. The savings realized usually depend also on the effect the sterilization process has on the available choices for materials and for the operations required before and after sterilization, including preparation and packaging. Seldom, however, can a cold sterilization process be wisely chosen on the basis of maximum assurance of achieving sterility.

From the microbiological standpoint, uniform conditions of chemical composition, temperature, and even pressure are of greater importance in cold sterilization techniques than in sterilization techniques performed at higher temperatures. This greater importance arises from the fact that the chemical, physical, and biological conditions which are lethal for one population of microorganisms may promote growth or a refractory state of dormancy in another. The conditions which distinguish the lethal from the dormancy-promoting environment for any one population, or even cell, may not differ much chemically.

Some types of chemical agents used in cold sterilization produce or favor the survival of strains of microorganisms which are resistant to sterilization at the concentrations and temperatures normally employed. This effect extends to the sterility tests for demonstrating process efficacy in that the nutritive requirements for populations or cells exposed to the sterilizing agent can be changed in perhaps significant ways.

Although sterilization of many materials and surfaces can be achieved at temperatures below 50°C. by processes based primarily on electromagnetic radiation, electron or particle beams, or even ultrasonic treatment, the following discussion will apply primarily to cold sterilization by sterilants based on germicidal chemical agents. Gases and liquids can be sterilized cold by separation processes based on filtration, centrifugation, or sedimentation. In a few applications electrostatic precipitation has been useful in sterilizing gases. In a few other applications, oscillations of the temperature through several cycles of freezing and thawing or long-term storage at temperatures capable of promoting germination but preventing proliferation of microorganisms have produced sterility. In a sense, these temperature-related processes resemble Tyndallization, a process of long standing in the practice of pharmacy. The process of drying will, under certain circumstances, sterilize surfaces.

The chemical sterilizing agents are frequently enhanced in their action by simultaneous application of one or another of the physical conditions promoting sterilization. Some chemical substances become sterilizing agents only when applied simultaneously with a suitable physical agent. Sterilization processes based on these agents will not be discussed further here.

To discuss cold sterilization quantitatively, a careful definition of the term sterilization will be useful. In a discussion of heat sterilization, the distinctions among the various practical meanings involve only differences of degree. The more strict meanings imply but a longer exposure to the specified temperature. In a discussion of cold sterilization, these distinctions involve differences in kind.

In the strictest sense, the concept of sterilization involves freeing an object from all living microorganisms. In the practical sense, however, sterilization processes must be evaluated and assessed on the basis of the methods available for demonstrating that the desired result has been attained. At present, these methods are all concerned ultimately with inferring the absence of living microorganisms from the failure of the object exposed to the process to produce a microbial population, growth, in certain standardized bacteriological media (World Health Organization, 1960). In the practical sense, then, sterilization is a process which destroys the demonstrable infective[3] potential of an object. This distinction between two concepts of sterilization, between a process which destroys all living microorganisms on or in an object and a process which eliminates the infective potential of the object, is important because practical processes can be demonstrated to be effective only when measured by the latter concept.

It is perhaps unfortunate that, operationally, infectivity is not a convenient property of an object. It relates the infective object to a second independent object which must be infected, if the infectivity is to be detected. Some species of microorganisms are fastidious about the environment in and the substrate on which they will proliferate. Some require human beings. Others require only human or primate cells. Yet others are content with only a

[3] As used here, infective does not involve the idea of pathogenicity.

nitrogen source, an energy source, and a few vitamins. There exist, most likely, yet-unidentified species which will infect neither animals nor any of the bacteriological culture media yet devised. Some of the algal and fungal populations grow so slowly, even at their optimum temperatures, that the infective potential of objects containing them is difficult to measure and yet populations of these species can destroy industrial and military materials (Greathouse and Wessel, 1954).

In pharmacy and medicine, sterilization, in the practical sense, means that an object or material has been processed to destroy all populations of pathogenic organisms, including those which produce only toxic products. In food technology, the term means that the material or equipment has been processed to destroy all those populations of organisms which can or could produce product spoilage. In interplanetary-spacecraft technology, the term means that the material, object, or enclosed space has been processed to remove or kill all living organisms to the extent that they are no longer detectable in standard culture media in which they have been previously demonstrated to proliferate. The actual objective in spacecraft technology is to kill or remove all living organisms to the extent that they can never be detected on another planet by any means whatsoever. Proof that this latter objective has been attained in any particular spacecraft sterilization is beyond the capability of presently available life-detection techniques.

Because of these differences in practical objectives, processes which are effective in sterilizing the objects of one technology may very well fail to sterilize those of another technology.

II. Sterilization of Surfaces of Solids

A. Cleaning

Because the effectiveness of any sterilization method depends upon the size of the microbial population to be destroyed, thorough cleaning of the surfaces to be sterilized is essential. A variety of effective surface-cleaning methods has been developed (Goodwin and Nichols, 1963) in connection with the manufacture of highly reliable missile components. While vapor degreasing and ultrasonic scrubbing are particularly useful tools, thorough scrubbing with detergent and water will reduce the size of a population of microorganisms on a surface by several orders of magnitude (Davis, 1960). Surkiewicz and Phillips (1948) report the results obtained from various cleaning methods used in removing bacterial spores from surfaces.

In addition to removing a large portion of the microbial population, thorough cleaning of a surface will remove particulate contamination which might contain live microorganisms protected from sterilization during exposure of the surface to chemical sterilants. The crystals of inorganic salts present the greatest resistance to diffusion of chemical sterilizing agents. In medical applications, the microorganisms inside a solid material or a crystalline particle are of little consequence if neither the material nor the particle is soluble in, or reactive with, body fluids. Even though pipettes or instruments contaminated with pathogenic microorganisms have been soaked in a sporocidal solution, they should be autoclaved to destroy any protected microorganisms before being handled by dishwashers. In spacecraft applications, on the other hand, all extraneous particles must be either removed or dissolved to expose contained microorganisms to the sterilant. Often populations of bacteria are heterogeneous with respect to resistance to chemical sterilants. Extraction of the cells or spores of these populations with the lipid solvents used in cleaning can change the degree of heterogeneity and make the population more nearly homogeneous in its resistance. The effect of the sterilant is thereby enhanced. Common vapor degreasing cleaning agents are also lipid solvents.

Davis (1960) points out that vegetative cells which cannot grow, either because of lack of nutrients or the presence of bacteriostats in their immediate environment, die, although sometimes slowly. Once the population is dead, sterilization has taken place and a chemical applied as a cleaning agent or bacteriostat on short exposures becomes, in effect, a sterilant in long exposures, under the appropriate conditions. Several highly effective bacteriostats are also effective detergents and serve both to remove microbial nutrients and cells from a surface and to suppress growth among the cells which remain.

An enormous number of germicides and germicidal detergents is available. Many are specified by trade names. Usually each has been developed for a particular application. In the design of the germicide, a particular type of object, environment, and types of microorganism and contamination were in mind. Usually the nature of the object and its normal use determine the species of microorganisms and the sizes of their populations to be destroyed. Even the significance of failure to destroy every cell of every species can be anticipated. Although each of these germicides can be highly effective under its intended conditions of use, none is equally useful or effective under all conditions of use.

Often the liquids used in cleaning are made sterilizing agents by adding to them certain sporocidal substances. The methods of using several liquid sterilants of this type have been discussed by Gremillion *et al.* (1959) and by Spaulding (1957). Opfell and coworkers (1961, 1962a,b) and Willard and Alexander (1964) have measured the effectiveness of formaldehyde and other alkylating agents dispersed in each of several common cleaning solvents in destroying populations of bacterial spores on the surfaces of typical spacecraft components.

B. Demonstrating the Effectiveness of Chemical Sterilants

In demonstrating the effectiveness of a chemical sterilant against a particular species of microorganism in a particular environment, it is essential that the test inoculum be in precisely the same environment as the microorganisms of the population to be destroyed. Royce and Bowler (1961) and Opfell *et al.* (1959) have shown that by an appropriate choice of surface or carrier for the test inoculum an exposure to gaseous ethylene oxide can be demonstrated to sterilize, or not to sterilize, at will. Certainly, a valid demonstration must be based on results and experiments imitating precisely the anticipated environment for each cell in the contaminating population and using microorganisms whose resistance to the sterilizing agent resembles that of the species in the contaminating population.

Recent reviews of the properties and applications of popular chemical sterilants have been presented by Bruch (1961), Opfell (1964), Phillips and Warshowsky (1958), Reddish (1957), and Sykes (1958). The reader is referred to these reviews for detailed information on chemical sterilants useful in various applications.

C. Monitoring a Sterilization Process

Once a particular process has been demonstrated to be effective, it is useful to show that this same process will also sterilize a large population of spores of species such as *Bacillus subtilis*, *Bacillus stearothermophilis*, or *Clostridium sporogenes* (Bruch, 1961) carried on a material of highly uniform properties like filter paper. Sterilization of such spore populations does not prove that an object simultaneously exposed to the same process is sterile. Failure of an established process to sterilize a standard spore inoculum is sufficient reason, however, to presume that errors can be and were made in the application of the process.

Information about the resistance of bacterial spores on filter paper (Grundy *et al.*, 1957) or on fabric (Phillips, 1961) exceeds that about any other carrier materials. Because of their reproducible results, commercial spore strips serve well as biological "reagents" for monitoring a sterilization process and are useful in many applications. In monitoring a sterilization process, the spores of *B. subtilis* are particularly useful because of the characteristic form and color of their colonies, their low pathogenicity, and the wealth of published information about their resistance and requirements for nutrients and incubation.

In many applications of sterilizing processes, however, standard spore inoculums, i.e., spore strips, are not useful. In the preparation of a sterile product, for example, it is illogical to expose that product at any time to a population of live microorganisms, particularly a population known to be resistant to the sterilizing agent in doses smaller than the nominal dose on which the sterilization process was established. An undetected error in the application of the process would produce nonsterile and possibly hazardous products. In some instances, of course, the test spore inoculum can be so completely segregated from the product that no hazard can exist. In recognition of the possibilities of human errors in applying the sterilization process or in packaging materials, good medical and pharmaceutical manufacturing technique will exclude all microorganisms, including standard spore inoculums, from the vicinity of the sterilizer or the product. The spore strip is not useful in showing that any particular sterilizer operated in any particular manner will sterilize a particular object other than the spore on the spore strip.

D. The Microorganism and Its Environments

The filter paper or fabric of the spore strip is not representative of most practically important environments. Some of the common sterilizing agents, e.g., formaldehyde, react with cellulose, thereby reducing the ambient concentration of the formaldehyde around the microorganisms below what would prevail if the environment contained only materials which did not react with or absorb the sterilizing agent.

The exhaustion of the sterilizing agent can be a very local effect because of a contaminant which accompanies the microorganism population. If the sterilizing agent reacts vigorously with the object to be sterilized, it will not be a useful sterilizing agent. Sometimes the contaminating material which accompanies microorganisms completely encases them, protecting them from chemical sterilizating agents. Typically crystalline materials (Abbott *et al.*, 1956; Royce and Bowler, 1961) protect microorganisms from the action of chemical sterilizating agents.

E. Protective Substances

Royce and Bowler (1961) have pointed out that bacterial spores dried from suspension in salt solution or culture broths are not always sterilized by exposure to ethylene oxide in concentrations and for periods of time adequate to sterilize the same numbers of the same spores dried from pure water. Phillips (1961) has suggested that with ethylene oxide and spores of *B. subtilis* var. *niger* more than just a physical effect may be involved in the protection provided by broth solids. Even though a large population of spores has been dried on a surface from a broth or saline suspension, it is not necessarily resistant to a chemical sterilant. Some materials will absorb both the water and the salt or protective substance while the spore is drying. Others will absorb only the water and still others, nothing at all. In each case the amount of the material from the suspension vehicle available to provide protection will be different. Some sterilants can destroy the protective effect of dried salt or of broth solids. Gilbert and co-workers (1964) have discussed the steps necessary to make dried bacterial spores susceptible to sterilization by ethylene oxide.

Phillips and Kaye (1949) have discussed the variety of chemical agents which will kill populations of spores dried on cotton fabric. Opfell *et al.* (1959) and Kelsey (1961) have found this environment to be perhaps the most favorable one for sterilizing bacterial spores. If the material providing the surface for the microbial populations is less hygroscopic or has physical or chemical properties very different from those of cellulose or if the microbial population was suspended in a less than completely volatile vehicle, a portion of the population will frequently survive exposures to ethylene oxide many times more severe than those reported as effective by Phillips (1961) or Ernst and Shull (1962a). The protective agents which might spare cells dried on other materials are readily absorbed by cellulose, leaving the microorganism exposed to the action of sterilizing agents.

For destroying a population of spores of *B. subtilis* var. *niger*, Ernst and Shull (1962a) have presented quantitative information on the relationship between the concentration of ethylene oxide and temperature and the effectiveness of a specific length of exposure to this gaseous sterilant. In a second paper (1962b), these same investigators report how the introduction of hygroscopic cotton into the environment in which ethylene oxide is acting can affect the thermochemical death time.

Royce and Bowler also found that proteins in the vehicle from which a bacterial suspension is dried provide relatively little protection against the sterilizing effect of ethylene oxide, whereas amino acids, sugars, and other broth ingredients, which crystallize on drying, effectively protect many microorganisms. Lactose is widely used to protect microorganisms during freeze-drying. Sometimes this sugar is used in the presence of milk proteins and sometimes not. The protective effects of the salts, sugars, and amino acids may be due to changes which take place inside the microorganism under conditions of high concentrations of these substances outside it.

Staphylococcus populations in the presence of the protective substances in broth are more effectively protected than are populations of other nonsporulating species or even the larger bacterial spores (Opfell and Duffy, 1964a; Royce and Bowler, 1961). The protective effect appears to be more than physical and involves the interaction of the cells, the protective substances, and the sterilizing agent. The resistance of *Staphylococcus* populations to drying is also affected by the presence of the same protective substances. *Staphylococcus epidermidis* populations dried on clean glass, Teflon, or aluminum surfaces from suspension in pure water die within a few hours (Opfell and Duffy, 1964a). From suspension in broth they die much more slowly. McDade and Hall (1963) reported that populations of *Staphylococcus aureus* dried from a broth culture on sutures would remain viable for several days, but Skaliy and Sciple (1964) reported that he was unable to detect *Staphylococcus* cells in a hospital room 1 day after an infected patient left the room. A population of *Staphylococcus* microorganisms which will survive drying well may also survive exposures to chemical sterilants. A population of S. *epidermidis* derived from an unknown source and contained in dust was found to survive an exposure to ethylene oxide more than enough to sterilize a standard large inoculum of *B. subtilis* var. *niger* spores. Another population was found to survive many months in solid propellant, and yet another population of this same species survived in a solid propellant formulation containing enough ethylene oxide to destroy an inoculum of spores of *B. subtilis* var. *niger* containing many thousands of spores per milliliter of propellant. A S. *epidermidis* inoculum will grow in broth containing a higher concentration of ethylene oxide than will an inoculum, of the same size, of spores of *B. subtilis* var. *niger*. On the other hand, a population of washed S. *epidermidis* cells in pure water will die within a few weeks.

F. Chemical Oxidizing Agents as Sterilants

Of all the chemical agents for sterilization, chlorine and solutions of hypochlorities are the best for many reasons. The reactivity of these agents reduces substantially the protective effects of most organic substances. When used in aqueous solution, the protective crystals of inorganic salts are often dissolved, thereby exposing the contained microorganisms to sterilization.

The very reactivity, so important in increasing effectiveness, restricts the range of materials and conditions to which these agents may be applied. Many materials are destroyed by exposure to chlorine or to the other powerful oxidizing sterilants, ozone and peracetic acid. These sterilants have their most useful applications in preparing tools and spaces for manipulations which require a sterile field or in preparing ducts for the transport of sterile fluids. The sterilization of isolators for rearing germfree animals (Trexler, 1964) is a typical application of peracetic acid.

The alkali solutions are also powerful and rapid-acting sterilants although they are often used at a temperature higher than those typical of cold sterilization techniques. It is unsound to make general statements comparing sterilizing effectiveness about the other chemical sterilizing agents. In some applications these agents can be highly effective and in others, not effective at all.

G. The Hazards in Extrapolating the Knowledge of Sterilant Effectiveness

Often, universal effectiveness as a sterilant is attributed to a chemical agent on the basis of dramatic effects shown by it in a few specific applications. To point out the possibilities for error in acting on such a premise the following example is illustrative. Royce and Bowler (1961) report that washing the slightly soluble antibacterial sulfonamides and penicillin salts reduced the bacterial population among crystals of them by at least a factor of two. Exposure of the unwashed crystals of these antibacterial powders to a standard ethylene oxide process reduced the population by several orders of magnitude and produced sterility in some of the powder samples. When the slightly soluble crystals were washed and dried before they were exposed to ethylene oxide, the bacterial population on them was relatively unaffected. Here, a bactericidal agent (in this case antibacterial crystals), was cleaned by washing with water and was then exposed to a powerful sterilizing agent, ethylene oxide; yet the initial population was only halved. The point is this: Sterilizing agents are not universally effective and their effects are not necessarily additive. In some instances they enhance each other's effects; in other instances they cancel them.

H. Liquid Sterilants

The advantages of liquid sterilants lie in their convenience. For many applications, in which the sterilant may evaporate or be rinsed away when its action is complete, they are inexpensive. In a few instances the liquid sterilant is sealed in or absorbed by the object sterilized. The long-term compatibility of the residual sterilant with the object then demands careful consideration. Often liquids act to sterilize surfaces more rapidly than do gas sterilants, but in no case should a liquid sterilant be presumed to act instantly. Hypochlorite and peracetic acid solutions are particularly rapid-acting liquid sterilants, but several minutes are required to produce sterile surfaces after they have been applied.

The rate of action of a liquid sterilant is usually dependent upon the concentration of the active chemical in the liquid. It also depends upon a variety of other factors, including temperature. Populations of one million spores of *B. subtilis* var. *niger* are destroyed within 90 minutes at room temperature by several of the alkylating agents when these agents are dissolved in common solvents at a concentration of only 5% (Opfell *et al.*, 1961, 1962a, b). Increasing the concentration of the agent in the solvent will usually increase the rate at which microorganisms are destroyed. The increase, however, is not necessarily linear.

Schabel (1957) reported the relative sterilizing effects of large numbers of chemical compounds with respect to two species of bacteria and one of virus. Phillips and Kaye (1949) have described the relative sterilizing effects of the alkylating agents. The fact that any one of these agents, when used pure, destroys populations of microorganisms does not imply that it will be effective when dispersed in a liquid vehicle.

When the liquid sterilant cannot be permitted to evaporate or to be rinsed away by an inert sterile fluid, chemical and physical stability of the sterilant becomes an important consideration. On long-term storage formaldehyde, even in methanol, polymerizes. Even though a large excess of one of the reaction products, methanol, is present, the autoxidation of formaldehyde to form both methanol and formic acid proceeds. In applications to electrical connectors for interplanetary spacecraft, undesirable corrosion might be expected.

Water or methanol solutions of ethylene oxide convert slowly, over several months' time, to solutions of ethylene glycol or of ethylene glycol monomethyl ether. Unlike those of formaldehyde, the ethylene oxide reaction products are not often corrosive to metals but they do have solvent properties different from those of mixtures of the reactants.

Among other liquid sterilants for surfaces, hypochlorite solutions are generally considered most satisfactory. The corrosive properties of these solutions impose far-reaching effects on the design of equipment to be sterilized by them. While hypochlorite solutions are generally useful in the dairy and food industries, they are unsuitable in certain specific processes in which even very small amounts of hypochlorite can ruin the product. To avoid this difficulty the food processer will use other sterilizing liquids, frequently caustic solutions. The processing equipment must then be designed to be compatible with these other liquid sterilants.

Jacobs (1960) discussed the dynamics of chemical sterilization with particular emphasis on phenols. Phillips and Warshowsky (1958), Reddish (1957), and Sykes (1958) presented thorough discussions of the properties of many chemical sterilizing agents.

Ethylene oxide is an effective sterilant in the liquid as well as in the gas phase. In the liquid phase it can be applied at higher concentrations, with the result that it acts much more rapidly than it does as a gas. Because ethylene oxide does not exist as a liquid at room temperature and atmospheric pressure, it must be diluted with another liquid to raise its boiling point above room temperature in order to prepare a liquid sterilant based on it. Water in excess of 77% will do this but less methanol or propylene oxide are required to produce the same effect. A fifty-fifty mixture of methanol and ethylene oxide will boil at about room temperature. This mixture is a particularly effective and useful sporocide because it leaves no residue on evaporation and is unreactive with a large variety of materials. Its stability on long-term storage has not been established, however. Equivalent concentrations of ethylene oxide in propylene oxide appears to be less effective sterilants than they are in methanol.

A 5% solution of freshly distilled monomeric formaldehyde in methanol is also a useful sterilant which is compatible with a large variety of materials. In methanol, formaldehyde is not as effective a sterilant as it is in water (Opfell *et al.*, 1961; Willard and Alexander, 1964). At the same time, however, it is less corrosive and when freshly prepared it leaves no deposit of paraformaldehyde, often an important consideration in spacecraft sterilization applications. The sterilizing and other properties of formaldehyde and its solutions were studied extensively by Nordgren (1939). Other liquid sterilants based on formaldehyde have been discussed by Reddish (1957) and by Sykes (1958).

I. Gaseous Sterilants

The amount of published information on the conditions required to sterilize surfaces by exposure to gaseous ethylene oxide now exceeds that for any other cold sterilization process. However, the information on the compatibility of ethylene oxide sterilants with various materials is, for the most part, limited to the observation that damage is negligible.

The particular advantages of gaseous agents in sterilizing surfaces are effectiveness of penetration and ease of removal of residual sterilant. Frequently, sterilization by a gaseous agent is less expensive than the alternative processes.

The penetration of a gaseous sterilizing agent is limited to those spaces available to it by the physical processes of diffusion, absorption, and solution. Gaseous sterilants cannot penetrate many solid materials, particularly crystalline materials. Diffusion into remote spaces often takes many hours (Opfell *et al.*, 1964) and completely through solid objects which absorb it, even longer.

In the use of the gaseous sterilants, particular care must be given to control of fire, explosion, and toxicity hazards. The engineering of safe methods of using ethylene oxide has been worked out. Several excellent reviews on sterilization by gaseous sterilants have recently been published by Bruch (1961), Mayr (1961), Perkins and Lloyd (1961), Phillips (1961), and Stierli *et al.* (1962). Because most of these reviews are readily available, the discussion here will be limited to a reiteration that the physical processes of diffusion, absorption, evaporation, and condensation as well as phase behavior often play determining roles in sterilization processes based on gaseous sterilants.

III. Internal Sterilization

A. Demonstrating the Effectiveness of Processes to Sterilize the Interiors of Solids, Liquids, and Gases

Most of the advantages, as well as the limitations, of cold sterilization techniques for surfaces apply in the sterilization of the interiors of solids, liquids, and gases. In particular, the chemical sterilizing agent must gain intimate access to every microorganism in the contaminating population in order to sterilize. Demonstration of process effectiveness includes proof of this access.

The distinction made earlier between the two concepts of sterilization is of particular importance in the proof that a solid has been sterilized internally. The demonstration of noninfectivity for, or disinfection of, the interior of a solid entails problems not present for gases, liquids, and the surfaces of solids, including powders. In order to demonstrate such noninfectivity, all the potentially viable microorganisms must be given access to the nutrient medium of the sterility test. If the solid is insoluble in all nonbactericidal solvents, it must be pulverized. The size of the particles produced by pulverization must be approximately that of the microorganisms themselves. Any process capable of producing such a degree of subdivision will also destroy many of the potentially viable cells.

Less pulverization will leave viable microorganisms entrapped in the interiors of the larger particles and these microorganisms might not have access to the nutrient medium. Some solids can be shown to contain microorganisms even though the particles are much larger than the individual microorganisms. This effect depends on the particular solid material. Solid propellant is one such material (Opfell and Duffy, 1964b).

Failure of a pulverized solid material to produce growth in a nutrient medium is not sufficient evidence that the interior of the intact solid was noninfective even for that medium.

Primary interest in techniques for cold sterilization of the interiors of solids has come from the requirement that planetary-impacting spacecraft be sterilized. This interest is relatively new and the technology for producing and demonstrating these sterile interiors is far behind that for other residences of microbial populations. In spite of these limitations, there are useful cold sterilization techniques for destroying microbial populations in the interiors of solids, liquids, and gases. They are discussed in the following sections.

B. Self-Sterilizing Formulations for Solids

The interiors of certain types of solids can be sterilized by the use of chemical sterilizing agents in the formulation of the material. The self-sterilizing property is important in those cases in which the material cannot be protected from contamination completely while it is in the uncured state. Formaldehyde, ethylene imine, and even ethylene oxide have been used to produce sterile greases (Opfell *et al.*, 1962a, b) and polymeric resins (Morelli, 1962). The use of chemical sterilants in formulations must not interfere to the detriment of the properties of the resulting solid material, however, and compatibility and effectiveness must be demonstrated as with any other sterilization technique.

The chemical sterilizing agents are often very reactive with the monomers of resins, uncured coatings, and uncured elastomers. They often polymerize. If these reactions proceed rapidly enough while the solid is curing the final state of the cure can be altered. The reaction of the chemical sterilizing agent with the ingredients will deplete its concentration and perhaps affect its ability to sterilize. The formulation of a self-sterilizing solid or grease must be based on knowledge of the nature of the reactions of the sterilizing agent with the ingredients and with the polymers in the solid as well as with the microbial population.

Certain gaseous sterilants, particularly ethylene oxide, diffuse into certain solids and dissolve in them. Exposure to these gases, under controlled conditions, can make the interior material of these solids noninfective when tested by any presently available testing technique. Demonstration of sterility, however, still has the difficulty discussed earlier. Moreover, care must be exercised in the sterility test to neutralize the residual sterilant just as in the case of self-sterilizing materials.

Long exposures to the gas are required, too, to permit the sterilizing agent to penetrate the solid completely. The useful properties of the solid may be seriously affected, but not necessarily, by saturation with the sterilant. The solid must be extremely homogeneous, too, because particles containing microorganisms protected from the action of the sterilizing agent would prevent sterilization from ever taking place. Diffusion of a sterilant into a solid propellant containing internally contaminated oxidizer crystals would never be sterilized by such a process. Polyethylene film, on the other hand, is readily penetrated by ethylene oxide and even permits sterilizing concentrations to be developed inside spaces completely enclosed by the film.

C. Self-Sterilizing Formulations for Liquids and Gases

The preparation of self-sterilizing formulations of liquids or of gases is a fundamentally simpler problem than it is of solids. The sterilant can be readily distributed in these fluids. Its concentration is easily measured. Many liquids are, by their very natures, germicidal to a broad spectrum of species of microorganisms. Acetone, for example, promptly kills populations of *S. epidermidis*. The killing effect may be simply the result of excessive removal of water from the microorganisms rather than of toxicity as such. Populations of spores of *B. subtilis* var. *niger*, on the other hand, are unaffected by even long storage in acetone. Phenol solutions (Jacobs, 1960) have been the standard by which other disinfectants have been measured. Yet, several species of microorganisms are not killed by these phenol solutions.

The alkylating agents, particularly formaldehyde, ethylene oxide, and β-propiolactone, have been used in preparing self-sterilizing liquids. Formaldehyde has been used traditionally in the preparation of immunizing agents. Certain of these immunizing agents are prepared by rendering liquid cultures of pathogenic microorganisms noninfective by the addition of appropriate and controlled amounts of formaldehyde. In the preparation of these immunization agents for injection into humans, many steps in addition to the destruction of infectivity are required, of course.

Ethylene oxide and β-propiolactone have been demonstrated to sterilize certain food products and human serum preparations. They have also been used to sterilize fermentation media. These liquids are self-sterilizing for limited periods of time after which the decay of the sterilant into nontoxic products has progressed far enough to make the liquid nontoxic and no longer sterilizing. The liquid is self-sterilizing during the period when it stands the greatest chance of becoming contaminated. Once packaged in a hermetic container, the self-sterilizing property is no longer required.

Some liquids provide starvation environments (Postgate and Hunter, 1963) for microorganisms. This environment, if maintained about the population of microorganisms long enough, will destroy it. This environment can be created either by excluding nutrients or by including bacteriostatic agents in the formulation of the liquid. In pharmaceutical preparations the bacteriostatic agents are called preservatives. These bacteriostats do not kill microorganisms outright but instead prevent reproduction and interfere with metabolism. In the absence of the bacteriostatic agents and the presence of many dead bacteria, cryptic growth of a few microorganisms can keep a liquid from becoming sterile through the starvation effect over even long periods of time. When bacterial spores are present in the contaminating population, they must be forced to germinate before bacteriostats have any promise at all of destroying them through starvation.

Two types of microbicide are available for the sterilization of gases. One is the true gaseous sterilant which, in effect, can make another gas self-sterilizing. The other is the quasi-gaseous sterilant (Phillips and Warshowsky, 1958) which is a mist formed of slightly volatile sterilizing agents. The true gaseous sterilant can be mixed with a compatible gas and will then remain dispersed in it. The quasi-gaseous sterilants use the processes of evaporation and condensation as well as bacterial toxicity in destroying aerial populations of microorganisms. Among the useful quasi-gaseous sterilants are solutions of β-propiolactone, formaldehyde, or peracetic acid in water.

It is often useful to disperse a quasi-gaseous sterilant at such a temperature that the particles of mist evaporate and then condense again on the contaminant particles to increase the rate sedimentation of these particles. The germicide acts then on the microorganisms on the surface on which they fall rather than in the air. Usually the air-borne microbial particles which must be precipitated in this way contain micrococci and are less than 1 micron in size. The bactericide can be one which is specially developed to kill micrococci.

IV. Statistical Aspects

Evidence that a particular process has been an effective one is at best statistical and is inferred from a repeated application of the process under carefully controlled and monitored conditions to a sequence of identical items or replicas. An item which will be used in a procedure or application requiring that it be sterile will never be tested for sterility before use. Evidence of its lack of infectivity will come after it has been used and will be the absence of infection in the items, the person, or the environment in which it was used.

The fact that a single replicate of this item, and not the item itself, failed to infect a test medium in a single sterility test is hardly sufficient evidence to support much confidence. Confidence in a process under proper control will naturally increase as the sequence of tests showing noninfectivity lengthens. A break in such a sequence requires explanation. The break may have been due to process failure or it may have been due to error in the sterility-test operator's technique. The cause of the break must be established in either case. If the process did indeed fail, all the product produced by that process is suspect. It is not possible to discriminate among batches of sterile and nonsterile items from a controlled process on the basis of statistical sampling and testing. The implication of this fact is the following. Confidence in a particular process, whether a cold sterilization technique or not, is soundly based only after a continuous sequence of successful applications of the process has been developed.

Cornfield and co-workers (1957) and Meier (1957) have discussed the statistical aspects of safety testing the Salk-process poliomyelitis vaccine. The statistical model constructed by Cornfield is a useful guide in designing a testing program to demonstrate effectiveness of a sterilization process. Bryce (1956), Knudsen (1949), Savage (1961), and the World Health Organization (1960) have presented particularly useful descriptions of the statistical as well as other requirements for meaningful sampling and quality control of sterilization processes.

In the demonstration of a particular sterilization procedure for an item assembled from a collection of components, replicas or samples of the final assembly must be used. The process must be demonstrated to be compatible with the functional objective of the item, whether it be a fluid or a device. In testing the compatibility and efficacy of a process with a particular design for an assembly or mixture, failure of any component in any failure mode independent of the interaction among the assembled components must be prevented. The failure mode may be failure to sterilize. In the preparation of a biological or a food product, for example, the bacterial population of each of the ingredients must be smaller than that which can cause failure of the component to be sterilized. In the fabrication of a spacecraft, the components must have been demonstrated individually to be sterilized by the process and they must be demonstrated to function properly after it.

V. Summary

In summary, cold sterilization techniques have the useful attributes of being compatible with many temperature- and radiation-sensitive materials. In many applications, a cold sterilization technique is less expensive to apply than one based on heat or radiation.

Each application of a cold sterilization technique must be demonstrated by an experimental program designed to provide enough statistical data to support an inference of both effectiveness and compatibility. Moreover, a careful analysis of the conditions and environments to which the material is exposed must show that no contamination could occur which cannot be reached by the sterilant or be detected.

Sterilization has been confused with disinfection in many discussions of these two subjects. Because of this confusion, the term sterilization means different things to different people. A process of disinfecting which may produce sterility in one person's frame of reference will fail to do so in another's because of the differences in the types of microbial contamination to be destroyed and which are therefore monitored. The ethylene oxide process is, for this reason, used and its effectiveness interpreted differently in spacecraft applications than in medical applications.

The demonstration of effectiveness of any sterilization process in destroying microbial populations in the interiors of many insoluble solid materials is extremely difficult, irrespective of the sterilization techniques applied. Culturing methods may be totally inadequate. When microorganisms are encased in these solid materials, even in the form of small particles on the surfaces of the other solids, chemical sterilization will generally be ineffective.

References

Abbott, C. F., Cockton, J., and Jones, W. (1956). *J. Pharm. Pharmacol.* **8**, 709-720.

Bruch, C. W. (1961). *Ann. Rev. Microbiol.* **15**, 245-262.

Bryce, D. M. (1956). *J. Pharm. Pharmacol.* **8**, 561-572.

Cornfield, J., Halperin, M., and Moore, F. (1957). *Public Health Rept. (U.S.)* **71**, 1045.

Davis, J. G. (1960). *J. Pharm. Pharmacol.* **12**, 29T-39T.

Ernst, R. R., and Shull, J. J. (1962a). *Appl. Microbiol.* **10**, 337-341.

Ernst, R. R., and Shull, J. J. (1962b). *Appl. Microbiol.* **10**, 342-344.

Gilbert, G. L., Gambert, V. M., Spiner, D. R., Hoffman, R. K., and Phillips, C. R. (1964). *Appl. Microbiol.* **12**, 496-503.

Goodwin, T. C., and Nichols, O. (1963). Laboratory-Industrial Cleaning Techniques and Materials, DDC Document No. AD 409 323.

Greathouse, G. A., and Wessel, C. J. (1954). "Deterioration of Materials." Reinhold, New York.

Gremillion, G. G., Hanel, H., and Phillips, G. B. (1959). "Practical Procedures for Microbial Decontamination." USA Chemical Corps Biological Laboratories, Fort Detrick, Frederick, Maryland.

Grundy, W. E., Rdzok, E. J., Remo, W. J., Sagen, H. E., and Sylvester, J. C. (1957). *J. Am. Pharm. Assoc. Sci. Ed.* **46**, 439-442.

Jacobs, S. E. (1960). *J. Pharm. Pharmacol.* **12**, Suppl., 9T-18T.

Kelsey, J. C. (1961). *In* "Recent Developments in the Sterilisation of Surgical Materials" (Department of Pharmaceutical Sciences of the Pharmaceutical Society of Great Britain and Smith & Nephew Research Limited, eds.), pp. 203-207. The Pharmaceutical Press, London.

Knudsen, L. F. (1949). *J. Am. Pharm. Assoc. Sci. Ed.* **38**, 332-337.

Mayr, G. (1961). *In* "Recent Developments in the Sterilisation of Surgical Materials" (Department of Pharmaceutical Sciences of the Pharmaceutical Society of Great Britain and Smith & Nephew Research Limited, eds.), pp. 90-97. The Pharmaceutical Press, London.

McDade, J. J., and Hall, L. B. (1963). *Am. J. Hyg.* **77**, 98-108.

Meier, P. (1957). *Science* **125**, 1067-1071.

Morelli, F. (1962). Research Summary No. 36-12, I, pp. 14-16. Jet Propulsion Laboratory, Pasadena, California.

Nordgren, G. (1939). "Investigations on the Sterilization Efficacy of Gaseous Formaldehyde." Munksgaard, Copenhagen.

Opfell, J. B. (1964). *In* "Life Sciences and Space Research" (M. Florkin and A. Dollfus, eds.), Vol. II, pp. 385-405. North-Holland Publ., Amsterdam.

Opfell, J. B., and Duffy, W. T. (1964a). Resistance of *Alpha* Organisms to Drying and to Sterilization by Ethylene Oxide, Task I, Final Summary Report on JPL Contract 950 740 (Mod. 1). Dynamic Science Corporation, South Pasadena, California.

Opfell, J. B., and Duffy, W. T. (1964b). Naturally Occurring Microbiological Flora from Normally Prepared Propellant Specimens, Task II, Final Summary Report on JPL Contract 950 740 (Mod. 1). Dynamic Science Corporation, South Pasadena, California.

Opfell, J. B., Hohmann, J. P., and Latham, A. B. (1959). *J. Am. Pharm. Assoc. Sci. Ed.* **48**, 617-619.

Opfell, J. B., Miller, C. E., and Hammons, P. N. (1961). Evaluation of Liquid Sterilants, Final Report on JPL Contract N1-143 452. Dynamic Science Corporation, South Pasadena, California.

Opfell, J. B., Miller, C. E., and Louderback, A. L. (1962a). Evaluation of Liquid Sterilants, Semifinal Report on JPL Contract N2-150 247. Dynamic Science Corporation, South Pasadena, California.

Opfell, J. B., Miller, C. E., Louderback, A. L., Koretz, R. L., and English, E. G. (1962b). Evaluation of Liquid Sterilants, Phases III-VII, Final Report on JPL Contract N2-150 247. Dynamic Science Corporation, South Pasadena, California.

Opfell, J. B., Wang, Y.-L., Louderback, A. L., and Miller, C. E. (1964). *Appl. Microbiol.* **12**, 27-31.

Perkins, J. J., and Lloyd, R. S. (1961). *In* "Recent Developments in the Sterilisation of Surgical Materials" (Department of Pharmaceutical Sciences of the Pharmaceutical Society of Great Britain and Smith & Nephew Research Limited, eds.), pp. 76-90. The Pharmaceutical Press, London.

Phillips, C. R. (1961). *In* "Recent Developments in the Sterilisation of Surgical Materials" (Department of Pharmaceutical Sciences of the Pharmaceutical Society of Great Britain and Smith & Nephew Research Limited, eds.), pp. 59-75. The Pharmaceutical Press, London.

Phillips, C. R., and Kaye, S. (1949). *Am. J. Hyg.* **50**, 270.

Phillips, C. R., and Warshowsky, B. (1958). *Ann. Rev. Microbiol.* **12**, 525-550.

Postgate, J. R., and Hunter, J. R. (1963). *J. Appl. Bacteriol.* **26**, 295-306.

Reddish, G. F., ed. (1957). "Antiseptics, Disinfectants, Fungicides, and Chemical and Physical Sterilization." Lea & Febiger, Philadelphia, Pennsylvania.

Royce, A., and Bowler, C. (1961). *J. Pharm. Pharmacol.* **13**, 87T-94T.

Savage, R. H. M. (1961). *In* "Recent Developments in the Sterilisation of

Surgical Materials" (Department of Pharmaceutical Sciences of the Pharmaceutical Society of Great Britain and Smith & Nephew Research Limited, eds.), pp. 190-198. The Pharmaceutical Press, London.
Schabel, F. M. (1957). *In Vitro* and *In Vivo* Evaluation of Sporocidal, Bactericidal, and Virucidal Chemicals, Report 4 (Final), Report 3385-803-4, DA 18-064-404-cml-188, ASTIA Document No. AD 149 727. Southern Research Institute, Birmingham, Alabama.
Skaliy, P., and Sciple, G. W. (1964). *Arch. Environ. Health.* **8**, 636-641.
Spaulding, E. H. (1957). *In* "Antiseptics, Disinfectants, Fungicides, and Chemical and Physical Sterilization" (G. F. Reddish, ed.), pp. 619-648. Lea & Febiger, Philadelphia, Pennsylvania.
Stierli, H., Reed, L. L., and Billick, I. H. (1962) Evaluation of Sterilization by Gaseous Ethylene Oxide, Public Health Monograph No. 68, Public Health Service Document 903. U.S. Govt. Printing Office, Washington, D. C.
Surkiewicz, B. F., and Phillips, C. R. (1948). Removal of *Bacillus globigii* Spores from Various Surfaces, ASTIA Document No. AD 222 726.
Sykes, G. (1958). "Disinfection and Sterilization." Van Nostrand, Princeton, New Jersey.
Trexler, P. C. (1964). *Sci. Am.* **211**, 64-88.
Willard, M., and Alexander, A. (1964). *Appl. Microbiol.* **12**, 229-233.
World Health Organization. (1960). *World Health Organ. Tech. Rept. Ser.* **200**.

Reprinted from *Ann. Rev. Microbiol.* **15**, 245–262 (1961)

4

GASEOUS STERILIZATION[1]

BY CARL W. BRUCH
Wilmot Castle Company, Rochester, New York

Gaseous sterilization, as it is presently used and understood, is a fortuitous outgrowth of the field of agricultural and industrial fumigation. During the period between World Wars I and II, gaseous compounds were developed to combat insect infestation in grain and grain products. Among the gaseous chemicals so developed were ethylene oxide and methyl bromide. Later, it was found that ethylene oxide reduced the microbial contamination of the treated foods, and this discovery led to the application and issue of patents concerning its formulation and use as a gaseous decontaminant and sterilant. By 1942, the use of gaseous ethylene oxide to reduce the microbial population of spices and gums had been described in several journals of food technology and manufacture. Early in World War II, the U. S. Government deemed it necessary to establish a biological warfare laboratory under the jurisdiction of the Chemical Corps of the U. S. Army. The use of gaseous fumigants as sterilants was reinvestigated by this group, and the results of their investigations with ethylene oxide were published by Phillips & Kaye in 1949 (1 to 4). Since their first paper gave a thorough review of the work on ethylene oxide prior to 1949, no attempt will be made to discuss these early reports. This review will cover much of the work of the past decade, particularly the past four years, and will overlap an extensive review published by Phillips (5) four years ago and a recent brief review by Phillips & Warshowsky (6). Because there is a tendency to become overly concerned with the medical applications of gaseous sterilization, the author will review the applications in the food industry where recent legislation by the federal government has curtailed the use of ethylene oxide on some products.

INTRODUCTION

Gaseous sterilization is the treatment of objects or materials with a chemical in the gaseous or vapor state to destroy all microorganisms with which they have been contaminated. The need for such a method of sterilization has developed from the use of many items that cannot be subjected to heat, radiation, or liquid chemical sterilization. The following advantages are noted: sterilization is at low temperatures thus avoiding damage to heat- and moisture-sensitive materials; objects or items can be terminally sterilized in their containers or packages; diffusion of some gaseous sterilants through containers of plastic, paper, or fabric eliminates problems of removal of sterilant; gaseous sterilants penetrate into areas not reached by liquids; sterilization by some gases takes place in the presence of large quantities of

[1] The survey of the literature pertaining to this review was completed in November, 1960.

organic matter; and it is possible to use simple equipment such as plastic or rubber bags and metal drums as sterilizing chambers. The disadvantages are as follows: the length of time for sterilization and aeration is much greater than with other methods; the flammability of some gases requires special operating procedures; toxicity hazards exist with most sterilizing gases; chemical analyses are occasionally necessary to determine residues or addition products formed during sterilization of some organic materials; corrosion or other forms of physical damage can occur from improper sterilizing procedures; and the cost of sterilization is much greater than with moist or dry heat. As a general rule, gaseous sterilization needs close control and supervision to insure effectiveness.

All of the compounds most actively employed in gaseous sterilization are alkylating agents. Brief sketches of some of the properties and the necessary requisites for their use as gaseous sterilants are presented for five alkylating agents in their decreasing order of use: (*a*) Ethylene oxide: C_2H_4O; b.p., 10.4°C.; flammability limits in air, 3.6 to 100 per cent by volume; requires dilution by inert gases, carbon dioxide, or chlorofluorohydrocarbons, for safe use; usual concentrations for sterilizing purposes, 400 to 1000 mg. per l.; requires relative humidity in the range of 25 to 50 per cent; has strong penetrating ability and moderate microbicidal properties; most versatile gas for sterilizing purposes. (*b*) Propylene oxide: C_3H_6O; b.p., 34.0°C.; flammability limits in air, 2.1 to 21.5 per cent by volume; may or may not require dilution with inert gases for safe use; acceptable concentrations for sterilizing purposes, 800 to 2000 mg. per l.; requires humidities in the range of 25 to 50 per cent; penetrating ability and microbicidal properties are less than those of ethylene oxide; frequently used as a substitute for ethylene oxide. (*c*) Formaldehyde: CH_2O; b.p., −21°C. for pure gas, but approximately 90°C. for formalin solutions; flammability limits in air, 7 to 73 per cent by volume, but this hazard is minimized by the large percentage of water usually present; usual concentrations for sterilizing purposes, 3 to 10 mg. per l.; requires high relative humidity, over 75 per cent; has weak penetrating ability but strong microbicidal properties; most commonly used as a surface sterilant. (*d*) Methyl bromide: CH_3Br; b.p., 4.6°C.; essentially non-flammable; usual concentrations for sterilizing purposes, about 3500 mg. per l.; requires moderate relative humidities in the range of 40 to 70 per cent; has strong penetrating ability but weak microbicidal properties; usually employed as a decontaminant for fungi or vegetative bacteria. (*e*) β-Propiolactone: $C_3H_4O_2$; b.p., 163°C.; no flammability hazard at room temperatures; usual concentrations for sterilizing purposes, 2 to 5 mg. per l.; requires high relative humidity, over 75 per cent; has weak penetrating ability but very strong microbicidal properties; essentially a surface sterilant.

The differences among gases as to penetrating ability and humidity requirements for microbicidal activity are striking and must be considered for any intended use of each of these compounds as sterilants. It should be noted that propylene oxide and methyl bromide are more commonly employed as gaseous decontaminants rather than as sterilants, i.e., they are used to destroy specific groups of organisms such as fungi, yeasts, coliforms, and salmonellae.

Other compounds which have microbicidal activity and which could be used in gaseous sterilization are epichlorohydrin, epibromohydrin, ethylene imine, ethylene sulfide, glycidaldehyde, propylene imine, chloropicrin, and ozone. Difficulty with commercial availability, increased toxicity, or lower microbicidal activity has prevented their practical development and use. Since most gaseous sterilization is carried out with ethylene oxide, this compound will be the focal point of this review.

Biochemistry of Gaseous Alkylating Agents Used in Sterilization

In 1949, Phillips (2) reported data obtained from studies with a group of gaseous alkylating agents which showed that microbicidal activity was directly related to the alkylating activity of each chemical. Thus, ethylene oxide, ethylene sulfide, and ethylene imine are active alkylating agents and have strong bactericidal activity, but cyclopropane, which has the same 3-membered ring structure, is not an alkylating agent and is inert microbiologically. Other compounds, e.g., methyl bromide, which are structurally quite different from ethylene oxide, but which possess similar activity as alkylating agents, were found to be active as vapor-phase bactericides. Later, Phillips (7) reported that bacterial spores, which are hundreds to thousands of times more resistant to heat and chemical disinfectants than are vegetative bacteria, were only slightly more difficult to kill with alkylating agents than were vegetative cells. He suggested that the ability to kill bacterial spores relatively easily was a general property of alkylating agents, which can act through alkylation of sulfhydryl, amino, carboxyl, hydroxyl, and phenolic groups.

Since 1946, there has been tremendous activity in research on the cytotoxic effects of alkylating agents, particularly the nitrogen and sulfur mustards. Because of the close relationship between growth inhibitory activity and tumor induction, representative compounds from other groups of alkylating agents have been tested for their cytotoxic activity. Various epoxides, ethylene imines, methanesulfonates, β-lactones, and diazo compounds have been investigated. These groups of alkylating agents have been referred to as "radiomimetic poisons" because in their biological effects they closely simulate ionizing radiations.

Since there is a wide variety of structures among these groups of alkylating agents, the only common feature is the ability to act as alkylating agents under physiological conditions. A further characteristic of all of these compounds is that they are electrophilic and most readily react with so-called nucleophilic (electron-rich) groups such as organic and inorganic anions, amino groups, and sulfide groups. It is convenient to picture the reactions as usually involving a carbonium ion (8). Esters, alkylated amines, ethers, thio ethers, and ammonium and sulfonium compounds are formed as a result of these reactions. Under physiological conditions there will be little or no reaction with undissociated acid groups or with ammonium cations since these are not nucleophilic (8).

Stacey *et al.* (9) have reacted bovine serum albumin under physiological conditions with different alkylating agents including *bis*-epoxypropylether and propylene oxide. While all the different types of alkylating agents esterify carboxyl groups, only the epoxides reacted extensively with the primary amino and imidazole groups provided by the side chains of lysine and histidine, respectively. Further experiments (9) with two model substances that have only one kind of reactive group, the polyacid, polymethacrylic acid, and the polybase, polyvinyl amine, confirmed the fact that, while all the reagents used esterify carboxyl groups, only the epoxides reacted extensively with the amino groups.

Contrary to these results, Fraenkel-Conrat (10) earlier had claimed that more than 50 per cent of the carboxyl groups of egg albumin and β-lactoglobulin were esterified by propylene oxide. His method of estimation consisted of a determination of the amount of basic dye which combines with the protein at pH 11.5 after standing for a least 24 hr. There is ample evidence to show that the ester groups in proteins are completely saponified under these conditions, and therefore this method of analysis cannot be used for determining esterification of carboxyl groups (11).

Windmueller *et al.* (12, 13) investigated the reaction of ethylene oxide with nicotinamide and nicotinic acid, and with histidine, methionine, and cysteine. These studies were directly related to the possible fate of these compounds when foods are fumigated with ethylene oxide. Ethylene oxide was found to react with nicotinamide in aqueous solution at 25°C. to yield, after acidification with HCl, N-(2-hydroxyethyl)-nicotinamide chloride. By a similar reaction, nicotinic acid is converted to the betaine of N-(2-hydroxyethyl)-nicotinic acid. Ethylene oxide reacted with imidazole or histidine to yield the corresponding 1,3-*bis*-(2-hydroxyethyl)-imidazolium derivative. With methionine or N-acetylmethionine, ethylene oxide hydroxyethylates the sulfur to yield the corresponding sulfonium derivatives. Likewise, double alkylation of the mercapto group of cysteine produces a sulfonium group. The primary amino groups of these amino acids also become alkylated, but esterification of carboxyl groups does not seem to be involved. Thus, all of the reactions involved hydroxyethylation of an atom with one or more lone pairs of electrons, either nitrogen or sulfur.

As a result of their work, Windmueller *et al.* (12) came forth with a hypothesis to explain the moisture requirements for ethylene oxide sterilization. Their proposal is that water facilitates proton reactions, and protons are required by an alkylating agent such as ethylene oxide in its reaction with tertiary nitrogen compounds. It is my opinion that whether an alkylating agent has a low or high relative humidity requirement for activity as a gaseous sterilant may also be related to whether the agent acts by first-order or second-order nucleophilic substitution reactions. Since this is a very complex subject, the reader is referred to the article by Price (14).

There is the possibility that alkylating agents produce their characteristic cytotoxic effects by enzyme inhibition. Phosphokinases, certain peptidases, choline oxidase, and acetylcholine esterase have proved to be among the most sensitive enzymes so far examined. The objection to the enzyme inhibition theory has been that the concentrations of alkylating agent required for inactivation do not appear to be achieved *in vivo* when cytotoxic effects can be demonstrated (15). All alkylating agents appear to react readily with sulfhydryl groups of proteins and enzymes although in the native protein not all sulfhydryl groups are accessible (9).

Alexander & Stacey (16) hold the view that the biologically important reaction of alkylating agents occurs with DNA (or possibly RNA) in nucleoproteins and modifies these in such a way that they become useless to the cell. The only way by which preformed DNA can be modified is by reaction with the phosphate groups, which constitute the Achilles heel of this substance. The predominant reaction of epoxides with DNA is one of esterification of the phosphate groups and follows second-order reaction kinetics (9). After long treatments with excess epoxide (propylene oxide and hexane bisepoxide), changes in the ultraviolet absorption spectrum are noticed. There is increased absorption at 270 mμ, which suggests reaction with groups other than phosphate, such as the amino group of guanidine or one of the ring nitrogens of the purines or pyrimidines (9). As a result of their investigations with both alkylating agents and radiation, Alexander & Stacey (16) feel that the biological damage of ionizing radiations and alkylating agents is initiated at the molecular level by an attack on the DNA moiety, although by different chemical reactions. It may be that the radiomimetic properties of alkylating agents account for the high microbicidal activity of these compounds and their consequent use as gaseous sterilants.

Biological Effects of Gaseous Alkylating Agents

During the past 15 years there has accumulated a vast amount of data which show that alkylating agents are mutagenic, that they damage the cytoplasm and nuclei of rapidly growing cells, and that they cause injury to the chromosomal mechanism of rapidly dividing cells. These effects are usually noted in cells that are exposed to near-lethal concentrations of these agents. The desired goal in gaseous sterilization is the lethal effect on microorganisms, and there is little interest in the biological events that occur during this disinfection process. Since mammalian cells are as liable as microorganisms to destruction by these chemicals, their toxic properties are of direct concern to man. Accordingly, a brief discussion of their mutagenicity, carcinogenicity, toxicity, and microbicidal properites is relevant.

The mutagenic action of alkylating agents has been recorded for bacteria, yeasts, molds, barley seeds, and root tips of leguminous seedlings. Strauss & Okubo (17) state that protein synthesis is not required for the fixation of potential mutations in *Escherichia coli* by the alkylating agents, ethyl sulfate and epichlorohydrin. Kölmark & Giles (18) tested six different monoepoxides as inducers of reverse mutations in a purple adenineless strain of *Neurospora crassa*. In general, they found that epoxy rings carrying side chains with strong electronegative properties are stronger mutagens than epoxy compounds with weak electronegative side chains. Ehrenberg & Gustafsson (19) have treated barley seeds with ethylene oxide and found it to be a mutagenic agent of equal or even greater efficiency than ionizing radiation; ethylene imine (20) is even more efficient as a mutagenic agent than ethylene oxide. β-Propiolactone causes reversions to growth factor independence and gene mutation in *N. crassa* (21) and produces chromatid aberrations in lateral root-tip chromosomes of *Vicia faba* (22). Iyer & Szybalski (23) have found β-propiolactone to be a very efficient mutagen for reversion to growth factor independence in *E. coli*.

After the discovery of the radiomimetic properties of alkylating agents, several of these compounds were tested for and were found to possess carcinogenic activity (24). These findings were not noticed by the technical people doing research in gaseous sterilization until the proposed use of β-propiolactone as a gaseous sterilant for enclosed spaces was questioned by federal regulatory agencies and their scientific advisors (25, 26). β-Propiolactone has been found to be an initiator of skin sarcomas and carcinomas in the mouse (27, 28, 29), and Wisely & Falk (30) have stated that single intradermal doses of 0.002 ml. in mice have caused sarcomas and squamous papillomas. The mention of the production of sarcomata in rats with diepoxybutane by Koller (31) and the confirmation if its carcinogenic activity by McCammon *et al.* (32) caused speculation that the monoepoxides, ethylene oxide and propylene oxide, would also be found carcinogenic. Walpole (24) has recorded the induction of sarcomata in rats after repeated injection of propylene oxide but not after treatment with ethylene oxide. He has concluded from his investigations that the presence in a molecule of one or more groups having alkylating function may result in carcinogenic activity. It certainly behooves the users and practitioners of gaseous sterilization not only to be concerned with the acute and chronic toxicity of gaseous alkylating agents but also to keep all contacts with these compounds to a minimum to prevent any concern about the possibility of long-term biological effects.

The acute toxicity of ethylene oxide and its irritant action on the skin and eyes are well known. Pure anhydrous liquid ethylene oxide does not produce primary injury to the dry skin of workers, but solutions of ethylene oxide have a vesicant action (33, 34) and may cause conjunctivitis if splashed in the eye (35, 36). Burns are particularly likely to occur when the solution is held in contact with the skin by clothing, gloves, and shoes. In common with many other skin irritants, ethylene oxide can produce sensitization (34).

Skin lesions can result from contact with ethylene oxide absorbed in sterilized rubber gloves and shoes (1, 37). Royce & Moore (37) have shown that immediately after overnight treatment in liquid ethylene oxide a piece of rubber weighing 1 gm. contained no less than 600 mg. of ethylene oxide. After sterilization in 10 per cent ethylene oxide gas, 1 gm. of rubber contained 15.4 mg. of the oxide; at 4 hr. there was 0.4 mg. remaining. A shoe can absorb up to 10 gm. of ethylene oxide during sterilization with this compound (38), and Beard & Dunmire (39) have used radioactive ethylene oxide to determine which parts of shoes are most retentive. Grundy *et al.* (40) have established that ethylene oxide gas absorbed during the sterilization of plastic intravenous injection equipment exerted a continuing sterilizing effect after the materials were removed from the sterilizer. These data point to the necessity of holding treated plastic and rubber materials at least 8 hr. or preferably a day before use.

Several recent papers have presented the results of animal experiments dealing with the acute and chronic effects of both ethylene oxide and propylene oxide vapors. When animals were subjected to repeated 7-hr. exposures to ethylene oxide vapor, 5 days a week, for 6 or 7 months, guinea pigs, rabbits, and monkeys tolerated 113 p.p.m., and rats aad mice tolerated 49 p.p.m. without adverse effects (41). A concurrent independent study (42) observed that dogs, rats, and mice exposed over a 6-month period to 100 p.p.m. of ethylene oxide exhibited no clinical signs of toxicity, but a few significant hematological changes were noted in one animal. These same investigators (42, 43) concluded from toxicity studies with propylene oxide that it was about one-third as toxic as ethylene oxide by inhalation and ingestion in all animal species studied. They recommended an industrial hygiene standard of 50 p.p.m. for ethylene oxide vapor and 150 p.p.m. for propylene oxide vapor. Those readers interested in the toxicity of other gaseous alkylating agents should consult the article by Rowe (44) on methyl bromide, the paper by Feazel & Lang (45) on β-propiolactone, and any good toxicology handbook for the toxicity of formaldehyde vapor.

Most of the available reports concerned with the microbicidal properties of gaseous alkylating agents present data that relate the physical factors of time, temperature, relative humidity, and concentration of gas to the destruction of a given population of microorganisms. Only the report of Loveless & Stock (46) on the inactivation of T_2 phage by aqueous alkylating agents describes in part how mono- and *bis*-epoxides react with a microorganism. Their data support many of the biochemical mechanisms of alkylating action previously discussed and may promote more basic research to learn how ethylene oxide inactivates microorganisms.

Ethylene oxide is effective against all microorganisms. The earlier literature containing references to its effect on many bacteria and molds as natural contaminants has been reviewed by Phillips & Kaye (1). Phillips (2, 7) was the first to quantitate the relative resistance of spore-forming and vegetative bacteria to ethylene oxide. He found that spores of *Bacillus globigii* (now *B. subtilis* var. *niger*) were only 2 to 6 times more resistant than vegetative cells from several bacterial species. Although no quantitative data are available for the relative resistance of *Mycobacterium tuberculosis* to ethylene oxide, several papers (47 to 50) have verified its destruction on contaminated materials. Friedl *et al.* (51) tested the sporicidal activity of ethylene oxide against five aerobic and five anaerobic spore-forming bacterial species employing the sporicide testing method of the Association of Official Agricultural Chemists. Dried spores, which were much more resistant to ethylene oxide than were wet spores, from all test organisms were destroyed after an 18-hr. exposure. Under their conditions, spores of *B. subtilis* and *Clostridium sporogenes* withstood a 6-hr. exposure, while spores of *B. globigii* and *B. anthracis* were killed in 30 min. No direct relation could be found between resistance to constant boiling HCl and to ethylene oxide. Although there have been occasional reports of the destruction of staphylococci only after prolonged exposure to ethylene oxide (52, 53), the data available from studies that were designed to compare the resistance of bacterial spores and staphylococci have shown bacterial spores to be more resistant (2, 50, 54, 55). Toth (56) has recorded aerobic sporeformers to be more resistant than vegetative bacteria, yeasts, and molds to destruction by ethylene oxide. Church *et al.* (57) have pointed out that populations of spores of some aerobic bacilli are heterogenous in their susceptibility to ethylene oxide and consist of a major component sensitive to ethylene oxide and a minor component resistant to ethylene oxide.

The sterilizing activity of ethylene oxide for viruses has been confirmed by several investigators. The following viruses have been inactivated by liquid ethylene oxide: vaccinia (47), influenza A and B (58), Newcastle disease virus (58), Theiler's mouse encephalomyelitis virus (58), MM mouse encephalomyelitis virus (58, 59), lymphocytic choriomeningitis virus (59), Eastern equine encephalomyelitis virus (59, 60), and foot-and-mouth disease virus (61, 62). The activity of gaseous ethylene oxide against 15 animal viruses was noted by Mathews & Hofstad (63), against foot-and-mouth disease virus by Savan (64), Callis *et al.* (65), and Fellowes (62), and against Columbia SK encephalomyelitis virus and vaccinia virus by Klarenbeek & van Tongeren (66).

The microbicidal properties of the other alkylating agents employed in gaseous sterilization have not been quantitated to the same extent as have those of ethylene oxide. Phillips (5) has adequately noted the bactericidal properties of gaseous formaldehyde. The sporicidal activity of methyl bromide against spores of *B. anthracis* has been documented by Kolb & Schneiter (67) and Kolb *et al.* (68) and against fungi by Munnecke *et al.* (69). Phillips (5) states that methyl bromide has one-tenth the activity of ethylene oxide or approximately the activity of 10 per cent ethylene oxide inerted with 90 per cent carbon dioxide by weight. Bruch & Koesterer (70) have quantitated the sporicidal activity of propylene oxide, which has about one-fourth the activity of ethylene oxide. The microbicidal properties of β-propiolactone are recorded in several papers from the U. S. Army Biological Warfare Laboratories (71, 72, 73). On a Ct_{90} basis (molar concentration of gas times the time for 90 per cent kill), β-propiolactone is approximately 25 times more active as a vapor-phase disinfectant than formaldehyde, 4000 times more active than ethylene oxide, and 50,000 times more active than methyl bromide (71).

To date, all evidence indicates that the effect of ethylene oxide or the other alkylating agents employed in gaseous sterilization is irreversible and microbicidal. However, Morpurgo & Sermonti (74) have demonstrated the reactivation by manganous chloride of spores of *Penicillium chrysogenum* inactivated by nitrogen mustard. They suggest that the site of the inactivation-reactivation process is in the cytoplasm of these spores. If their work is confirmed, this effect should be sought following the inactivation of organisms by other alkylating agents.

Physical Handling and Mode of Use of Gaseous Sterilants

Sterilization with gaseous ethylene oxide is a function principally of the concentration of gas, time of exposure, and temperature of exposure. Humidity must be known and controlled within certain limits, i.e., a certain minimal amount of moisture must be present for sterilization to occur. The degree of contamination constitutes another important variable since organisms protected by layers of dense organic material such as dried pus, blood, and serum or entrapped within crystals of salt or the dried solids from thick microbial suspensions can resist destruction by this method. The molecules of gas plus some molecules of added water or of water already present in the material must be in contact with an organism for inactivation to occur.

As a result of the report by Kaye & Phillips (4), it is generally accepted that ethylene oxide sterilization proceeds better at relative humidities of from 25 to 50 per cent than at humidities approaching saturation. These data support the empirical use of ethylene oxide in the presence of no added moisture by food processors (52, 75, 76, 77). These processors rely on the available water present in the dried powders or flakes to provide the necessary water for the inactivation reaction. The difficulties experienced in the destruction of excessively desiccated organisms (4, 63) can be traced to the lack of water in the cells or to the inability of added water to penetrate the dry cells. Opfell *et al.* (78) have shown that the absence of hygroscopic substances in the drying menstruum of spores of *B. globigii* increased the resistance of these spores to sterilization by ethylene oxide. Znamirowski *et al.* (55) have claimed that lack of humidity control was responsible for the inefficiency of a commercially available ethylene oxide sterilizer, but an analysis of their methods and data indicates that entrapment of spores in salt crystals provides a more likely explanation for the failure to achieve sterility.

Ethylene oxide concentrations are usually expressed as milligrams per liter (mg. per l.) or ounces per 1000 cubic feet of chamber space. In a series of experiments with ethylene oxide at concentrations of 22 to 884 mg. per l. and temperatures of 5 to 37°C., Phillips (2) found that the death rate was logarithmic, that doubling the concentration of ethylene oxide roughly halved the time required for sterilization, and that the temperature coefficient of the reaction was 2.7 for each rise of 10°C. Although the exact time for sterilization depends on the volume of the load, the nature of the materials and their degree of contamination, our laboratory employs 720 mg. per l. for 8 hr. at 100°F. (37.7°C.) or for 4 hr. at 130°F. (54.4°C.) for a load of clean plastic items in a 24-cubic foot sterilizer. These times are increased several fold for loads of greater volume in larger sterilizers.

Any gaseous sterilization process should be controlled by the use of biological indicators placed in the most difficult article or location in an article to be sterilized. Spores from any of several spore-forming bacterial species can be employed, but unpublished data from our laboratory have shown that spores from certain strains of *B. subtilis* and *C. sporogenes* are highly resistant. Friedl *et al.* (51) have also described these two organisms as being highly resistant to destruction by ethylene oxide. The use of spores with high heat resistance is not necessary since no correlation has been found between resistance to heat and gaseous sterilization. The concentration of organisms used should be reasonable (not greater than 1×10^6 spores dried on a 2-in. by $\frac{1}{4}$-in. filter paper strip) because physical protection from dense concentration can result. Royce & Bowler (79) have recently reported the use of a chemical control device that has been correlated against biological inactivation by ethylene oxide. This device requires sorption and penetration of its plastic package by ethylene oxide before the gas can react with the chemical reagents.

Although the penetration and diffusion of ethylene oxide through materials such as flour, spices, and layers of paper, clothing and blankets has been documented in past reviews (1, 5, 6), much more data are needed on the sorption by and penetration through many plastic films and articles. Among the inexperienced, it is not uncommon to attempt to sterilize articles wrapped in plastic films that are nearly gas- and moisture-proof. Waack *et al.* (80) have determined the permeability constants for several polymer films to ethylene oxide, methyl bromide, and other gases. Results of their studies showed that polyethylene and rubber hydrochloride (see original article for trade names) were most permeable to ethylene oxide, whereas cellulose acetate, polyvinylidene chloride, and polyester were less permeable to ethylene oxide in the order listed. Dick & Feazel (81) in the development of flexible plastic chambers for ethylene oxide sterilization tested the relative permeability of several plastic films and found cellophane, polyvinyl alcohol, and polyester impermeable to ethylene oxide under their test conditions. The results of Lloyd & Thompson (82) with wrapping materials such as cellophane, polyvinylidene chloride, polyethylene and laminated polyester indicated that polyvinylidene chloride was the most difficult and polyester rather difficult to penetrate with ethylene oxide. Unpublished data from our laboratory indicate that polyethylene, which is highly permeable to ethylene oxide, has a low transmission rate for water vapor, but since the humidity requirement for ethylene oxide sterilization is low, enough water vapor is usually present in the packages to allow satisfactory sterilization.

Although liquid ethylene oxide is stable to detonating agents (36), the vapor is explosive and will propagate a flame at concentrations ranging from 3.6 per cent by volume in air to 100 per cent ethylene oxide (36, 83). This flammability problem can be avoided by dilution with inert gases such as carbon dioxide (84) or chlorofluorohydrocarbons (83, 85). Definite nonflammable compositions have been formulated, and many of these gaseous mixtures are commercially available. This safety is achieved at a considerable loss in potency since about 90 per cent of these mixtures is diluent. This loss of potency is less for the chlorofluorohydrocarbon mixtures (11 per cent by weight ethylene oxide and equal parts by weight of dichlorodifluoromethane and trichloromonofluoromethane) since the concentration of ethylene oxide attained with these mixtures at 1 atm. pressure is almost three times that obtained with carbon dioxide mixtures (10 per cent ethylene oxide by weight).

A wide variety of equipment has been used for ethylene oxide treatments. Any gas-tight container can be employed although rigid chambers similar to laboratory autoclaves are usually used. The use of large vacuum chambers from which air is first removed before pure ethylene oxide is admitted has been described for the decontamination of bulk food materials (52, 75, 76, 77, 86, 87). The conversion of ordinary laboratory autoclaves (49, 88, 89) and the use of plastic bags (81, 89), tarpaulins (38, 89), and metal drums (38, 89) have been reported. Specially designed, automatic equipment is now commercially available (90, 91, 92). Recently, in West Germany, commercial equipment has become available that employs the 10 per cent ethylene oxide-90 per cent carbon dioxide mixture at pressures of 3 to 6 atm. and temperatures of 35 to 65°C. (50, 93). This procedure has been called the "Mainz sterilization method" and appears to have few advantages over the processes that employ the chlorofluorohydrocarbon mixtures at much lower pressures and at similar ethylene oxide concentrations.

The physical handling and mode of use of other gaseous sterilants can be given only brief mention. The sterilization of rooms or large spaces with formaldehyde has been reviewed before (5), and its recent use in disinfecting chambers has been detailed by several European workers (94, 95, 96). The employment of β-propiolactone as a surface sterilant in small chambers, rooms, or buildings has been cited in several recent publications (25, 26, 71, 97, 98). Propylene oxide (70, 99) and methyl bromide (67, 68, 69) are utilized in the same type of equipment as ethylene oxide.

Medical Applications of Gaseous Sterilization

It has been documented in past reviews that ethylene oxide will sterilize hospital bedding, plaster of Paris bandages, various articles of clothing and footwear, plastic and rubber laboratory items, ophthalmic instruments, catheters, cystoscopes, bronchoscopes, forceps, extractors, scalpel blades and holders, clinical thermometers, dental and root canal files, and penicillin in powder or solution. These accepted uses and the newer applications for ethylene oxide sterilization in hospital practice have also been discussed by Spaulding *et al.* (100), Freeman & Barwell (54), and Thomas (101).

Recent applications are included in the reports of Skeehan (102) and Linn (103), who have sterilized ophthalmic instruments in a small, table-model, ethylene oxide sterilizer. This same model of sterilizer has been criticized as being inefficient (104), and another group (100) has doubled the manufacturer's recommended exposure time. Other new or confimed applications are the sterilization of blankets (53), urological instruments (105), plastic intravenous injection equipment in commercial packages (40), ampules for anesthesia (106), procaine hydrochloride tablets (107), and the decontamination of blankets by the addition of ethylene oxide to plastic bag containers (108). Additional uses that are known to the reviewer include the sterilization of surgical rubber gloves, sutures, plastic syringes, disposable needles, oxygen tents, inhalation equipment, cameras, and photographic film.

A new application that has received much attention is the sterilization of pump-oxygenators. Spencer & Bahnson (109) modified a standard steam autoclave to sterilize a completely assembled pump-oxygenator with the ethylene oxide-chlorofluorohydrocarbon mixture. McCaughan *et al.* (110) made a 61-cubic ft. stainless steel chamber which employs the ethylene oxide-chlorofluorohydrocarbon mixture at a concentration of 180 to 200 mg. per l. Completely reliable sterilization of an assembled vertical screen pump-oxygenator was obtained at 16-hr. exposure at room temperature and ambient humidities. Bracken *et al.* (111) have used large polyvinyl chloride bags and the 10 per cent ethylene oxide-90 per cent carbon dioxide mixture to sterilize a heart-lung machine. They eventually hope to simplify the sterilization technique by discarding the plastic bag altogether and to maintain an adequate concentration of ethylene oxide in the machine by a slow trickle, i.e., the oxygenator would become its own sterilizing chamber.

To the reviewer's knowledge gaseous formaldehyde is very seldom used in the United States to sterilize hospital equipment and supplies or to fumigate hospital rooms. However, in Great Britain the committee on formaldehyde disinfection of the Public Health Laboratory Service has recently submitted a lengthy report on disinfection of hospital items by gaseous formaldehyde (95). This committee concluded that formaldehyde gas could not be recommended for disinfection of fabrics contaminated with smallpox virus or anthrax spores, nor was it really suitable for the disinfection of articles contaminated with tubercle bacilli. Contrary to these findings Caplan (96) has reduced the incidence of infections in a surgical ward by the regular disinfection of blankets and bedside curtains with formaldehyde vapor. Thomas *et al.* (53) compared sterilization of blankets by several methods. Although they list boiling as the simplest way of "sterilizing" blankets, ethylene oxide was considered a more promising sterilizing agent than formaldehyde, which, in normal use, allowed the survival of non-sporulating organisms. Phillips (5) in past reviews has noted the deficiencies of formaldehyde disinfection (condensation of gas and lack of penetration) and has pointed out how superior ethylene oxide is for many of these hospital applications.

Another gaseous alkylating agent that is felt to have potential applications in the hospital field is β-propiolactone. Like formaldehyde, this gas is non-penetrating and essentially a surface sterilant. After Hoffman & Warshowsky (71) detailed its microbicidal properties and mentioned its use to decontaminate a barracks, several reports on its use in hospital rooms followed (25, 26, 27). In general, these reports have shown that rooms can be treated and put back into use within 24 to 48 hr. The commercial development of this application has been hindered by the discovery of the carcinogenic properties of this compound on mouse skin as previously discussed. An additional limited application is the sterilization by the lactone of surfaces of unwrapped ophthalmic instruments in plastic sacks, desiccators, and plastic or metal boxes (98).

Agricultural and Industrial Applications of Gaseous Sterilization

Although gaseous sterilization with ethylene oxide had its birth in the food industry, much of the information regarding this application has remained a trade secret or has been listed briefly in patents. Very little information has been published in the United States during the past decade that describes new applications for ethylene oxide sterilization in this field. Some data on existing and known uses were presented by Hall (86), Pappas & Hall (87), and Coretti (112) verifying the destruction of thermophiles, yeasts, and molds in food ingredients. What is new and what has brought a sharp turn of events in this field has been the examination of the treated foods toxicologically and the promulgation of regulations by governmental agencies regarding acceptable levels of addition products and residues.

The first reference to nutritional damage of foods treated with ethylene oxide was presented in the paper by Hawk & Mickelsen (113), who noted severe growth depression in weanling albino rats when their diet, either stock or purified, had been exposed to the gas. Thiamine was indicated to be one of the factors, though not the only one, destroyed by this treatment. Oser & Hall (114) followed with evidence that when dried yeast and a rat diet composed of natural products were exposed to ethylene oxide according to a commercial method, there was no significant destruction of thiamine, riboflavin, nicotinic acid, pantothenic acid, or choline. There was an indication that some folic acid and pyridoxine were destroyed. The reviewer cannot agree with their objections that the levels of treatment used by Hawk & Mickelsen were too severe since gas concentrations in food sterilization can range from 300 to 1000 mg. per l. (75, 76, 115) and Griffith & Hall report the use of 1600 mg. per l. in one of their patents (116).

Further work by Bakerman *et al.* (117) has shown that various vitamins were destroyed when mixtures of the B vitamins suspended in starch were exposed to ethylene oxide. Practically all of the thiamine and large amounts of riboflavin, pyridoxine, niacin, and folic acid were destroyed when choline chloride was present; there was no destruction of pantothenic acid, biotin, or vitamin B_{12}. The effect of ethylene oxide on thiamine was due in part to the increase in pH in the presence of choline chloride; the destructive effect of ethylene oxide on thiamine solutions at pH 9 has also been shown by Diding (107). This alkalinity may explain the destruction of thiamine but cannot explain the destruction of niacin, riboflavin, or folic acid.

Windmueller *et al.* (118) observed that exposure of casein to very high concentrations of ethylene oxide resulted in essentially complete destruction of histidine and methionine determined by rat feeding studies and microbiological assays. As a result of their work, Mickelsen (119) ran microbiological assays on purified diets exposed to ethylene oxide under conditions that he previously described (113) and found that 22 per cent of the histidine and 17 per cent of the methionine were destroyed.

The realization that a tertiary nitrogen group was common to six of the labile nutrients prompted Windmueller *et al.* (12) to investigate the reaction of ethylene oxide with pyridine and the closely related nicotinamide and nicotinic acid. The destructive action of ethylene oxide on histidine, methionine, cysteine, and lysine was also studied in model systems in which the individual amino acids or amino acid derivatives were treated with ethylene oxide in aqueous solution (13). Nutritional damage by ethylene oxide treatment appears to be correlated with the electrophilic hydroxyethylation of an atom with one or more lone pairs of electrons, either nitrogen or sulfur.

With the passage in 1958 of the Food Additives Amendment to the U. S. Food, Drug and Cosmetic Act, the use of direct and indirect food additives not approved by the U. S. Food and Drug Administration was to be halted after March 6, 1960, although temporary extensions until March 6, 1961, could be granted. Ethylene oxide is considered a direct additive to foods treated with it and has been granted temporary clearance until March 6, 1961, for use in dried fruits, ground spices, dried mushrooms, and edible gums (120, 121). The objection to the use of ethylene oxide stems not only from the destruction of vitamins and amino acids but also from the known toxicity of ethylene and diethylene glycols that are almost invariably formed in small quantities as the hydrolytic residues from ethylene oxide sterilization of foods. Thus, the food industry has started to search for new sterilants, is reexamining other compounds such as propylene oxide and methyl bromide, and is developing new chemical procedures for residue determinations.

Gordon *et al.* (122) fumigated a prune with C_{14}-ethylene oxide and determined the main sites of alkylation. They found over 50 per cent of the total radioactivity to be combined with insoluble hydroxyethyl cellulose in the prune skin, about 30 per cent as hydroxyethylated sugars in the pulp, 10 per cent as alkylated proteins and amino acids, and 3 per cent as glycols. A similar study has been carried out by Winteringham and associates (123, 124, 125) with C_{14}-methyl bromide and wheat flour. The data from these papers indicate that no toxic products per se are formed, but only animal feeding studies could confirm this supposition.

Other new uses for gaseous sterilants in the agricultural field include the sterilization of dried gelatin and dried eggs by ethylene oxide or its mixture with propylene oxide or methyl bromide (126). Although Adam (127) has confirmed the destruction of salmonellae in egg powder by this method, he urges caution in the adoption of this technique because of possible toxicological and nutritional effects. The decontamination of various seeds with ethylene oxide has been described by Steinkraus *et al.* (128), and the destruction of fungi in barley seeds by propylene oxide has been recorded by Tyner (129). McBean & Johnson (130) and Nury *et al.* (131) have reported the preservation of prunes with propylene oxide, and Bruch & Koesterer (70) have utilized propylene oxide to decontaminate flaked and powdered foods.

While sterilization of powders is a problem in the pharmaceutical industry, many of the details of their techniques are kept as trade secrets. Bullock & Rawlins (132) have detailed the sterilization of kaolin powder mixtures by gaseous formaldehyde moving through the powders at constant flow rates or constant gas concentrations. They showed that the death rate of spores of *B. subtilis* is a function of the amount of formaldehyde permeating the powders in unit time and that humidities over 85 per cent are required for this process. A similar apparatus was used by Abbott *et al.* (133) to expose crystals formed from liquids contaminated with spores of *B. subtilis* to sterilization by gaseous formaldehyde and ethylene oxide. Neither of these gases could sterilize crystals which had spores entrapped in the crystal matrix. The static sterilization of talc powder in powder cans by the injection of propylene oxide or ethylene oxide has been listed in a recent patent by Masci (134).

Other recently noted applications for formaldehyde include the decontamination of microbiological laboratories (135) and incubators in egg hatcheries (136). These uses for formaldehyde will eventually be assumed by β-propiolactone vapor. Several investigators have demonstrated the decontamination of large industrial laboratories with this compound (25, 26). The full usefulness of β-propiolactone will not be achieved until its toxicity is further defined.

Future

After an attempt at some representation of the total picture of the field of gaseous sterilization, a projection into the future reveals many bright areas contrasted with some uncertain areas which need delineation and clarification. On the promising side is the fact that the use of ethylene oxide in the hospital and medical field will grow. The increasing use of disposable plastic materials requires their sterilization by a "cold" method. As specialized apparatus such as heart-lung machines become more prevalent in hospitals, the installation of permanent gaseous sterilization equipment will follow. The problems of staphylococcal contamination in many hospitals has forced numerous "infections committees" to consider sterilization of blankets, linens, and mattresses with ethylene oxide and even decontamination of patients' rooms with β-propiolactone or formaldehyde. Thus, the potential applications for gaseous sterilization look very bright and hopeful in this area.

In contrast, the future of gaseous sterilization in the food and agricultural field is certainly cloudy and befuddled. Although the use of gaseous chemicals as fumigants (destruction of insects and fungi) is a permanent part of the agricultural scene, the application of these same gaseous chemicals for sterilization of food or materials that may come into contact with foods remains to be cleared with governmental regulatory agencies. It may well be that the use of the available gaseous sterilants will have to be closely controlled with respect to the type of foods treated and the degree of decontamination that would be acceptable. Certainly, the presence of pathogenic staphylococci and salmonellae in many dried foods necessitates some remedial action. Part of the uncertainty regarding gaseous sterilization of food results from lack of knowledge of possible toxic or damaging effects, but, as more information is accumulated about the toxicological, cytotoxic and tumor-inhibiting effects of alkylating agents, the present difficulties will certainly be resolved.

LITERATURE CITED

1. Phillips, C. R., and Kaye, S., *Am. J. Hyg.*, **50,** 270–79 (1949)
2. Phillips, C. R., *Am. J. Hyg.*, **50,** 280–88 (1949)
3. Kaye, S., *Am. J. Hyg.*, **50,** 289–95 (1949)
4. Kaye, S., and Phillips, C. R., *Am. J. Hyg.*, **50,** 296–306 (1949)
5. Phillips, C. R., in *Antiseptics, Disinfectants, Fungicides, and Sterilization*, 746–65 (Reddish, G. F., Ed., Lea & Febiger, Philadelphia, Pa., 975 pp., 1957)
6. Phillips, C. R., and Warshowsky, B., *Ann. Rev. Microbiol.*, **12,** 525–50 (1958)
7. Phillips, C. R., *Bacteriol. Revs.*, **16,** 135–38 (1952)
8. Ross, W. C. J., *Ann. N. Y. Acad. Sci.*, **68,** 669–81 (1958)
9. Stacey, K. A., Cobb, M., Cousens, S. F., and Alexander, P., *Ann. N. Y. Acad. Sci.*, **68,** 682–701 (1958)
10. Fraenkel-Conrat, H. L., *J. Biol. Chem.*, **154,** 227–38 (1944)
11. Alexander, P., *Advances in Cancer Research*, **2,** 1–72 (1954)
12. Windmueller, H. G., Ackerman, C. J., Bakerman, H., and Mickelsen, O., *J. Biol. Chem.*, **234,** 889–94 (1959)
13. Windmueller, H. G., Ackerman, C. J., and Engel, R. W., *J. Biol. Chem.*, **234,** 895–99 (1959)
14. Price, C. C., *Ann. N. Y. Acad. Sci.*, **68,** 663–68 (1958)
15. Philips, F. S., *Pharmacol. Revs.*, **2,** 281–323 (1950)
16. Alexander, P., and Stacey, K. A., *Ann. N. Y. Acad. Sci.*, **68,** 1225–37 (1958)
17. Strauss, B., and Okubo, S., *J. Bacteriol.*, **79,** 464–73 (1960)
18. Kölmark, G., and Giles, N. H., *Genetics*, **40,** 890–902 (1955)
19. Ehrenberg, L., and Gustafsson, A., *Hereditas*, **43,** 595–602 (1957)
20. Ehrenberg, L., Lundquist, U., and Strom, G., *Hereditas*, **44,** 330–36 (1958)
21. Smith, H. H., and Srb, A. M., *Science*, **114,** 490–92 (1951)
22. Swanson, C. P., and Merz, T., *Science*, **129,** 1364–65 (1959)
23. Iyer, V. N., and Szybalski, W., *Appl. Microbiol.*, **6,** 23–29 (1958)
24. Walpole, A. L., *Ann. N. Y. Acad. Sci.*, **68,** 750–61 (1958)
25. Spiner, D. R., and Hoffman, R. K., *Appl. Microbiol.*, **8,** 152–55 (1960)
26. Bruch, C. W., *Am. J. Hyg.*, **73,** 1–9 (1961)
27. Walpole, A. L., Roberts, D. C., Rose, F. L., Hendry, J. A., and Homer, R. F., *Brit. J. Pharmacol.*, **9,** 306–23 (1954)
28. Roe, F. J. C., and Salaman, M. H., *Brit. J. Cancer*, **9,** 177–203 (1955)
29. Roe, F. J. C., and Glendenning, O. M., *Brit. J. Cancer*, **10,** 357–62 (1956)
30. Wisely, D. V., and Falk, H. L., *J. Am. Med. Assoc.*, **173,** 1161 (1960)
31. Koller, P., *Heredity*, **6,** suppl., 181–96 (1953)
32. McCammon, C. J., Kotin, P., and Falk, H. L., *Proc. Am. Assoc. Cancer Research*, **2**(3), 229–30 (1957)
33. Sexton, R. J., and Henson, E. V., *J. Ind. Hyg. Toxicol.*, **31,** 297–300 (1949)
34. Sexton, R. J., and Henson, E. V., *Arch. Ind. Hyg. Occupational Med.*, **2,** 549–64 (1950)
35. McLaughlin, R. S., *Am. J. Ophthalmol.*, **29,** 1355–62 (1946)
36. Hess, L. G., and Tilton, V. V., *Ind. Eng. Chem.*, **42,** 1251–58 (1950)
37. Royce, A., and Moore, W. K. S., *Brit. J. Ind. Med.*, **12,** 169–71 (1955)
38. Fulton, J. D., and Mitchell, R. B., *U. S. Armed Forces Med. J.*, **3,** 425–39 (1952)
39. Beard, H. C., and Dunmire, R. B., *Arch. Ind. Health*, **15,** 167–69 (1957)
40. Grundy, W. E., Rdzok, E. J., Remo, W. J., Sagen, H. E., and Sylvester, J. C., *J. Am. Pharm. Assoc., Sci. Ed.*, **46,** 439–42 (1957)
41. Hollingsworth, R. L., Rowe, V. K., Oyen, F., McCallister, D. D., and Spencer, H. C., *Arch. Ind. Health*, **13,** 217–27 (1956)
42. Jacobson, K. H., Hockley, E. B., and Feinsilver, L., *Arch. Ind. Health*, **13,** 237–44 (1956)
43. Rowe, V. K., Hollingsworth, R. L., Oyen, F., McCallister, D. D., and Spencer, H. C., *Arch. Ind. Health*, **13,** 228–36 (1956)
44. Rowe, V. K., *Pest Control*, **25**(9), 18–27 (1957)
45. Feazel, C. E., and Lang, E. W., *Soap Chem. Specialties*, **35**(10), 113–21 (1959)
46. Loveless, A., and Stock, J. C., *Proc. Roy. Soc. (London), B.*, **150,** 423–45 (1959)
47. Wilson, A. T., and Bruno, P., *J. Exptl. Med.*, **91,** 449–58 (1950)
48. Kaye, S., *J. Lab. Clin. Med.*, **35,** 823–28 (1950)
49. Newman, L. B., Colwell, C. A., and

Jameson, E. L., *Am. Rev. Tuberc. Pulmonary Diseases*, **71**, 272–78 (1955)
50. Lammers, T., and Gewalt, R., *Z. Hyg. Infektionskrankh.*, **144**, 350–58 (1958)
51. Friedl, J. L., Ortenzio, L. F., and Stuart, L. S., *J. Assoc. Offic. Agr. Chemists*, **39**, 480–83 (1956)
52. Rauscher, H., Mayr, G., and Kaemmerer, H., *Food Manuf.*, **32**, 169–72 (1957)
53. Thomas, C. G. A., West, B., and Besser, H., *Guy's Hosp. Repts.*, **108**, 446–63 (1959)
54. Freeman, M. A. R., and Barwell, C. F., *J. Hyg.*, **58**, 337–45 (1960)
55. Znamirowski, R., McDonald, S., and Roy, T. E., *Can. Med. Assoc. J.*, **83**, 1004–6 (1960)
56. Toth, L. Z., *Arch. Mikrobiol.*, **32**, 409–10 (1959)
57. Church, B. D., Halvorson, H., Ramsey, D. S., and Hartman, R. S., *J. Bacteriol.*, **72**, 242–47 (1956)
58. Ginsberg, H. S., and Wilson, A. T., *Proc. Soc. Exptl. Biol. Med.*, **73**, 614–16 (1950)
59. Hartman, F. W., Kelly, A. R., and LoGrippo, G. A., *Gastroenterology*, **28**, 244–56 (1955)
60. Bucca, M. A., *J. Bacteriol.*, **71**, 491–92 (1956)
61. Tessler, J., Barber, L., and Fellowes, O. N., *Bacteriol. Proc.* (*Soc. Am. Bacteriologists*), 70 (1959)
62. Fellowes, O. N., *Ann. N. Y. Acad. Sci.*, **83**, 595–608 (1960)
63. Mathews, J., and Hofstad, M. S., *Cornell Vet.*, **43**, 452–61 (1953)
64. Savan, M., *Am. J. Vet. Research*, **16**, 158–59 (1955)
65. Callis, J. J., Tessler, J., Fellowes, O. N., and Poppensiek, G. C., *Bacteriol. Proc.* (*Soc. Am. Bacteriologists*), 22 (1957)
66. Klarenbeek, A., and van Tongeren, H. A. E., *J. Hyg.*, **52**, 525–28 (1954)
67. Kolb, R. W., and Schneiter, R., *J. Bacteriol.*, **59**, 401–12 (1950)
68. Kolb, R. W., Schneiter, R., Floyd, E. P., and Byers, D. H., *Arch. Ind. Hyg. Occupational Med.*, **5**, 354–64 (1952)
69. Munnecke, D. E., Ludwig, R. A., and Sampson, R. E., *Can. J. Botany*, **37**, 51–58 (1959)
70. Bruch, C. W., and Koesterer, M. G., *J. Food Sci.* (In press)
71. Hoffman, R. K., and Warshowsky, B., *Appl. Microbiol.*, **6**, 358–62 (1958)
72. Dawson, F. W., Hearn, H. J., and Hoffman, R. K., *Appl. Microbiol.*, **7**, 199–201 (1959)
73. Dawson, F. W., Janssen, R. J., and Hoffman, R. K., *Appl. Microbiol.*, **8**, 39–41 (1960)
74. Morpurgo, G., and Sermonti, G., *Genetics*, **44**, 1371–81 (1959)
75. Griffith, C. L., and Hall, L. A., *U. S. Pat. 2,189,947* (Feb., 1940)
76. Griffith, C. L., and Hall, L. A., *U. S. Pat. Re. 22,284* (March, 1943)
77. Baer, J. M., *U. S. Pat. 2,229,360* (Jan., 1941)
78. Opfell, J. B., Hohmann, J. P., and Latham, A. B., *J. Am. Pharm. Assoc., Sci. Ed.*, **48**, 617–19 (1959)
79. Royce, A., and Bowler, C., *J. Pharm. and Pharmacol.*, **11**, Suppl., 294T–98T (1959)
80. Waack, R., Alex, N. H., Frisch, H. L., Stannett, V., and Szwarc, M., *Ind. Eng. Chem.*, **47**, 2524–27 (1955)
81. Dick, M., and Feazel, C. E., *Modern Plastics*, **38**(3), 148–50, 226, 233 (1960)
82. Lloyd, R. S., and Thompson, E. L., *Gaseous Sterilization with Ethylene Oxide*, 1–21 (American Sterilizer Co., Erie, Pa., 21 pp., 1958)
83. Haenni, E. O., Affens, W. A., Lento, H. G., Yeomans, A. H., and Fulton, R. A., *Ind. Eng. Chem.*, **51**, 685–88 (1959)
84. Jones, G. W., and Kennedy, R. E., *Ind. Eng. Chem.*, **22**, 146–47 (1930)
85. Kaye, S., *U. S. Pat. 2,891,838* (June, 1959)
86. Hall, L. A., *Food Packer*, **32**(12), 26–28, 47 (1951)
87. Pappas, H. J., and Hall, L. A., *Food Technol.*, **6**, 456–58 (1952)
88. Skeehan, R. A., Jr., King, J. H., Jr., and Kaye, S., *Am. J. Ophthalmol.*, **42**, 424–30 (1956)
89. Schley, D. G., Hoffman, R. K., and Phillips, C. R., *Appl. Microbiol.*, **8**, 15–19 (1960)
90. Perkins, J. J., *Principles and Methods of Sterilization*, 325–33 (Charles C Thomas Co., Springfield, Ill., 340 pp., 1956)
91. Stryker, W. H., *Hosp. Manage.*, **85**(3), 74–77 (1958)
92. Kaye, S., and Darker, G. D., *Bacteriol. Proc.* (*Soc. Am. Bacteriologists*), 22–23 (1957)
93. Gewalt, R., and Fischer, E., *Münch. med. Wochschr.*, **101**, 563–65 (1959)

94. Adam, W., *Z. Hyg. Infektionskrankh.*, **144,** 117–24 (1957)
95. Committee on Formaldehyde Disinfection of the Public Health Laboratory Service, *J. Hyg.*, **56,** 488–515 (1958)
96. Caplan, H., *Lancet*, **I,** 1088–89 (1959)
97. Woodward, M. F., and Clark, A. B., *U. S. Armed Forces Med. J.*, **11,** 459–63 (1960)
98. Allen, H. F., and Murphy, J. T., *J. Am. Med. Assoc.*, **172,** 1759–63 (1960)
99. Atherton, F. R., *Australasian J. Pharm.*, **40,** 1192–95 (1959)
100. Spaulding, E. H., Emmons, E. K., and Guzara, M. L., *Am. J. Nursing*, **58,** 1530–31 (1958)
101. Thomas, C. G. A., *Guy's Hosp. Repts.*, **109,** 57–74 (1960)
102. Skeehan, R. A., Jr., *Am. J. Ophthalmol.*, **47,** 86–89 (1959)
103. Linn, J. G., Jr., *Arch. Ophthalmol.*, **62,** 619–25 (1959)
104. Walter, C. W., and Kundsin, R. B., *J. Am. Med. Assoc.*, **170,** 1543–44 (1959)
105. Boden, O., *Z. Urol.*, **53,** 49–53 (1960)
106. Hallowell, P., Murphy, J. T., and Mangiaracine, A. B., *Anaesthesiology*, **19,** 665–70 (1958)
107. Diding, N., *Pharm. Acta Helv.*, **35,** 582–87 (1960)
108. Lammers, T., Day, H., Koernlein, M., and Seibel, M., *Z. Hyg. Infektionskrankh.*, **146,** 236–43 (1960)
109. Spencer, F. C., and Bahnson, H. T., *Bull. Johns Hopkins Hosp.*, **102,** 241–44 (1958)
110. McCaughan, J. S., Jr., McMichael, H., Schuder, J. C., and Kirby, C. K., *Surgery*, **45,** 648–54 (1959)
111. Bracken, A., Wilton-Davies, C. C., and Weale, F. E., *Guy's Hosp. Repts.*, **109,** 75–80 (1960)
112. Coretti, K., *Fleischwirtschaft*, **9,** 183–90 (1957)
113. Hawk, E. A., and Mickelsen, O., *Science*, **121,** 442–44 (1955)
114. Oser, B. L., and Hall, L. A., *Food Technol.*, **10,** 175–78 (1956)
115. Griffith, C. L., and Hall, L. A., *U. S. Pat. 2,107,697* (Feb., 1938)
116. Griffith, C. L., and Hall, L. A., *U. S. Pat. 2,189,949* (Feb., 1940)
117. Bakerman, H., Romine, M., Schricker, J. A., Takahashi, S. M., and Mickelsen, O., *J. Agr. Food Chem.*, **4,** 956–59 (1956)
118. Windmueller, H. G., Ackerman, C. J., and Engel, R. W., *J. Nutrition*, **60,** 527–37 (1956)
119. Mickelsen, O., *J. Am. Dietet. Assoc.*, **33,** 341–46 (1957)
120. Anonymous, *Federal Register*, **25,** 3525–26 (1960)
121. Anonymous, *Federal Register*, **25,** 5338–39 (1960)
122. Gordon, H. T., Thornberg, W. W., and Werum, L. N., *J. Agr. Food Chem.*, **7,** 196–200 (1959)
123. Winteringham, F. P. W., Harrison, A., Bridges, R. G., and Bridges, P. M., *J. Sci. Food Agr.*, **6,** 251–61 (1955)
124. Bridges, R. G., *J. Sci. Food Agr.*, **6,** 261–68 (1955)
125. Winteringham, F. P. W., *J. Sci. Food Agr.*, **6,** 269–74 (1955)
126. Mayr, G., and Kaemmerer, H., *Food Manuf.*, **34,** 169–70 (1959)
127. Adam, W., *Deut. Lebensm. Rundschau*, **54,** 110–11 (1958)
128. Steinkraus, K. H., Crosier, W. F., and Provvidenti, M. L., *Proc. Assoc. Offic. Seed Analysts, 49th Meeting*, 159–66 (1959)
129. Tyner, L. E., *Phytopathology*, **48,** 177–78 (1958)
130. McBean, D., and Johnson, A. A., *Food Preserv. Quart.*, **17,** 48–51 (1957)
131. Nury, F. S., Miller, M. W., and Brekke, J. E., *Food Technol.*, **14,** 113–15 (1960)
132. Bullock, K., and Rawlins, E. A., *J. Pharm. and Pharmacol.*, **6,** 859–76 (1954)
133. Abbott, C. F., Cockton, J., and Jones, W., *J. Pharm. and Pharmacol.*, **8,** 709–20 (1956)
134. Masci, J. N., *U. S. Pat. 2,809,879* (Oct., 1957)
135. Hundemann, A. S., and Holbrook, A. A., *J. Am. Vet. Med. Assoc.*, **135,** 549–53 (1959)
136. Bierer, B. W., *J. Am. Vet. Med. Assoc.*, **132,** 174–76 (1958)

Reprinted from *Biotechnology and Bioengineering* **10**, 1–31 (1968)

5

Sterilization with Gaseous Ethylene Oxide: A Review of Chemical and Physical Factors

ROBERT R. ERNST and JOHN E. DOYLE,
Research Laboratory, Castle Company, Rochester, New York 14623

Summary

Although the basic parameters for ethylene oxide sterilization are established, it is sometimes difficult to attain in practice where the principal limiting factor is moisture availability. There are situations which can limit or enhance the dynamics of sterilization. Such factors, if overlooked, could upset experiments and lead to erroneous conclusions, or defeat the sterilization process entirely. Such are, namely: stratification effects, diffusion barriers, moisture-reducing effects, polymerization, and temperature distribution gradients.

Introduction

Fumigation is almost as old as civilization itself. The application of ethylene oxide as a fumigant several decades ago set the stage for ethylene oxide to become one of the two major sterilizing agents of the present time. Like many new concepts, the ethylene oxide sterilization process is both highly praised by many and severely condemned by others. Since there is no overall panacea for sterilization, let us recognize the fact that all processes have limitations, and sterilization processes are not excluded.

Consideration of many factors leads one to an appreciation of the fact that cold sterilization with ethylene oxide (EO) or any other sterilizing gas is exceedingly more complex than the classical steam process. Whereas sterilization with steam is concerned with a biphasic mixture of two components, the EO system can be a triphasic complex of five components.

Many of the parameters of EO sterilization have already been mentioned in the basic work of early investigators in this field. However, many interrelationships have been overlooked by novices in the application of basic data to the sterilization process. The result has been discouragement, discontent, and the publication of papers denouncing the process on the basis of results obtained because of ignorance of many of the intricacies involved in the successful process.

The principal limitation in ethylene oxide sterilization seems to be diffusion and how the diffusion of moisture, gas, and heat are limited by protective effects provided by the state of materials to be sterilized and by dynamic changes occurring in and surrounding their contaminated sites. In addition, there are other factors which can further limit or enhance the dynamics of sterilization. Such factors if overlooked could upset experiments and lead to erroneous conclusions, or defeat the sterilization process entirely.

Basic Parameters

Since most of the basic work on gaseous ethylene oxide was done at temperatures and pressures below those set by commercial sterilizer manufacturers, Ernst and Shull[1] attempted to expand the knowledge of basic parameters to higher temperatures and pressures or concentrations. Investigating the relationships of temperature and concentrations, results were in general agreement with Phillips,[2] but revealed a very interesting new phenomenon.

The fact that the system was found to be basically a first-order reaction was reconfirmed by Ernst and Shull[1] and El Bisi et al.[3] However, Ernst and Shull discovered that kinetics went beyond first order to zero order with respect to high ethylene oxide concentrations at higher treatment temperatures. Within low temperature ranges the average Q_{10} for the range of concentrations tested agreed with Phillips' 2.74. The thermochemical death curves depicted in Figure 1 show that each concentration reflected its own Q_{10} at the lower temperatures, and the straight lines representing the first-order kinetics converged with the straight line representing zero with respect to concentration. At temperatures above those represented by the points of intersection, concentration was no longer a limiting factor. In the zero-order region the Q_{10} was found to be 1.80 as a minimal limit. This is in close agreement with El Bisi[3] who recorded a Q_{10} of 1.5. Opfell[4] had previously noted also that doubling the ethylene oxide concentration in his system had negligible added effect.

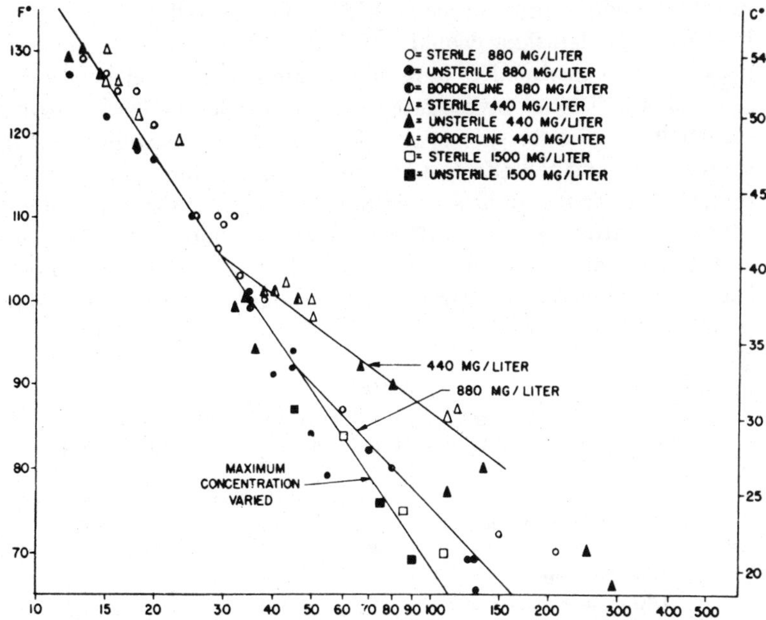

Fig. 1. Thermochemical death time curves for spores of *Bacillus subtilis* var. *niger*.

Before leaving Figure 1, note that the thermochemical death time for the sterilization of exposed surfaces with EO in a prehumidified environment of 40% relative humidity (RH) at 130°F. can be accomplished in a time equivalent to sterilization with saturated steam at 250°F. In agreement with the majority of investigators in the field, the principal limiting factor to sterilization does not appear to be ethylene oxide concentration at commercial sterilizing temperatures, but moisture. Ernst and Shull[5] indicated how barriers to the effective diffusion of moisture could limit ethylene oxide effectiveness even when working in the zero-order concentration region, and what influence temperature, and the means of providing moisture, had on the system. They found that severely dried barrier materials create a greater demand for humidification, and that prehumidification under a previously evacuated environment facilitates shorter sterilization times over the use of a humidity "conditioned" gas.

"Carrier" materials used as supporting media for microbial populations; materials which could act as barriers to the diffusion of moisture such as proteinaceous debris, and crystallizable salts; and how such preparations would affect the resistance of a microbial population to gaseous EO were investigated (Ernst and Doyle[6]).

Ernst and Doyle[6] investigated various carrier materials used as supporting media for spores, the effect due to the cleanliness of the spores used, and the effect of severe drying. From Table I a wide range of resistance can be seen with no consistent differences between spores on hard or porous surfaces. What we noticed however, was a large zone of partial survival, especially in the last three carriers listed. We believe this large zone was due to the lack of proper cleaning of the spores.

TABLE I

Effect of Various Carriers on the Resistance of *Bacillus* var. *niger* (10^5 spores/unit) to Ethylene Oxide (1200 mg./l. at 40% RH, 130°F.)[a]

Carrier material	Total survival, min.	Partial survival, min.
Bibulous paper	3	<5
Chromatography paper	3	<5
Nylon film	—	<10
Polypropylene film	—	<10
Aluminum foil	—	<10
Nylon fabric	—	>10
Wax paper	—	>10
Rubber glove film	—	>10
Aclar film	—	>10
Poly(vinyl chloride) film	4	<25
100% Acetate fabric	5	>45
Heavy paper	—	<1 hr.
Acetate–Rayon fabric	45	>1 hr.

[a]Spore suspension washed 2 times in distilled water.

However, Table II shows the effect of various carriers on the survival of a carefully cleaned preparation of *Bacillus subtilis* spores. Once again there was little difference as to whether the carrier was absorbent or non-absorbent. Extremely high resistance due to any carrier was not observed with these spores.

Since the cleanliness of a spore suspension seemed to be an important aspect of the relative resistance of spores to EO it was investigated further. Since hard surfaces have been reported to

TABLE II

Effect of Various Carriers on the Resistance of *Bacillus* var. *niger* (10^6 spores/unit) to Ethylene Oxide (1200 mg./l. at 40% RH, 130°F.)[a]

Carrier material	Total survival, min.	Partial survival, min.
Yellow sponge ("Ivalon")	5	<15
Reinforced cellulose	5	<15
100% Cotton fabric	5	<15
100% Rayon fabric	5	<15
Aluminum foil	5	<15
Chromatography paper	5	<15
100% Acetate fabric	<5	<5
Rick-rack	<5	<15
Glass tubing	<5	<10
Wax paper	<5	<10
Polyethylene film	<5	<10
Balsa wood	5	<10
Acetate–Rayon satin	5	<10
Rubber glove film	<5	>15

[a]Spore suspension washed 8 times in distilled water.

create a greater resistance than porous surfaces, aluminum foil carriers were compared with porous paper carriers. Also because desiccation has been reported by Gilbert et al.,[7] and Phillips[8] to increase the resistance of spores and even defeat their sterilization it was decided to investigate this aspect also.

Strips made from five suspensions of spores were divided, half being dried and kept at room temperature, the other half being desiccant-dried under vacuum over calcium sulfate at room temperature until ready for experimentation. Hence, there were air-dried and desiccant-dried aluminum foil and paper carriers contaminated with spores of 10^6 unit of varying degrees of cleanliness as shown by the number of resuspensions reflecting the washing procedure in distilled water. Figure 2 summarizes the experimental results.

Considering the aluminum carriers, one can readily see that if the suspension is not cleaned at all, an extreme resistance is obtained, probably due to occlusion of the spores in the dried media constituents. With one washing the broad region of partial survival attained indicates that some spores were being randomly protected.

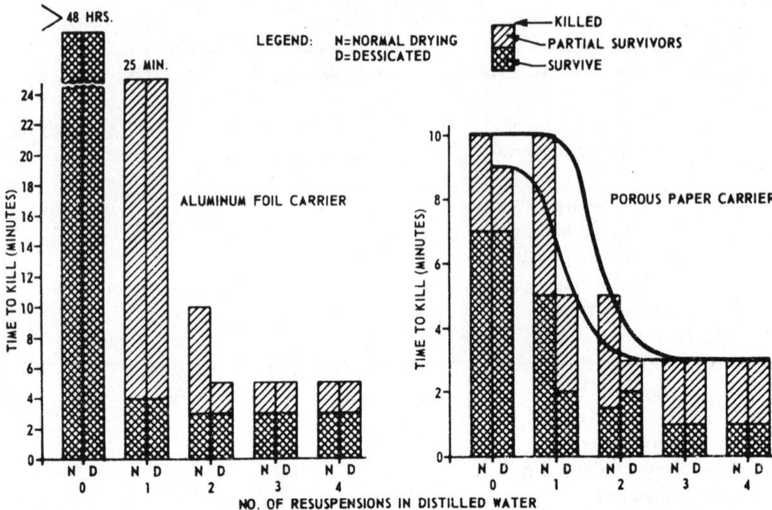

Fig. 2. Effect of relative cleanliness on the resistance of *Bacillus subtilis* var. *niger* to gaseous ethylene oxide.

With a second washing there was still some effect of the inadequate washing of the suspension, however only on the undesiccated carriers. After the third washing the resistance levels off to 3 min. total survival and $4^1/_2$ min. total inactivation. The partial survival zone is approximately only $^1/_2$ min. Desiccation had little effect on the resistance of the spores.

With the porous paper carrier the effect of the relative cleanliness of the spore suspension can also be seen. Complete resistance to EO was not obtained, however, even with the suspension which was not washed at all. The desiccated carriers were less resistant than the normally dried carriers when they had been washed up to two times. Upon further washing, spores on either undesiccated or desiccated strips had equal resistance.

In comparing the aluminum foil carrier (a hard surface) with the paper carrier (porous surface), the cleanliness of the spore suspension used greatly determined any difference in resistance. In every degree of cleanliness the aluminum foil resulted in a greater resistance than the porous paper, with the difference in resistance becoming quite small after three washings.

Desiccation of spores appears not to play a major role under these experimental conditions. Spores were desiccated by all possible means of heat and high vacuum and combinations thereof. Even at 10% RH little difference in resistance between desiccated and undesiccated spores were observed, although the time for sterilization for both was increased.

Figure 3 shows a model comparing thermal chemical death time curves of a clean spore crop with a dirty spore crop. If the spore crop is clean, the region of partial survivors is narrow. If the spore crop is unwashed, then the region of partial survivors is broad. Carriers inoculated with an unwashed spore suspension are randomly protected by crystals, organic material, or both.

Ernst and Shull[5] demonstrated a definite advantage of prehumidification over simultaneous or post-humidification with respect to diffusion barriers. Eltronics relative humidity (RH) probes were sealed in polyethylene bags and RH measurements were recorded. The result is shown in Figure 4. Prehumidification takes place in the sterilizer for a selected period of time after an evacuation to approximately 26 in. Hg negative pressure. Steam is pulsed into the chamber until a preset RH controller in the chamber is satisfied. This level of RH is maintained until the hot sterilizing gas is admitted to the chamber. This figure shows how the humidity rises and levels

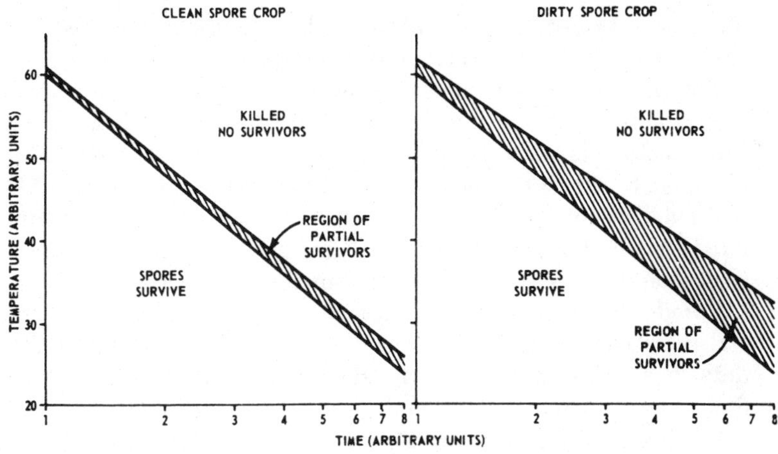

Fig. 3. Model of thermochemical death time curves for *Bacillus subtilis* var. *niger* spores.

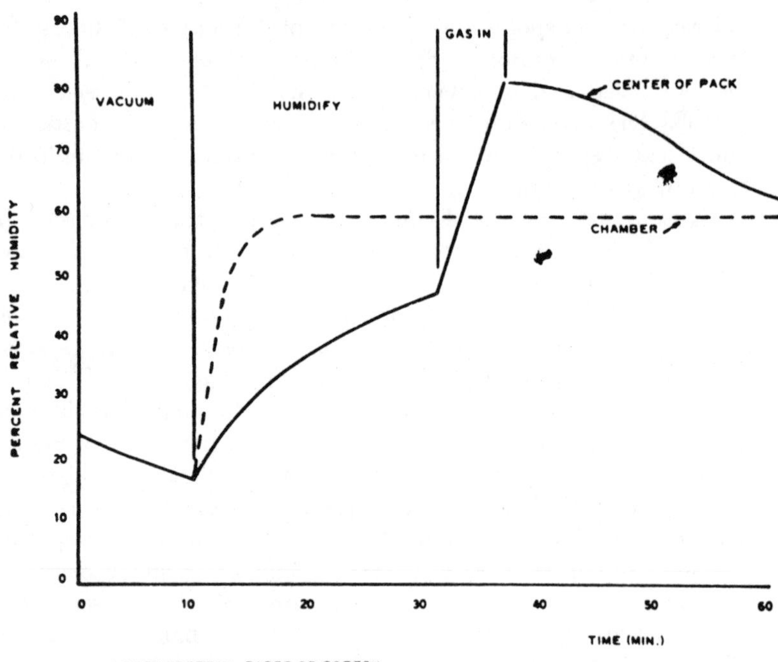

Fig. 4. Moisture penetration characteristics with prehumidification.

off in the chamber space. Then as the hot gas is admitted to the chamber the RH inside the bag rises sharply.

The principle of prehumidification under vacuum is to provide a deep penetration of moisture into moisture-hungry materials. Thus, the moisture is strategically located to enhance the dynamics of diffusion. Since it probably forms thin films on barriers with a diffuse molecular dispersion outward therefrom, it is least likely to be interfered with by the penetrating sterilizing gas, but will be carried with the gas and before it into the contaminated sites.

Paradoxically, there are conflicting opinions as to actual optimum RH requirements in the ethylene oxide process. Kaye and Phillips[9] data show an optimal RH in the vicinity of 33%; whereas Ernst and Shull,[5] Perkins and Lloyd,[10] and Mayr[11] presented data to show that sterilizing efficiency increased with increased RH. A conflict does not actually exist. The methods or test procedures were entirely different and represented diverse conditions. Phillips' optimal low-level RH requirement was based on work where microorganisms and their carrier materials were allowed to equilibrate with respect to their RH environment. In this case the optimal was determined at 33% RH at 25°C. Efficiency dropped off sharply below 20% RH and dropped more gradually as RH was increased beyond 40%. On the other hand, Ernst and Shull, Perkins and Lloyd, and Mayr presented data under conditions which were below equilibrium with respect to moisture content versus RH environment.

A model system was proposed by Ernst and Doyle[6] which would logically explain why an optimal RH is indicated under experimental conditions, whereas a high RH is generally required in practice. It is hypothesized that water molecules carry ethylene oxide to reactive sites. In practice either water or EO increases the permeation of the other through plastic films depending upon their polar or nonpolar character.

The fact that ethylene oxide acts as a "carrier" for moisture through nonpolar, and normally hydrophobic films having low moisture permeations was frequently observed in the Castle Process Laboratory. When a sealed polyethylene bag was placed into a sterilizer conditioned to 130°F. in a high relative humidity, little if any moisture diffused through the polyethylene film. However, on addition of EO to this system, globules of water were found on the inside of the polyethylene bag indicating that EO acted as the carrier for the diffusion of moisture through the polyethylene film. Conversely, water aids the permeation of ethylene oxide through polar type films (e.g., nylon and cellophane) which normally allow water to readily permeate but are slow to diffuse EO.

The model system is portrayed in Figures 5 and 6. Spores are characterized with respect to their immediate environment and relative moisture content as compared with the gross environment surrounding them with respect to available moisture. The arrows represent the dynamic exchange of moisture. In Figure 5 the "contaminated sites" are represented as having equal amounts of moisture, but are not in equilibrium with their gross environment. On the left is represented a relatively low environmental moisture with respect to the site. The exchange of moisture is outward, away from the spore. In practice this condition is very limiting to the sterilization process. On the right is shown the opposite effect of a high environmental moisture. The dynamic exchange of water is

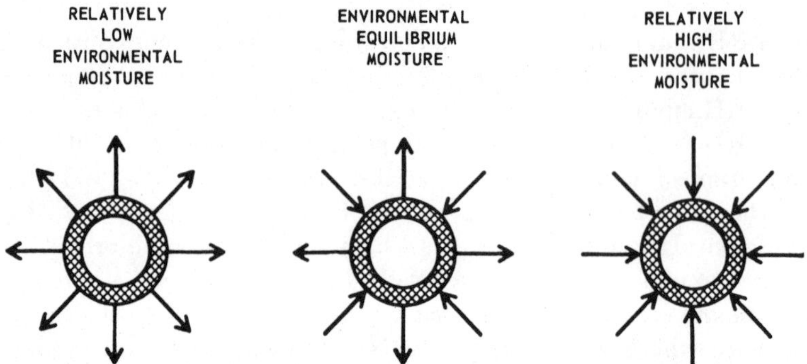

Fig. 5. Model representing the dynamic exchange of water by bacterial spores unequilibrated and equilibrated with their environmental moisture.

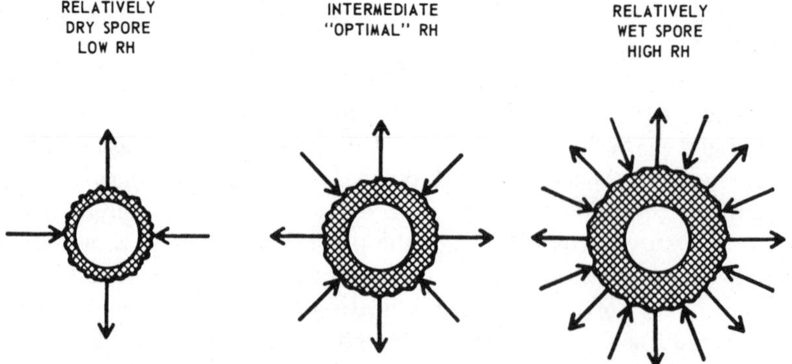

Fig. 6. Model representing the dynamic exchange of water by bacterial spores equilibrated to different levels of environmental moisture.

primarily toward the site. This represents the most ideal situation in practice. In the center is represented the equilibrium (steady-state) condition which is intermediate in effectiveness. Figure 6 is the second part of the model showing in all three cases situations where the spore and its immediate environment (the site) is in equilibration with its surroundings with regard to moisture exchange. Represented on the left is a relatively dry site in low environmental moisture under steady-state conditions. There is little exchange of moisture in and out of the spore. In practice we know this situation is very limiting for sterilization. On the right, the opposite situation shows a relatively wet site in an environment of high available moisture and equilibrated therewith, representing a high rate of interchange of moisture between the site and its surroundings. It was suggested by Phillips[8] that a zone of high moisture would have a diluting effect on EO reducing its availability to the cell, especially when the EO environment is minimal. The model represented by the central figure would agree with the optimal RH designated by Phillips.

Experience has shown that, although Phillips' basic parameter is correct, for all practical purposes it is more realtistic to base sterilization processes on the first consideration for two primary reasons: (*1*) Usually sterilization processes are carried out at higher than ordinary room temperatures. This produces a condition which, as described above, presents materials to be sterilized which are moisture deficient with respect to an established RH environment. (*2*) Usually materials to be sterilized, except for exposed surfaces, have wrapping, matrices, and the like which present diffusion barriers. And even though the optimal 33% RH is desirable at the site of bacterial surfaces, a much higher than optimal level must exist to achieve this goal. Fick's diffusion law applies here where, all other factors being constant, the rate of diffusion across a barrier is directly proportional to the concentration gradient across the barrier (the gradient in this case being moisture in the sterilizer versus moisture at the bacterial site).

$$m = \Delta A(C_2 - C_1)t/h$$

where m = mass of substance diffused; Δ = coefficient of diffusion; A = cross-sectional area; $(C_2 - C_1)$ = concentration gradient across a thickness, h; t = time.

The diffusion law is a theoretical consideration. In practical situations there are molecular interactions which seriously interfere with diffusion through membranes and into materials. For example, if heat-sealed bags of plastic film which contain air are subjected to an environment which is evacuated, they will expand and an internal pressure can be exerted by the air attempting to diffuse out. Sterilizing under negative pressure (which is done with pure EO) presents a severe limitation for diffusion of moisture and EO through such bags.

Organic matter itself will not ordinarily defeat the sterilization process as was shown in Tables I and II, unless in-solid or in-crystal protection (occlusion) is severe enough to completely stop diffusion of moisture and EO (Royce and Bowler[12]).

Figure 7 shows the occlusion of spores of *Bacillus subtilis* in crystals of calcium carbonate. The crystals are approximately 10 μ on a side and up to 100 spores are occluded per crystal. Paper spore strips were prepared each containing 10^3 of the occluded spores. Figure 8 shows the result of EO exposure under zero-order conditions. The free spores are readily killed, but the protected spores are not harmed even after 2 weeks exposure. Microbial contamination occluded in crystals cannot be sterilized by EO unless the crystal structure can be broken down by rehydration or by dissolving. The same calcium carbonate-occluded spores were resistant to thermal destruction in steam at 250°F. for over $2^1/_2$ hr., although these unoccluded spores would normally be killed in a fraction of a minute under the same conditions.

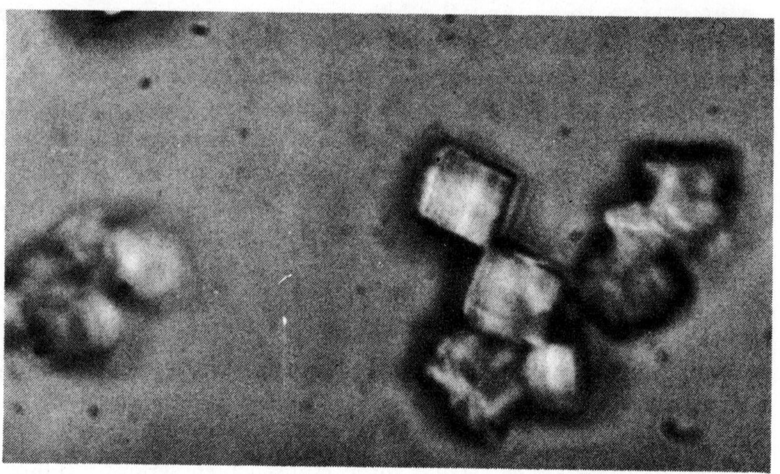

(*a*)

Fig. 7. Phase contrast photomicrographs of crystals and various stages of dissolution: (*a*) crystals prior to addition of 0.1*N* HCl. The unoccluded spores in the field are out of phase in order to get a sharp view of the crystals; (*b*) crystals in the process of dissolving, approximately 1 min. after addition of 0.1*N* HCl; (*c*) clumped spores that are left after the crystals are dissolved, approximately 5 min. after addition of 0.1*N* HCl.

Temperature Variations

To measure variations of temperature three iron–constantan thermocouples were positioned in an electrically heated rectangular sterilizer. These were placed $^1/_2$ in. from the metal floor and ceiling of the sterilizer: (*1*) at the front, center, bottom, near the door;

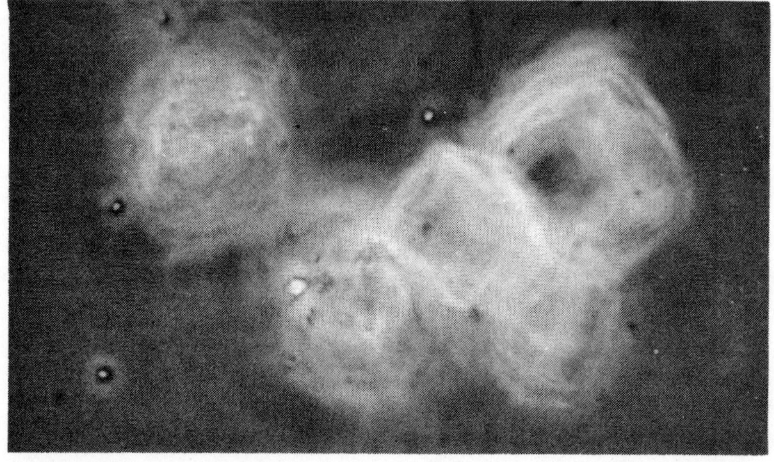

(*b*)

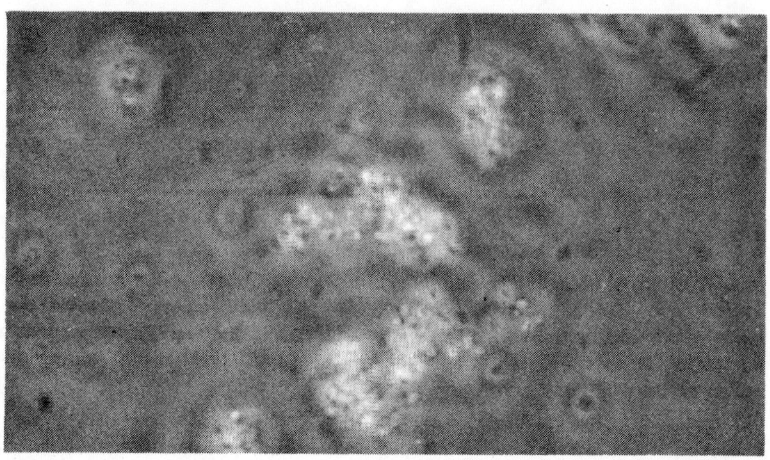

(*c*)

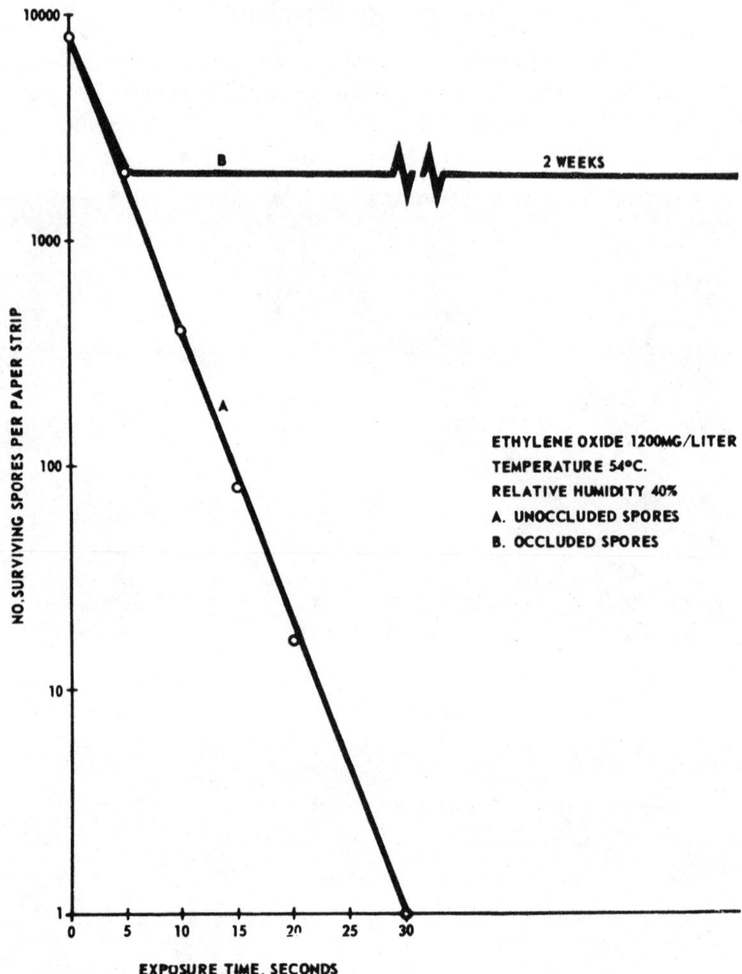

Fig. 8. Effect of occlusion of *Bacillus subtilis* var. *niger* spores on resistance to ethylene oxide (1200 mg./l. at 40% RH, 130°F.): (*A*) survivor curve based on the starting number and sterilization time of 8 × 10³ spores dried on chromatography grade paper; (*B*) spores occluded in crystals of calcium carbonate, suspension dried on chromatography grade paper.

(*2*) at the rear, bottom, near the back header; (*3*) at the rear, upper region, near the back header. The temperature was measured and recorded on a commercial potentiometric temperature recorder.

Figures 9–12 represent the temperature changes reflected by expansion, compression, environmental positional effects, and the influx of three cold sterilant mixtures in their liquid state to the heated chamber.

Figure 9 shows the temperature changes occurring upon the introduction of cold sterilant to the warm empty vessel. In this case 20% EO diluted in CO_2 vaporizes and absorbs heat from the sterilizer jacket. Thus, there is an initial rise in temperature at all points. Then a separation occurs where the top rear environment shows a decided elevation to a maximum peak, whereas the two bottom positions show a depression. The bottom rear temperature is severely depressed by about 65°F. In 4 min. the sterilizer has attained maximum pressure and no more sterilant is being admitted. As liquid-to-gas expansion occurred during initial influx of the sterilant, the effect of cooling the immediate piping and wall at the admission port allowed the ethylene oxide to separate out as a liquid leaving the cold CO_2 to compress the residual warm air upward. The warming up period which follows is due to heating of the revaporized EO. Temperature equilibrium is not attained for nearly 60 min. The normal gradient characteristic of the sterilizer is shown in the latter portion of the curve.

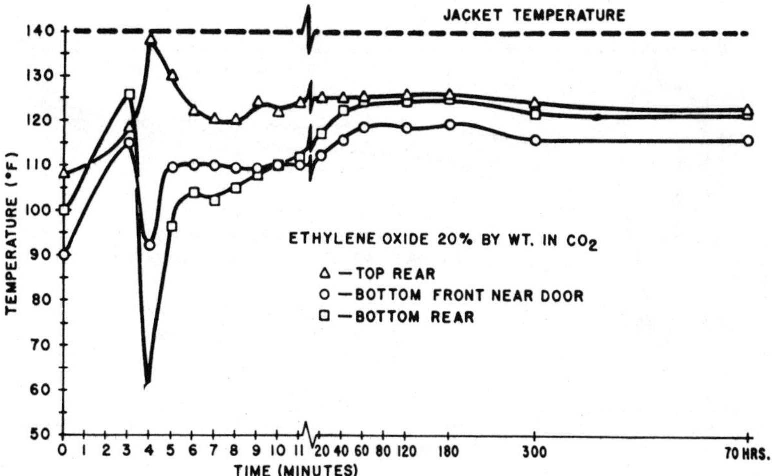

Fig. 9. Temperature changes upon introduction of unheated sterilant to a heated rectangular sterilizer.

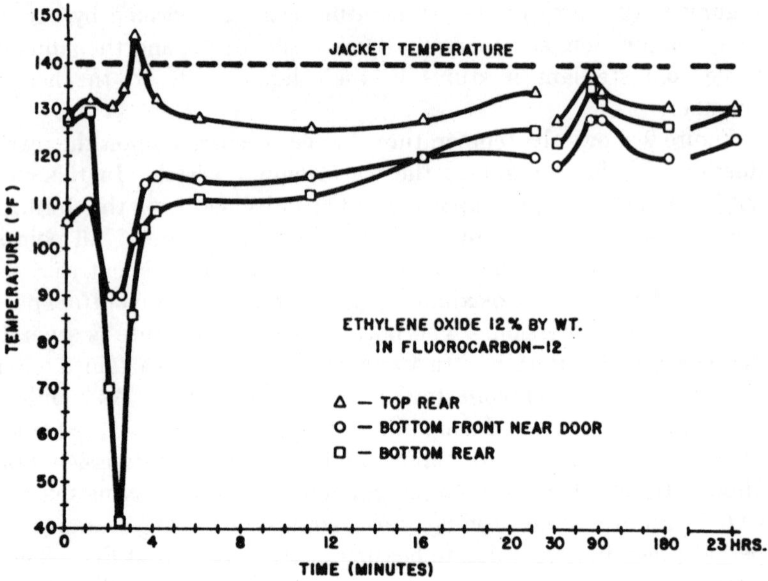

Fig. 10. Temperature changes upon introduction of unheated sterilant to a heated rectangular sterilizer.

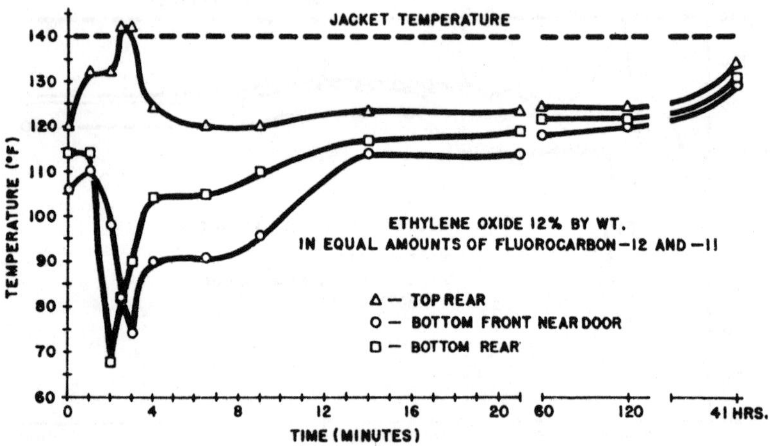

Fig. 11. Temperature changes upon introduction of unheated sterilant to a heated rectangular sterilizer.

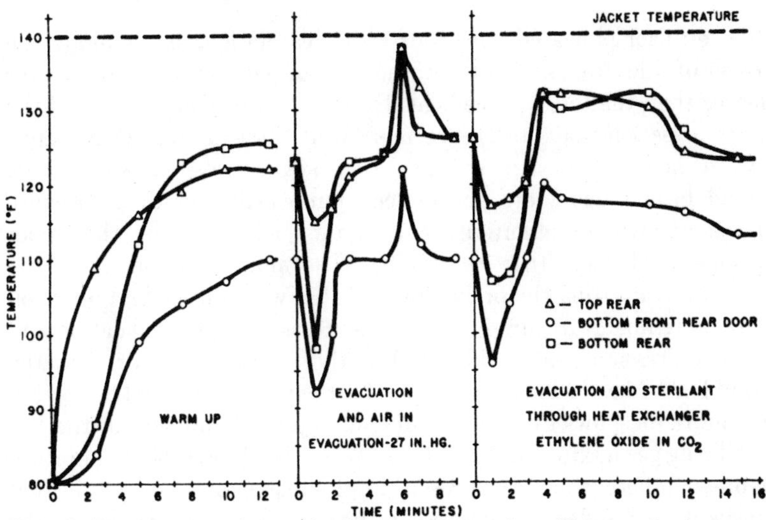

Fig. 12. Temperatures changes in different phases of sterilizing cycles in heated rectangular sterilizer.

In Figure 10 the temperature depression is much more severe for this EO mixture, which is 12% by weight or 27.3% by volume in fluorocarbon-12 (F-12). The temperature is depressed in this case 90°F.

Figure 11 of EO (12% by wt. or 28% by vol.) in equal amounts of fluorocarbon-11 and fluorocarbon-12 (F-11 and F-12) sterilant shows a temperature depression less than that reflected by the (F-12) mixture alone, but it is 65°F., similar to the CO_2 mixture. One principal difference is the much greater depression of the lower front temperature near the door, which was not nearly so great in the former cases.

Since (F-11) is a relatively high-boiling liquid, it tends to remain as a liquid and flow as such toward the front of the sterilizer, as it is influenced by the inflowing gas. The F-11 will tend to carry with it F-12 and EO dissolved in it. The revaporization is much slower compared to the other mixtures. This is reflected in the greater temperature difference and the much longer time for recovery.

Figure 12 shows temperature changes in different phases of sterilizing cycles in the electrically heated rectangular sterilizer. The section at the left shows warm-up at the three thermocouple positions. Characteristically, the coolest position is the bottom near the door which levels off about 15°F. cooler than the warmest position. Since this sterilizer is heated with four strip heaters lengthwise along the center of sides, top, and bottom, the bottom tends to heat to a greater degree than the top. Since heat dissipates more rapidly upward the bottom section tends to absorb more heat than the top which tends to lose heat to the atmosphere. In a steam-jacketed vessel there would be a much more pronounced temperature gradient because the steam will preferentially rise in the jacket heating the upper regions much more than the lower. The middle section shows the effect of evacuating the preheated chamber with subsequent addition of room temperature air. Note the depression due to evacuation and the compression peaks which follow the admission of air, and the rapid loss of heat which is absorbed by the metal walls. The section on the right shows evacuation and subsequent admission of the hot sterilizing gas mixture (EO in CO_2). Note the absence of temperature depression here which was present in previous figures when unheated sterilant was added. Compression peaks are not as intense as the air peaks in the other sections. This is probably due to a difference in the speed of gas admission.

Gas Concentration Changes, Stratification, and Gas Densities

Gas sampling points were incorporated within 1 in. of both the top and bottom near the back header of the same sterilizer. Prior to the admission of sterilant the vessel was evacuated to 27 in. Hg negative pressure.

The samples were analyzed by gas chromatography utilizing a Perkin Elmer #154 Vapor Fractometer. The CO_2–EO mixture was separated on a Teflon base $^1/_4$ in. × 2 m. column containing Carbowax 1500. F-11 and F-12 mixtures were separated on a di-2-ethyl hexyl sebacate on chromosorb column having the same dimensions.

Figures 13–15 portray the gas concentration changes in per cent on the ordinate at various time intervals after admission of the unheated sterilant to the heated rectangular sterilizer. Figure 13 shows the variations in per cent of components including air. The sterilant is 20% EO in CO_2. The EO concentration rose initially in the bottom samples whereas the CO_2 fell. Air was also initially low in the bottom sample, but initially fairly high at the top. The stratification here was not very severe and equilibration occurred within a relatively short period of time although temperature equilibrium required nearly 60 min. to attain. The test system was pressurized to only slightly above atmospheric pressure. Under these conditions 12–13% residual air is expected theoretically. This amount of air is very critical when it is stratified to a great degree as can be seen in Figure 14. Assuming the same degree of starting vacuum, the addition of sterilizing gas mixtures to higher total pressures will reduce the volume of residual air. However, the attempt to sterilize at sub-atmospheric pressures is extremely hazardous with respect to the amount of residual air volume. For example, having evacuated to 26 in. Hg, sterilizing with pure EO at 1000 mg./l. will leave approximately 23% by volume residual air. It has been found in practice that it is very difficult to mix gases dissimilar in weight and molecular energy (temperature).

Figure 14 shows the concentration changes in per cent of components by the unheated admission of liquid sterilant (EO—12% by weight, 27.3% by volume in F-12). Here is shown how extreme stratification can be. Initially all of the air was seen in the top samples at 40% by volume, and none was observed in the bottom samples. Late sampling of the bottom region does not adequately reflect the extreme effect of a high per cent and flammable range of

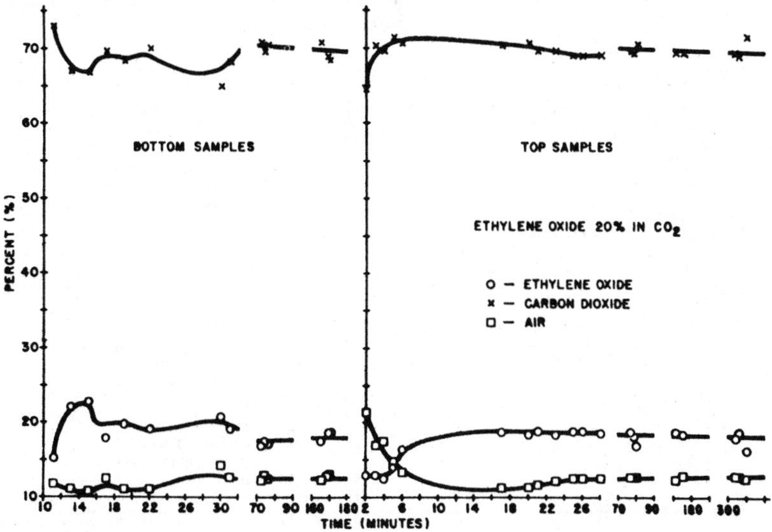

Fig. 13. Gas concentration changes after admission of cold sterilant to heated rectangular sterilizer.

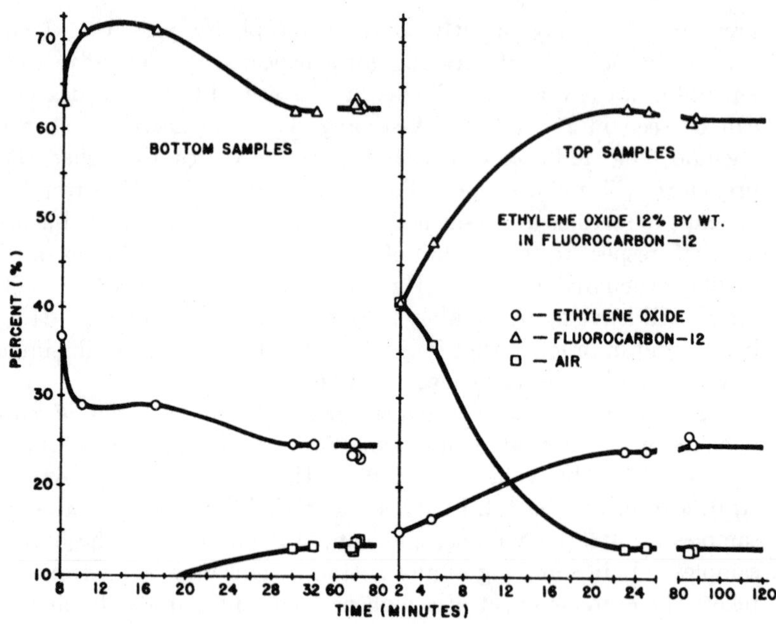

Fig. 14. Gas concentration changes after admission of cold sterilant to heated rectangular sterilizer.

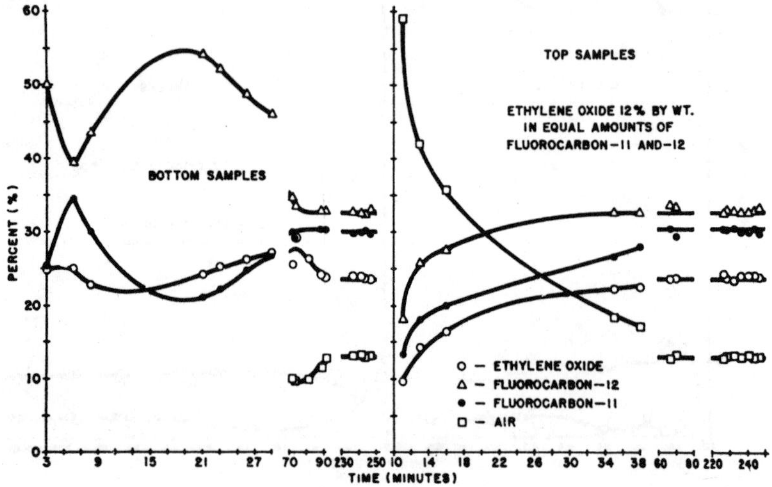

Fig. 15. Gas concentration changes after admission of cold sterilant to heated rectangular sterilizer.

ethylene oxide. This flammable range extends for nearly 30 min. to the equilibration point.

Figure 15 shows how concentration changes with the third sterilizing mixture (EO 12% by wt., 28% by vol. in equal amounts of F-11 and F-12). It was mentioned previously that high-boiling F-11 will remain liquid after sufficient cooling of pipe and walls occur by the vaporizing liquid. This component (F-11) will carry dissolved in it large amounts of EO and F-12. Thus, the cooling effect is extended for a longer time and covers a larger area, as was observed. A greater gas density gradient occurs, therefore, and stratification is much more severe. True equilibration does not occur until almost 1 hr. after admission of the sterilizing mixture. This mixture does not appear to initially pass through the flammable range since the EO tends to remain blanketed by the two inerting agents.

Figure 16 is a photograph of a plastic surgical isolator initially developed by Walter Reed Army Hospital, constructed by Curtiss-Wright Corporation, and is now being used in actual surgical procedures at Albert Einstein School of Medicine. Castle Laboratory developed the sterilization procedure for this unit. The isolator is

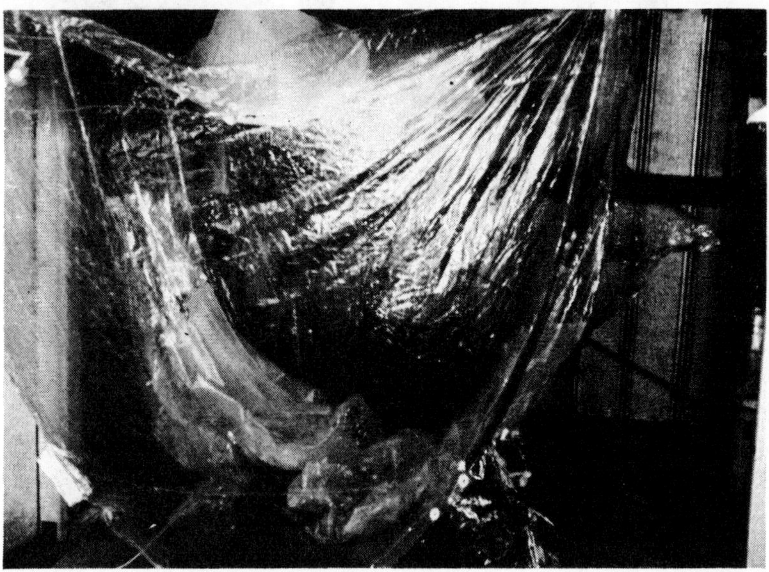

Fig. 16. Surgical isolator expanded with air.

hanging from a rack as it normally would after removal from its container expanded with filtered air.

Figure 17 is another photograph of the isolator. The isolator is not filled with water. It is the EO–F-12 mixture. A comparison of Figures 16 and 17 demonstrates the extreme differences in vapor density that would be expected comparing EO–F-12 mixture with an approximate vapor density of 4 with air. Thus, stratification is a

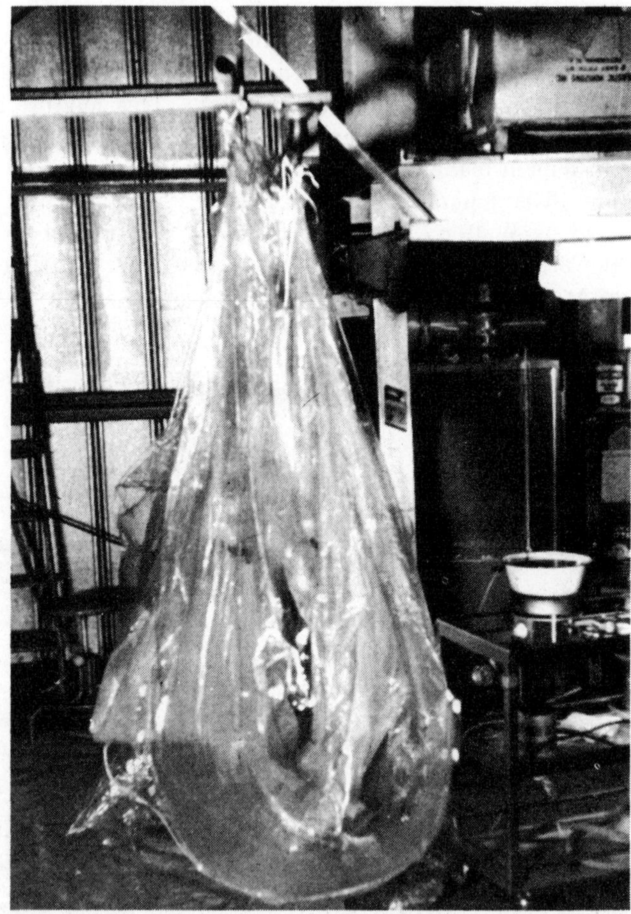

Fig. 17. Surgical isolator expanded with sterilant–ethylene oxide–fluorocarbon mixture.

serious hazard to be considered. Despite extreme vapor density differences gases will eventually diffuse into each other in a closed sterilizer. However, stratification is minimized when prevaporized preheated sterilizing mixtures are added to the chamber. Furthermore, stratification is not the only effect to be noted by the manner in which sterilants are added to chambers. Moisture and EO may not only be reduced in concentration, but nearly depleted if the sterilant is added as a cold liquid expanding to the gaseous state.

Coincident with the extreme temperature depression and slow recovery to equilibrium conditions by the unvaporized liquids, as the liquids are impelled into a warm sterilizer and they refrigerate its interior, moisture is condensed and frozen out on the cold surfaces produced.

Figure 18 shows a research program sterilizer. Various conditions of temperature, pressure, and gaseous atmospheres can be programmed and what is going on can be observed by the flow chart, recorders, and observation windows. In Figure 19 the cold influx of sterilizing mixture (in this case EO–F-12) is seen inside the sterilizer chamber. The vapor cloud is the result of the condensing water vapor initially present in the sterilizer being entrained by the inflowing sterilant gases. In the photograph taken at a later interval (Fig. 20), the

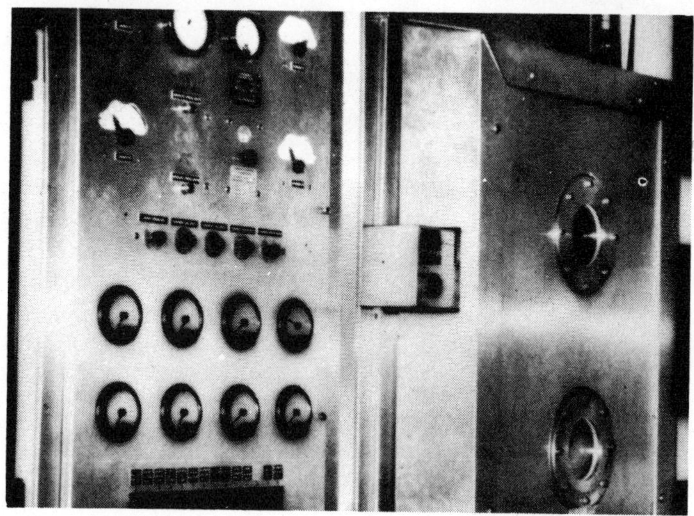

Fig. 18. Research program sterilizer (courtesy of Castle Company).

vapor cloud can no longer be seen, but some of the liquid components are decidedly running off at the point of entry. In Figure 21 a greater liquid run-off and pronounced icing is seen on the diffusion disk.

Expansion Tank Systems

Another pitfall is exemplified by the expansion tank system. These systems were originally designed for EO–CO_2 mixtures.

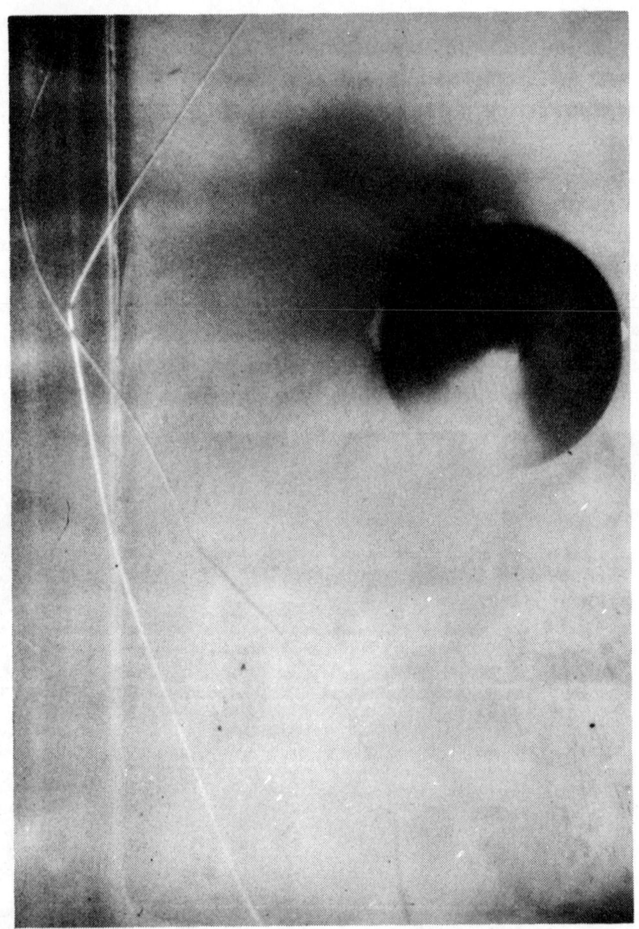

Fig. 19. Sterilant expanding gas influx to sterilized chamber.

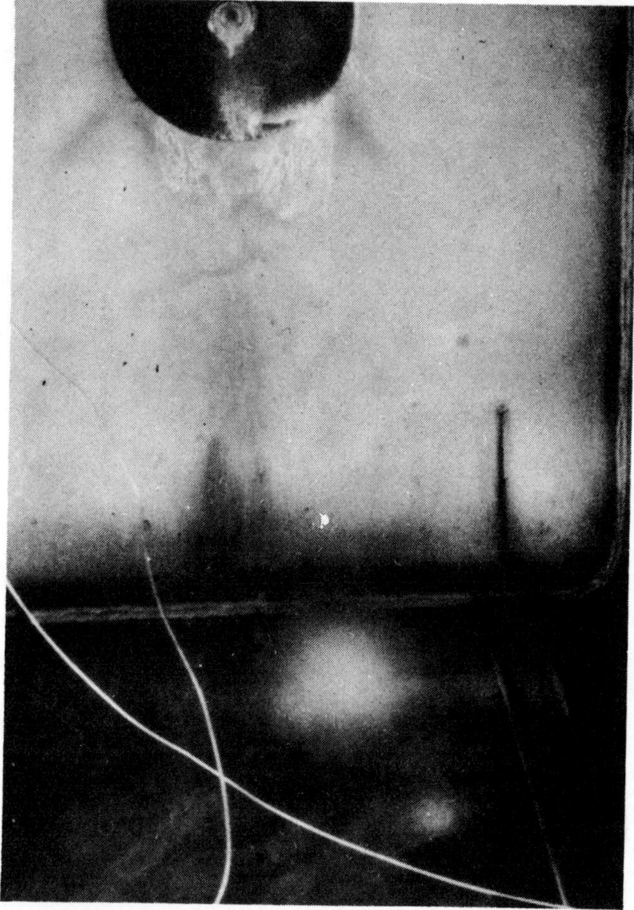

Fig. 20. Sterilant liquid running from entry diffusion plate.

Cylinders of this mixture are normally at pressures of about 800 psig. When the liquid contents of such cylinders are depleted, a residual fraction of almost pure CO_2 compressed gas remains weighing as much as 8 lb. and representing about 13% of the original contents. Furthermore, as the contents are used, there is a region of liquid emission which may pass through a flammable range. In order to obtain a more economical usage and to keep the concentration of EO constant, these cylinders were depleted into an expansion tank

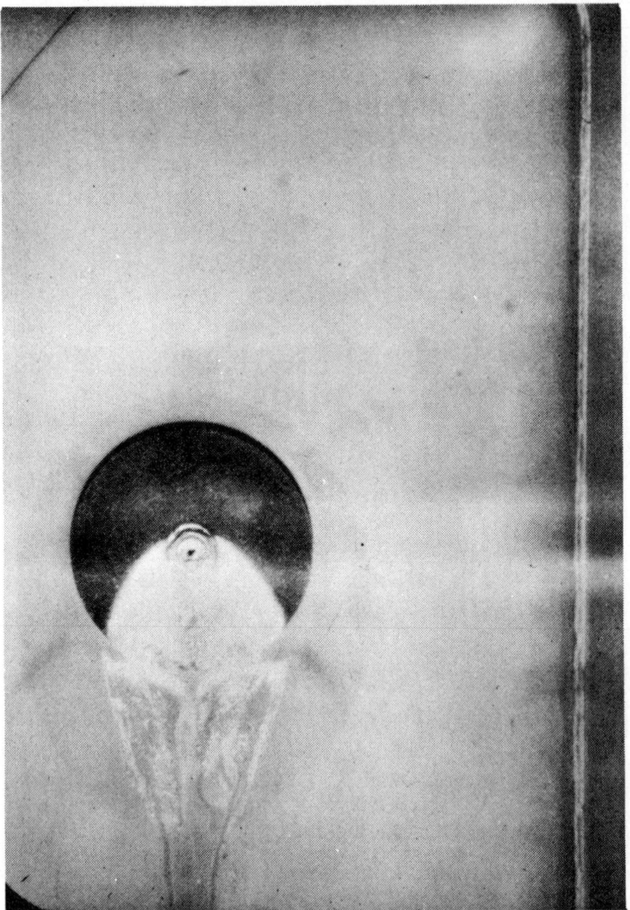

Fig. 21. Icing of diffusion plate due to cooling by sterilant expanding into chamber space.

which is shown in Figure 22. In the bottom section there are coils heated with steam. As the liquid is introduced into the expansion tank it is revaporized and kept in a gaseous state. One bad feature here is the tendency to create ideal conditions for rapid polymerization. As the sterilizer is fed gas from the expansion tank its internal pressure drops to a point where it demands more gas by means of a pressure-sensitive switch. Liquid sterilant enters the expansion tank from the cylinder attached to the gas-metering station to produce a situation similar to that observed when cold gas was introduced into a sterilizing chamber. The EO gas already in the tank condenses as the liquid introduced into the chamber expands, producing a cold region near the point of admission which was observed as a frosted area on the outside of the tank near the lower section. This indicated that pure liquid EO was flowing down the inside of the chamber, which collected at the bottom where it eventually revaporized. This characteristic is analogous to what was observed in the sterilizer with respect to the depletion of water vapor.

In a specific practical situation where an expansion tank supplied both a small and a large sterilizer the difference in volumes was a factor of 8. Gas chromatography samples taken at intervals under varying circumstances revealed a very disturbing situation. The expansion tank was unable to supply all the gas required by the large sterilizer. A drop in expansion tank pressure initiated the transfer of liquid sterilant from the supply cylinders to the expansion tank. Condensation of the EO took place as described in the previous paragraph. The tendency then under this dynamic condition would be to draw CO_2 from the tank preferentially.

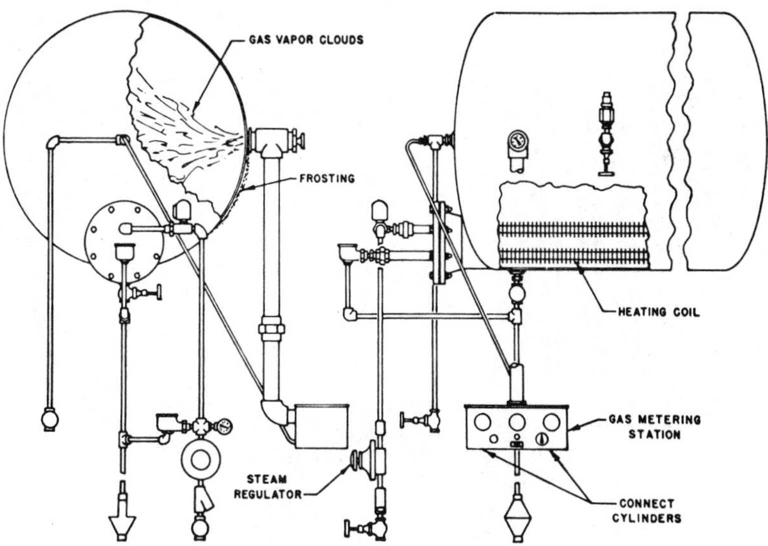

Fig. 22. Expansion tank and controls.

In this specific case it was found that the final EO concentration in the large sterilizer went as low as 3% by volume. On the other hand, as the expansion tank was allowed to acquire heat, the liquid EO revaporized in a CO_2-deficient atmosphere. If on a subsequent sterilization the small sterilizer was used, there was not sufficient volume in the small sterilizer to produce the foregoing result in the expansion tank. Samplings from this sterilizer showed concentrations of EO in excess of 45%. Thus, the very thing that was thought to be avoided was enhanced.

Hazardous flammable concentrations were built up, polymerization was maximized, and the operators were deluded. They did in fact use the small sterilizer to determine sterilizing conditions, and extrapolated these results for sterilization of large commercial loads going of course unknowingly from experimental concentrations of 45% or higher to applied 3% concentrations of EO.

Figure 23 shows a heat exchanger which if used knowledgeably will minimize the hazards discussed. It is a concentric tube within a tube helix. Steam enters at the top and flows through the outside tube down to a trap. EO enters at the bottom through the inner tube and out at the top to the sterilizer. Polymerization is minimized due to reduced retention time. Providing vaporization and heat to the gas prior to admission to the sterilizer maximizes mixing,

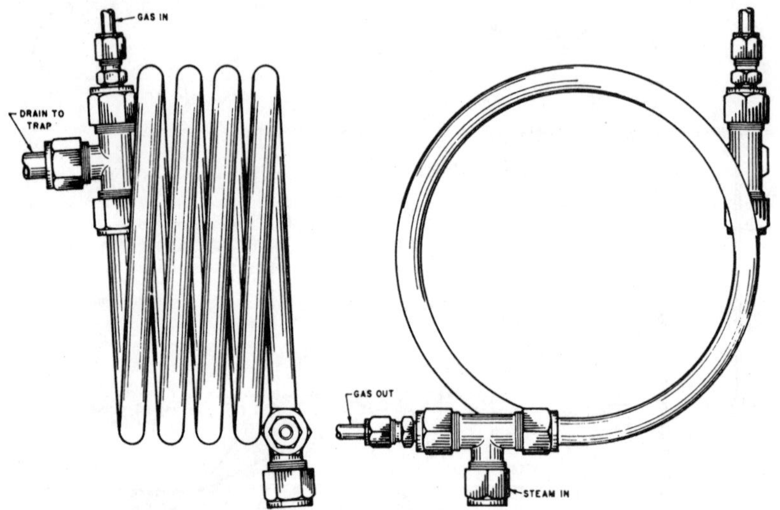

Fig. 23. Heat exchanger assembly.

heat transfer, and minimizes stratification. Stratification, temperature distribution, and diffusion problems become more severe as sterilizers increase in size.

Polymerization Effects

Polymerization can be a severe limitation of EO. According to Baize[13] it is initiated by steel, stainless steel, glass, lead, and zinc. There are many other polymerization catalysts such as anhydrous chloride of tin, iron, and aluminum, carbonate, acids and alkali. Polymerization rates increase under increased temperature, pressure, and in the presence of water vapor. Gas transmission lines can become clogged and valves may cease functioning by its accumulation, and it can cause severe damage to unprotected materials. The exercise of intelligent caution and care will alleviate this hazard. EO polymerization is noted in many forms: (*1*) as a white powder (Fig. 24) where water has a tendency to accumulate by condensation, such as near the relatively cool door, (*2*) as a straw colored oily liquid which appears in the piping associated with steam under heat and pressure. The oily liquid eventually continues to polymerize to form the "chewing" gum solid shown in Figure 25. The

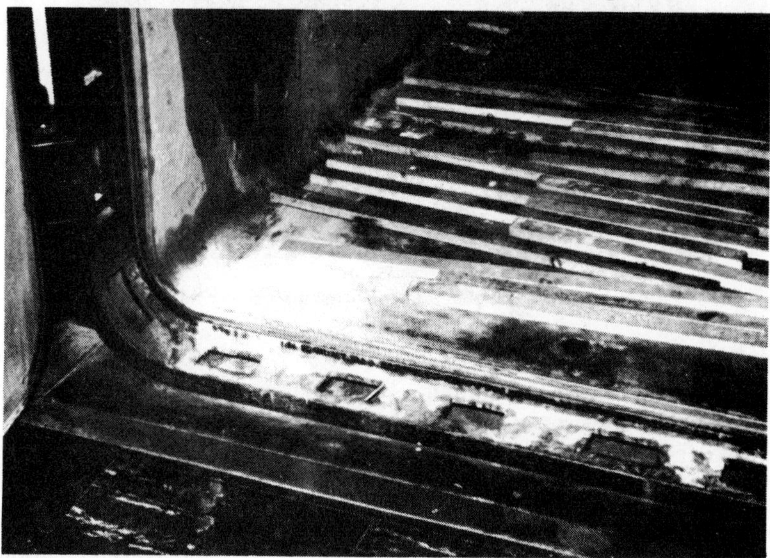

Fig. 24. White polymer formed from ethylene oxide in presence of condensate.

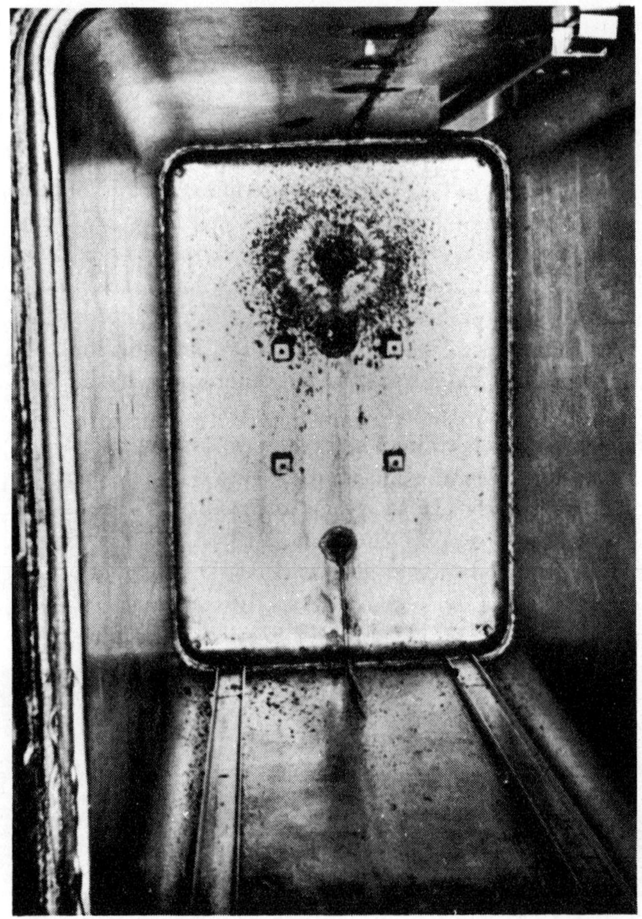

Fig. 25. Craters of polymer formed on sterilizer and shield.

polymer is usually water soluble. Good maintenance will keep accumulations to a minimum. Plastic covers on sterilizable items will adequately protect them from damaging polymers.

Conclusion

Basic parameters for ethylene oxide gaseous sterilization have been defined for the inactivation of bacterial spores. The overall reaction kinetics are first order; but with respect to concentration dependence, the reaction reverts to zero for higher treatment temperatures. For each treatment EO concentration there is a temperature conversion point above which increasing the concentration does not reduce the inactivation time.

Diffusion of moisture into the immediate environment of the contaminating microbe was implicated as the primary limiting factor of the gaseous sterilization process with ethylene oxide. A model system was proposed which would logically explain why an optimal relative humidity (RH) is indicated under certain conditions, whereas a high RH is generally required in practice. It is hypothesized that water molecules carry ethylene oxide to reactive sites. In practice either water or EO served to increase the permeation of the other through plastic films depending upon their polar or nonpolar character.

There are situations which can limit or enhance the dynamics of sterilization. Such factors, if overlooked, could upset experiments and lead to erroneous conclusions, or defeat the sterilization process entirely. Such are, namely: stratification effects, diffusion barriers, moisture-reducing effects, polymerization, and temperature distribution gradients.

References

1. R. R. Ernst and J. J. Shull, *Appl. Microbiol.*, **10**, 337 (1962).
2. C. R. Phillips, *Am. J. Hyg.*, **50**, 280 (1949).
3. H. M. El Bisi, R. M. Vondell, and W. B. Esselen, *Bacteriol. Proc., Am. Soc. Microbiol.*, 1963, p. 13.
4. J. B. Opfell, J. P. Hohman, and A. B. Latham, *J. Am. Pharm. Assoc.*, **48**, 617 (1959).
5. R. R. Ernst and J. J. Shull, *Appl. Microbiol.*, **10**, 342 (1962).
6. R. R. Ernst and J. E. Doyle. Paper presented at the 64th Annual Meeting of the American Society for Microbiology, 1964.
7. G. L. Gilbert, V. M. Gambill, D. R. Spiner, R. K. Hoffman, and C. R. Phillips, *Appl. Microbiol.*, **12**, 496 (1964).
8. C. R. Phillips, "The sterilizing properties of ethylene oxide," in *Sterilization of Surgical Materials*, Pharmaceutical Press, London, 1961, p. 59.
9. S. Kaye and C. R. Phillips, *Am. J. Hyg.*, **50**, 296 (1949).
10. J. J. Perkins and R. S. Lloyd, "Applications and equipment for ethylene oxide sterilization," in *Sterilization of Surgical Materials*, Pharmaceutical Press, London, 1961, p. 78.
11. G. Mayr, "Equipment for ethylene oxide sterilization," in *Sterilization of Surgical Materials*, Pharmaceutical Press, London, 1961, p. 90.
12. A. Royce and C. Bowler, *J. Pharm. Pharmacol.*, **13**, 87T (1961).
13. T. H. Baize, *Ind. Eng. Chem.*, **53**, 903 (1961).
14. R. R. Ernst, "Physical-chemical factors in gaseous sterilization with ethylene oxide," paper presented at American Chemical Society Meeting, *Abstracts*, 13Q (1964).

Received March 3, 1967

Reprinted from *Appl. Microbiol.* **16**, 1742–1744 (1968) *Printed in U.S.A.*

6

Limitations of Thioglycolate Broth as a Sterility Test Medium for Materials Exposed to Gaseous Ethylene Oxide[1]

JOHN E. DOYLE, WILLIAM H. MEHRHOF, AND ROBERT R. ERNST

Research Laboratory, Castle Company, Rochester, New York 14623

Received for publication 31 July 1968

Although ethylene oxide is a reliable sterilizer, the process may be limited by diffusion. Thus, situations may exist where microorganisms are protected from the sterilizing gas. It is possible that the exterior of a substance may be sterilized, whereas the interior is not. We investigated three general types of materials in which this limitation of diffusion could occur: the bore of glass and plastic tubing, the center of cotton balls, and plastic adhesive film/paper backing interface. These materials were contaminated as close to their geometric center as possible with *Bacillus subtilis* var. *niger* spores occluded in crystals of sodium chloride. After exposure of the contaminated materials (except aluminum foil) to ethylene oxide, thioglycolate broth (a standard sterility-test medium) indicated sterility, whereas Trypticase Soy Broth indicated nonsterility. It is likewise possible that aerobic microorganisms, surviving in or on material after exposure to dry heat or steam sterilization processes, would not be recovered by thioglycollate broth. Entrapped aerobic organisms will probably not grow out in the low oxygen tension zone of an anaerobic medium such as thioglycollate broth. It is recommended than an aerobic medium such as Trypticase Soy Broth be used concurrently with thioglycolate broth for sterility testing.

A significant contribution to microbiological control was made by Brewer (3) when he developed a liquid medium capable of supporting both aerobic and anaerobic growth. Many modifications have been made since then (10, 11). The final result was the thioglycolate broth now recommended as a standard sterility test medium by the United States Pharmacopeia, the National Formulary, the National Institutes of Health, and the Food and Drug Administration.

Ethylene oxide is a reliable sterilizing agent, but its action is extremely complex (6). The principal concomitant factors are moisture availability and diffusion, that is, the diffusion of ethylene oxide, moisture, and heat into the contaminated sites.

In addition, in situations where microorganisms are protected from the sterilizing process, such as occlusion in crystals (1, 4) or contact with protective agents (7), either may react with the moisture or the ethylene oxide, thus preventing inactivation.

[1] Presented at the 68th Annual Meeting of the American Society for Microbiology, Detroit, Mich., 5-10 May 1968.

This study was performed to determine whether viable aerobic microorganisms present in materials after exposure to ethylene oxide will grow out in thioglycolate broth.

MATERIALS AND METHODS

Organism. Bacillus subtilis var. *niger* 356 S.C. no. 4 N.R. Smith strain was used (12).

Culture methods. The culturing methods have been described previously (4).

Preparation of test materials. The following materials were investigated: aluminum foil (3.81 by 0.63 cm), aluminum foil (3.81 by 0.63 cm) rolled up in the center of cotton balls (Johnson & Johnson, New Brunswick, N.J.), Teflon tubing (0.083-cm outside diameter by 11.4 cm; Cadillac Plastic & Chemical Co., Detroit, Mich.), glass melting-point capillary tubing (0.8 to 1.2 mm, inside diameter, by 100 mm) Kimble no. 34502 (Will Scientific Inc., Rochester, N.Y.), and plastic surgical adhesive film (1.27 by 1.27 cm, Vi-Drape; Parke, Davis & Co., Detroit, Mich.).

Initially, the test materials were inoculated with *B. subtilis* var. *niger* spores in isotonic saline. Later, a similar suspension containing 1% hydroxyethylcellulose to bind the inoculum and salt crystals to the test materials was used.

The test materials were inoculated with 10^5 spores

per test material with one drop from a syringe and a 25-gauge needle (a reproducible 0.01-ml inoculum).

Glass and Teflon tubing were inoculated in the following manner. The droplet inoculum was placed on polyethylene film; then the tubing was placed over the drop so that the inoculum was drawn into the tubing by capillary action and into the center of the tubing by suction.

The plastic surgical adhesive film was inoculated as follows. The paper backing was removed, and the inoculum was placed on the adhesive side of the film. The paper backing was replaced after the inoculum dried. This provided protected organisms at the plastic film/paper backing interface.

All materials were dried at 55 C until visibly dry. Salt crystals always formed upon drying.

Ethylene oxide procedures. Procedures similar to those described by Ernst and Shull (8) were used. Ethylene oxide conditions were determined that would sterilize all portions of the materials except the protected area in the geometrical center. The spore count was repeatedly reduced from 10^5 to 10^3 per test piece, as ascertained by standard plate count procedures after 1 hr of exposure to 1,200 mg of ethylene oxide per liter at 40% relative humidity and 54 C. High resistance of spores inoculated from isotonic saline on aluminum foil was also obtained by Beeby and Whitehouse (2). Similar material contaminated with 10^5 *B. subtilis* var. *niger* spores in distilled water was inactivated under these conditions in 10 min; therefore, 1-hr exposure times were used throughout this study. In this way, nonsterile materials (10^3 spores per test piece) were obtained in approximately their geometric center.

Recovery methods. After exposure to the ethylene oxide process, half of the exposed samples were transferred to Thioglycollate Medium (BBL) and half to Trypticase Soy Broth (BBL) and incubated at 32 C for 14 days. At least 200 pieces of each test material were treated in this manner.

RESULTS

The initial test pieces were inoculated with *B. subtilis* var. *niger* spores dried from isotonic saline. Although there was a distinct difference in recovery from Thioglycollate Medium and Trypticase Soy Broth, there was a relatively high percentage of recovery in Thioglycollate Medium with the aluminum foil in the center of the cotton balls and with the glass capillary tubing (Table 1). The data are reported as percentage of recovery, derived from the number of pieces producing growth divided by the number of pieces tested.

Salt crystals containing occluded spores may have been dislodged from the inoculated surfaces during manipulation. Thus, protection from ethylene oxide sterilization could have been occasionally produced near or close to the exterior of the material, and internal contamination was not truly represented. Therefore, a suspension containing hydroxyethylcellulose was used to bind the inoculum to the test pieces.

TABLE 1. *Comparison of recovery of viable organisms after exposure to ethylene oxide*[a]

Test material[b]	Percentage of recovery	
	Trypticase soy broth	Thioglycolate broth
Aluminum foil	100	100
Aluminum foil in center of cotton balls	100	27
Teflon tubing	100	0
Glass capillary tubing	100	50
Plastic surgical adhesive film/paper backing	100	10

[a] After 1 hr of exposure to 1,200 mg of ethylene oxide per liter at 40% relative humidity and 54 C.

[b] Each test piece was contaminated with 10^5 *B. subtilis* var. *niger* spores in isotonic saline (reduced to 10^3 spores per test piece after ethylene oxide exposure).

TABLE 2. *Comparison of recovery of viable organisms after exposure to ethylene oxide*[a]

Test material[b]	Percentage of recovery	
	Trypticase soy broth	Thioglycolate broth
Aluminum foil only	100	100
Aluminum foil in center of cotton balls	100	0
Glass capillary tubing	100	0
Plastic surgical adhesive film/paper backing	100	10

[a] After 1 hr of exposure to 1,200 mg of ethylene oxide per liter at 40% relative humidity and 54 C.

[b] Each test piece was contaminated with 10^5 *B. subtilis* var. *niger* spores in isotonic saline and 1% hydroxyethylcellulose (reduced to 10^3 spores per test piece after ethylene oxide exposure).

Growth from these materials developed in the Trypticase Soy Broth but not in the Thioglycollate Medium (Table 2).

DISCUSSION

In these experiments, thioglycolate broth did not support growth of *B. subtilis* var. *niger* spores when entrapped or held, so that the organisms could not be released into an environment in which they will grow, i.e., containing high oxygen tension.

One of the principal functions of thioglycolate broth is to produce a low oxygen tension zone in which anaerobes will grow. However, strict aerobic organisms held in this zone probably will not grow. It is possible that aerobic organisms that are least accessible to an ethylene oxide process will not grow when cultured in thioglycolate broth. Many disposable materials processed with ethylene oxide are composed of absorbent materials, such as cotton, plastic tubing materials, and plastic film/paper interface materials.

It is possible that materials exposed to dry heat or steam-sterilizing conditions may fail to show growth when cultured into thioglycolate broth. For example, there are limitations of time, heat transfer, and in the case of steam, air pockets, superheat, etc., that can exist in material resulting in nonsterility in the center (5).

Koesterer (9) reported that Trypticase glucose yeast extract broth (an aerobic medium) gave better recovery than thioglycolate broth from soil exposed to dry heat. Perhaps the surviving organisms were heat-fixed to the particles of soil and unable to grow in the low oxygen tension zone of thioglycolate broth.

It is recommended that an aerobic medium, such as Trypticase Soy Broth, be used concurrently with thioglycolate broth in sterility testing.

LITERATURE CITED

1. Abbott, C. R., J. Cockton, and W. Jones. 1956. Resistance of crystalline substances to gas sterilization. J. Pharm. Pharmacol. **6**:709–721.
2. Beeby, M. M., and C. E. Whitehouse. 1965. A bacterial spore test piece for the control of ethylene oxide sterilization. J. Appl. Bacteriol. **28**:349–360.
3. Brewer, J. H. 1940. Clear liquid mediums for the "aerobic" cultivation for anaerobes. J. Am. Med. Assoc. **115**:598–600.
4. Doyle, J. E., and R. E. Ernst. 1967. Resistance of *Bacillus subtilis* var. *niger* spores occluded in water-insoluble crystals to three sterilization agents. Appl. Microbiol. **15**:726–730.
5. Ernst, R. R. 1968. Sterilization by heat, p. 703–740. *In* C. A. Lawrence and S. S. Block (ed.) Disinfection, sterilization, and preservation. 1st ed. Lea & Febiger, Philadelphia.
6. Ernst, R. R., and J. E. Doyle. 1968. Sterilization with ethylene oxide: a review of chemical and physical factors. Biotech. Bioeng. **10**:1–31.
7. Ernst, R. R., and J. E. Doyle. 1968. Limiting factors in ethylene oxide gaseous sterilization. Develop. Ind. Microbiol. **9**:293–296.
8. Ernst, R. R., and J. J. Shull. 1962. Ethylene oxide gaseous sterilization. I. Concentration and temperature effects. Appl. Microbiol. **10**:337–341.
9. Koesterer, M. G. 1964. Thermal death studies on microbial spores and some considerations for the sterilization of spacecraft components. Dev. Ind. Microbiol. **6**:268–276.
10. Linden, B. A. 1941. Fluid thioglycollate medium for the sterility test. Natl. Inst. Health Bull. Bethesda, Md.
11. Pittman, M. 1946. A study of fluid thioglycollate medium for the sterility test. J. Bacteriol. **51**:19–32.
12. Smith, N. R., R. E. Gordon, and F. E. Clark. 1952. Aerobic spore forming bacteria. U.S. Dept. Agr. Monograph No. 16.

Editor's Comments on Papers 7 through 10

7 **Sykes:** *The Sporicidal Properties of Chemical Disinfectants*

8 **Portner and Hoffman:** *Sporicidal Effect of Peracetic Acid Vapor*

9 **Trujillo and David:** *Sporostatic and Sporicidal Properties of Aqueous Formaldehyde*

10 **Stonehill, Krop, and Borick:** *Buffered Glutaraldehyde: A New Chemical Sterilizing Solution*

These four papers show the sporostatic and sporicidal properties of individual chemical agents generally accepted as chemical sterilizers. These articles were selected from a wide list of publications; it was felt that sufficient information and references could be gleaned from them to satisfy the needs of scientists seeking information in this area. As an example, the paper by Stonehill, Krop, and Borick was the first to be published that showed the biological and chemical properties of aqueous, alkaline glutaraldehyde; but at last count over forty papers presenting the scientific aspects of glutaraldehyde had been published.

Reprinted from *J. Appl. Bacteriol.* **33**, 147–156 (1970)

7

(Symposium on Bacterial Spores: Paper XII)

The Sporicidal Properties of Chemical Disinfectants

G. Sykes

Microbiology Laboratory, Boots Pure Drug Co. Ltd., Nottingham, England

Contents

1. Introduction

Almost without exception any study of disinfection includes a statement to the effect that bacterial spores 'are difficult to kill' or 'are much more resistant than are vegetative cells', or that 'disinfectants are ineffective or unreliable in their action against bacterial spores'. And often it is added that 'the reason for the high resistance is unknown'. These statements are broadly true for many of the commoner disinfectants and antiseptics, but there are important exceptions and these are of practical significance in controlling the level of microbial contamination in situations where other methods, e.g. heat, cannot be used. These exceptions, being sporicidal agents, come within the definition of sterilizing agents, but with the exception of those used in the gaseous or vapour state (see below), they are used only very rarely for this purpose because of the obvious difficulty of removing them at the end of the treatment.

In this contribution I shall consider the sporicidal properties of a number of the better known substances and preparations, together with some of the factors influencing their activities, and finally discuss the nature of spore resistance.

2. Experimental Methods

(a) *Organisms*

In the experiments to be described 4 aerobic sporeforming bacilli were variously used. They were *Bacillus stearothermophilus* (the strain used for checking the efficacy of steam sterilization), *B. subtilis* var. *niger* (the strain used for checking the efficacy of ethylene oxide sterilization), *B. pumilus* NCIB 8982 and *B. subtilis* (an unidentified laboratory strain): no anaerobe was included. Each culture was grown on nutrient agar at the appropriate temperature and for a suitable time until nearly all of the cells had become phase bright spores. The growths were then harvested in ¼ strength Ringer's solution, washed 3 times and finally suspended in 15% glycerol in water (to prevent germination) and stored at 4°: each suspension contained 10^7–10^8 cells/ml.

(b) *Test methods*

Disinfection tests were made, generally at ambient temperature, by inoculating 0·1 ml of the spore suspension into 5 ml of the chosen disinfectant dilution in water and determining the number of surviving viable spores at appropriate intervals by either (a) filtering 1 ml of the mixture through a membrane, washing the membrane through with ¼ strength Ringer's solution (with an inactivating agent added where necessary) and then resuspending the washed cells and determining the viable count by the drop-plate method, or (b) by sampling 1 ml of the mixture, preparing from it decimal dilutions in ¼ strength Ringer's solution (with an inactivating agent added when necessary) and again determining the viable count by the drop-plate method. No attempt was made to assess the influence of added organic matter.

Preliminary experiments showed that heat activation at 70° for 10 min before treatment with a disinfectant did not affect the resistances of the cells to the disinfectant and that heat activation after the treatment did not affect the ultimate recoveries of viable cells. In the main experiments, therefore, no heat activation was used.

(c) *Heat resistances of cultures*

As a matter of interest, but not as a major part of the investigations, the heat resistances of some of the spore preparations were determined. To do this, the spores were washed free from glycerol, suspended in ¼ strength Ringer's solution and distributed in 2 ml amounts into all-glass ampoules. The ampoules were immersed in a water bath at the selected temperature and after different time intervals one was withdrawn to determine the number of survivors.

The most sensitive culture was the unnamed strain of *B. subtilis* which survived 80° for 4 h without any loss in viability but suffered a 10^7 reduction in count after 2 h at 95° and was totally inactivated after a few min at 100°. In contrast, *B. stearothermophilus* showed only a 30% reduction in count after 2 h at 95° and 50% reduction after 2 h at 100°.

3. Sporicidal Activities of Disinfectants

Of the wide range of antibacterial agents more readily available only a few can be regarded as reliably sporicidal. They are the chlorine releasing compounds, iodine, formaldehyde, ethylene oxide, glutaraldehyde and acid alcohol. And to these may be added, although less frequently encountered, the strong mineral acids, β-propiolactone, propylene oxide and other heterocyclic, 3-membered ring compounds, and acrolein. Most of these compounds are used in aqueous solution, but ethylene oxide, propylene oxide and β-propiolactone are used entirely in the gaseous or vapour state and formaldehyde in both. Each compound or formulation has its own conditions in terms of pH value, solvent, humidity, etc., for optimum activity, and each is affected to a greater or less extent by organic soiling materials.

It is axiomatic that the concentration of a disinfectant is important in determining its activity, but there is no fixed value relating the concentrations of different compounds and formulations with their rate of kill. Each has its own dilution coefficient, or concentration exponent, and there is no theoretical basis from which to calculate this value: it can only be determined experimentally.

Temperature can also have a profound effect on the lethal activity of a disinfectant and on its rate of kill. Some examples are given in a later section, but one of particular interest is the heat + bactericide process of the British Pharmacopoeia used for sterilizing certain solutions for injection. In this, the solution is heated for 1 h at 80° in the presence of a bactericide such as chlorocresol or phenylmercuric nitrate. Such compounds, at the concentrations employed, are only mildly bactericidal at room temperature but at the elevated temperatures can kill moderate numbers of resistant bacterial spores within the time specified.

(a) *The chlorine releasing compounds*

This group of compounds includes the inorganic hypochlorites, the organic chloramine compounds, the chlorinated isocyanuric acids (e.g. ACL59) and dichlorodimethylhydantoin. The activities of all these are influenced considerably by pH value, although the isocyanuric acids are very much less affected in this respect than are the other compounds. According to Ortenzio & Stuart (1959), the chlorinated isocyanuric acids differ only slightly in their activities over the pH range 6–10, but the chloramines and dichlorodimethylhydantoin can vary as much as 500–1000-fold over the same pH range. Somewhat lower figures were quoted for sodium hypochlorite by Tilley & Chapin (1930) who found that 2 p/m of available chlorine at pH 4 had the same activity against anthrax spores as had 100 parts at pH 10, and by Brazis *et al.* (1958) who found 1·9 p/m at pH 6·2 to be equivalent to 450 p/m at 10·5 in killing the spores of *B. subtilis* var.

TABLE 1

Sporicidal activities of chlorine releasing compounds against B. subtilis *var.* niger

Available Cl_2 (p/m)	pH value	Sporicidal activity of		
		Hypochlorite	Chloramine-T	ACL 59
100	'Natural'*	10^4 kill in 1 h	No kill in 24 h	10^4 kill in 30 min
	Buffered (pH 7·0)	10^4 kill in 5 min	10^1 kill in 24 h	10^4 kill in 1 h
1000	'Natural'*	10^4 kill in 10 min	10^2 kill in 24 h	10^5 kill in 5 min
	Buffered (pH 7·0)	10^5 kill in 30 sec	10^5 kill in 24 h	10^5 kill in 5 min

The original inoculum was *c.* 4 × 10^5 spores/ml of solution.
* 'Natural' pH values of the solutions: hypochlorite, 9–10; chloramine-T, *c.* 8; ACL 59, 6–6·5.

niger and *B. anthracis*, the lethal time in both instances being 90 min. The apparent equiresistances of the two spore cultures is coincidental.

Another factor determining the sporicidal activities of these compounds is the speed with which the chlorine is released. Because of this, solutions of the different compounds, even though having the same total available chlorine, can differ markedly in their speed of kill. Thus, in a typical experiment (Table 1) chloramine-T, even at 1000 p/m of available chlorine was relatively inactive against the spores of *B. subtilis* var. *niger* whereas ACL 59 and sodium hypochlorite were rapidly lethal. ACL 59 was the more effective at its 'natural', unbuffered pH value of 6–6·5 (against hypochlorite with a value of 9–10), but significantly less rapidly active in solutions buffered to pH 7.

(b) *Iodine*

Iodine can be used in aqueous solution (with potassium iodide as the solubilizing agent), in alcoholic solution or as an iodophor. The last is not a compound of iodine, but a mixture of iodine with a surface active agent which acts as the carrier and as the solubilizer for the iodine; the iodine is released slowly from the mixture and is active whilst the solution remains coloured. In a manner similar to that of the chlorine releasing compounds, the activity of an iodine solution depends on the vehicle in which it is dissolved and, therefore, presumably on its availability, or accessibility, to the site of action within the spore. To illustrate this 1% solutions of iodine in water and in alcohol were compared for their sporicidal activity with a commercially available iodophor, Betadine, which also contains 1% of available iodine using two different spore suspensions (Fig. 1). The slopes of the curves obtained, especially with the more

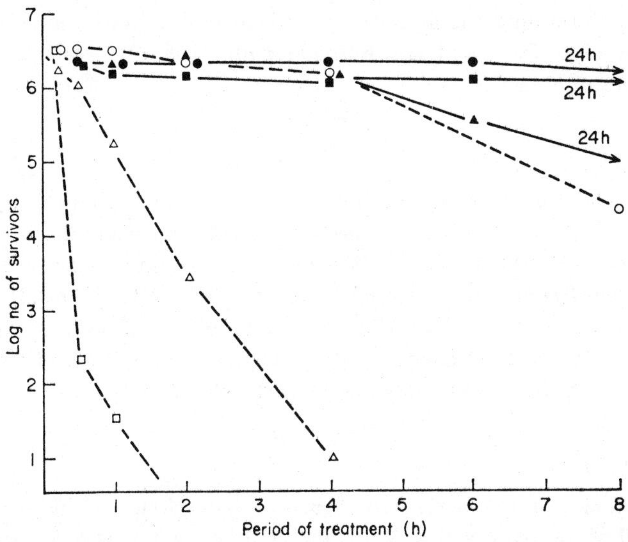

Fig. 1. Sporicidal activities of iodine solutions against *B. subtilis* and *B. pumilus*. Open symbols, *B. subtilis* spores; closed symbols, *B. pumilus* spores; circles, alcoholic iodine, 1%; triangles, aqueous iodine, 1%; squares, Betadine, 1% av. iodine.

sensitive *B. subtilis* spores, show clearly the much more rapid action of an aqueous solution over an alcoholic one and the even greater activity of the iodophor. Against the more resistent spores of *B. pumilus*, the latter difference was not maintained, but here the spores exhibited a much greater overall level of resistance than did those of the *B. subtilis* culture.

(c) *Gaseous sporicidal agents*

Brief reference must be made to the sporicidal activities of the gaseous sterilizing agents, in particular, formaldehyde, ethylene oxide and β-propiolactone.

(i) *Formaldehyde*

Formaldehyde in its gaseous state has long been known as an effective bactericidal agent. Its activities were described in detail by Nordgren (1939) and many of the points were subsequently confirmed in an investigation by the Public Health Laboratory Service Committee on Formaldehyde Disinfection (*Report*, 1958). In this Report attention was drawn to the finding that bacterial spores are only a little more resistant than are vegetative cells to formaldehyde vapour, and a factor of 2 or 3 was quoted from a limited number of experiments. This confirms the earlier findings of Phillips (1952) who stated that although bacterial spores are usually 'hundreds or thousands of times more resistant to chemical disinfectant than are vegetative bacteria' the differences with formaldehyde and other alkylating agents are much smaller, and he gave ratios for formaldehyde of 2–15 and for ethylene oxide of 2–6. Relative humidity is important in determining the activity of formaldehyde: Nordgren (1939) quoted a minimum RH of *c.* 50% and the Formaldehyde Committee (*Report*, 1958) gave optimum values of 80–90%.

(ii) *Ethylene oxide*

Ethylene oxide is used extensively for sterilizing apparatus and equipment which cannot be sterilized by heat; it is also used for sterilizing certain drugs which are not affected adversely by the action of ethylene oxide. Again, the activity of ethylene oxide is influenced considerably by RH: below *c.* 30% RH the activity falls away considerably and the optimum value ranges between 30 and 90%, depending on the physical state of the organism being treated. The various methods of treatment have already been described in some detail (see Sykes, 1965).

(iii) *β-Propiolactone*

This compound is said to be much more active than ethylene oxide as a bactericidal and sporicidal agent (Hoffman & Warshowski, 1958) but it is not used extensively because of its allegedly carcinogenic and other physiologically undesirable properties (Wiseley & Falk, 1960; Searle, 1961). Maximum activity occurs at RH *c.* 80% and at this level a concentration of 1·5 mg/l of air will kill 99% of a spore population dried on cloth in a few minutes.

(d) *Other compounds and preparations*

Although the commoner types of disinfectant and antiseptic can rightly be claimed to be effective against the nonsporing bacteria when used under the right conditions, with a few exceptions they are notoriously lacking in sporicidal activity. This lack of activity, even at relatively high concentrations, contrasts remarkably with the much lower concentrations effective in relatively short time, often measured in minutes, against the nonsporing bacteria (Table 2).

TABLE 2

Activities of various disinfectants against sporing and nonsporing bacteria

Disinfectant (and conc. tested)	Organism*	Sporicidal activity	Recommended normal use dilution
Phenol (5 %)	ST	< 50 % kill in 15 days	1–5 %
	SN	97 % kill in 15 days	
White coal tar disinfectant (5 %)	ST	60 % kill in 5 days	1 %
	SN	93 % kill in 4 days	
A chloroxylenol preparation (undiluted)	SN	75 % kill in 6 days	Up to 5 %
Tego 103G (1 %)	SN	10^4 kill in 7 days	1 %
(2 %)	SN	10^2 kill in 24 h	
Benzalkonium chloride (1 %)	SN	No kill in 4 days	Up to 0·1 %
Domiphen bromide (1 %)	P	70 % kill in 24 h	Up to 0·05 %
Chlorhexidine digluconate (2 %)	ST	No kill in 5 days	Up to 0·05 %
	SN	96 % kill in 6 days	
Amyl-*m*-cresol (10 % in 70 % alcohol)	SN	80 % kill in 4 days	Up to 0·01 %
Glutaraldehyde (2 %)	SN	10^6 kill in 1 h	2 %, only as a sporicide
Hydrochloric acid (1 % in 70 % alcohol)	ST	10^6 kill in 5 h	Only as a sporicide
	SN	10^4 kill in 4 h	

* ST, *B. stearothermophilus*; SN, *B. subtilis* var. *niger*; P, *B. pumilus* spores.

The white coal tar disinfectant quoted, a so called high coefficient fluid having a Rideal-Walker value of 20–22 and a Chick-Martin value of *c.* 4, is typical of this group of disinfectants. Similarly the chloroxylenol preparation is typical of this group of antiseptic preparations now on the market. The Tego range of products, recommended for use in dairying, brewing and in animal houses, are formulated with ampholytic surface active agents, usually high molecular weight amino acids, as their active agents. Benzalkonium chloride and domiphen bromide are typical of the quaternary ammonium group of compounds and chlorhexidine digluconate is a well known skin disinfectant. Amyl-*m*-cresol, first described by Coulthard (1931), is used in a variety of antiseptic preparations.

In contrast to the inefficacy of the compounds just mentioned, glutaraldehyde is outstanding. It is necessary to use it in an alkaline solution with the addition of 1 % of sodium carbonate in order to obtain maximum activity, and a commercial preparation of this type is available. It is used extensively in hospitals and in other situations, and its antibacterial properties have been described in detail by Rubbo, Gardner & Webb (1967) and reviewed by Borick (1968).

Perhaps insufficient attention has been given to the value of acid alcohol as a sporicidal and sterilizing agent. This property of relatively low concentrations of the mineral acids, and to a less extent of Na and K hydroxides, in alcohol to kill the most resistant bacterial spores was first discovered by Coulthard & Sykes (1936). It is an interesting property because neither the acids at the concentrations employed nor the alcohol have any sporicidal activity, but the mixture is relatively rapid in its action. Hydrochloric acid alone, for example, must be used at a concentration of 2·5 N, i.e. *c.* 9% in water, to be effective within 1 h (Borick, 1968), whereas in 70% alcohol a 1% solution is lethal within 4 h.

This high resistance to the individual components and the complementary sensitivity to the mixture gives some indication of the complexity of the structure of the bacterial spore as a whole.

(e) *Effect of temperature*

Temperature has a considerable influence on the rate of kill of micro-organisms, including bacterial spores, by all types of bactericidal agents. The change in rate of kill is not uniform for every compound, each having its own temperature coefficient. To illustrate this the spores of *B. pumilus* were subjected to treatment by 4 different preparations: Betadine, Chloramine-T, Tego 103G and domiphen bromide. Treatments were at 3 temperatures, 25, 37 and 50°, and the differences in type of response (Figs 2 and 3) are significant. With Tego and Betadine there was a marked increase in activity at 37° compared with that at 25° and an even greater increase at 50° (with Betadine it was almost dramatic), and there was no delay in the initiation of the killing process. In contrast, Chloramine-T and domiphen bromide showed no change in activity at 37° compared with 25°, the rate of kill at both temperatures being almost negligible. After

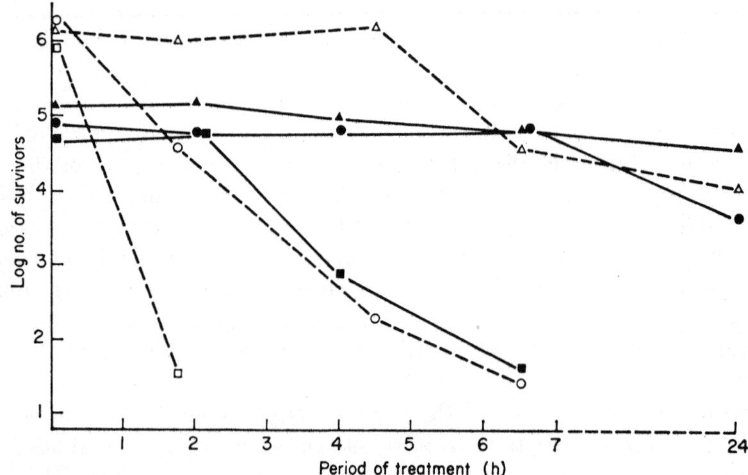

Fig. 2. Effect of Tego 2% (w/v) and domiphen bromide 1% (w/v) on *B. pumilus* at 25°, 27° and 50°.

Closed symbols, domiphen bromide treated spores; open symbols, Tego treated spores. Triangles, at 25°; circles, at 37°; squares, at 50°.

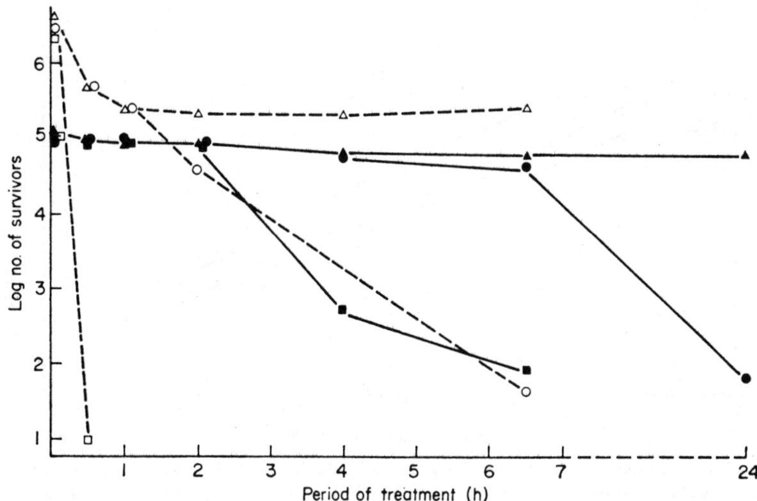

Fig. 3. Effect of Betadine (1% available I_2) and chloramine-T (2000 p/m av. Cl_2) on *B. pumilus* spores at 25°, 37° and 50°. Closed symbols, chloramine-T treated spores; open symbols, Betadine treated spores. Triangles, at 25°; circles, at 37°; squares, at 50°.

a few hours, however, the spores at 37° became more susceptible and a measurable rate of kill was established. When the temperature was raised to 50° there was still a delay in the initiation of the lethal action, but it was limited to *c.* 2 h, after which there was a substantial rate of kill such that after $6\frac{1}{2}$ h the survivor level was only *c.* 10^{-4} of the original.

The results with these 4 preparations (chosen fortuitously) indicate at least 2 pathways of attack on the viability of a spore. With Betadine and Tego the attack would appear to be direct and without a lag, thus indicating an immediate penetration to the sensitive areas of the cell. With Chloramine-T and domiphen the lag period before any sensible kill takes place suggests a prereaction or re-orientation within the cell coat before penetration takes place to the sensitive nuclei.

4. Germination and Sensitivity

There are numerous references in the literature (see Halvorson, Vary & Steinberg, 1966) to the physiological and other changes which take place in the spore at the point of germination. These changes include losses in the dipicolinic acid and calcium contents of the cell, loss of heat resistance, increased permeability to dyes and loss of refractility and optical density. To these can also be added a loss in resistance to chemical disinfectants.

To illustrate: washed spores of *B. pumilus* were suspended in a Trypticase-soya broth to induce germination. At intervals up to 1 h samples were removed and immediately examined under the phase contrast microscope to assess the proportion of phase bright cells present. This determination was made by two operators and the mean approximate percentage was recorded. Simultaneously, the resistance of the suspension to 70% alcohol and to 5% phenol solution was determined, the disinfecting period in

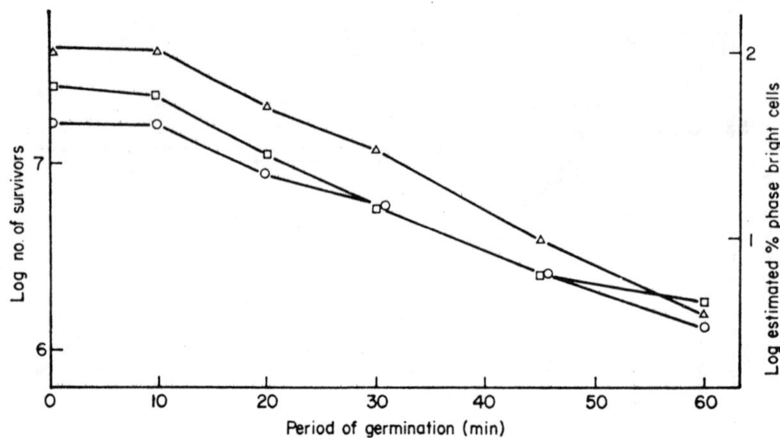

Fig. 4. Phase appearance and resistance to 70% alcohol and 5% phenol of germinating *B. pumilus* spores. Squares, phenol treated cells; circles, alcohol treated cells; triangles, phase bright cells.

each instance being 15 min. The results (Fig. 4) showed a very close relationship between the resistance of the culture and the percentage of phase bright cells present.

5. The Nature of the Resistance of Spores

Other papers in this symposium have described the complexity of the bacterial spore and the intracellular changes which take place during sporogenesis and during germination. Even so, the nature of spore resistance and the mechanism of such resistance is still an enigma. It seems most probable, however, that any germination or lethal process takes place within the endospore and not at the cortical surface, although the latter is not entirely ruled out. On this assumption, therefore, it is essential that any

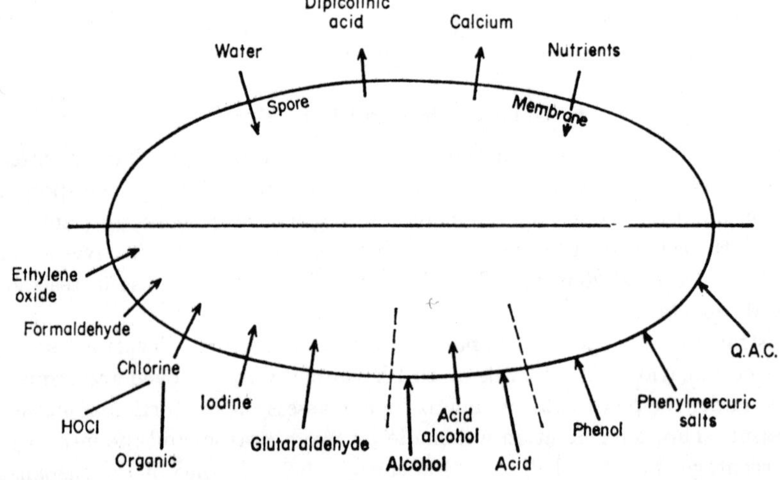

Fig. 5. The permeability of the bacterial spore membrane to nutrients and disinfectants.

agent inducing germination or having a lethal effect must be able to penetrate this membrane.

In view of the high resistance imparted to the cell, at least in part, by this membrane it is interesting to consider some of its physical properties.

For the germination cycle, it must be able to allow the passage of water and of growth factors into the cell and of dipicolinic acid and calcium out of the cell. For disinfection, it allows the passage of substances such as chlorine, iodine, formaldehyde, glutaraldehyde and ethylene oxide, but not the ingress of the nonlethal agents such as the phenols, the quaternary ammonium compounds (even though they are highly surface active) or the ampholytic compounds. Moreover, this latter group of preparations, although unable to kill the spore, can prevent its germination, because even after long contact with these compounds the spores are still able to grow when placed in a more favourable situation. If, of course, germination had been possible under these circumstances a suicidal situation would have obtained, in which the cells in the presense of antibacterial agent would have lost their protective mechanism and thus have rendered themselves susceptible to the action of that agent.

6. Acknowledgement

My thanks are due to Sandra Humphreys for her enthusiastic and reliable work at the bench.

7. References

Borick, P. M. (1968). Chemical sterilizers (chemosterilants). In *Advances in Applied Microbiology*, vol. 10. Eds W. W. Umbreit & D. Perlman. London: Academic Press.

Brazis, A. R., Leslie, J. E., Kablet, R. W. & Woodward, R. L. (1958). The inactivation of spores of *Bacillus globigii* and *Bacillus anthracis* by free available chlorine. *Appl. Microbiol.* **6,** 338.

Coulthard, C. E. (1931). The disinfectant and antiseptic properties of amyl-meta-cresol. *Br. J. exp. Path.* **12,** 331.

Coulthard, C. E. & Sykes, G. (1936). The germicidal effect of alcohol. *Pharm. J.* **137,** 79.

Halvorson, H. O., Vary, J. C. & Steinberg, W. (1966). Developmental changes during the formation and breaking of the dormant state in bacteria. *Ann. Rev. Microbiol.* **20,** 169.

Hoffman, R. K. & Warshowsky, B. (1958). *Beta*-propiolactone vapor as a disinfectant. *Appl. Microbiol.* **6,** 358.

Nordgren, G. (1939). Investigation on the sterilization efficiency of gaseous formaldehyde. *Acta path. microbiol, scand.* Suppl. XL.

Ortenzio, L. F. & Stuart, L. S. (1959). The behavior of chlorine-bearing organic compounds in the A.O.A.C. available chlorine germicidal equivalent concentration test. *J. Ass. off. agric. Chem.* **42,** 630.

Phillips, C. R. (1952). Relative resistance of bacterial spores and vegetative bacteria to disinfectants. *Bact. Rev.* **16,** 135.

Report of the Committee of Formaldehyde Disinfection of the Public Health Laboratory Services (1958). Disinfection of fabrics with gaseous formaldehyde. *J. Hyg., Camb.* **56,** 488.

Rubbo, S. D., Gardner, Joan F. & Webb, R. L. (1967). Biocidal activities of glutaraldehyde and related compounds. *J. appl. Bact.* **30,** 78.

Searle, C. E. (1961). Experiments on the carcinogenicity and reactivity of β-propiolactone. *Br. J. Cancer* **15,** 804.

Sykes, G. (1965). *Disinfection and Sterilization.* 2nd ed. London: E. & F. N. Spon.

Tilley, F. W. & Chapin, R. M. (1930). Germicidal efficiency of chlorine and the N-chloro derivatives of ammonia, methylamine and glycine against anthrax spores. *J. Bact.* **19,** 295.

Wiseley, D. V. & Falk, H. L. (1960). Beta-propiolactone is a carcinogen. *J. Am. med. Ass.* **173,** 1161.

Reprinted from *Appl. Microbiol.* **16**, 1782–1785 (1968)

Printed in U.S.A.

8

Sporicidal Effect of Peracetic Acid Vapor

DOROTHY M. PORTNER AND ROBERT K. HOFFMAN

Department of the Army, Fort Detrick, Frederick, Maryland 21701

Received for publication 9 August 1968

The sporicidal activity of peracetic acid (PAA) vapor at 20, 40, 60, and 80% relative humidity (RH) and 25 C was determined on *Bacillus subtilis* var. *niger* spores on paper and glass surfaces. Appreciable activity occurred within 10 min of exposure to 1 mg of PAA per liter and 40% or higher RH. The sporicidal rate decreased from the optimum at 80% RH to a slight effect at 20% RH. Spores on an impermeable surface were more difficult to kill than those on a porous one, probably because the cells tend to pile up on an impermeable surface and the vapor penetrates poorly through the layer of covering cells.

Numerous studies (3–5, 7, 8, 10) have shown that peracetic acid (PAA) in aqueous solution is an effective germicide against a wide spectrum of microorganisms. On the other hand, information about the vapor-phase bactericidal activity of PAA is very limited and seems to be confined to a brief study by Greenspan et al. (4).

The corrosiveness of PAA has limited its practical application as a disinfectant. However, because PAA itself is not adsorbed onto surfaces and its decomposition products (acetic acid, water, and oxygen) are nontoxic and free-rinsing, PAA has found wide application as a surface decontaminant for foods (5, 6, 9). Spraying dilute solutions of PAA until a fog forms has been an effective means of sterilizing equipment used in gnotobiotic studies (1, 11).

The accumulation of liquid PAA and moisture produced from spraying a dense fog may be undesirable because of corrosion or other damaging effects. Therefore, it is possible that PAA vapor may be used instead of the fog. Because of the extreme reactiveness and considerable volatility of PAA, the study reported here was undertaken to determine the effectiveness of PAA vapor against bacterial spores, on porous and impermeable surfaces, at various relative humidities (RH).

Materials and Methods

Preparation of test samples. An aqueous stock spore suspension of *Bacillus subtilis* var. *niger* was used to contaminate filter-paper discs [5/8 inch (1.58 cm) in diameter] and glass squares [0.5 by 0.5 inch (1.27 by 1.27 cm)]. The contaminated samples were conditioned for 4 days in desiccators maintained at 25 C and at constant RH of 80, 60, and 40% by saturated salt solutions of ammonium sulfate, sodium bromide, and chromic acid, respectively. Samples were conditioned at 20% RH in the laboratory during the winter months when the ambient RH was constantly low as indicated by a hygrothermograph.

Exposure to PAA. The 86-liter test chamber shown in Fig. 1 was fabricated for vapor-phase decontamination studies. Prior to spraying PAA, the RH within the test chamber was adjusted to the same RH used to precondition the samples, either by spraying water into the chamber to raise the RH or by blowing dry air in to lower it. No adjustment was needed for tests conducted at 20% RH because the RH in the test chamber and the laboratory was the same. The RH within the test chamber was monitored with a humidity-sensing element (El-tronics, Inc., Warren, Pa.).

The commercial grade of PAA solution is composed of approximately 40% peracetic acid, 5% hydrogen peroxide, 39% acetic acid, 1% sulfuric acid, and 15% water, w/w. A direct spray UCTL atomizer (2) was used to spray 0.5 ml of the undiluted solution into the test chamber. To allow time for the vapor concentration to stabilize, the test samples were not exposed to the vapor until 30 min after spraying. (Note the rapid initial drop in concentration in Fig. 2.) Furthermore, the fan in the test chamber was run throughout the test period to insure uniform distribution of the PAA vapor. For each exposure period, 16 contaminated samples (8 paper, mounted on pins; 8 glass, laid on wire screen) were placed on an aluminum tray then quickly inserted into the middle of the chamber (Fig. 1). All samples were exposed to PAA vapor at 25 ± 2 C and the same RH that was used for conditioning them. Individual exposure periods ranged from 75 sec to 80 min.

PAA concentration. The concentration of PAA in the chamber was determined at periodic intervals during each exposure period by drawing 500 ml of the chamber air through 20 ml of 20% buffered potassium iodide. The optical density was measured at 500 nm with a spectrophotometer, and the concentration was read from a standard curve prepared by plotting optical densities against known weights of PAA. This method is specific for PAA.

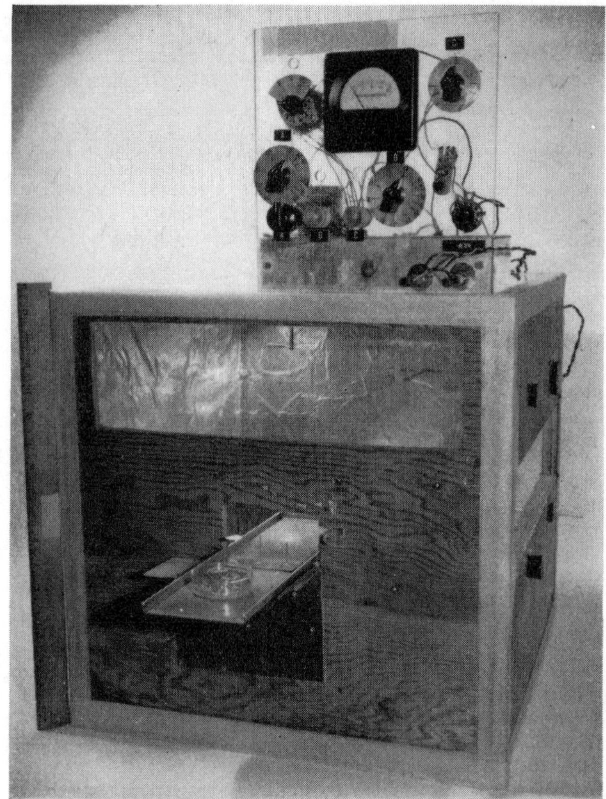

FIG. 1. *Test chamber used for vapor-phase decontamination studies.*

Method of asssy. After exposure to PAA vapor, the samples were transferred to sterile, stoppered plastic tubes containing 10 ml of 0.01% sodium thiosulfate solution, to neutralize excess PAA, with about 0.5 g of sand, to aid in removal of spores; the samples were then shaken vigorously. To insure that an estimate of the number of organisms could be obtained for each exposure period regardless of population size, duplicate 2.5- and 1-ml portions from each tube were plated directly and the remainder was used for serial dilutions. Pour plates were prepared with Trypticase soy agar and were counted after 72 hr of incubation at 32 C. At each exposure period, conditioned samples not exposed to PAA vapor were also assayed in the manner described above. The solution of sodium thiosulfate used in these tests had no observable effect upon the viability of the spores.

The precision of counting a small population is increased by plating a large portion of the sample. One can also be confident that sterility is being attained when no colonies appear on any of the plates prepared from over 70% of the suspending fluid of the sample.

RESULTS AND DISCUSSION

The results are summarized in Table 1. Because an exceptionally high value occasionally appeared among the individual sample counts for given conditions, which were otherwise of the same order of magnitude, the data are expressed by geometric rather than arithmetic means to represent more truly the relationships among the samples. For many of the test samples assayed per exposure period, no organisms were recovered from the part (70%) of the sample that was plated. The frequency of this occurrence is also given in Table 1 as another indication of vapor activity.

Most of the spore population was killed with PAA vapor within a few minutes at 40% or higher RH. At 20%, only a slight reduction occurred on paper and none occurred on glass after 80 min of exposure.

The apparently faster sporicidal action on paper than on glass is probably the result of distribution. The spores in a drop of water spread over a large surface area when placed on a porous material; thus, they are not as likely to pile up on one another as the liquid evaporates. When a similar drop of suspension begins to dry on an impermeable surface, however, there is a tendency for the organisms to collect and pile up

TABLE 1. *Effectiveness of PAA vapor against B. subtilis var. niger spores on paper and glass at various RH values*[a]

Exposure to PAA (min)	80% RH		60% RH		40% RH		20% RH	
	No. of organisms per sample[b]	No. of samples sterile[c]	No. of organisms per samples[b]	No. of samples sterile[c]	No. of organisms per sample[b]	No. of samples sterile[c]	No. of organisms per samples[b]	No. of samples sterile[c]
Paper surface								
0[d]	816,000		831,000		658,000		275,000	
1.25	676	0	—[e]	—	—	—	—	—
2.5	1	5	1,390	0	—	—	—	—
5	<1	12	14	2	7,270	0	—	—
10	<1	14	2	7	24	2	171,000	0
20	0	16	1	8	7	1	117,000	0
40	—	—	<1	12	<1	8	129,000	0
80	—	—	—	—	<1	13	26,000	0
Glass surface								
0[d]	813,000		971,000		709,000		290,000	
1.25	5	7	—	—	—	—	—	—
2.5	2	7	216	1	—	—	—	—
5	<1	13	88	2	33,600	0	—	—
10	<1	13	38	0	1,530	0	218,000	0
20	<1	10	4	6	2,330	0	153,000	0
40	—	—	2	7	623	0	327,000	0
80	—	—	—	—	143	0	267,000	0

[a] Approximately 1 mg of PAA/liter.
[b] Each entry is the geometric mean of 16 samples, except at 20% RH which is based on 8 samples.
[c] Based on plating 70% of each sample. With 80, 60, and 40% RH, 16 test samples were assayed; wit 20% RH, 8 test samples were assayed.
[d] Control, no exposure to PAA.
[e] Not tested.

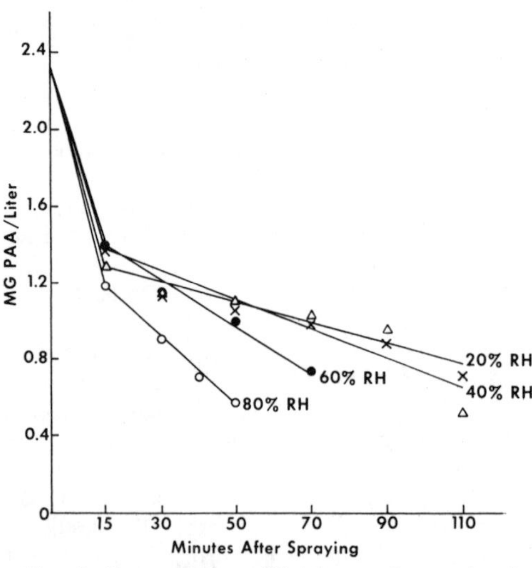

FIG. 2. *Concentration of PAA vapor in test chamber as a function of time and RH.*

at the periphery of the drop. Such a pileup of cells provides protection for the spores underneath from the lethal action of a poorly penetrating vapor like PAA.

The data for the activity of PAA against spore on glass show a rapid initial death rate, then a decrease and leveling off of the curve. The contaminated surfaces were not inserted into the chamber until 30 min after spraying the PAA; by this time, the initial rapid concentration drop (Fig. 2) had taken place and the period of gradual decrease with time had begun. The gradual concentration drop is not sufficient, however, to account for the slower rate of killing with time. Greenspan et al. (4) concluded that PAA vapor-phase sterilization is only dependable with clean surfaces. Trexler and Reynolds (11) believed that dirt was the cause for their difficulty in sterilizing animal cages with a fog of PAA. The surfaces used in this study were clean, but the high concentration of spores on the small sample area of the impermeable surface may have had an effect similar to that of dirt. The outer layer of spores killed during the initial exposure may physically protect the remaining viable spores. Because PAA vapor apparently does not penetrate well its power as a germicide seems to be limited to exposed microorganisms.

The results of this study indicate that, at RH values between 40 and 80%, PAA vapor ca appreciably reduce spore contamination on both porous and impermeable surfaces within 10 min. However, the optimal sporicidal activity occurs at 80% RH, and no appreciable activity occurs at a low (20%) RH. The level of microbial contamination and the cleanness of the surface, as well as the RH, are undoubtedly factors that determine whether sterility is achieved by treatment with PAA vapor.

Acknowledgments

We thank F. M. Wadley for help in interpretation of the data and T. E. Nappier for technical assistance.

Literature Cited

1. Barrett, J. P., Jr. 1959. Sterilizing agents for Lobound flexible film apparatus. Proc. Animal Care Panel **9**:127–133.
2. Decker, H. M., L. M. Buchanan, L. B. Hall, and K. R. Goddard. 1962. Air filtration of microbial particles. Public Health Serv. Publ. No. 953. U.S. Government Printing Office, Washington, D.C.
3. Gershenfeld, L., and D. E. Davis. 1952. Effect of peracetic acid on some thermoaciduric bacteria. Am. J. Pharm. **124**:337–342.
4. Greenspan, F. P., M. A. Johnsen, and P. C. Trexler. 1955. Peracetic acid aerosols. Chem. Specialties Mfrs. Assoc. Proc. Ann. Meeting **42**:59–64.
5. Greenspan, F. P., and D. G. MacKellar. 1951. The application of peracetic acid germicidal washes to mold control of tomatoes. Food Technol. **5**:95–97.
6. Hartman, P. A., and F. Carlin. 1957. Peracetic acid treatment of eggs. Poultry Sci. **34**:673–675.
7. Jones, L. A., R. K. Hoffman, and C. R. Phillips. 1967. Sporicidal activity of peracetic acid and β-propiolactone at subzero temperatures. Appl. Microbiol. **15**:357–362.
8. Kline, L. B., and R. N. Null. 1960. The virucidal properties of peracetic acid. Am. J. Clin. Pathol. **33**:30–33.
9. Lowings, P. H. 1956. The fungal contamination of Kentish strawberry fruits in 1955. Appl. Microbiol. **4**:84–88.
10. Merka, V., F. Sita, and V. Ziker. 1965. Performic and perpropionic acids as disinfectants in comparison with peracetic acid. J. Hyg. Epidemiol. Microbiol. Immunol. (Prague) **9**:220–226.
11. Trexler, P. C., and L. I. Reynolds. 1957. Flexible film apparatus for rearing and use of germfree animals. Appl. Microbiol. **5**:406–412.

Reprinted from *Appl. Microbiol.* **23**, 618–622 (1972) *Printed in U.S.A*

9

Sporostatic and Sporocidal Properties of Aqueous Formaldehyde

RALPH TRUJILLO AND THOMAS J. DAVID

Planetary Quarantine Department, Sandia Laboratories, Albuquerque, New Mexico 87115

Received for publication 28 December 1971

Aqueous formaldehyde is shown to exert both sporostatic and sporocidal effects on *Bacillus subtilis* spores. The sporostatic effect is a result of the reversible inhibition of spore germination occasioned by aqueous formaldehyde; the sporocidal effect is due to the temperature-dependent inactivation of these spores in aqueous formaldehyde. The physicochemical state of formaldehyde in solution provides a framework with which to interpret both the sporostatic and sporocidal properties of aqueous formaldehyde.

Although the bacteriostatic effects of aqueous formaldehyde appear to be well recognized (2), the effect of aqueous formaldehyde on spore germination does not appear to have been investigated. Such a study would seem necessary to distinguish between the sporostatic and sporocidal properties of aqueous formaldehyde for disinfectant purposes, especially in light of a recent study (5) on the reversible inhibition of spore germination by low levels of aliphatic or aromatic alcohols, which suggested that aldehydes also may reversibly inhibit the spore germination process. Furthermore, the temperature-dependent nature of the bacteriocidal activity of formaldehyde in aqueous solution has been described (2, 4); yet a complimentary study on the temperature-dependent nature of the sporocidal activity of aqueous formaldehyde has not been undertaken. This communication investigates the capacity of aqueous formaldehyde to inhibit the germination of *Bacillus subtilis* spores and establishes that the inactivation of these spores by aqueous formaldehyde is a highly temperature-dependent process.

MATERIALS AND METHODS

The *B. subtilis* var. *niger* spores used in this investigation were prepared by an active-culture technique described previously (5). The spores were suspended in 95% ethanol at a concentration of 3×10^9 spores per ml and were stored at −10 C.

The aqueous formaldehyde was prepared by refluxing 5 g of para-formaldehyde (Matheson, Coleman & Bell) in 80 ml of deionized water until a clear solution was obtained (approximately 1.5 hr). The aqueous formaldehyde solution was then made up to 100 ml in a volumetric flask and stored at 31 C. The formaldehyde concentration was determined by using the phenylhydrazine hydrochloride-potassium ferricyanide method (1) and reading the absorption at 515 nm.

The effect of aqueous formaldehyde on spore germination was studied by pipetting the ethanol suspension of spores into calibrated Bausch & Lomb Spectronic 20 tubes and removing the ethanol under vacuum. A 5-ml amount of Trypticase soy broth (4% w/v, BBL), containing the aqueous formaldehyde at various concentrations, then was added to the tubes containing the spores. Insonation of these tubes for 20 sec in an ultrasonic bath (Turco Products, Inc., 20 amp, 250 v) resulted in complete suspension of these spores in the germinating medium. The spore suspensions then were incubated at 30 C. Periodically, the cultures were shaken, and optical density determinations were made with a Bausch & Lomb Spectronic 20 colorimeter. The viable-spore concentration in each suspension was determined after each experiment by serially diluting a given spore suspension and plating out on Trypticase soy agar (4% w/v). The plates were incubated at 31 C for 4 to 5 days to ensure sufficient time for colony development.

The inhibition of spore germination was shown to be reversible by removing the inhibiting aqueous formaldehyde from the spore environment via membrane filtration (Millipore Corp., type HA, 0.45 μm) and resuspending the spores in germinating media free from inhibiting additive. The resuspended spores germinated. A similar study was carried out using ethylene glycol (Fisher Scientific Co.) as the inhibiting additive. In all studies, the spore suspensions were incubated at 30 C.

The effect of temperature on spore viability in aqueous formaldehyde was determined by pipetting the ethanol spore suspension into screw cap vials (25 mm inside diameter by 95 mm high) and removing the ethanol under vacuum. Each temperature study consisted of three such vials, to which was added 8 ml of either sterile, deionized water or a 1% (w/v) formaldehyde solution. After addition of the appropriate solutions, the vials were insonated in an ultrasonic bath for 30 sec to achieve complete suspension of the spores. One vial containing spores in 1% aqueous formaldehyde was allowed to remain at room temperature (24 C), while the remaining two vials, containing the spores suspended in either 1% aqueous formaldehyde or sterile, deionized water, were placed in a Blue M constant-temperature water bath at a given temperature controlled to ± 0.1 C. The temperatures studied were 24, 30, 40, 50, 55, and 60 C. Samples were withdrawn periodically, serially diluted, and plated out using Trypticase soy agar (4% w/v, BBL). The plates were incubated at 31 C for 4 to 5 days to ensure sufficient time for outgrowth. Dilution bottles containing either 0.5% sodium sulfite or ammonium chloride were used to serially dilute spore suspensions in two different experiments in an effort to neutralize the formaldehyde and, perhaps, reverse the formaldehyde-induced inactivation.

Those spore suspensions subjected to heating in 1% formaldehyde at 50, 55, and 60 C were tested for sterility by pipetting 0.1 ml from each suspension into separate dilution bottles containing 100 ml of sterile Trypticase soy broth (4% w/v). After 5 days of shaking at 24 C, a 1-ml sample was removed from each solution and pipetted into separate dilution bottles containing 100 ml of sterile Trypticase soy broth (4% w/v). All broth solutions were gently shaken for a total of 10 days and were visually inspected for turbidity daily.

RESULTS

The process of spore germination can be followed by observing the changes in optical density for a spore suspension as a function of time (3). Fig. 1 illustrates the data obtained when spores of *B. subtilis* var. *niger* were exposed to germinating media in the absence and presence of aqueous formaldehyde at 30 C. Increasing the formaldehyde concentration in the germinating media caused a decrease in the extent of spore germination. A plot of the extent of germination as a function of formaldehyde concentration is presented in Fig. 2. From such data it was possible to obtain an extrapolated value of approximately 0.8% as the level of aqueous formaldehyde required to completely inhibit germination of *B. subtilis* var. *niger* spores.

The spore suspensions containing the various formaldehyde concentrations (Fig. 1) were serially diluted and plated on Trypticase soy agar. The colony counts obtained from the spore suspensions exposed to aqueous formaldehyde were nearly a log lower than those obtained from the control spore suspension (12×10^7 spores per ml) not exposed to formaldehyde. For example, the 0.0938% formaldehyde solution, which allowed complete germination, yielded a spore concentration of 3.6×10^7 spores per ml, while the 1.5% formaldehyde solution, which caused complete inhibition of germination, yielded a spore concentration of 1.6×10^7 spores per ml. The remaining formaldehyde solutions had spore concentrations between these two values. The initial optical density of both the control and 0.0938% formaldehyde solution was 0.66 at 625 nm.

These results suggested that the inhibition of spore germination by aqueous formaldehyde was reversible, and a study to test this possibility was undertaken. *B. subtilis* spores were suspended in germinating medium containing no added formaldehyde (solution A) and 2.5% formaldehyde (solution B). After 1 hr, spore suspension B was passed through a membrane filter and suspended in germinating medium containing either a 2.5% formalde-

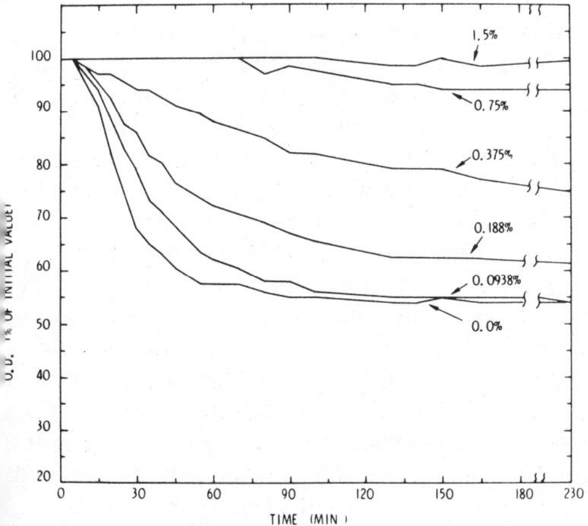

FIG. 1. *Effect of various concentrations of aqueous formaldehyde on the germination of Bacillus subtilis spores.*

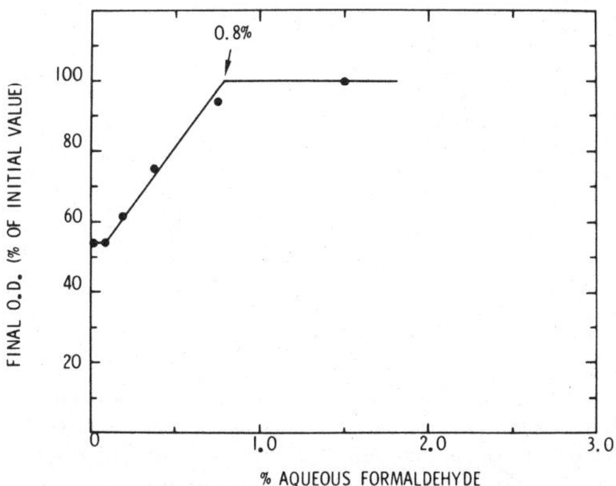

FIG. 2. *Inhibition of spore germination by aqueous formaldehyde. Arrow indicates the extrapolated aqueous-formaldehyde concentration required for 100% inhibition of spore germination.*

hyde (solution C) or no added formaldehyde (solution D). Fig. 3 shows that the inhibition of spore germination by aqueous formaldehyde is reversible, since the resuspended spores germinated in media containing no formaldehyde, whereas the spores resuspended in media containing formaldehyde did not germinate. The initial optical density of both solutions A and D was 0.61, whereas the viable spore concentration in solution A was determined to be 9.4 $\times 10^7$ spores per ml and that of solution D was 4.5 $\times 10^5$ spores per ml. These results indicate that formaldehyde can exhibit both sporostatic and sporocidal properties since aqueous formaldehyde can reversibly inhibit spore germination (sporostatic property) and decrease survival levels (sporocidal property).

The sporocidal property of aqueous formaldehyde was observed to be strongly dependent on temperature; in fact, a synergistic response was observed for the inactivation of *B. subtilis* spores on exposure to aqueous formaldehyde at elevated temperatures. Heating an aqueous suspension of *B. subtilis* spores from 30 C to 60 C for 4 hr did not result in spore inactivation, whereas spores suspended in a 1% formaldehyde solution exhibited less than a log reduction in population after 4 hr at 24 C. However, the combination of 1% formaldehyde and heat (30 to 60 C) resulted in the extensive spore inactivation illustrated in Fig. 4. The inactivation of spores by heat and dilute formaldehyde may be characterized as a synergistic

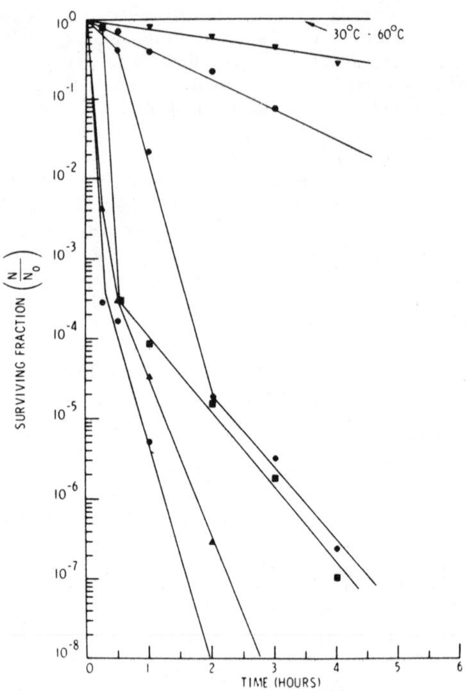

FIG. 4. *Inactivation of B. subtilis spores suspended in 1% formaldehyde and heated at 24 C (▼), 30 C (●), 40 C (✚), 50 C (■), 55 C (▲), and 60 C (●). Heating aqueous spore suspensions from 30 C to 60 C for four hours did not inactivate the B. subtilis spores. N/N_0 refers to the ratio of viable spores at a given time (N_0).*

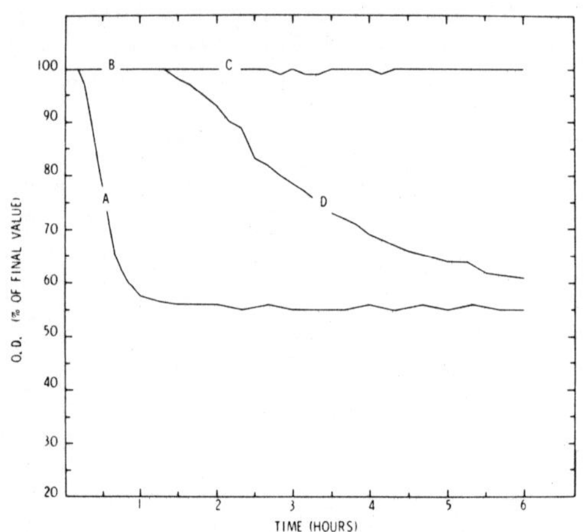

FIG. 3. *Reversibility of the aqueous formaldehyde-induced inhibition of spore germination. Spores were suspended in Trypticase soy broth with (A) no additive and (B) 2.5% aqueous formaldehyde. After 70 min, spore suspension B was passed through a membrane filter and resuspended in Trypticase soy broth containing (C) 2.5% aqueous formaldehyde and (D) no additive.*

inactivation, because the rate of inactivation for spores exposed to both agents simultaneously is greater than the rate of spore inactivation due to heating at a given temperature in the absence of aqueous formaldehyde plus the inactivation rate due to 1% formaldehyde at 24 C. Those spores suspended in 1% formaldehyde at a concentration of 10^8 spores per ml were completely inactivated on heating to 55 or 60 C for 4 hr. Sterility was determined by direct colony count and incubation in broth for 10 days, as described previously. Dilution bottles containing either 0.5% sodium sulfite or ammonium chloride were used to serially dilute spore suspensions in two different experiments, in an effort to neutralize the formaldehyde and, perhaps, reverse the formaldehyde-induced inactivation. No difference in survival level was observed between these experiment and those in which formaldehyde-treated spores were not exposed to these chemicals.

DISCUSSION

A previous study established that the germination of bacterial spores can be inhibited reversibly by low concentrations of either aliphatic or aromatic alcohols (5). The present investigation indicates that aqueous formaldehyde can also reversibly inhibit the spore-germination process. Structurally and chemically an aldehyde is different from an alcohol, yet both appear to affect spore germination in a similar manner. Insight into why formaldehyde should act as an alcohol in its effect on spore germination may be obtained from basic chemical considerations. Gaseous formaldehyde rapidly reacts with water to form a monohydrate, methylene glycol, $CH_2(OH)_2$, which subsequently forms a series of low-molecular-weight, polymeric hydrates or polymethylene glycols, having the type formula, $HO(CH_2O)_nH$. The reaction of formaldehyde with water is shown in Fig. 5.

It has been determined (6) that at 30 C a 2%-formaldehyde solution contains 0.001% formaldehyde monomer and 99.999% methylene glycol and polymers of methylene glycol. In other words, formaldehyde in water is 99.999% in the form of a di-alcohol (methylene glycol) or polymeric di-alcohols. Therefore, formaldehyde acts like an alcohol in reversibly inhibiting spore germination because, in aqueous solution, formaldehyde exists essentially as a di-alcohol. That di-alcohols per se can inhibit spore germination was shown in a study in which ethylene glycol (10% v/v) reversibly inhibited the germination of *B. subtilis* var. *niger* spores.

The contention that aqueous formaldehyde reversibly inhibits spore germination (Fig. 4), because in solution formaldehyde essentially exists as a di-alcohol and alcohols are known to reversibly inhibit spore germination, invites interesting comparisons. For example, Table 1 compares the physical and sporostatic properties of ethanol and aqueous formaldehyde (methylene glycol). Calculations based on the data in Table 1 reveal that nearly identical amounts of ethanol and methylene glycol are required to inhibit the germination of a single *B. subtilis* var. *niger* spore (column A). This result suggests that these additives, of comparable molecular weight, steric volume, and chemical substituents, are interacting with

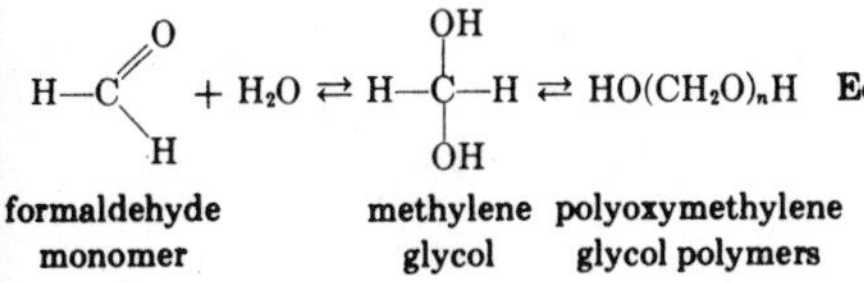

$$H{-}C(=O){-}H + H_2O \rightleftarrows H{-}C(OH)_2{-}H \rightleftarrows HO(CH_2O)_nH \quad \textbf{Equation 1}$$

formaldehyde monomer — **methylene glycol** — **polyoxymethylene glycol polymers**

Fig. 5. *Reaction of formaldehyde with water.*

Table 1. *Comparison of the physical and sporostatic properties of ethanol and methylene glycol*

Additive	Structure	Mol wt	Germination inhibiting concn	Column A[a]
Ethanol	$CH_3{-}CH_2{-}OH$	46.07	1.4%[b]	1.46×10^{12}
Methylene glycol	$HO{-}CH_2{-}OH$	48.03	0.8%	1.0×10^{12}

[a] Figures in this column refer to the calculated number of atoms of additive required to inhibit one *B. subtilis* var *niger* spore. Calculated from the germination-inhibiting concentration, inhibited spore concentration (1×10^8 spores per ml), and Avogadro's number.

[b] Data obtained from reference 5.

the spore in the same manner to inhibit spore germination, perhaps by combining with spore enzyme(s) required for spore germination. The observation that the rate of reversal of spore inhibition by aqueous formaldehyde is approximately five times slower (Fig. 3) than that observed for ethanol suggests that, whereas both additives may be interacting with the same spore component and with the same stoichiometry, they do so in different manners.

A further difference between alcohol and aqueous formaldehyde is that exposure of spores to formaldehyde results in decreased spore survival levels, whereas exposure of spores to alcohol is not sporocidal. For example, spore suspensions A and D in Fig. 4 both achieved essentially the same extent of germination, and yet the viable spore concentration in solution A was 9.4×10^7 spores per ml and that of solution D was 4.5×10^5 spores per ml. Both of these spore suspensions had the same initial optical density of 0.61. These two observations, (i) that the inhibition of germination occasioned by a formaldehyde solution was fully reversible on removal of the aqeuous formaldehyde from the spore environment, and (ii) that the survival level of the formaldehyde-treated, resuspended spores (suspension D) was more than 100 times lower than the control levels, strongly imply that the sporostatic and sporocidal properties of aqueous formaldehyde are not related.

The equilibrium between formaldehyde and its hydrate forms (see Fig. 5) may also serve as the basis for understanding the synergistic inactivation of spores by heat and aqueous formaldehyde (Fig. 4). It is suggested that, whereas the inhibition of spore germination is due to methylene glycol, the inactivation of spores is a result of an irreversible reaction between the free formaldehyde monomer present in a formaldehyde solution and the spores suspended in such a solution. The equilibrium between formaldehyde monomer and its diol form in water (methylene glycol) is not greatly affected by changes in temperature up to 60 C (6). Therefore, the extreme temperature dependence observed for the inactivation of spores in aqueous formaldehyde may be a result of the increased rate of reaction between free formaldehyde monomer and the spores with increasing temperature. Consistent with such an interpretation is the observation that spores suspended in 1% formaldehyde solution and heated to 50, 55, or 60 C all exhibited approximately the same survival level after treatment for 30 min, and thereafter had different rates of inactivation (Fig. 4). This result can be understood if one assumes that sufficient thermal energy was present at 50 to 60 C to allow the equilibrium concentration of formaldehyde monomer to be completely utilized in combining with and inactivating a certain fraction of the total spore population. The subsequent differences in spore inactivation rate from 50 to 60 C could then reflect the influence of temperature on the reestablishment of the equilibrium between formaldehyde monomer and methylene glycol in an aqueous formaldehyde solution.

ACKNOWLEDGMENTS

The technical assistance of C. Edward Leonard is gratefully acknowledged.

This work was conducted under contract no. W-12,853, Planetary Programs, Office of Space Science and Applications, NASA Headquarters, Washington, D.C.

LITERATURE CITED

1. Hanson, N. W., D. A. Reilly, and H. E. Stagg (ed.). 1965. The determination of toxic substances in air—a manual of ICI practice, p. 131–134. W. Heffer and Sons, Cambridge.
2. Sykes, G. 1967. Disinfection and sterilization, 2nd ed., p. 345–346. Spon, London.
3. Sussman, A. S., and H. O. Halvorson. 1966. Spores: their dormancy and germination, p. 133–139. Harper and Row, Publishers, New York.
4. Tilley, F. W. 1945. The influence of changes in concentration and temperature upon the bactericidal activity of formaldehyde in aqueous solutions. J. Bacteriol. **50**:469–473.
5. Trujillo, R., and N. Laible. 1970. Reversible inhibition of spore germination by alcohols. Appl. Microbiol. **20**:620–623.
6. Walker, J. F. 1964. Formaldehyde, 3rd ed., p. 59–62. American Chem. Soc. Monograph Series, Reinhold Publishing Corp., New York.

Reprinted with permission from the *Am. J. Hosp. Pharm.* **20**, 465–485 (1963)

BUFFERED GLUTARALDEHYDE

10

a new chemical sterilizing solution

by A. A. STONEHILL, S. KROP, and P. M. BORICK

► THE NEED FOR A RAPID ACTING, SIMPLE TO USE, safe, aqueous chemical solution for the complete disinfection or sterilization of medical, dental and hospital instruments has been apparent for some time. Many chemical compounds have been proposed, tested, and found wanting in some aspect. Phenols, chlorinated phenols, the lower alkanols such as ethyl and isopropyl alcohol, and the quaternary ammonium compounds have been used, but none were rapidly sporicidal.[1]

The value of a chemical agent can best be measured by (a) its ability to kill spores rapidly such as *Clostridium sporogenes, Clostridium tetani, Bacillus subtilis,* and *Bacillus pumilis;* (b) its activity in the presence of organic matter; (c) its activity in relatively low concentrations; (d) its lack of corrosive and toxic properties. Heretofore, no chemical disinfectant has been found which contained all of these attributes.

Formaldehyde solutions have been found to be sporicidal but they possess the inherent undesirable properties of irritation, skin sensitization and vapor toxicity which make them inappropriate for use as chemical disinfectants.

Our objective was to develop a full range, quickly-acting sporicidal agent that would have none of the undesirable properties of formaldehyde. A systematic study of various aldehydes culminated in the development of a buffered dialdehyde solution* that is capable of killing resistant spores in three hours or less, when tested by the rigid AOAC method[2] recommended by the U. S. Department of Agriculture. This buffered solution has been found to be of particular advantage in the rapid sterilization of many hospital, dental and surgical items that are difficult or incapable of being safely sterilized by other means.[3]

Chemistry

The active chemical in the buffered dialdehyde solution is glutaraldehyde. It is a saturated dialdehyde of

A. A. STONEHILL, Ph.D., S. KROP, Ph.D., and P. M. BORICK, Ph.D. are associated with Research Division of Ethicon, Inc., Somerville, N. J.

*CIDEX® aqueous activated dialdehyde solution.

the following formula: $CHO\text{-}CH_2\text{-}CH_2\text{-}CH_2\text{-}CHO$; molecular weight is 100.12. In contrast to formaldehyde, which is a simple aldehyde, glutaraldehyde has two active carbonyl groups. Under proper conditions these two groups, either singly or together, undergo most of the typical aldehyde reactions to form acetals, cyanohydrins, oximes, and hydrazones. Through a crosslinking reaction, the carbonyl groups react with protein.

Aqueous solutions of glutaraldehyde are mildly acid in reaction. In this acid state they are not sporicidal. Only when the solution is buffered by suitable alkalinating agents to a *p*H of 7.5 to 8.5, does the solution become antimicrobially active.

In the acid state, the glutaraldehyde solution is stable for long periods of time, when stored in closed containers in a cool place. However, when rendered alkaline, the glutaraldehyde gradually undergoes polymerization and loses activity. Above *p*H 9, the polymerization proceeds comparatively rapidly. In the *p*H range of 7.5 to 8.5, the polymerization reaction is slowed down considerably, so that full antimicrobial activity is maintained for at least two weeks.

To provide greater utility to the activated or buffered glutaraldehyde solution, it has been found convenient to add, in addition to the alkaline buffer, a surface tension depressant, an anti-corrosive compound, and a non-staining water soluble dye, D. & C Green No. 8. From a practical viewpoint, this is best accomplished by preparing a dry powder blend of these chemicals and packaging them in a tightly closed vial, which is attached to the container of unactivated glutaraldehyde solution. To activate the glutaraldehyde solution, it is merely necessary to add the contents of the vial to the aldehyde solution and shake gently until dissolved.

The minimum concentration of aqueous glutaraldehyde that has been found to be rapidly sporicidal is two percent. To buffer this concentration of glutaraldehyde to the required alkaline range, the addition of 0.3 percent of sodium bicarbonate is necessary. Although other alkalinating agents may be employed, the alkali metal bicarbonates, such as sodium bicarbonate, have given best results.

The purpose of the dye is to indicate the addition of buffer salts to the activated glutaraldehyde solution. Before the addition of the buffer-dye combination, the unactivated glutaraldehyde solution is colorless; after the addition, the solution turns a characteristic fluorescent green.

Microbiological Evaluation

Non-Sporeforming Bacteria. Tests using two percent activated glutaraldehyde solution were conducted against nonsporeforming bacteria using the Millipore Filter Method.[4] Test microorganisms included *Micrococcus pyogenes* var. *aureus*, American Type Culture Collections (ATCC 6538),

Table 1. Bactericidal Action Exhibited by 2 Percent Activated Glutaraldehyde Solution Using the Millipore Filter Method

	Aqueous			Alcoholic		
	Tested Initially	Tested One Week After Activation	Tested Two Weeks After Activation	Tested Initially	Tested One Week After Activation	Tested Two Weeks After Activation
Staphylococcus aureus ATCC 6538	All Less Than Two Minutes			All Less Than Two Minutes		
Proteus vulgaris ATCC 6380						
Escherichia coli ATCC 6880						
Pseudomonas aeruginosa ATCC 10145						
Diplococcus pneumoniae Type III*						
*Serratia marcescens***						
Streptococcus pyogenes ATCC 12384						
Klebsiella pneumoniae ATCC 132						
*Micrococcus lysodeikticus****						
Escherichia coli (T phage) ATCC 1303						

* Dr. Nungester, University of Michigan
** Source, Department of Microbiology, Rutgers University
*** Source, Ohio State University

Table 2. Bactericidal Activity Shown with Activated Glutaraldehyde Solution Against **Ps. aeruginosa** by the Use-Dilution Method

Concentration of Glutaraldehyde Parts Per Million	Time In Minutes	Microorganism Surviving
22	0.5	0
22	2	0
22	6	0
22	17	0
22	60	0

Proteus vulgaris (ATCC 6380), *Escherichia coli* (ATCC 6880), *Pseudomonas aeruginosa* (ATCC 10145), *Diplococcus pneumoniae* (W. Nungester, University of Michigan), *Serratia marcescens* (Rutgers University), *Streptococcus pyogenes* (ATCC 12384), *Klebsiella pneumoniae* (ATCC 132), *Micrococcus lysodeitikus,* (Ohio State University), and *Escherichia coli* (T-phage strain). All of the test bacteria were in contact with the glutaraldehyde solution for less than two minutes, transferred directly to the appropriate culture media after exposure and incubated at 37°C for 48 hours.

The microbiological effectiveness of 2 percent activated glutaraldehyde solution is shown in the data presented. Only a short period of time was necessary to destroy various vegetative bacterial cells as can be seen in Table 1. Activated glutaraldehyde solution was destructive to both gram-positive and gram-negative bacteria in less than 2 minutes contact time, the shortest time interval employed. Even the highly resistant gram-negatives; *e.g., Pseudomonas* and *Proteus,* were inactivated in less than two minutes.

The high degree of bactericidal activity demonstrated in Table 1 prompted us to determine the minimal inhibitory concentration necessary for the inactivation of *Pseudomonas aeruginosa.* In order to determine the minimal inhibitory concentration necessary for activity against vegetative cells, the 2 percent activated glutaraldehyde solution was also tested by the use-dilution method of Ortenzio and Stuart[5] (1961) against *Pseudomonas aeruginosa* ATCC 10145. Cultures were incubated at 37°C and results read after 72 hours.

It was shown that this microorganism could not be recovered after 30 seconds exposure to 22 ppm activated glutaraldehyde solution. See Table 2.

Sporeforming Bacteria. A high degree of sporicidal activity with activated glutaraldehyde solution was demonstrated against the spores of *Bacillus subtilis, Bacillus globigii, Clostridium tetani* and *Clostridium welchii* by Chandler, Pepper, Dondershine and Borick (1963).[10] Rapid sporicidal action with *Bacillus megaterium* was shown by Dr. O. Wyss[6] and its activity compared with other disinfectants. The efficiency of activated glutaraldehyde solution was compared with Lysol and a 2 percent formaldehyde preparation contained in 65 percent isopropanol and 3 percent methanol.

Two percent activated glutaraldehyde solutions were compared with other sporicidal agents. See Table 3. The spores of *Bacillus megaterium* were readily inactivated by glutaraldehyde solutions. Neither 2 percent cresol nor 2 percent formaldehyde was able to destroy all of the cells in four hours. It will also be noted that 2 percent activated glutaraldehyde solutions were able to destroy all spores within two hours, two weeks after activation of the test solutions.

The sporicidal activity of 2 percent activated glutaraldehyde solution in the presence of blood serum was also compared with that of a commercially available 8 percent formaldehyde formulation. Nine parts of activated glutaraldehyde solution or the formaldehyde solution were mixed with one part of human blood serum and tested for activity by the AOAC pennycylinder method. Bacterial spores included in the above test method were *Bacillus globigii, Bacillus subtilis, Clostridium tetani* and *Clostridium welchii* received from the U. S. Department of Agriculture.

Table 4 gives a comparison of activated glutaraldehyde solution with 8 percent formaldehyde solution when one part of human blood serum was added to nine parts of the test material. Both solutions showed a high degree of sporicidal activity in the presence of blood serum by the AOAC pennycylinder method.

Tuberculocidal Activity. The tuberculocidal activity of 2 percent glutaraldehyde was evaluated by Dr. E. Spaulding[7] and Dr. M. Shelanski.[8] Tubercle bacilli were shown to be destroyed by activated glutaraldehyde solution as they could not be recovered by Shelanski on Lowenstein-Jensen medium or recovered from guinea pigs nor could they be grown on Petragnani slants by Spaulding.

Fungicidal Activity. The fungicidal activity of 2 percent activated glutaraldehyde solution was compared with various commercially available preparations by testing against *Trichophyton interdigitale* ATCC 640 using the AOAC proce-

Table 3. Sporicidal Action of Activated Glutaraldehyde Solution as Compared with Other Disinfectants Using **B. megaterium** as the Test Microorganism. Results Shown Below Represent Numbers of Surviving Organisms.

	Contact Time					
	0	10 min.	30 min	1 hour	2 hours	4 hours
2% Activated glutaraldehyde freshly mixed	3980	1650	250	4	0	0
2% Activated glutaraldehyde 2 weeks later	3980	2570	300	19	0	0
1% Saponated cresol	3700	3040	3600	2400	2300	2200
2% Saponated cresol	3650	2900	3040	3030	2680	1320
2% Formaldehyde	4010	3150	2300	1920	20	10
Control (water)	4080	4000	3990	4050	3960	3940

Survivor counts above x100.

Table 4. Sporicidal Action of Nine Parts of 2 Percent Activated Glutaraldehyde Solution or 8 Percent Formaldehyde* with One Part of Human Blood by the AOAC Pennycylinder Method

	2% Activated Glutaraldehyde	Formaldehyde
	Aged 18 Hours (Time Required to Kill in Hours)	
B. globigii	2-3	>3
B. subtilis	2	>3
Cl. tetani	<2	<1
Cl. welchii	2-3	<1
	Aged 2 Weeks	
B. globigii	<1	<1
B. subtilis	3	<1
Cl. tetani	<2	>6
Cl. welchii	2	2

* Purchased as commercial preparation.

Table 5. Fungicidal Activity Exhibited by Various Commercially Available Preparations Using **T. interdigitale** ATCC 9533 and Employing the AOAC Procedure

PRODUCT	CONCENTRATION TESTED	RESISTANCE OF FUNGAL SPORES
		(Time In Minutes)
Activated Glutaraldehyde Solution	2%	<5
Zephiran®	1:1000	5
Amphyl®	2%	<5
Ioclide	200 ppm free I_2	<5
Mercuric oxycyanide	1:1000	>15
Bard-Parker®	Full Strength	<5
Wescodyne®	75 ppm free I_2	<5
Phenol control	1:45	<10
Phenol control	1:60	>15

dure of Ortenzio (1960). Results indicate that the glutaraldehyde solution was able to inhibit growth of *Trichophyton interdigitale* in less than 5 minutes, the time interval tested by us. This is in contrast to a 1:60 phenol dilution which required more than 15 minutes as well as other preparations which ranged in activity from that of glutaraldehyde to phenol (See Table 5).

Virucidal Activity. The virucidal activity of glutaraldehyde was carried out by Dr. M. Klein[9] and the results were reported by Chandler *et al.*[10] Polio types 1 and 2, Coxsackie B-3, Influenza A-2 and Mouse Hepatitis (MHV3) were shown to be killed within 10 minutes exposure to the test solution.

Toxicology

Toxicological study was designed to obtain data by which to assess the relative hazards of "equicidal"* solutions of glutaraldehyde and of formaldehyde.

Systemic Toxicity

Acute. Albino mice and rats were used for the acute toxicity determinations. Formaldehyde and activated glutaraldehyde solutions were diluted with physiological saline so that the volume administered did not exceed 0.5 ml. for intravenous, and 1.0 ml. for oral administration to mice and 5.0 ml. for oral administration to rats.

a. *Intravenous.* Glutaraldehyde and formaldehyde solutions were administered intravenously to albino mice and rats in groups of ten animals for each dose, after preliminary dose range-finding. Simultaneously, the acute intravenous toxicity of formaldehyde was determined in the same manner. The results appear in Table 6. Symptoms of toxicity appeared in a few minutes at doses approaching the LD_{50}, and consisted of pallor, gasping, convulsions, and depression. Survivors were depressed for one to two hours, *i.e.*, spontaneous motor activity was decreased; recovery was complete. Autopsy of fatalities revealed hemorrhagic lung congestion; sacrificed survivors autopsied at various periods during recovery exhibited no effects grossly. The symptoms of poisoning, their time course, and the post-mortem findings were similar for glutaraldehyde and for formaldehyde. The acute intravenous LD_{50} for mice was estimated at 15 and 54 mg. for glutaraldehyde and formaldehyde respectively; for rats, 9.8 and 45 mg./Kg. respectively.

* "Equicidal" as applied here, roughly equates 2 percent activated glutaraldehyde solution with 8 percent formaldehyde in bactericidal and sporicidal power.

Table 6. Acute Intravenous Toxicity of Glutaraldehyde and Formaldehyde in Albino Mice and Rats

SPECIES	LD_{50} GLUTARALDEHYDE	LD_{50} FORMALDEHYDE
Mice	15.0 mg./Kg.	54.0 mg./Kg.
Rats	9.8 mg./Kg.	45.0 mg./Kg.

b. *Oral.* Glutaraldehyde and formaldehyde solutions were administered to albino rats and mice by stomach tube. After preliminary dose range-finding tests, doses were given to groups of ten animals each. The results appear in Table 7. Symptoms of poisoning were similar to those after intravenous administration to mice, but required longer to develop. Gross post-mortem examination revealed irritation of the gastrointestinal tract, the more intense (hemorrhagic) irritation occurring with the higher doses. Many animals exhibited lung congestion resembling that following intravenous administration, and congestion of the abdominal viscera. The oral LD_{50} in mice was 352 mg. and 305 mg. for glutaraldehyde and formaldehyde respectively; in rats it was 252 mg. and 451 mg. respectively.

c. *Percutaneous.* Rabbits and rats receiving single and multiple applications of glutaraldehyde as a 2 percent aqueous solution exhibited no evidences of systemic effects even in the cases in which irritation was produced upon daily application for approximately one month. The effects upon the skin appear in the section on local effects, following.

d. *Inhalation.* Inhalation of vapors by mice and rats from 2 percent activated aqueous glutaraldehyde solutions evaporating freely at room temperature in a closed system for periods up to four hours produced no symptoms and animals sacrificed immediately after exposure and at varying intervals after exposure showed no effects grossly. Formaldehyde evaporating from "equicidal" 8 percent aqueous solutions under identical conditions produced signs of respiratory tract irritation in the animals clinically and evidence of severe lung injury at sacrifice after the exposure. Table 8 summarizes the data. Higher concentrations of both compounds in the evaporating aqueous solutions produced more effects, which were uniformly much more severe with formaldehyde.

Subacute and Chronic. Observations on subacute and chronic effects of glutaraldehyde in albino rabbits were made only (a) after single and daily cutaneous applications of aqueous solutions for periods up to six weeks and (b) after single applications of aqueous solutions to the conjunctiva. Applications to the closely clipped skin of 0.5 ml. of solution, spread with a soft brush and allowed to dry, were made to a given area. There were no symptoms suggesting systemic toxicity, *i.e.*, resulting from skin penetration and accumulation to toxic levels, in any of the animals. These effects are described in the section on local effects following.

Table 7. Acute Oral Toxicity of Glutaraldehyde and Formaldehyde in Albino Mice and Rats

SPECIES	LD_{50} GLUTARALDEHYDE	LD_{50} FORMALDEHYDE
Mice	352 mg./Kg.	305 mg./Kg.
Rats	252 mg./Kg.	451 mg./Kg.

Table 8. Acute Inhalation Toxicity of Glutaraldehyde (GA) and Formaldehyde (FA) Vapors in Mice and Rats

Animal Species	*Compound*	*Concentration and Volume/Liter of Air Space*	*Exposure Time (hours)*	*Mortality Died/ Exposed (7 days later)*	*Immediate Effects*	*Delayed Effects*	*Comments*
Rats	GA	aqueous-2%-1.5 ml.	4	0/12	none. slightly more restless than controls	initial weight loss in 5/12, regained in 1-2 days	pneumonitis in 10/12, as in controls
Rats	FA	aqueous-2%-1.5 ml.	4	1/8	moderate dyspnea, restlessness, pawing of face	weight loss in 6/8, progressive deterioration	lungs grossly hemorrhagic at autopsy
Rats	FA	aqueous-8%-1.5 ml.	4	3/4	one died in 2 hours; restlessness, gasping, rhinorrhea, severe dyspnea	2/3 survivors died 1-4 days post implantation	lungs deeply hemorrhagic grossly at autopsy
Rats	H_2O Control	aqueous-8%-1.5 ml.	6	0/3	1/3 slight rhinorrhea	1/3 initial weight loss, regained in 3 days	pneumonitis in 2/3
Rats	H_2O Control	aqueous-8%-1.5 ml.	4	0/16	none	1/16 initial weight loss, regained in 2 days	pneumonitis in 1/4
Mice	GA	aqueous-2%-1.5 ml.	4	0/5	none	2/5 initial weight loss, regained	pneumonitis in 2/4
Mice	FA	aqueous-2%-15. ml.	4	0/12	pawing of face; "wheezing"	6/12 initial weight loss, regained slowly	pneumonitis in 1/5
Mice	FA	aqueous-8%-1.5 ml.	6	3/3	3/3 died in 1-5 hours	- - - -	stomach and intestines air-filled; lungs deeply hemorrhagic
Mice	H_2O Control	aqueous-8%-1.5 ml.	4	0/2	none	2/2 weight loss, regained in 7 days	pneumonitis in 6/11
Mice	H_2O Control	aqueous-8%-1.5 ml.	6	0/11	none	none	

Local Effects

Skin. Aqueous solutions of 2 percent activated glutaraldehyde and of 8 percent formaldehyde were applied daily for six weeks to the clipped dorsal skin of 20 albino rabbits, 0.5 ml. of each for comparison in the same animal. The solutions were spread with a soft brush and allowed to remain until "dry". The application sites were examined daily prior to repetition of the day's application and the extent of reaction noted. Table 9 summarizes the findings. Faint yellow staining of the skin and hair appeared after the first application of 2 percent activated glutaraldehyde solution which gradually became more intense and gradually turned to a golden brown over the six week period of application. The discoloration interfered with good estimation of erythema, which in any case appeared to be no more than questionable. The discoloration persisted up to 35 days after application ceased. A mild "rash" appeared early during the application in some animals receiving both glutaraldehyde and formaldehyde, in most cases disappearing despite continued application of the solutions. Formaldehyde of equal concentration produced definite erythema. An "equicidal" aqueous formaldehyde (8 percent) produced a severe erythematous reaction with edema after one to two daily applications with necrosis and eschar formation in seven to ten days; the eschar pealed off leaving the site scarred. A 25 percent aqueous concentrate of glutaraldehyde produced a similarly intense reaction.

Eye. Irritation of the eye by aqueous solutions of glutaraldehyde and of formaldehyde was determined in five albino rabbits by single installation of 0.1 ml. into one conjunctival sac of each animal, the other sac serving as control. Effects were noted at two hours and then daily thereafter. In some instances, washing with 5 ml. of water followed the instillation of the 25 percent concentrate of glutaraldehyde. Two percent aqueous glutaraldehyde caused a severe reaction consisting of inflammation, lachrymation, and edema which required seven to eight days for complete recovery. Formaldehyde of equal concentration produced a milder reaction requiring three to four days for recovery. Eight percent formaldehyde (equicidal with 2 percent activated glutaraldehyde) produced a very severe reaction requiring seven to forty-five days for recovery. Table 10 summarizes the results.

Gastrointestinal Tract. Observations on the gastrointestinal effects by local action were made incidental to determinations of systemic toxicity by oral administration and have been described in a preceding section of this report.

Urinary Tract. Observations on the effects of aqueous activated glutaraldehyde solutions on the mucosa of the urethra and bladder were confined to those arising from careful passage and retention of catheters which had been immersed in sporicidal (2 percent) concentrations of activated glutaraldehyde solutions. Comparisons of effects of unrinsed, rinsed-with-water, and control catheters (trauma controls) were made in dogs under light pentobarbital anesthesia. Catheters were permitted to remain in place six to eight hours, after which gross examination of urethra and bladder was made at necropsy followed by examination of stained microscopic sections. Three dogs were used for each treatment and two dogs as trauma controls. No effects attributable to the presence of residual glutaraldehyde were noted, *i.e.*, the effects of trauma, which were mild and variable, were as great as those due to the "treated" catheters.

Respiratory Tract. Observations on certain aspects of the effects of vapors on the respiratory tract have been described in a preceding section of this report. In addition, observations have been made on the effect of residual 2 percent activated glutaraldehyde solution adhering to endotracheal tubes on the mucosa of the pharynx and trachea of dogs under pentobarbital anesthesia. Rubber endotracheal tubes were immersed, then removed from the solution, allowed to drain freely and passed into the trachea to within approximately one inch of the bronchial bifurcation (three dogs). Tubes similarly treated but rinsed with water (three dogs) and tubes treated with water alone prior to intubation of the trachea served as controls (two dogs). There was no evidence that the residual glutaraldehyde exerted an action on the mucosa beyond that of the (mechanical) trauma produced by the control tubes.

Summary of Toxicological Effects

The acute systemic toxicity of glutaraldehyde has been studied in rats and mice, and the local effects in rabbits and dogs. The compound is slightly to moderately toxic. A 2 percent aqueous solution is slightly irritant to the skin and severely irritant to the eye, being less so than an "equicidal" formaldehyde solution. Precautions for handling and using are simple and consist in limiting contact with tissues, prompt washing of exposed body parts with water, and avoidance of inhalation, *i.e.*, precautions are identical in kind with those for safe use of formaldehyde. Eye contact with the solution should, after prompt irrigation with water, be reported to a physician.

Table 9. Effects of Daily Aqueous Glutaraldehyde (GA) and Formaldehyde (FA) Solution Applications on the Skin of Albino Rabbits

Compound and Concentration	*No. Days Applied*	EFFECTS		
		Erythema	*"Rash"*	*Scarring*
GA 2%	7	spotty, mild; questionable	slight to moderate; reversible	pin-point, questionable; clearing despite further application
	42	no further intensification of effects, except discoloration		
FA 2%	7	mild, distinct	slight to moderate; reversible	as for GA 2%
	42	as for GA 2%, except no discoloration		
FA 8%	1-2	severe with edema		
	7-10			marked, with hard eschar
	14	application stopped; scarring after eschar sloughed off		

Table 10. Effect of Aqueous Glutaraldehyde (GA) and Formaldehyde (FA) on the Eye of Albino Rabbits (single application - five rabbits each)

COMPOUND AND CONCENTRATION	EFFECTS		
	IRRITATION		
	SCORE (MAX. = 110)	RATING	RECOVERY
GA 2%	17	Severe	7-8 days
FA 8%	96	Severe	7-45 days
FA 2%	10	Moderate	3-4 days

Other Advantages

In addition to its remarkable bactericidal activity, activated glutaraldehyde solution has the following advantages:

1. Its aqueous solution has no deleterious effect on the cement or the lenses of such medical instruments as bronchoscopes, cystoscopes, telescopes, etc. A cystoscope was immersed for a total of 125 immersions of three hours duration each in activated glutaraldehyde solution without any ill effects to the lens system. A bronchoscope was immersed for two continuous weeks in activated glutaraldehyde solution. At the end of this period, the bulb lighted, the lens system was unaffected and there was no sign of corrosion of the metal parts. This test was repeated on the same instrument for two more weeks with the same satisfactory results. An Englehard Exam Telescope was completely immersed in activated glutaraldehyde solution for 16 days. There was no evidence of harmful effect to the optical system, lens cement, or plastic eye-piece.

2. It does not interfere with the electrical conductivity of rubber anesthesia equipment. Anesthesia black rubber corrugated breathing tubes and face masks were tested for conductivity in accordance with Recommended Safe Practices for Hospital Operating Rooms as recommended in Bulletin No. 56 issued by National Board of Fire Underwriters. After initial conductivity tests, the equipment was immersed completely in activated glutaraldehyde solution for three hours, followed by rinsing in a full stream of running tap water. The equipment was then air dried for one day and finally dried for 30 minutes under high vacuum. There

Table 11. Conductivity of Anesthesia Equipment

Anesthesia black rubber corrugated breathing tubes and face masks were tested for conductivity in accordance with Recommended Safe Practices for Hospital Operating Rooms using Conductivity Test Kit, Model F-2, distributed by Herman H. Sticht Co., Inc. After initial conductivity testing, the anesthesia equipment was immersed completely in activated CIDEX solution for 3 hours, followed by rinsing in a full stream of running tap water. The equipment was then air dried for one day with an occasional shaking off of water droplets and finally dried for 30 minutes under high vacuum. *The conductivity measured as electrical resistance (in ohms) is shown.* The maximum electrical resistance for anesthesia rubber tubes and parts is 1,000,000 ohms (National Board of Fire Underwriters).

	Resistance In Ohms			
Anesthesia Equipment	*Initial*	*After 1st Cidex Immersion*	*After 2nd Cidex Immersion*	*After 3rd Cidex Immersion*
Large black rubber corrugated breathing tube — 31″ long	125,000	70,000	60,000	80,000
Small black rubber corrugated breathing tube — 13″ long	325,000	180,000	180,000	200,000
Adult face mask (Ohio Chem. Inc.)				
soft rubber	400,000	400,000	300,000	370,000
hard rubber	30,000	25,000	25,000	30,000
Small adult face mask (Ohio Chem. Inc.)				
soft rubber	1,000,000	400,000	450,000	600,000
hard rubber	40,000	30,000	45,000	25,000
Adult face mask (Air Shield, Inc.)				
soft rubber	4,000,000	1,000,000	300,000	280,000
hard rubber	45,000	40,000	45,000	45,000

was no *adverse change* in the conductivity of the equipment (See Table 11).

3. It does not affect the markings on clinical thermometers. Several rectal and oral clinical thermometers from two manufacturers were immersed in activated glutaraldehyde solution for two weeks. At the end of this time, there was no effect on the colored markings.

4. Its low surface tension permits easy penetration and permits easy rinsing. A large corrugated breathing tube, a small breathing tube, a rubber and a plastic endotracheal tube were sterilized in activated glutaraldehyde solution for three hours, allowed to drain for one minute and rinsed in a full stream of running water. Within 30 seconds of rinsing, the glutaraldehyde content was reduced on the average to less than 8 parts per million (See Tables 12 and 13).

5. It is non-corrosive. Dental picks, burrs, mirrors, diamond point drills; surgical instruments such as biopsy instruments, Gigli saws, stainless scissors, pick-up forceps, eye needle holders, were not corroded after having been immersed in buffered glutaraldehyde solution for two weeks.

6. It does *not affect* rubber and plastic articles. Rubber and plastic catheters, O.R. rubber pads, rubber suction tubings, endotracheal tubes, plastic airways, polyethylene tubing and esophageal bougies exhibited no deleterious effects after two weeks immersion in buffered glutaraldehyde solution.

7. It is non-corrosive to aluminum foil suture packets. Aluminum foil suture packets were forcibly immersed in buffered glutaraldehyde solution for 30 days at 100°F. There was no corrosion of the aluminum foil at the end of this period.

8. It does not coagulate blood, and therefore makes the cleaning of blood-covered instruments easier. Buffered aqueous glutaraldehyde solution, and an alcoholic formaldehyde solution were individually mixed with whole human blood in a 4 to 1 ratio. The aqueous glutaraldehyde solution did not coagulate the blood, the alcoholic formaldehyde solution did coagulate the blood.

9. It has a low vapor pressure—22 millimeters of mercury, as compared to 24 millimeters of that of water. It is, therefore, no more volatile than water and will not evaporate as quickly as the more volatile alcoholic solutions. Also, because of its low vapor pressure it tends to keep odor permeation to a minimum, as compared to formaldehyde vapors which are highly volatile causing irritating fumes to permeate the area.

10. It does not affect the sharpness of cutting instruments. A surgical scissor and a surgical nail clipper were immersed repeatedly in buffered glutaraldehyde solution for two weeks with no effect on the cutting edge.

Table 12. Hospital Breathing Items Were Sterilized in Aqueous Cidex Solution for Three Hours, Allowed to Drain For One Minute and Rinsed in a Full Stream of Running Tap Water

	Residual Glutaraldehyde (ppm)			
	Running Water Rinse Time			
Hospital Item	15 sec.	30 sec.	60 sec.	120 sec.
Large 32″ Corrugated Rubber Breathing Tube	–	10	7	5
Small 13″ Corrugated Rubber Breathing Tube	–	8	7	4
Forregger No. 22 Red Rubber Endotracheal Tube	2	1	–	–
Davol No. 3 White Plastic Endotracheal Tube	2	1	–	–
Portex White Plastic Endotracheal Tube	1	1	–	–
Forregger 28F Brown Fiber Endotracheal Tube	9	6	–	5

11. It has active buffering capacity. Normal carry-over of extraneous fluid adhering to washed and rinsed instruments will not interfere with antimicrobial activity.

Discussion

Buffered glutaraldehyde solution most nearly fulfills the criteria for the ideal instrument germicide as set forth by Dr. E. M. Spaulding in 1957.[11] He stated:

> The perfect instrument germicide is not likely to be found or created as will be seen by examining the following arbitrary criteria for an ideal solution:
>
> 1. Produces rapid sterilization of instruments which have been mechanically cleansed but still carry a few tubercle bacilli, spores or virus particles.
> 2. Retains a major portion of its activity in the presence of body protein and does not coagulate it.
> 3. The quantity of germicide remaining on instruments after immersion does not irritate tissues.
> 4. No irritating fumes or unpleasant odor.
> 5. Does not corrode metal, damage rubber goods or dissolve cement mountings of lens systems.
> 6. Low cost.
>
> The first criterion listed is the primary one, the others secondary. For example, safety should not be sacrificed; whereas the risk of tissue irritation can be avoided by rinsing in sterile water after disinfection. If the user chooses to ignore the risk of spore and tubercle bacillus contamination, any one of many available solutions will be satisfactory. On the other hand, if emphasis is placed upon protection against tuberculosis, the number to choose from is much smaller. And those who demand a sporicide are limited, for the time being at least, to aqueous and alcoholic formalin solutions.

A careful comparison of his criteria with the properties reported here for buffered glutaraldehyde solution would tend to indicate that the criteria have been met.

Based on the satisfactory results obtained in our laboratories, an extensive test-in-use program was initiated in a number of hospitals, including large medical teaching hospitals, located all over the country. These hospitals have conducted their own bacteriological tests, investigated the effect of the activated glutaraldehyde solution on expensive lens instruments such as bronchoscopes, and noted the reaction of personnel as regards skin irritation, odor, ease of handling and practical utility.

These tests have been going on for over a year. Although the evaluations are still continuing a sufficient number of reports have been received confirming the rapid cidal effectiveness of the activated glutaraldehyde solution, its inertness against the lens and cement of various examining scopes, and its lack of irritating odor, non-irritation of skin, and ease of handling.

Conclusions

1. A satisfactory sporicidal chemical solution has been developed for the rapid sterilization of surgical, dental and hospital instruments.

2. Common non-sporeforming bacteria are killed within two minutes after immersion.

3. *Mycobacterium tuberculosis* is killed within ten minutes. This is the more remarkable because it is one of the few *non-alcoholic solutions* that possesses this important property.

4. Bacterial spores are killed within three hours when tested by the rigid AOAC method for spores.

5. The buffered glutaraldehyde solution was non-corrosive to metal instruments, did not harm lens instruments nor their cement systems.

6. The buffered 2 percent glutaraldehyde solution is slightly to moderately toxic. It is slightly irritant to the skin and severely irritant to the eye, being less so than formaldehyde in concentrations of equal antiseptic action.

Table 13. The Following Hospital Items Were Totally Immersed in Aqueous Cidex for Three to Five Hours

	Residual Glutaraldehyde (ppm)				
	Number of Rinses*				
Hospital Item	1st	2nd	3rd	4th	5th
Large 32" Corrugated Rubber Breathing Tube	300	24	8	7	6
Small 13" Corrugated Rubber Breathing Tube	100	14	13	6	5
Rubber Rebreathing Bag	79	7	4	12	Nil
Rusch 20 Tracheal Tube	33	27	6	5	–
Tragger 28F Brown Plastic Endotracheal Tube	31	5	Nil	–	–
Tragger 22 Red Rubber Endotracheal Tube	19	5	Nil	–	–
Davol No. 3 White Plastic Endotracheal Tube	15	4	Nil	–	–
Portex White Plastic Endotracheal Tube	15	5	Nil	–	–

* Immersed in 500 ml. of water, except corrugated rubber tube which was immersed in 1,000 ml. water. Each item was rinsed and drained three times in each immersion bath, and allowed to drain for one minute before transferring to second immersion bath and subsequent baths.

References

1. Lamy, P. P. and Flack, H. L.: A Review of Some Agents for Hospital Infection Control, *Am. J. Hosp. Pharm.* *19*:473 (Sept.) 1962.
2. Official Methods of Analysis of the Assoc. Off. Ag. Chem. 1960, 9th Ed., pp. 67-69.
3. U. S. Patent No. 3016 328.
4. Millipore Filter Corp., Watertown, Mass.
5. Ortenzio, L. F. and Stuart, L. S.: Adaptation of the Use-Dilution Method to Primary Evaluations of Disinfectants, *J. Assoc. Off. Ag. Chem.* *44*:416-421 (1961).
6. Wyss, C. and Spaulding, E., University of Texas, personal communication.
7. Temple University, personal communication.
8. Industrial Biology Research and Testing Laboratories, personal communication.
9. Temple University, personal communication.
10. Chandler, V. L., R-E Pepper; F. Dondershine and P. M. Borick. Activated Glutaraldehyde, A New Sporicidal Agent. In Press.
11. Spaulding, E. M.: Chemical Disinfection of Medical and Surgical Materials, in Reddish, G. F., ed.: *Antiseptics, Disinfectants, Fungicides, and Chemical and Physical Sterilization,* Philadelphia, Lea & Febiger, 1957, pg. 642.

Editor's Comments on Papers 11, 12, and 13

11 Russell: *Resistance of Bacterial Spores to Heat, Disinfectants, Gases and Radiation*

12 Schmidt and Winicov: *Detergent/Iodine Systems*

13 Steiger-Trippi: *Classical and Modern Methods of Antimicrobial Treatment*

The article by Russell describes the resistance of bacterial spores to various chemical and physical agents and shows that spores which offer a high degree of resistance to one process are not necessarily insensitive to another.

Schmidt and Winicov describe the preparation of iodine concentrates, which were among the earliest substances to be used in antimicrobial destruction.

Steiger-Trippi considers the pros and cons of classical and modern methods of antimicrobial treatment and discusses a wide variety of subjects related to this area.

Reprinted from *Manufacturing Chemist & Aerosol News* **36**, 38–45 (1965)

Resistance of bacterial spores to heat, disinfectants, gases and radiation

11

A D Russell BPharm PhD MPS
Welsh School of Pharmacy

Bacterial spores are generally far more resistant than vegetative cells to certain processes designed to achieve sterilisation or disinfection. This fact has an important application in both (a) the methods of sterilisation of certain pharmaceutical and medicinal products, such as injections, eyedrops, sutures, surgical dressings, etc, and (b) the food industry, where spoilage of products may occur because of, for example, the presence of heat-resistant organisms which have survived a heat sterilisation process. This, in turn, leads to the problem of determining whether any spores survive a given treatment; this subject was reviewed by Schmidt[1] and more recently by Harris[2] and Russell[3], both of whom stressed the importance of the post-treatment medium (the recovery medium) and incubation temperature, on the recovery of damaged sporing and non-sporing organisms. Adequate means of neutralising or inactivating chemical agents to which organisms have been exposed must also be considered in determining the degree of bacterial susceptibility (Russell[3]; Russell and Gilbert[4]).

The purpose of this paper has been to assess the resistance or susceptibility of bacterial spores to certain chemical and physical processes. No attempt has been made to carry out a fully comprehensive survey of the literature in an article of this length, since the field is obviously a wide and varied one.

HEAT

Mathematical considerations

In an excellent paper, Kelsey[5] considered the findings of various authors on the resistance of bacterial spores of various species to moist heat. When thermal death time (the time to kill at a particular temperature) was plotted on a log scale against temperature (°C), a straight line was produced (fig 1) the slope of which is the Z-value. This is defined as the number of degrees of temperature per tenfold increase of time. Based on this, Kelsey[5] showed that if a Z-value of 10°C is assumed, and a survival of 5 minutes at 121°C is taken, then extrapolating the line shows that a survival time of about 10 hours at 100°C is to be expected (fig 2, 0—0). Similarly, if a Z-value of 10°C is assumed, and a survival time of 2 minutes at 121°C is taken, a survival time of about 250 minutes at 100°C is to be expected (fig 2, ●—●). This is of use in accepting an organism as a test of the autoclaving process.

Two other values frequently used in heat-resistance studies are the F-value and D-value. The F-value is the time in minutes required to kill all spores in a suspension at 250°F (121°C) (fig 3). Fields and Finley[6], for example, estimated the F-value of stored spores of *Bacillus stearothermophilus* strain 1518 to be 7 minutes, and the Z-value to be 12°F, whereas the F-value for new spores was >18 minutes, so that ageing of the spores caused a decrease in spore resistance. On the other hand, Kelsey[7] working with other strains of *B.stearothermophilus* showed that spore papers could be stored for at least six months without any alteration in LD_{50} (measured in minutes).

D-value (also known as D_{10} value, decimal reduction time or DRT) is the time in minutes required to reduce the number of spores in a suspension by 90 per cent, *ie* to 10 per cent of the original number, at a given temperature. It is also used in heat studies on non-sporing bacteria: see, for example, White[8]. Ley and Tallentire[9] recently described the survival curves of *B.megaterium* spores in water at 100°C, and of *B.stearothermophilus* spores at 115°C; the inactivation of these appears to follow an exponential law, apart from an initial *increase* in the number of colony-forming units with the latter organism (see the later description of 'Heat activation'). The probability of existence of survivors can be calculated from the survival curves by first obtaining the D-value. The linear plot can be expressed as $\log_{10}N/N_0 = kD$, in which N_0 is the initial number of viable cells, N the number of cells surviving a treatment D, and k is a constant equal to the slope of the curve.

Inactivation factor (IF) represents the degree of reduction in

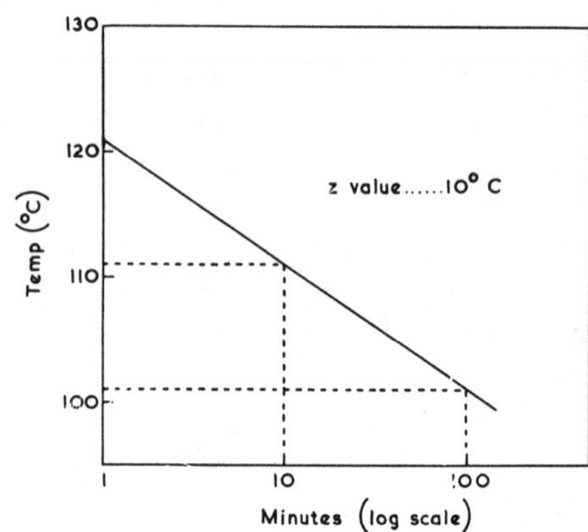

Fig 1. Thermal death time (log scale) plotted against temperature

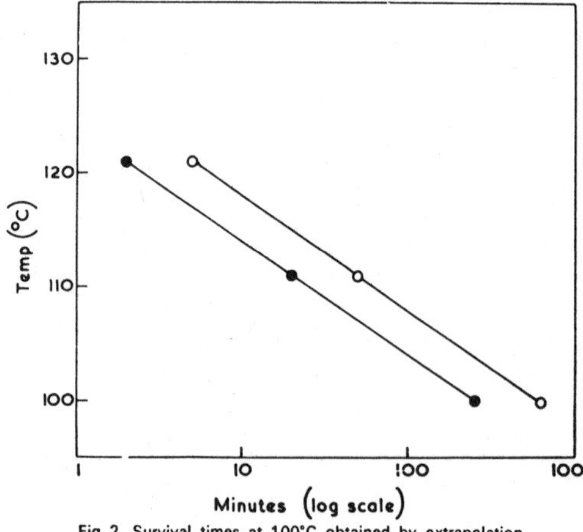

Fig 2. Survival times at 100°C obtained by extrapolation

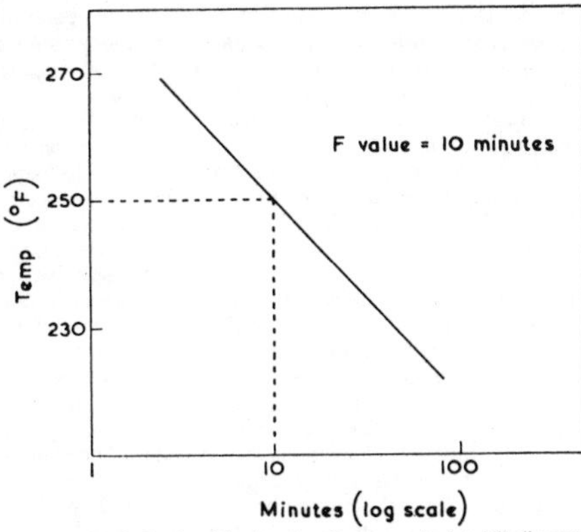

Fig 3. F-value (the time in minutes required to kill all spores in a suspension at 250°C)

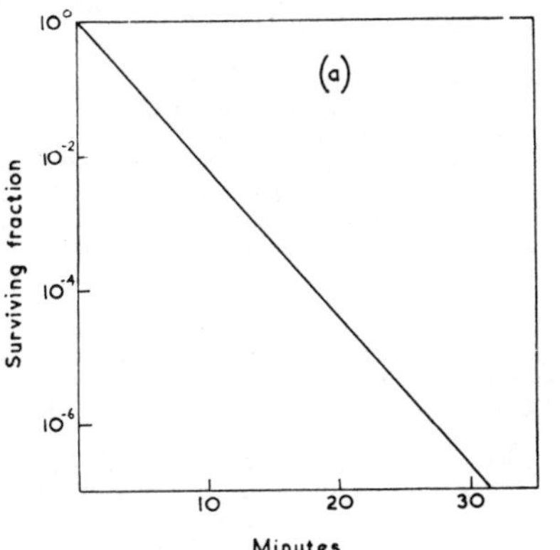

Fig 4a. Exponential death curve. D-value is $4\frac{1}{2}$ min and IF is 10^7

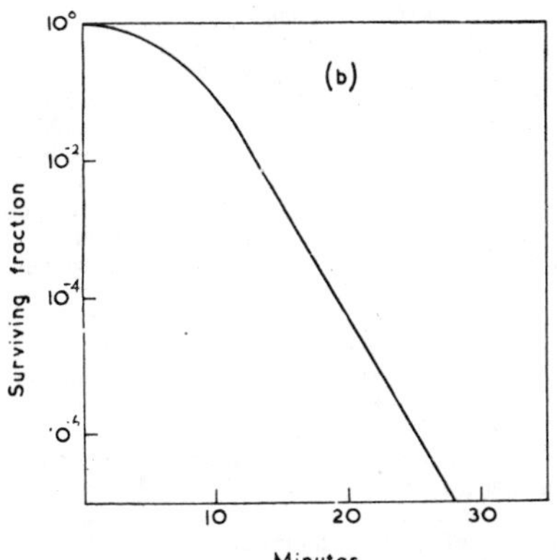

Fig 4b. Initial shoulder followed by exponential death curve. D-value is 3 min and IF (calculated) is 10^9

the number of viable spores and is obtained by dividing the initial viable count by the final viable count, *ie* IF = N_0/N.

Frequently, the IF is calculated from the D-value, although this is open to criticism (Powell[10]), *eg* two hypothetical death-curves of spores at a certain temperature are considered in fig 4, (a) showing an exponential death curve, and (b) an initial shoulder, followed by an exponential death curve.

From fig 4a, D-value = $4\frac{1}{2}$ minutes. Thus, the number of log cycles (= treatment dose/D-value) is $31\frac{1}{2}/4\frac{1}{2} = 7$. Therefore IF = 10^7. Alternatively, IF = $N_0/N = 10^7/1$ (or $10^0/10^{-7}$) = 10^7.

From fig 4b, the D-value from the straight portion of the graph is 3 minutes. Thus, the number of log cycles is $28/3 \simeq 9$ so that when calculated in this way, the IF = 10^9. This, however, is true only if the line is perfectly straight and goes through the origin. The true IF is $N_0/N = 10^7/1$ (or $10^0/10^{-7}$) = 10^7. (Apart from the initial lag, the rate of killing in b is, of course, greater than in a.)

As Powell[10] has pointed out, the D-value approach can give a false picture, and this is also the case in irradiation sterilisation, which is discussed in a later section.

Heat activation and deactivation

Shull and Ernst[11] found that the thermal death curves of dried spores of *B.stearothermophilus* in saturated steam showed three phases: a sharp initial rise in viable count, followed by a low rate of death which gradually increased, and the final phase of logarithmic death at maximal rate (see also Humphrey and Nickerson[12]). The initial phase was due to 'heat activation' of the spore population. Curran and Evans[13, 14] were the first to show that sublethal heat could induce dormant spores to germinate, and this phenomenon was referred to as heat activation. It has since been observed by many other workers, although not all spores are capable of being so activated.

Conversely, Finley and Fields[15] observed heat-induced dormancy (decreased plate counts, or deactivation) to occur when spores of two strains of *B.stearothermophilus* were subjected to sublethal temperatures of 100°C or less. This phenomenon was, however, transient, for when the spores were subjected to a more drastic heat treatment (105 to 115°C), true activation resulted.

Susceptibility of spores to moist heat

The resistance of bacterial spores to moist heat varies with each strain, *eg* some strains of *B.subtilis* spores are heat-sensitive, being rapidly destroyed at 100°C, whereas others withstand boiling for several hours (Wilson and Miles[16]). Similarly, *B. megaterium* spores are reported to be highly resistant to moist heat[16] or highly sensitive (Rode and Foster[17]). *B.anthracis* is destroyed after 10 minutes at 100°C, and *B.stearothermophilus* requires 12 minutes at 121°C.

There is a similar variation with the anaerobic spore-formers, *eg Cl.botulinum* spores can withstand boiling for some hours, *Cl.welchii* may be destroyed by boiling in less than 5 minutes (Headlee[18]) or may be fairly resistant to higher temperatures (see Kelsey[5]). *Cl. tetani, Cl.oedematiens* and *Cl.septicum* spores may all be fairly highly resistant to moist heat temperatures above 100°C.

Susceptibility of spores to dry heat

Less information is available about the resistance of bacterial spores to dry heat, although Koch and Wolfhügel[19] were the first to show that dry heat was less effective in destroying bacteria than moist heat; they also found that $1\frac{1}{2}$ hours at just over 100°C destroyed vegetative organisms, whereas for spores a dry heat temperature of 140°C for 3 hours was required. Gerhards[20], in work on the thermal death point of bacteria in fan ovens, stated that 140°C for 1 hour was sufficient, so that the higher temperatures specified for sterilisation of articles are due to the wide variation of temperature within ovens (Darmady and Brock[21]). However, to ensure sterility with dry heat, Darmady *et al*[22] recommended that the holding time at a selected temperature should be $1\frac{1}{2}$ times that time required to kill all *Cl.tetani* spores at a temperature 10°C lower, *eg* if a sterilising temperature of 160°C is to be used, then a holding time of $1\frac{1}{2}$ times the sterilising time at 150°C will be required, which is $1\frac{1}{2} \times 30 = 45$ minutes (see table 1).

Cl.tetani was found by *Darmady et al*[22] to be the most resistant of all organisms to dry heat, and a non-toxigenic strain has been suggested as being a suitable indicator of dry heat sterilisation.

There is not necessarily any correlation between resistance to dry heat and resistance to moist heat, *eg B.stearothermophilus*

Table 1. Time-temperature relationships for dry heat sterilisation (after Darmady *et al*[22])

Temp °C	Mins to kill *Cl.tetani* spores	Holding time (mins) in sterilisation process	BP recommended holding time (mins)
150	30	—	60
160	12	45	60
170	5	18	—
180	1	7½	—
190	—	1½	—

is highly resistant to the latter, but not particularly so to the former, process. Nevertheless, this organism, *B.subtilis* spores, and samples of earth have been used for testing gas ovens (Patrick *et al*[23]).

O'Brien and Parish[24] heavily contaminated liquid paraffin, almond oil and olive oil with a spore-containing mixture of earth, hay and faeces, which contained spores resistant to dry heat at 140°C for 1 hour, and found that heating at 150°C for 1 hour satisfactorily sterilised the oils, whereas Tyndallisation could not be relied upon to ensure sterilisation.

Water activity and heat resistance of spores

As defined by Murrell[25], water activity (a_w) = equilibrium relative humidity (ERH)/100. Thus, a_w values can vary from 0.00 to 1.00.

Bullock and Keefe[26], in a detailed investigation into bacterial survival in systems of low moisture content, showed that spores of *B.subtilis* remained viable in oils, fats and liquid paraffin for over two years. Obviously, this fact is of importance in considering the sterilisation of these products by dry heat. Similarly, Bullock and Tallentire[27] found that when powders containing *B.subtilis* spores were exposed to atmospheres of increasing humidity, a definite sequence of events occurred:

(i) Below a certain moisture content, the spores remained viable and heat resistant;

(ii) Over a certain range of moisture uptake, the spores lost their heat resistance, but retained their viability;

(iii) At a still higher moisture content, both heat resistance and viability were lost.

Spores of *B.subtilis* were found to remain viable and heat-resistant in a dry peptone powder for long periods of time. In peptone powders containing up to 30 per cent of moisture the spores remained viable and heat-resistant; with a moisture uptake of 50 per cent the majority of the spores lost their heat resistance but remained viable; when the moisture uptake was 80 per cent, there was a loss of both heat resistance and viability, and these effects took place more rapidly at 100 per cent relative humidity.

Bullock and Tallentire[27] concluded that spores in a dry powder underwent no change over long periods, and Murrell[25] stated that spores heated in anhydrous oils or fats might have a heat resistance similar to that in the dry state.

The subject of water activity and thermoresistance has recently been re-investigated by Marshall, Murrell and Scott[28], who showed that freeze-dried spores of *B.megaterium, B.stearothermophilus, Clostridium bifermentans* and *Cl.botulinum* did not survive well under extremely dry or very moist conditions, and that for maximum retention of viability and of heat-resistance, storage in air or in vacuum at a_w values of 0.2 to 0.8 was required.

Dipicolinic acid, cations, and heat resistance of spores

Powell[29] found that about 5 to 15 per cent of the dry weight of spores was composed of dipicolinic acid (DPA) and that when

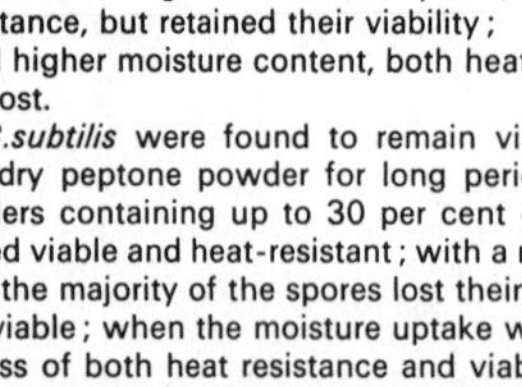

```
              H
              C
           //   \
        HC        CH
        |         ||
   HOOC-C         C-COOH
          \\    /
              N
```

Pyridine-2,6-dicarboxylic acid (dipicolinic acid, DPA)

spore germination took place, DPA was released with a loss of heat resistance.

El-Bisi and Ordal[30] found that higher growth temperatures markedly enhanced the thermal resistance of the spores of *B.coagulans* var. *thermoacidurans*, an important food spoilage organism. Continuing this work, Lechowich and Ordal[31] showed that, in *B.subtilis*, elevated sporulation temperatures led to increased contents of DPA, Ca, Mn and Mg, and an increased heat resistance, whereas in *B.coagulans*, higher sporulation temperatures gave a decreased content of DPA. However, the ratio of total cation content to DPA increased as thermoresistance increased, which supported the conclusion (Halvorson[32]) that the chelated form of DPA is responsible for thermoresistance of spores. On the other hand, Walker, Matches and Ayres[33] concluded from their work on the chemical composition and heat resistance of some aerobic bacterial spores that, while Ca^{++}, Mg^{++} and DPA play an important role in determining thermal resistance, 'other factors need to be included before a full explanation of thermal stability of spores can be made'. Curran[34] also reported that the specific function of minerals in sporulation and thermostability had not then been well explained.

Lechowich and Ordal[31] showed that spores of *B.coagulans* produced at 45°C possessed nearly 80 times as much DPA, 4.5 times as much Ca^{++} and three times as much Mn^{++} as vegetative cells* produced at the same temperature, and that whereas vegetative cells were rapidly destroyed at 80°C, spores were killed only after exposure for 75 minutes at 98.5°C.

Heat-sensitive spores are produced when sporulation occurs in a Ca^{++}-deficient medium. Slepecky and Foster[35] found that replacement of Ca^{++} in part by other cations gave spores which were less thermoresistant but which resembled those with a normal Ca^{++} content in morphology, etc. Tallentire and Chiori[36] investigated the heat resistance of *B.megaterium* spores grown on a medium containing varying quantities of divalent metallic cations, and confirmed earlier reports that thermoresistance depended on the concentration of these cations in the sporulation medium.

From the work of Rode and Foster[17], it is apparent that DPA is built up during sporulation and released during germination. The strain of *B.megaterium* used by Rode and Foster was rapidly killed at 85°C, and thus is less resistant to moist heat than the majority of strains of this organism.

This loss of viability was associated with a lack of DPA retained in the spores: thermal loss of DPA occurred only upon the death of the cell.

Thermophilic spore papers and the testing of sterilisers

Kelsey[5] drew attention to the dangers of using spore preparations of inadequate resistance for testing the efficiency of autoclaves, and later[7] published details of the preparation and standardisation of spore papers of *B.stearothermophilus* of known heat resistance. Kelsey postulated that it was reasonable to assume that the slope of the dose-response curve was characteristic of the strain and that it would remain reasonably constant at least for some months. The LD_{50} (in minutes) could thus be used to characterise a batch of spore papers and a minimum LD_{50} could be required from a batch made from that particular strain. An LD_{50} of 4½ to 6½ minutes at 121°C appeared to be the recommended resistance.

Recovery of heated spores

Early investigations on the heat-resistance of bacterial spores were made by Morrison and Rettger[37, 38], who showed that the response or behaviour of aerobic spore-forming organisms after heating was dependent on the environmental conditions; tomato-juice agar and yeast extract broth were found to have a stimulatory effect on the germination of these heat-treated spores, whereas the use of nutrient broth as the recovery medium frequently resulted in a much delayed initiation of growth. Curran and Evans[39] later reported similar findings, in that enrichment substances incorporated in culture media were essential for the accurate enumeration of bacteria previously exposed to highly lethal factors. Olsen and Scott[40] studied the heat resistance of strains of *Cl.botulinum*, and showed that various media which gave equivalent counts of unheated spores gave divergent

* Vegetative cells are supposed to be devoid of DPA

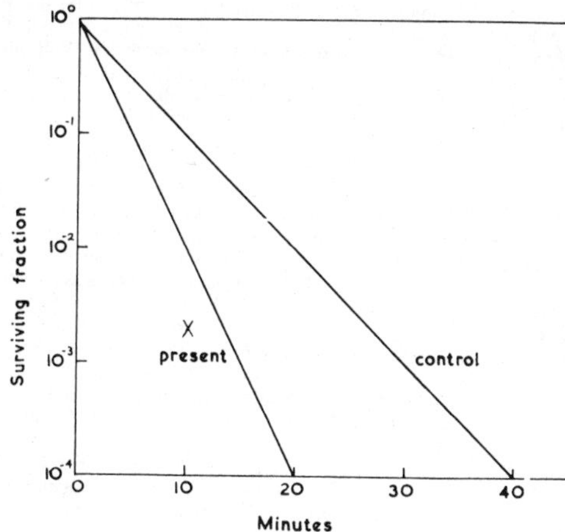

Fig 5. D-value for control (no chemical present) and in presence of substance X

estimates of the number of survivors following heat treatment; the addition of soluble starch increased markedly the recovery of these heated spores.

Schmidt[1] has reviewed the resistance of bacterial spores, with particular emphasis on spore germination and its inhibition.

Chemicals which reduce the heat resistance of bacterial spores

Anderson and Michener[41] and Lewis, Michener, Stumbo and Titus[42] showed that nisin and subtilin reduced the heat resistance of spores of the *Clostridium* strain PA 3679. Subsequently, Michener, Thompson and Lewis[43, 44] compared the number of spores of this organism surviving a particular heat treatment in the presence and absence of various substances, and expressed the results as the percentage reduction in the D-value of the spores caused by the substance under test. In the theoretical example provided (fig 5), assuming a logarithmic response, the D-value for the control (no chemical present) at the temperature used is 10 minutes. In the presence of a substance X, the D-value is 5 minutes, so that there has been a 50 per cent reduction in the D-value. Reductions in the D-value of <20 per cent were not considered significant. The degree of D-value reduction obviously depended on the concentration of substance employed. Of the antibiotics tested, only subtilin and nisin gave a D-value reduction of >45 per cent; of several common disinfectants, only hydrogen peroxide, formaldehyde and silver nitrate were active, whereas calcium hypochlorite, potassium permanganate and merthiolate were inactive. Of several epoxides, ethylene oxide (200 ppm) and propylene oxide (1,300 ppm) were included in those which gave D-value reductions of about 50 per cent. The significance of this work was the possibility of reducing the severity of heat processes for canned foods by including chemical additives; the authors stressed that they were aware of the need for further experimental work to be carried out, particularly with regard to demonstrating lack of toxicity of any chemical(s) which possessed the essential activity against spores of food spoilage organisms.

Bose and Roy[45] investigated the effect of different substances on the heat resistance of *B.subtilis* spores at 110°C. Moist heat alone killed practically all the spores within 6 minutes; sodium chloride at concentrations of one per cent increased somewhat the rate of kill, as did calcium chloride at a concentration of 0.189 per cent. A 55 per cent sucrose concentration slightly increased the rate of death as compared with the control. No data were provided as to whether the differences were significant.

Bose and Roy[46] subsequently investigated the effect of various spices on the heat resistance of *B.subtilis* spores at 105°C. The spices used were chillies, turmeric, coriander, cumin and mustard. The first four whole powders, when used in aqueous suspensions, were more effective than their ether—or alcohol-soluble fractions. Chillies and mustard oil were particularly effective in reducing the heat resistance of the spores.

CHEMICALS

Several early investigators considered that various chemicals were sporicidal, *eg* Koch[47] proposed that mercuric chloride had a rapid and lethal effect on the spores of *B.anthracis,* whereas Geppert[48] using an improved and more logical technique found that this action was sporostatic and not sporicidal. Subsequent research has amply confirmed these findings, and it has been shown that spores are generally resistant to various disinfectants. It is thus logical, when considering bactericidal activity, to assess the efficiency of a substance as a sporicide, *eg* Berry[49] considered that a disinfectant should be tested against a variety of organisms including spores, in the presence and absence of organic matter.

Reports on sporicidal tests have been published by Friedl and his co-workers (Ortenzio, Stuart & Friedl[50]; Friedl[51]; and Friedl[52]). The method is based on testing the disinfectant against dried spores on suture loops or on porcelain rings. The recovery medium is a thioglycollate medium. The spores tested are strains of *B.subtilis* and *Cl.sporogenes,* selected on account of their resistance to constant boiling hydrochloric acid (the reference substance).

A recent rapid evaluation of disinfectants has been published by Mossel[53]. In this method, a mixed suspension of various vegetative bacteria, a spore (*B.cereus*) and yeast (*Sacch. cerevisae*), are treated with the disinfectant for 5 minutes at 20°C. A 1 ml sample is then transferred to a sterile 'universal' neutralising solution, and the number of survivors determined in infusion and in selective agar. A disinfectant is considered satisfactory if it effects at least 5 decimal reductions* (percentage of organisms killed equals at least 99.999) in the non-sporing bacteria and the yeast. If less than five DRs with *B.cereus* are effected, the disinfectant may still be considered effective, but if the manufacturer of the substance claims it to be sporicidal, a minimum of five DRs in the viable spore count is also required.

Hare, Raik and Gash[54] described a method in which an overnight culture of the organism was spread evenly over the outer surface of the flat base of special tubes and allowed to dry. The tube was then immersed in the disinfectant solution for a specified time, the antibacterial substance removed by tap-water, and the number of survivors determined by apposing the film to the surface of a solid nutrient medium.

The main problem associated with the viable counting of surviving spores is the fact that allowance must be made for the spore to germinate, and for the vegetative cell thus produced to multiply to produce a colony. This was the basis of the method adopted by Loosemore and Russell[55] and Russell and Loosemore[56] in determining the sporicidal activity of phenol at 37°C and at higher temperatures.

The effect of individual substances on bacterial spores will be considered next.

Mercurials

In an excellent paper, Brewer[57] has reviewed the role of mercurials as antiseptics. He posed the question of whether mercury compounds could prevent the germination of spores in the animal body, and attempted to evaluate this by injecting a freshly prepared mixture of *Cl.tetani,* of constant virulence, and the mercurial into white mice and noting the number of deaths which occurred over a period of time. In the absence of antiseptic, the animals died of tetanus within 4 days. A further series of experiments was conducted in which the spores were injected into white mice, followed at various time intervals by the antiseptic under test; it was found that organic mercury compounds could prevent infection with spores, even though administered one hour after injection of the organisms. It seems likely that these compounds exert a sporostatic rather than sporicidal action, for Brewer[58] had earlier reported that spores would remain viable even when suspended in the market strength of mercurials for several years, and Morton, North and Engley[59] have shown that spores and vegetative cells may still be infectious while in a state of bacteriostasis. Berry, Jensen and Siller[60] showed that phenylmercuric nitrate (PMN) at a concentration of 0.001 per cent w/v

* One decimal reduction (DR) means that 10 per cent of the original number remain viable, *ie* 90 per cent are killed

was effective at 98°C in destroying the spores of a strain of *B.subtilis*, and this work was later incorporated into the pharmacopoeial method of sterilising injections, 'Heating with a bactericide', although criticisms of this have been put forward. Thus, Davison[61] found that relatively low concentrations of bacterial spores (of *B.cereus*) could survive the process of heating with 0.002 per cent PMN at 98 to 100°C. The screw-capped bottles used, however, were closed with a rubber liner, and since it is known that PMN is absorbed into rubber, this could be one reason for the results obtained.

Phenols

Kronig and Paul[62] investigated the effect of various chemicals against anthrax spores dried on garnets. Chick[63] found that their results could be represented by a straight line when $\log_{10}$ of bacteria surviving was plotted against time. Chick[63] went on to show that a similar logarithmic order of death was obtained with anthrax spores treated with five per cent w/v phenol.

However, phenol at ordinary temperatures is not normally considered as being an effective sporicidal agent (Sykes[64]). Coal-tar fluids, also, are almost inactive against bacterial spores. Cook[65] stated that the information available on this subject was but little, but since then Lund[66] and Loosemore and Russell[55] have shown that even phenol concentrations as high as 2.5 to 5.0 per cent w/v have little lethal effect on *B.subtilis* spores at 25°C or 37°C. Reddish[67] found that *B.cereus* suspensions heated at 80°C for 15 minutes (to remove vegetative cells) before exposure to 5 per cent phenol at 25°C were far more sensitive to the phenol than spores which had not suffered an initial pre-heating. The reason, presumably, is that certain spores can be heat-activated (see under 'Heat'), thus rendering them liable to germinate. Phenol itself is lethal to germinated spores, *eg* Fernelius[68] used 1 per cent phenol to selectively kill germinated spores of *B.anthracis*. Similarly, in contrast to its low sporicidal activity, only low concentrations of phenol are required to inhibit growth of the spores in nutrient broth (*ie* germination followed by division of the vegetative cells); *eg* Loosemore[69] found that, depending on the number of spores present, the sporostatic concentration of phenol against *B.subtilis* was 0.1 to 0.2 per cent, and Sykes and Hooper[70] found a concentration of 0.25 per cent to be effective against their organism.

The effectiveness of phenol as a general bactericidal agent is known to be influenced by various factors such as pH and temperature (Bennett[71]), and it has been found that its activity against *B.subtilis* spores is also affected by such variables. Thus, Sykes and Hooper[70] reported that whereas these spores remained viable in 0.5 per cent phenol for two weeks at pH 7.5, they were killed within 8 days by 0.1 per cent phenol at pH 3 and 4. Using a pH range of 5.8 to 8.1, Loosemore[69] also showed that phenol was more effective at an acid than at an alkaline pH.

At high temperatures, the sporicidal activity of phenol is greatly accelerated, *eg* Berry, Jensen and Siller[60] found that 5 per cent phenol at 80°C or one per cent at 98°C killed a heat-resistant strain of *B.subtilis* spores within 15 minutes. A more recent investigation has amply confirmed the increased sporicidal action of phenol at elevated temperatures (Russell and Loosemore[56]). Berry *et al*[60] also showed that 0.2 per cent w/v chlorocresol (p-chloro-m-cresol, BP) was rapidly lethal to *B.subtilis* spores at 98°C, and suggested the use of this substance in parenteral injections, as it was quite stable to heat and towards light. This method was later adopted by the British Pharmacopoeia in the process of 'Heating with a bactericide'. Davies and Davison[72], however, found that relatively low concentrations of bacterial spores (of *B.subtilis*) could survive this process.

Loosemore and Russell[73] investigated the effect of various phenol concentrations on the oxygen uptake of *B.subtilis* spores in glucose at 37°C and found that in the absence of phenol, the amount of O_2 taken up by the cells increased with time. It was suggested that this was due to the germination of the spores in glucose (a known germination stimulant), whereas in the phenol range of 0.25 to 5.0 per cent tested, germination could not proceed, with the result that no, or very little, oxygen was taken up. It is interesting to note the closeness of the concentration of 0.25 per cent in inhibiting O_2 uptake with that of 0.2 per cent phenol quoted earlier (Loosemore and Russell[55]) as being the sporostatic concentration against large numbers of *B.subtilis*. The conclusion above is in agreement with the findings of Lund[66] that phenol inhibits a stage in the germination process; this point will be returned to shortly. It appears from the work of Wolf and Mahmoud[74] on the germination and enzymic activities of spores of *B.subtilis* and *B.cereus* at low temperatures that certain enzymes are activated and diffuse into the medium during the course of germination.

Germination may be defined (Lund[66]) as the changes which occur between the mature resting spore and the vegetative cell at its first stage of division. This process may be subdivided into (i) the initiation stage, in which the spores lose their refractility ('bright' spores becoming 'dark' spores) and heat resistance, and become readily stainable; (ii) the outgrowth stage in which the spores swell, and the vegetative cells which are released elongate and finally divide. Lund[66] found that 0.2 to 2.5 per cent phenol inhibited the initiation stage in germination, whereas cetrimide allowed initiation to proceed but inhibited outgrowth. Rode and Foster[17] showed that after 64 hours treatment at 4°C, 5 per cent phenol was very effective in inducing the release of DPA from the spores of *B.megaterium*. Spores that had lost all or most of their DPA as a result of such treatment retained full refractility, *ie* were 'bright' spores. Wolf and Mahmoud[74] had earlier suggested that sporicidal substances exerted their effect in two stages: (a) inducement of germination, followed by (b) toxicity to the germinated spore. Such a proposition could, of course, explain the *lack* of sporicidal activity of phenol and cetrimide, since neither allows germination to proceed.

Alcohols

Ethyl alcohol is rapidly lethal to non-sporing bacteria, but alcohol in all concentrations is ineffective as a germicidal agent towards spore-forming bacteria (Gershenfeld[75]; Klarmann[76]).

When used at the same concentration, isopropyl alcohol is a more effective bactericide than ethyl alcohol, but is more or less inactive against bacterial spores.

Chlorhexidine

Chlorhexidine is more effective against Gram-positive than Gram-negative bacteria, but is inactive against mycobacteria, and against bacterial spores.

Quaternary ammonium compounds

The quaternary ammonium compounds (QACs) are not considered as being sporicidal substances. Cetrimide, however, inhibits a stage in the germination process of *B.subtilis* spores (Lund[66]), as already described. Benzalkonium chloride is cited by Klarmann[77] as being effective as a sporostatic substance against various *Clostridia*, *eg* the bacteriostatic dilutions of this substance against *S.typhi*, *E.coli*, *K.aerogenes* were 1 : 256,000, 1 : 64,000 and 1 : 16,000, respectively, and against each of four *Clostridia* species (*Cl. welchii*, *Cl.tetani*, *Cl.histolyticum* and *Cl.oedematiens*) 1 : 200,000. Klarmann and Wright[78] stressed that the QACs were not capable of killing the spores of resistant *Clostridia* and of *Bacillus anthracis*, and that publications which put forward an opposing view were based upon failure to control adequately sporostasis in the subcultures.

Iodine and iodophors

Iodine in aqueous or alcoholic solution is a most effective germicide, which is rapidly lethal to vegetative bacteria and also to spores (Gershenfeld and Witlin[79]; Gershenfeld[80]; Report[81]). Polyvinyl pyrrolidine and other surface-active agents solubilise iodine to form compounds, the iodophors, which retain the germicidal activity of iodine, but not its disadvantages. Lawrence, Carpenter and Naylor-Foote[82], for example, found that 1,000 ppm of available iodine destroyed *B.subtilis* spores in six to 10 hours; the lethal time increased to about 24 hours with available iodine concentrations down to 500 ppm. The germicidal activity of an iodophor is that of the free iodine present.

Davis[83] has described the factors affecting the use of iodophors and their advantages compared with aqueous solutions of iodine.

Hypochlorites

The antibacterial activity of the hypochlorites is due primarily to the release of hypochlorous acid, HClO. Hare *et al*[54] showed tha

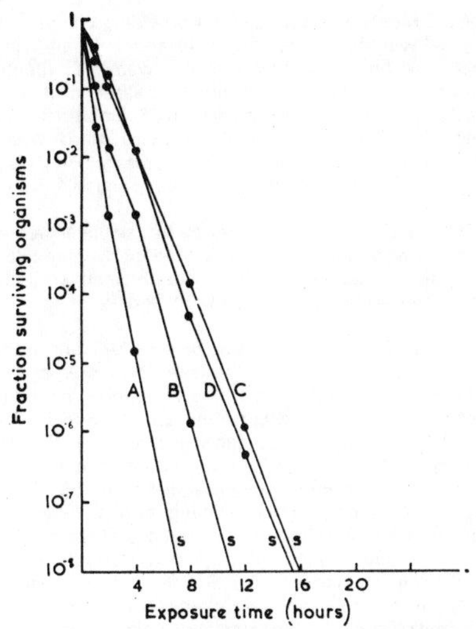

Fig 6. *B subtilis* spores on cotton patches, exposed to ethylene oxide 120 mg/litre at 25°C (s = sterile)

Per cent RH, dried and conditioned	Per cent RH, exposed
A 33	33
B 50	50
C 75	75
D 98	98

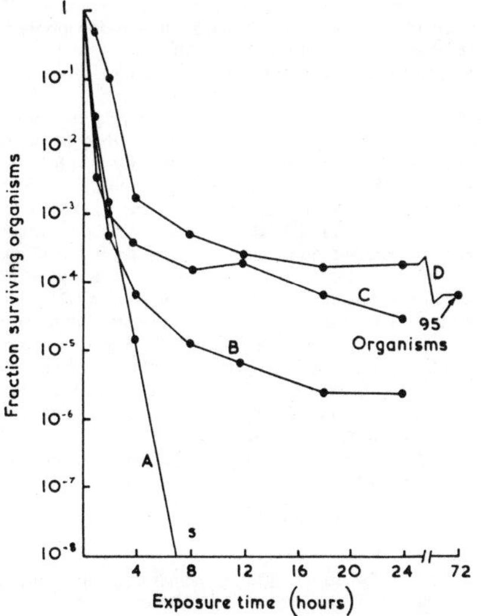

Fig 7. *B subtilis* spores on cotton patches, exposed to ethylene oxide 120 mg/litre at 25°C (s = sterile)

Per cent RH, dried and conditioned	Per cent RH, exposed
A 33	33
B 22	22
C 11	11
D<1	<1

(Figs 6 and 7 are reproduced by kind permission of Dr C. R. Phillips and the Editor, Pharmaceutical Press, London)

sodium hypochlorite was lethal to dried non-sporing pathogens within $\frac{1}{2}$ to $2\frac{1}{2}$ minutes; the hypochlorites have much less activity against bacterial spores (Report[81]), and a long period of contact may be necessary to demonstrate any death of the spores.

Dyes

Triphenylmethane dyes, which include brilliant green and crystal violet (its crude form is gentian violet), and the acridines (*eg* aminacrine, acriflavine, proflavine) have been adequately reviewed by McCulloch[84] and Sykes[64].

The triphenylmethane dyes are selectively bacteriostatic against Gram-positive bacteria; this activity includes a growth-inhibitory effect on bacterial spores.

The acridines are generally more effective against the more nutritionally-exacting species (including *Clostridia* species) than they are against the less exacting species.

Formaldehyde

Formaldehyde solution is rapidly sporicidal, according to Ortenzio, Stuart and Friedl[50], against *B.subtilis* but not *Cl.sporogenes*. Their technique has, however, been criticised by Klarmann[85], who obtained survival of spores of this organism, *Cl.perfringens* and *Cl.tetani* even after exposure for 8 hours; Klarmann also found that *B.subtilis* spores survived a 4 hour exposure to eight per cent formaldehyde solution provided that the factor of sporostasis in the subculture medium was controlled. Klarmann[76] further stated that any sporicidal action was slow.

This latter point has lately been re-emphasised (Report[81]): solutions containing 5 to 10 per cent formaldehyde in alcohol are slowly sporicidal, although against vegetative organisms formaldehyde is rapidly lethal.

Formaldehyde is also an effective germicide when in the vapour phase, but requires a high degree of humidity to exert its effect.

GASES

Most of the research on the antibacterial effect of gases has been carried out with ethylene oxide. Original work (Phillips and Kaye[86]; Phillips[87]; Kaye[88]; Kaye and Phillips[89]; Kaye *et al*[90]) showed that this gas had a wide antimicrobial spectrum, including a sporicidal action. The sterilising efficiency of ethylene oxide is related to the concentration of the gas, the time of exposure, the temperature and the relative humidity, the moisture content of the materials, and the sorptive capacity of the materials (Phillips[87, 91]; Phillips and Warshowsky[92]; Thomas[93]; Kelsey[94]; Bruch[95]; Sutaria and Williams[96]; 'British Pharmacopoeia', 1963). An example of the relationship between temperature, time and concentration, based on the results of Phillips[87] is given in table 2.

Table 2. Activity of ethylene oxide against *B.globigii* spores

Concn. of ethylene oxide (mg/l)	Time (hours) to kill 99-99.9 per cent spores at 25°C	37°C
22.1	10	4
44.2	8	2
88.4	4	1—2
442	1	$<\frac{1}{2}$
884	1	$<\frac{1}{2}$

The 'British Pharmacopoeia' (1963, page 1164) states that the temperature coefficient is about 2.7 for each 10°C rise in temperature, which is equivalent to 1.104 for each °C rise.

Vegetative organisms are less resistant than are spores, but the difference in resistance is less than that found in sterilisation by dry or moist heat (Phillips[97]; Thomas[93]).

A factor of great importance in ethylene oxide sterilisation is relative humidity; *eg* Friedl, Ortenzio and Stuart[98] investigated the sporicidal activity of ethylene oxide against the spores of five *Bacilli* species and five *Clostridia* species by the AOAC sporicide test. Their results confirmed the sporicidal activity of the gas, and also demonstrated its greater effect on wet spores than on completely dried spores, in which case prolonged exposure periods were required for a lethal effect to be observed.

A more extensive investigation was published by Phillips[91], who showed that spores dried on hard and impermeable objects, such as glass and metal, were more difficult to sterilise when thoroughly dry than spores dried on porous materials such as paper or cloth. Additional experiments, with *B.subtilis* var *niger* (*B.globigii*) were also made in which small clean cotton patches seeded with spores, were dried and maintained at a specified relative humidity before being exposed to ethylene oxide gas at the same or different rh at 25°C. Examples of the results obtained by subsequent viable counting are given in figs 6, 7. At rh values of 33 per cent and above, the order of death was exponential (fig

6); at rh values below 33 per cent, however, there was no simple exponential response (fig 7). Further, *B.globigii* spores became increasingly resistant to ethylene oxide by dehydration within an hour or less. Perkins and Lloyd[99] stated that the resistance of bacteria to ethylene oxide depended on (a) the growth phase of the organism, *ie* spore or vegetative cell, (b) the number of spores or cells present, (c) the state of hydration of the organisms. It was shown that if the rh was increased to 55 to 60 per cent and a 'dwell' period allowed, after the introduction of moisture into the sterilising chamber, solid surfaces would absorb sufficient moisture and so render the contaminants susceptible to the gas. It was also pointed out that humidification of a chamber to a rh of 20 to 40 per cent at 54°C was not sufficiently effective to render the dried organisms on those surfaces susceptible to the gas.

Propylene oxide, C_3H_6O, is less microbiocidal than ethylene oxide (Bruch[95]). Acceptable concentrations for sterilising purposes are 800 to 2000 mg/l. Bruch and Koesterer[100] found that the lethal power of propylene oxide vapour decreased with increasing relative humidity. Himmelfarb, El-Bisi, Read and Litsky[101], however, who investigated the activity of propylene oxide vapour against various sporing and non-sporing organisms, reported the reverse effect. Of the organisms tested (see table 3 for a summary), *B.subtilis* spores were the most resistant, whereas *B.stearothermophilus* spores were less resistant than certain non-sporing organisms.

Table 3. Bactericidal activity of propylene oxide vapour (after Himmelfarb *et al*[101])

Organism	Approximate D-values (mins) at rh (%) of				
	1	52	65	80	98
E.coli	24	10	6		
Ps.aeruginosa	19	8			
S.aureus	155	59	18	12	8
Strept. faecalis	110	25	8	8	
B.stearothermophilus	112	50	31	22	15
B.subtilis	974	357	117	63	54

β-Propiolactone (BPL): Curran and Evans[102] showed that β-propiolactone rapidly killed resistant bacterial spores in water,

```
CH2 ———————— CH2
 |            |
 O ————————— CO
```

milk and nutrient broth. Its sporicidal activity was greatly enhanced by increases in temperature. BPL is a colourless liquid at room temperatures; in its vapour-phase it is more active as a bactericide than ethylene oxide, and requires a rh of 75 per cent; in aqueous solutions, BPL hydrolyses to products which are not bactericidal (Extra Pharmacopoeia, Supplement 1961, p 81).

IRRADIATION

Bacterial spores are more resistant to ionising radiations than are vegetative cells (Summer[103]; Powell[10, 104]; Powell and Bridges[105]). Powell[104] pointed out that micro-organisms showed a wide range of susceptibility to ionising radiations, and that rapidly developing cells were highly sensitive; this means that spores will thus be more resistant than vegetative bacteria. Although this type of response is similar to susceptibility to heat, there is apparently no relationship between heat-resistance and radiation-resistance, *eg B.stearothermophilus* is highly resistant to moist heat, but only fairly resistant to radiation. The radiation-sensitivity of various bacteria is shown in table 4, which has been constructed from the data of Powell[10, 104] and Darmady *et al*[106].

Table 4. Lethal doses of ionising radiations

Organism	Dose (Mrads) to kill
S.aureus	0.1–0.5
Ps.pyocyanea	0.1–0.5
E.coli	0.5–1.0
B.stearothermophilus	1.0–1.5 or 1.0–2.0
B.pumilis	1.5–2.5
Cl.welchii	1.5–2.5
Cl.botulinum	About 4.5

B.pumilis is among the most resistant of aerobic spore-formers to radiation, and is now used for checking sterilisation (Powell[10]; Ley and Tallentire[9]). At 2.5 Mrads, an inactivation factor (IF) of 10^{10} to 10^{12} is obtained, although Fuld, Proctor and Goldblith[107] found that with *Cl.sporogenes* an IF of only 10^7 was obtained at this dose. However, the results of Darmady *et al*[106] indicated that a dose of 2.5 Mrads was adequate for providing complete safe which agreed with the conclusions of Artandi and van Winkle[1(

Another resistant organism which warrants attention *Cl.botulinum*, the elimination of which is essential if foods a to be satisfactorily sterilised by irradiation (Schmidt[109]). Cloust and Sangster[110] have stated that for those foods where th organism is a hazard, an IF of 10^{12} is necessary. They also sta that doses as high as 4.5 Mrads may be required for adequa security.

Powell[10] has criticised the tendency to calculate theoretica from D-values what IFs would be obtained from a particular dos since, as shown under 'Heat' the number obtained would be tr only if the line were perfectly straight and went through t origin.

Dow[111] investigated the effect of gamma-radiation at vario doses up to 2 Mrads on 3,500 dressings infected with *B.subti* spores at numbers ranging from 10^2 to 10^8 spores in multiples 10, and showed that with 2 Mrads there was a reduction in viab count of approximately 8 decades. Hunter[112] included filt paper strips of *B.pumilis* in disposable hypodermic syring which were then exposed to gamma-radiation of 2.5 Mrads, ar found that there was no rejection of syringes due to faulty sterilis tion. These two examples provide illustrations of the medical ar pharmaceutical applications of irradiation sterilisation; certa surgical dressings are listed by the 'British Pharmaceutical Code (1963)' as being sterilised by this method, and the 'Britis Pharmacopoeia' (1963) includes ionising radiations as one methc for sterilising powders.

Powers and co-workers (Powers, Webb and Ehret[113]; Power Webb and Kaleta[114]) showed that the sensitivity of bacteri spores to γ- and x-radiation was greater when spores we irradiated in oxygen than in its absence (anoxic condition). similar response has been noted by other workers (Tallentire ar Davis[115]; Tallentire and Dickinson[116]; Burt and Ley[117]; Ley ar Tallentire[9]). Burt and Ley [117], for example, showed that the D value of spores of *B.pumilis* E.601 suspended in phosphate buffe and irradiated under anoxic conditions was 0.306 Mrad whereas spores aerated during irradiation had a D-value of 0.17 Mrads.

Tallentire and Davis[115] described experiments in whic damage, induced in spores by irradiation in oxygen, increase after irradiation. In their experiments, very dry *B.subtilis* spore irradiated in oxygen and subsequently stored under oxygen die during this post-treatment storage, whereas spores irradiate under reduced pressure did not die off during post-irradiatic storage under reduced pressure. Thus, the presence of oxyge after irradiation increased the lethal damage caused by energ absorption (Tallentire and Dickinson[116]). Powers *et al*[113, 114] hav demonstrated that post-irradiation treatments influenced th survival of organisms x-irradiated anoxically. Further work on th post-irradiation effect of oxygen was carried out by Tallentire an Dickinson[116]: samples of kaolin powder contaminated wi *B.subtilis* spores were irradiated under vacuum at 22°C and the stored in controlled gaseous atmospheres at 25°C. Colony coun were made at intervals, and the slopes of dose/survivor curve were estimated from:

$$\text{surviving fraction} = e^{-kD}$$

where k is the slope, D the dose in Krad (see also Ley an Tallentire[9], under Section 1, 'Mathematical considerations'). Th higher the value of k, the greater is the lethal effect. The highe value of k (0.045 $Krad^{-1}$) was obtained with post-irradiatio storage of spores in oxygen for 48 hours, and the lowest value c k (0.01 $Krad^{-1}$) with identical oxygen treatment but preceded b exposure to nitric oxide for 15 minutes. Tallentire and Dickinson[1 also found that the development of the post-irradiation oxyge effect could be arrested by removing the oxygen, but could b restarted by readmitting oxygen to the dried spore system. On th other hand, treatment with nitric oxide between exposures t oxygen prevented further development of the oxygen effect.

Proctor, Goldblith, Oberle and Miller[118] irradiated *B.subtil* 6051 under different conditions, and found that the mea inactivation dose was affected by the irradiation atmosphere an the substrate. More recently. Burt and Ley[117] attempted to simula conditions met in practice by comparing the resistance to gamm radiation of spores of *B.pumilis* strain E.601 dried in air fror various media on to several insoluble supporting substances (glass, Perspex, polystyrene, aluminium or stainless steel) or one soluble surface in the form of polyvinyl alcohol film, with that of *B.pumilis* spores suspended in nutrient broth or in buffer solution under both aerated and anoxic conditions. The radiation resistance of air-dried spores was found to be more or less independent of the media from which they were dried, and was only influenced when the supporting medium was soluble (*ie* by polyvinyl alcohol) when higher D-values, in Mrads, were obtained; this effect is probably due to local anoxic conditions with the spores being trapped in the film during drying since (as stated earlier) the D-value of the organism irradiated under anoxic conditions in buffer was much higher than that obtained when the spores were aerated during irradiation in buffer. Burt and Ley[119] subsequently compared the effect on spores of *B.pumilis* E.601 of radiation doses given in fractions at various storage intervals, with doses delivered continuously. There was no significant difference between the D-values obtained using various treatments.

The nature of bacterial inactivation by radiation has been discussed by Thornley[120]. Increased resistance to radiation during sporulation of *B.cereus* was found to parallel an increase in cystine-rich compounds (Vintner[121]) which occurred in the spore coat, and which may act as protective agents.

CONCLUSIONS AND SUMMARY

This paper has attempted to describe the resistance of bacteria spores to various chemical and physical agents. Spores which are highly resistant to one process are not necessarily insensitive to another process.

The detailed applications to medicine and pharmacy of the various sterilisation processes and chemical disinfectants listed have not been discussed, since it is felt that these are outside the scope of the present article, and the interested reader is referred to the recent summary by Kelsey[122] on 'Sterilisation and Disinfection Techniques and Equipment'.

REFERENCES

1 C. F. Schmidt, *Ann. Rev. Microbiol.*, 1955, **9**, 387
2 N. D. Harris, *J. appl. Bact.*, 1963, **26**, 387
3 A. D. Russell, *Lab. Pract.*, 1964, **13**, 114
4 A. D. Russell & R. J. Gilbert, *Manufacturing Chemist & Aerosol News*, 1964, **35** (2), 42
5 J. C. Kelsey, *Lancet*, 1958, i, 306
6 M. L. Fields & N. Finley, *University of Missouri Agr. Exp. Station Res. Bull.*, 1962, 807
7 J. C. Kelsey, *J. clin. Path.*, 1961, **14**, 313
8 H. R. White, *J. appl. Bact.*, 1963, **26**, 91
9 F. J. Ley & A. Tallentire, *Pharm. J.*, 1964, **193**, 59
10 D. B. Powell, Symposium, 'Sterilisation of Surgical Materials', 1961, p 9, London, Pharmaceutical Press
11 J. J. Shull & R. R. Ernst, *Appl. Microbiol.*, 1962, **10**, 452
12 A. E. Humphrey & J. T. R. Nickerson, *Appl. Microbiol.*, 1961, **9**, 282
13 H. R. Curran & F. R. Evans, *J. Bacteriol.*, 1944, **47**, 437
14 H. R. Curran & F. R. Evans, *J. Bacteriol.*, 1945, **49**, 335
15 N. Finley & M. L. Fields, *Appl. Microbiol.*, 1962, **10**, 231
16 G. S. Wilson & A. A. Miles, 'Topley & Wilson's Principles of Bacteriology & Immunity, 1964', vol. 1, 5th ed. Arnold, London
17 L. J. Rode & J. W. Foster, *J. Bacteriol.*, 1960, **79**, 650
18 M. R. Headlee, *J. inf. Dis.*, 1931, **48**, 468
19 R. Koch & G. Wolfhügel, *Mitt. Gesundh Amte*, 1881, **1**, 301
20 G. A. Gerhards, *Arch. Hyg., Berl.*, 1952, **136**, 457, cited by E. M. Darmady & R. B. Brock, ref. 21
21 E. M. Darmady & R. B. Brock, *J. clin. Path.*, 1954, **7**, 290
22 E. M. Darmady, K. E. A. Hughes & J. Jones, *Lancet*, 1958, ii, 766
23 E. A. K. Patrick, R. H. Wharton, K. Prentis & A. G. Signy, *J. clin. Path.*, 1961, **14**, 62
24 R. A. O'Brien & H. J. Parish, *Quart. J. Pharm. Pharmacol.*, 1935, **8**, 94
25 W. G. Murrell, *Austral. J. Pharm.*, 1964, May 30th
26 K. Bullock & W. G. Keefe, *J. Pharm. Pharmacol.*, 1951, **3**, 717
27 K. Bullock & A. Tallentire, *J. Pharm. Pharmacol.*, 1952, 4, 917
28 B. J. Marshall, W. G. Murrell & W. J. Scott, *J. gen. Microbiol.*, 1963, **31**, 451
29 J. F. Powell, *Biochem. J.*, 1953, **54**, 210
30 H. M. El-Bisi & Z. J. Ordal, *J. Bacteriol.*, 1956, **71**, 1; 1956, **71**, 10
31 R. V. Lechowich & Z. J. Ordal, *Canad. J. Microbiol.*, 1962, **8**, 287
32 H. O. Halvorson, in 'The Bacteria', 1960, Vol. 4, Eds. I. C. Gunsalus & R. Y. Stanier. Academic Press, London
33 H. W. Walker, J. R. Matches, & J. C. Ayres, *J. Bacteriol.*, 1961, **82**, 960
34 H. R. Curran, 'Spores', 1957, ed. by H. O. Halvorson. Am. Inst. Biol. Sci.
35 R. Slepecky & J. W. Foster, *J. Bacteriol.*, 1959, **78**, 117
36 A. Tallentire & C. O. Chiori, *J. Pharm. Pharmacol.*, 1963, **15**, 148T
37 E. W. Morrison & L. F. Rettger, *J. Bacteriol.*, 1930, **20**, 299
38 E. W. Morrison & L. F. Rettger, *J. Bacteriol.*, 1930, **20**, 313
39 H. R. Curran & F. R. Evans, *J. Bacteriol.*, 1937, **34**, 179
40 A. M. Olsen, & W. J. Scott, *Nature*, 1946, **157**, 337
41 A. A. Anderson & H. D. Michener, *Food Technol.*, 1950, **4**, 188
42 J. C. Lewis, H. D. Michener, C. R. Stumbo, & D. S. Titus, *J. Agr. Food Chem.*, 1954, **2**, 298
43 H. D. Michener, P. A. Thompson & J. C. Lewis, *Appl. Microbiol.*, 1959, **7**, 166
44 H. D. Michener, P. A. Thompson & J. C. Lewis, *Agric. Res. Service, U.S. Dept. of Agric.*, 1959, Western Utilisation Res. & Development Div. ARS 74-11
45 A. N. Bose & A. K. Roy, *J. sci. industr. Res.*, 1959, **18C** (12), 248
46 A. N. Bose & A. K. Roy, *J. sci. industr. Res.*, 1960, **19C** (11), 277
47 R. Koch, *Mitt. Gesundh Amte*, 1881, **1**, 1
48 J. Geppert, *Berl. Klin. Wehnschr.*, 1889, **26**, 789
49 H. Berry, *J. Pharm. Pharmacol.*, 1951, **3**, 689
50 L. F. Ortenzio, L. S. Stuart & J. L. Friedl, *J. Ass. Off. Agric Chem.*, 1953, **36**, 480
51 J. L. Friedl, *J. Ass. Off. Agric Chem.*, 1957, **40**, 759
52 J. L. Friedl, *J. Ass. Off. Agric. Chem.*, 1960, **43**, 386
53 D. A. A. Mossel, *Lab. Pract.*, 1963, **12**, 898
54 R. Hare, E. Raik & S. Gash, *Brit. med. J.*, 1963, i, 496
55 M. Loosemore & A. D. Russell, *J. Pharm. Pharmacol.*, 1963, **15**, 558
56 A. D. Russell & M. Loosemore, *Appl. Microbiol.*, 1964, **12**, 403
57 J. H. Brewer, *Ann. N. Y. Acad. Sci.*, 1950, **53**, 211
58 J. H. Brewer, *J. Am. Med. Assoc.*, 1948, **137**, 858
59 H. E. Morton, L. L. North & F. B. Engley, *J. Am. Med. Assoc.*, 1948, **136**, 36
60 H. Berry, E. Jensen & F. K. Siller, *Quart. J. Pharm. Pharmacol.*, 1938, **11**, 729
61 J. E. Davison, *J. Pharm. Pharmacol.*, 1951, **3**, 734
62 B. Kronig & T. Paul, *Z. Hyg. Infekt. Kr*, 1897, **25**, 1
63 H. Chick, *J. Hyg. Camb.*, 1908, **8**, 92
64 G. Sykes, 'Disinfection and Sterilisation', 1964, 2nd Ed. Spon. London
65 A. M. Cook, *J. Pharm. Pharmacol.*, 1960, **12**, 19T
66 B. M. Lund, *Ph. D. Thesis*, University of London, 1962
67 G. F. Reddish 1950. Cited by C. F. Schmidt, ref. 1
68 A. L. Fernelius, *J. Bacteriol.*, 1960, **79**, 755
69 M. Loosemore, *M. Pharm. Thesis*, University of Wales, 1964
70 G. Sykes & M. C. Hooper, *J. Pharm. Pharmacol.*, 1954, **6**, 552
71 E. O. Bennett, *Adv. Appl. Microbiol.*, 1959, **1**, 123
72 G. E. Davies & J. E. Davison, *Quart. J. Pharm. Pharmacol.*, 1947, **20**, 212
73 M. Loosemore & A. D. Russell, *J. Pharm. Pharmacol.*, 1964, **16**, 817
74 J. A. Wolf & S. A. Z. Mahmoud, *J. appl. Bact.*, 1957, **20**, 124
75 L. Gershenfeld, *Amer. J. Med. Sci.*, 1938, **195**, 358
76 E. G. Klarmann, *Amer. J. Pharm.*, 1959, **131**, 86
77 E. G. Klarmann, in 'Medicinal Chemistry', 1960, 2nd Ed., p 1109. Edited by A. Burger. Interscience Publishers Inc.
78 E. G. Klarmann & E. S. Wright, *Amer. J. Pharm.*, 1950, **122**, 330
79 L. Gershenfeld & B. Witlin, *Ann. N Y. Acad. Sci.*, 1950, **53**, 172
80 L. Gershenfeld, 'Antiseptics, Disinfectants, Fungicides & Sterilisation. Ed. by G. F. Reddish. Kimpton, London
81 Report, 'Use of Disinfectants in Hospitals', 1965, Report by Public Health Laboratory Service Committee. *Brit. Med. J.*, i, 408
82 C. A. Lawrence, C. M. Carpenter & A. W. C. Naylor-Foote, *J. Amer. pharm. Ass., Sci. Ed.*, 1957, **46**, 500
83 J. G. Davis, *J. appl. Bact.*, 1962, **25**, 195
84 E. C. McCulloch, 'Disinfection & Sterilisation', 1945, Kimpton, London
85 E. G. Klarmann, *Amer. J. Pharm.*, 1956, **128**, 4
86 C. R. Phillips & S. Kaye, *Amer. J. Hyg.*, 1949, **50**, 270
87 C. R. Phillips, *Amer. J. Hyg.*, 1949, **50**, 280
88 S. Kaye, *Amer. J. Hyg.*, 1949, **50**, 289
89 S. Kaye & C. R. Phillips, *Amer. J. Hyg.*, 1949, **50**, 296
90 S. Kaye, H. F. Irminger & C. R. Phillips, *J. Lab. Clin. Med.*, 1952, **40**, 67
91 C. R. Phillips, 'Symposium, Sterilisation of Surgical Materials', 1961, p 59, Pharmaceutical Press, London
92 C. R. Phillips & B. Warshowsky, *Ann. Rev. Microbiol.*, 1958, **12**, 525
93 C. G. A. Thomas, *Guy's Hosp. Rep.*, 1960, **109**, 57
94 J. C. Kelsey, *J. clin. Path.*, 1961, **14**, 59
95 C. W. Bruch, *Ann. Rev. Microbiol.*, 1961, **15**, 245
96 R. H. Sutaria & F. H. Williams, *Pharm. J.*, 1961, **186**, 311
97 C. R. Phillips, *Bact. Rev.*, 1952, **16**, 135
98 J. L. Friedl, L. F. Ortenzio & L. S. Stuart, *J. Ass. Off. Agric. Chem.*, 1956, **39**, 480
99 J. J. Perkins & R. S. Lloyd, 'Symposium, Sterilisation of Surgical Materials', 1961, p 76, Pharmaceutical Press, London
100 C. W. Bruch & M. G. Koesterer, *J. Food Sci.*, 1961, **26**, 428
101 P. Himmelfarb, H. M. El-Bisi, R. B. Read, & W. Litsky, *Appl. Microbiol.*, 1962, **10**, 431
102 H. R. Curran & F. R. Evans, *J. inf. Dis.*, 1956, **99**, 212
103 W. Summer, *Manufacturing Chemist*, 1952, **23**, 451
104 D. B. Powell, *Manufacturing Chemist*, 1959, **30**, 435
105 D. B. Powell & B. A. Bridges, *Research*, 1960, **13**, 151
106 E. M. Darmady, K. E. A. Hughes, M. M. Burt, B. M. Freeman, & D. B. Powell, *J. clin. Path.*, 1961, **14**, 55
107 G. J. Fuld, B. E. Proctor & S. A. Goldblith, *Int. J. appl. Radiat.*, 1957, **2**, 35
108 C. Artandi & W. van Winkle, *Nucleonics*, 1959, **17**, 86
109 C. F. Schmidt, *Int. J. Appl. Rad. & Isotopes*, 1963, **14**, 19
110 J. G. Clouston & D. F. Sangster, *Austral J. Pharm.*, 1964, June 30th
111 J. Dow, 'Symposium, Sterilisation of Surgical Materials', 1961, p 61, Pharmaceutical Press, London
112 C. L. F. Hunter, 'Symposium, Sterilisation of Surgical Materials', 1961, p 32, Pharmaceutical Press, London
113 E. L. Powers, R. B. Webb & C. F. Ehret, *Exp. Cell Res.*, 1959, **17**, 550
114 E. L. Powers, R. B. Webb, & B. F. Kaleta, *Proc. Natl. Acad. Sci., U.S.*, 1960, **46**, 984
115 A. Tallentire & D. J. G. Davis, *Exp. Cell Res.*, 1961, **24**, 148
116 A. Tallentire & N. A. Dickinson, *J. Pharm. Pharmacol.*, 1962, **14**, 127T
117 M. M. Burt & F. J. Ley, *J. appl. Bact.*, 1963, **26**, 484
118 B. E. Proctor, S. A. Goldblith, E. M. Oberle & W. C. Miller, *Radiat. Res.*, 1955, **3**, 295
119 M. M. Burt & F. J. Ley, *J. appl. Bact.*, 1963, **26**, 490
120 M. J. Thornley, *J. appl. Bact.*, 1963, **26**, 334
121 V. Vintner, *Nature*, 1961, **189**, 589
122 J. C. Kelsey, *Hosp. & Hlth. Mgmt*, 1964, **27**, 606

Reprinted from *Soap Chem. Specialties* **43**, 61–64 (1967)

12

Detergent/Iodine Systems

*By W. Schmidt and M. Winicov**
West Chemical Products, Inc.
Long Island City, N.Y.

IT is now almost 20 years since the value of polyvinylpyrrolidone as a detoxifying agent was first documented in the United States (1), and since polyvinylpyrrolidone and, subsequently, nonylphenol ethoxylates were documented as of value in reducing the toxicity of iodine and for the purpose of formulating high dilution iodine products (2,3,4). The importance of the iodine complexing involved has been little understood either by the industry or by the regulatory agencies. As will be demonstrated later in this report, inadequate complexing in commercial products can result in a significant drop in iodine levels. Our laboratory has concluded analytical examination of over 100 commercial brands of iodine disinfectants. Less than 50% met their label guarantee for available iodine as received, and only approximately one half of those met the guarantee after two weeks storage at 50°C., i.e., simulating what may be expected of normal shelf life. Most of these deficiencies could be traced to formulation with unstable concentrates.

In the early development of this complexed iodine field, many workers literally depended on their noses and on the starch-iodine test for measuring differences in iodine complexing between one class of complexing agents and another. Neither of these methods is satisfactory, and some early workers, failing to notice an iodine odor or failing to recognize that certain polymer or detergent concentrations interfered with the starch-iodine test, believed they had the ultimate in iodine complexation. In reality, the degree of iodine complexing can vary bv several orders of magnitude without necessarily being discernible by either of these tests. The degree of iodine complexing and the manufacturing methods are important considerations in product formulation for the following reasons:

(1) The more complexed the iodine, the more shelf stable the product.
(2) The more complexed the iodine, the less resistance from new users on the basis of odor.
(3) Highly complexed iodine is essentially non-irritating to the skin and can therefore be handled by less skilled personnel.
(4) Freedom from unknown, undesirable iodinated detergents and detergent fragments.
(5) Highly complexed iodine products are substantially free of the corrosive effects characterizing equivalent free iodine concentrations.

Definitions

In order to clarify what is meant by the various terms used in the field, the following definitions are proposed. It is thought that the adoption of these definitions would minimize misunderstandings.

Total Iodine: *The iodine value that is obtained after an oxidative procedure such as oxygen combustion (5) or treatment with concentrated nitric acid in a Carius tube (6). This is the true total amount and includes all forms of iodine. Ordinarily, this is the same as the actual formula iodine, since iodine vaporization losses during manufacture are usually negligible.*

Volhard Iodine: *The iodine value that is obtained by treating the composition with a reducing agent such as sulfite, and then titrating by the Volhard procedure. This has been called "total iodine," but this designation is incorrect and misleading since it fails to take into account iodine in some samples or products which has formed carbon-iodine bonds. The Volhard procedure determines the elemental iodine plus inorganic iodine content. Other halides interfere with this analysis.*

Available Iodine: *The iodine value that is obtained by direct titration with thiosulfate. This value is frequently termed "titratable" or "titrable" iodine, but this term is not preferred since other iodine analyses involve titrations.*

Complexed Iodine: *That portion of the available iodine which is bound by detergent and iodide and is directly titratable with thiosulfate.*

Free Iodine [I_2] or uncomplexed iodine: *That portion of the available iodine which is not complexed. This value can best be determined by distribution of iodine between the aqueous (product) phase and an organic solvent such as heptane. The D.C. procedure given in this report can be used to determine the free iodine.*

Importance of iodine complexing little understood by either industry or regulatory agencies. Inadequate complexing in commercial products can result in significant drop in iodine levels, authors say.

* Paper presented during 53rd midyear meeting, Chemical Specialties Manufacturers Association, Chicago, May 16, 1967.

Previous publications (7,8,9) dealing with detergent-iodine formulations described the usual procedure for making such concentrates, that is, heating the mixture for several hours during which time the iodine dissolves and reacts with the detergent. After such processing (Table 1) the concentrate may be analyzed for available iodine by direct thiosulfate titration, and for available iodine and iodide by the conventional Volhard method. Using this procedure with ethoxylated alkylphenols we found that the Volhard iodine content was consistently lower than the formula amount. Furthermore, on storage at room temperature (and more rapidly at 100° or 120°F.) the Volhard iodine continued to drop, along with the available iodine. We checked this result by analyzing laboratory and commercial samples for total iodine by oxygen combustion and found that the anticipated formula amount of iodine was indeed present. This proved that there was a significant amount of iodinated detergent or iodinated detergent fragments. Products made from cooked concentrates having limited shelf lives likewise had limited shelf lives unless considerable "overages" were used in making the product.

In other experiments, (Table 2) controls were prepared in which elemental iodine was dissolved in an iodide solution (46% aqueous hydriodic acid) and added to the detergent with stirring but without heating, i.e., cold. We found that regardless of detergent type, these "cold process" concentrates did not develop any measurable amounts of iodinated detergents; that is they showed essentially no loss of total iodine or available iodine even after storage for several weeks at 50°C. The cold process was obviously the method of choice. The improved stability and quality of the concentrate and resultant products dictates the use of the more expensive iodide. Unless the iodide is put in to begin with, elemental iodine will react with detergent in varying ways to form both carbon-iodine bonds and iodide. As the iodide accumulates, the reaction slows down, but not before a considerable amount of iodine has been "lost" in reacting with the detergents and in some cases fragmenting the detergent. In the absence of added iodide, the iodine will continue to react with the detergent in the manner described above at room temperature and in aqueous products made from concentrates. The relative amounts of carbon-iodine and iodide that form cannot be predicted easily; it is best to prevent unnecessary chemical reaction by adding iodide during the manufacturing process.

$$x\ \text{Detergent} + [I_2] + y\ I^- \rightleftarrows [\text{Detergent}_x \bullet I_2 \bullet I^-_y] \quad \text{Equation 1}$$

The extra iodide was found to exert a profound effect on iodine complexing (10, 11). The problem was to measure the differences accurately. Previous investigators (12) used petrolatum equilibration for the purpose of measuring the amount of thermodynamically free Iodine, $[I_2]$, in a detergent-iodine solution, but failed to take into consideration the effect of iodide on the measurements, and the disadvantage in working with petrolatum. Our method is based on the familiar physical chemistry relationship that the distribution of a common solute such as iodine between two mutually immiscible solvents (heptane and aqueous complexer in this case) is a reproducible characteristic for the solute and solvents involved at a specified temperature. For "ideal" solutions, and where the amount of solute used is small compared with its maximum solubility, the ratio of concentration of solute in the solvents is a constant, independent of the relative amounts of solvent or the amount of solute. Although the iodine solutions with which we are concerned do not properly fall into the "ideal" class, they are sufficiently close to this goal to give physical meaning to the distribution values obtained. Iodine distributes between the heptane and aqueous detergent phase in a ratio of about 30 to 1. The qualitative relationship between the detergent, iodine and iodide can be represented by equation 1.

The subscripts x and y are used because the molar relationships between the detergent, iodine and iodide may vary according to detergent type. In the case of a product containing about 15% detergent (nonylphenol + 10 EO), 1.75% I_2, and 0.75% I^-, the equili-

Table 1. Cooked Iodine Concentrates

Cooked Concentrates	Formula	% Iodine by Analysis Total	Volhard	Available
a) WL 2958 immediately after prepn.	28.0	28.0	24.74	21.21
b) WL 2958 after 2 wks. storage @ 50°C.	28.0	28.0	23.85	18.94
c) Commercial "cooked" Product A	—	27.6	25.08	20.70
d) Product B, ~ 2 years after manuf.	—	28.3	22.90	18.65

a) Laboratory batch of ethoxylated nonylphenol cooked 4 hrs. @ 50°C. with 28% elemental iodine.
c) Fresh commercial 20% available iodine product. Formula iodine not known.
d) Commercial 20% available iodine sample stored close to 2 years at room temperature. Not analyzed originally.

Table 2. Cold Process Iodine Concentrates

Cold Process Concentrates	Formula	% Iodine by Analysis Total	Volhard	Available
a) West Concentrate 20S	28.1	28.2	28.0	21.00
b) Above Conc. after 2 wks. @ 50°C.	28.1	28.2	28.1	21.05
c) West Clean Front Concentrate	29.0	29.0	29.0	21.45
d) Above Conc. after 2 wks. @ 50°C.	29.0	29.0	29.0	21.40
e) Above Conc. after 6 months @ room temp.	29.0	29.0	29.0	21.41

a) Formula based on ethoxylated nonylphenol.
c) Formula based on ethoxylated linear nonylphenol.

Table 3

% Ethoxylated Nonylphenol (10 - 11 EO)	Per-cent I_2	Distribution Coefficients (At Indicated Percent I^-) 0.2 I^-	0.4 I^-	0.65 I^-	0.90 I^-	1.40 I^-
5	1.0	25	38	53	68	—
10	1.0	40	100	193	310	478
15	1.0	60	190	526	1,250	2,162
20	1.0	75	204	1,210	4,350	6,300

Table 4

Percent Deterg.	Percent Iodine	Percent Iodide	Distribution Coefficients (with indicated detergents*) L62	P65	P85
10.6	1.1	0.45	166	117	123
10.6	1.1	0.65	292	212	253
10.[illegible]	1.1	0.95	572	377	480

* Polyethoxypolypropoxypolyethoxyethanol

brium lies far to the right. The measurement of the complexing is described below. The fact that the equilibrium lies far to the right does not prevent titration of the elemental iodine component by thiosulfate since dissociation is rapid. The uncomplexed, thermodynamically free iodine, $[I_2]$, which is on the left side of the equation is the portion of the iodine which is free to vaporize, irritate, react with starch, etc. This alone is the iodine component which will equilibrate with the heptane layer. Since the small amount of iodine present as $[I_2]$ is increased 30-fold in the heptane layer, it can be determined with a high degree of accuracy. In poorly complexed systems a considerable amount of iodine is extracted into the solvent thereby changing the iodine concentration in the aqueous phase. On the other hand, highly complexed systems are hardly extracted. Visually, a 1.75% iodine product can give results ranging from a dark purple heptane phase (a relatively uncomplexed iodine product) to a colorless heptane phase (a highly complexed iodine product). For analytical purposes the iodine in the solvent phase is determined spectrophotometrically.

The Method

The distribution coefficient (D.C.) is determined by adding 1.00 ml of standardized test solution containing between 0.05 and 5.0% iodine to a 50 ml graduated cylinder containing 25 mls purified n-heptane. The temperature of the heptane is brought to 25 $\pm 1°C$. The cylinder is stoppered and shaken vigorously by hand for one minute during which time the aqueous solution suspends in the heptane as a uniform haze. The solution is then allowed to stand a minute or two, and the temperature adjustment and shaking are repeated. For best results the solution should settle for an hour before the iodine determination.

The amount of iodine in the heptane layer is determined colorimetrically at 520 mμ, the absorption peak; the relationship between light absorption and iodine concentration in this solvent is linear throughout the range of one to 25 mg per 100 mls. The distribution coefficient is calculated by the following formula:

$$\text{D.C.} = \frac{\text{mg I remaining in aq. phase}}{\text{mg I in heptane}} \times \frac{\text{mls heptane}}{\text{mls aq. phase}}$$

Using the Beckman DU spectrophotometer with 1.00 cm cells, an absorption of 0.142 corresponds to 1.00 mg iodine extracted by 25 mls heptane. Values so obtained are readily reproducible to within 10% and frequently to within 1%.

The D.C. as defined here parallels iodine complexing in that the greater the complexing, the higher the D.C. number. For a given available iodine concentration the D.C. values are dependent upon the iodide and detergent levels. Simple regulation of these factors can result in a thousand-fold or more difference in complexing as shown in Table 3. "Cooked" iodine products characteristically contain only from 0.2 to 0.3 parts of iodide for every one part of titratable iodine.

Table 4 shows the D.C. values for some additional detergents at different iodide levels. Table 5 shows the effect of changing the detergent concentration at constant iodide content.

Dilutions of Complexed Iodine Products

A satisfactorily complexed iodine product is one which is characterized by a D.C. number in the range of about 150 to 300 for 1.75% available iodine content. When such a product is diluted in

Table 5

Percent Deterg.	Percent Iodine	Percent Iodide	Distribution Coefficients (with indicated detergents*) L62	P65	P85
8.1	1.1	0.45	119	90	90
10.6	1.1	0.45	166	117	123
15.6	1.1	0.45	265	182	205

* Polyethoxypolypropoxypolyethoxyethanol

Table 6. Relative Color of Different Detergent Iodine Compositions at 25, 12½, and 6 ppm Iodine

	Relative Color (Absorbance units) 25 ppm	12½ ppm	6 ppm	Peak Position @ 25 ppm
a) Ethoxylated alkylphenol	.660	.160	.025	385 mμ
b) Ethoxylated linear alcohol	.820	.300	.105	390 mμ

a) Ethoxylated nonylphenol (10-11 EO)
b) Octadecyl alcohol + 20 EO

water, the complex dissociates — i.e. the equilibrium in Equation 1 is shifted to the left, so that the free iodine increases at the expense of complexed iodine. At recommended use dilution iodine concentrations of 25-75 ppm available iodine, practically all of the iodine is free (90-100%), thereby insuring rapid germicidal action. It is possible to complex iodine so thoroughly that such dilutions contain mostly complexed iodine, (10, 11) but this would not necessarily be desirable for a detergent-sanitizer. Extremely complexed iodine solutions of the latter type are useful in certain pharmaceutical (11, 13) or prolonged contact situations where skin irritation and loss of iodine must be kept to a minimum.

It is well known that one of the main advantages of detergent-iodine products is the visual indication of the presence of iodine, hence germicidal activity, at the high use dilutions employed in the field. Commonly recommended dilutions call for 25-75 ppm available iodine. At these concentrations most detergents appear to be equivalent, since there is an adequate yellow to amber coloration. Iodine is an effective germicide at concentrations much below 25 ppm, but the visual indicator property falls off rapidly below this point. At 12½ ppm concentration, different detergents may behave differently. However, outstanding iodine colors can be obtained with certain ethoxylated linear alcohols, with which iodine concentrations of 6 ppm or even lower can be seen. At these iodine levels, some detergents rival starch as an iodine indicator.

For the purpose of illustration, two compositions are reported, in which the detergent/available iodine/iodide ratio was 10/1/0.4. These samples were diluted to provide aqueous concentrations of 25, 12½, and 6 ppm and the color of the solution was read at the absorption peak in a 1 cm cell on a Beckman spectrophotometer. The absorbance readings and absorption peak are shown in Table 6. These readings are essentially proportional to the relative amount of color that the eye can see, i.e., the color which carries over into the visible region starting at 400 mμ.

Summary

Iodine concentrates and products are now manufactured by a "cold process" in which a solution of iodine and iodide are added to unheated detergent. Products prepared by this process are extremely stable with respect to available iodine content and are unique in that essentially no organic carbon-iodine bonded fragments are formed. The addition of iodide has a profound effect on detergent-iodine complexing. A practical method for determining the degree of complexing by means of distribution coefficient (D.C.) has been developed. Certain nonionic detergents intensify iodine color at concentrations below 10 ppm, rivalling starch as an iodine indicator. Analytical differentiation of "Total Iodine," "Volhard Iodine" and "Available Iodine" as described in this paper can serve as a guide for better manufacturing methods, as well as for better regulatory enforcement.

Bibliography

1) Shelanski, H. A., and A. Cantor, U. S. Pat. Appl. Serial No. 135,520, Dec. 28, 1949 (U. S. 2,675,341; 1954).

2) Shelanski, H. A., U. S. Pat. Appl. Serial No. 135,519, May 19, 1950 (U. S. 2,739,922; 1956).

3) Shelanski, H. A., U. S. Pat. Appl. Serial No. 163,082, Dec. 28, 1949 (U. S. 2,931,777; 1960).

4) Cantor, A., and H. A. Shelanski, *Soap & San. Chems.* 27 No. 2, 133 (Feb., 1951).

5) Shoniger, W., *Mikrochim., Acta, 1955,* 123; *1956,* 869.

6) White, L. M., and G. E. Secor, *Anal. Chem.* 22 1047 (1950).

7) Sutton, M. G., and M. M. Reynolds (to West Laboratories), U. S. Patent No. 2,759,869 (1956).

8) Brost, G. A., and F. Krupin, *Soap & Chem. Spec., 33* No. 8, 93 (Aug. 1957).

9) Bartlett, P. G., and W. Schmidt, *Appl. Microbiol., 5* 355 (1957).

10) Winicov, M. W., and W. Schmidt (to West Laboratories), U. S. Patent No. 3,028,299 (1962).

11) Cantor A., and M. W. Winicov (to West Laboratories), U.S. Patent No. 3,028,300 (1962).

12) Allawala, N. A., and S. Riegelman, *J. Am Pharm. Assoc.,* Sci. Ed. *42* 396 1953).

13) Cantor, A., and M. W. Winicov, (to West Laboratories) U.S. Patent No. 3,177,114 (1965).

Reprinted from Soap and Chemical Specialties *for August, 1967*

Reprinted with permission from the *Am. J. Hosp. Pharm.* **21**, 11–21 (1964)

classical and modern methods of ANTIMICROBIAL TREATMENT

13

by Kurt Steiger-Trippi

► I WOULD LIKE TO MENTION BRIEFLY THE CLASSICAL sterilization methods even though my audience consists of hospital pharmacists who, routinely, as well as in the course of research, deal with sterilization problems.

We will find ourselves dealing in conflicting terms if we are confined to the generally recognized definition of "sterilization methods" and discuss under this key-word procedures which do not *necessarily* lead to sterility. "Sterile," as you know, means: free of all living microorganisms. The emphasis is placed on "all." Therefore, a sterilization method must destroy vegetative microorganisms, spores, fungi, viruses as well as larger organisms like trichinae, plasmodia, etc.

It has been known for decades that certain soil spores can survive treatment with live steam for 10 and more hours, or that viruses frequently pass through ordinary bacterial filters, *e.g.* the Jena G5-suction filters or the asbestos-cellulose sterilization filters. Thus, such methods should not be designated as "sterilization methods." The *Austrian Pharmacopoeia IX* employs the expres-

Kurt Steiger-Trippi, Ph.D. was formerly Director of Pharmacy Service at the Canton's Hospital and Professor of Pharmacy at the Swiss Federal Institute of Technology in Zurich. He is now with J. R. Geigy A.G., Basle, Switzerland.

Presented at the Section of Hospital Pharmacists, Fédération Internationale Pharmaceutique, Vienna, September 1962.
Translated by Otmar M. Netzer-Büchel, Pharm. D., 1640 South Jackson, North Chicago, Illinois.

sion "Entkeimung"* and the *Swiss Pharmacopoeia* will use in the future the term "antimicrobial treatment" instead of the misleading concept "sterilization method." As a matter of fact, there is actually, with the exception of combustion, no procedure which guarantees the destruction of *all* microorganisms. Until recently, the treatment of objects with saturated steam at 120°C for 15-20 minutes was also considered as classical, effective sterilization. Kurzweil[1] reported in 1957 on extremely thermoresistant spores which were resistant to steam at 100°C for 8 days and which required for killing autoclave treatment at 120°C for 30-40 minutes, or at 134°C for 2-3 minutes. Recently, there was even a report on actinomycetes which could be destroyed only after 15-20 minutes exposure to saturated steam at 140°C.[2] Perhaps tomorrow an even more resistant microorganism will be found. The change in terminology from "sterilization methods" to "Entkeimung"** or to "antimicrobial treatment" is, therefore, justified. Professor Fust proposed the following definition for the *Pharmacopoeia Helvetica VI*:

By antimicrobial treatment is understood the use of procedures whose purpose is to free drugs, materials or utensils from microorganisms.

If you, as hospital pharmacists, would consider the antimicrobial treatment methods, then, contrary to the research bacteriologist, you would not only give your attention to a procedure which shows the greatest possible power of destruction, but for the purpose of evaluation, you would also have to take other criteria into account.

Criteria for Evaluation of Antimicrobial Treatment Methods

1. Antimicrobial effect.
2. Influence on the chemical and physical stability of the material to be sterilized.
3. Is it possible to carry out the method on the finished, packaged form of the preparation (ampul, tube, dusting can, etc.)?
4. Economy.
5. Health hazards for the personnel.

If these criteria were not important, then we could employ effective, true sterilization methods: Dry heating until complete charring, or heating in saturated steam at 150°C for 30 minutes. Since, however, practically all pharmaceutical active ingredients from glucose to the enzymes, are thermolabile, we have to depend on antimicrobial procedures which provide the greatest safety with regard to the microbial aspect and at the same time cause the least damage to the preparation.

The *Austrian Pharmacopoeia IX*, 1960 takes into account the high thermoresistance of spores. Thus, it specifies, for example, as the antimicrobial treatment for thermostable infusion solutions, heating in saturated vapor at 140°C for 20 minutes. The question arises immediately as to whether the other criteria mentioned were also taken into consideration. Undoubtedly, one intends with such a provision to guarantee the patient greater safety against infections caused by injections and infusions. In order to determine the necessity of increased safety, the question has to be answered if at any time and anywhere, infections from injections or infusions occurred because these preparations were contaminated in *spite of correct manufacturing and autoclave treatment*. If such cases can be cited, then this would call for more rigorous antimicrobial treatment and all economic considerations must take second place. However, if there are no such cases, then treatment at 140°C for 20 minutes is of rather theoretical interest and those in authority will have to decide on the following:

—if the possibility of the dissolution of components from stoppers used on infusion and multiple dose containers, and

—if the considerable financial expenditure required by this modern antibacterial treatment, and

—if the provision to treat sodium chloride infusion solutions more rigorously than glucose solutions, etc., are in correct proportion to the gain in safety for the patient after long experience has demonstrated that aqueous solutions for injection and infusion which were correctly prepared and autoclaved at 120°C for 20 minutes were never contaminated. Furthermore, one should not disregard the fact that the best antimicrobial treatment becomes illusive if the solution, following the treatment, flows through less well treated tubing since such infusion tubings usually are fairly heat sensitive and, therefore, will not be exposed to a temperature of 140°C.

Since the highly resistant microorganisms are apathogenic, the *Pharmacopoeia Helvetica VI* pro-

*This expression cannot be translated (verbal translation: de-germination).

**In the following the term is translated as antimicrobial treatment.

poses for antimicrobial treatment an exposure to 135°C for 3 minutes. This is only a *possible* method, *i.e.* the manufacturer of infusion solutions is not bound to this particular method. Apparently, the Swiss Federal Pharmacopoeia Commission considers autoclave treatment for 20 minutes at 120°C sufficiently safe because it exempts the manufacturer by its soon to be adopted regulations from carrying out sterility tests if the manufacturer can prove, by means of automatic temperature recording devices, that the coldest point in the product was indeed kept at 120°C for 20 minutes.

A heating period of 20 minutes at 140°C destroys, at least to some extent, many of the most commonly used active ingredients. Personally, I am convinced that primary attention has to be given to the preservation of the active ingredient because the risk of non-sterility after autoclaving for 20 minutes at 120°C drops to zero if proper techniques in the manufacture of the infusion solutions are employed.

In these typical pharmaceutical research and development problems, only the close teamwork of the bacteriologist, the analyst, the physician and the businessman with the research pharmacist can lead to their successful conclusion. Certain special problems will require consultation with the engineer and, possibly, with the physicist.

Classical Methods of Antimicrobial Treatment

Tightly-sealed, dry containers cannot be sterilized by autoclaving at 120°C for 15 minutes since the steam vapor just does not reach the microorganisms. If there is no water present in the container, then this treatment is essentially dry heating at 120°C for 15 minutes. The same holds true for substances which are not miscible with water, such as camphorated oil and petrolatum. These are well known facts. But what is the situation in the case of substances and objects into which the vapor, by overcoming a certain resistance, can penetrate only with difficulty?

Antimicrobial Treatment of Equipment

Doctor Flury,[3] one of my co-workers, has for years investigated experimentally the success of antimicrobial treatment of equipment by autoclaving. This work was carried out in the Pharmacy Department at the Hospital of the Canton of St. Gall as well as in the Galenical Department of the School of Pharmacy at the Swiss Federal Institute of Technology (Eidg. Techn. Hochschule, Zurich). The items were smeared either directly with soil which contained spores (vapor resistance more than 12 hours), or the soil containing the spores was placed in amounts of 50 mg. into gauze pouches and then transferred into the equipment. The sterility test was carried out with thioglycollate broth.

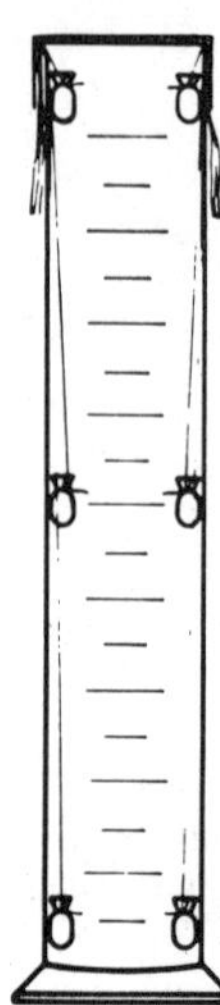

Figure 1. Graduated cylinders (height 30 cm.) with pouches placed at different levels. Cover: parchment paper. The pouches, at the bottom, in contrast to the upper ones, do not become sterile by autoclaving.

Graduated Cylinders

Gauze pouches, each filled with 50 mg. of soil which contained spores, were autoclaved in regular 250 ml. graduated cylinders 30 cm. in height which were covered with ordinary parchment paper (Fig. 1).

In dry, upright cylinders, the spores in the lower layers were not killed, whereas sterility was achieved in the middle and top layers. Pre-evacuation of the autoclave down to 65 mm. Hg *did not suffice* to induce sterility. If, however, 2 ml. of water were placed in the cylinders or if the cylinders were placed upside-down to allow the escape of the warmed air, and the rising of the vapor in the cylinder, then perfect sterilization was achieved. The upper pouches were sterile in each instance (Fig. 1).

Ophthalmic Solution Bottles

Since today ophthalmic solutions are only dispensed if they are sterile and contain a preservative, each pharmacy keeps a supply of sterile dropper bottles. The question arises: Do we reach positive sterility inside the containers with autoclave treatment at 120°C for 15 to 20 minutes? Certainly not if we use closed, dry bottles. However, if we take each bottle apart so that the steam comes in contact with all parts, then we will obtain sterility.

Positive sterility was reached for type A bottles when the pre-evacuation autoclave method was used. Without pre-evacuation the steam cannot penetrate through

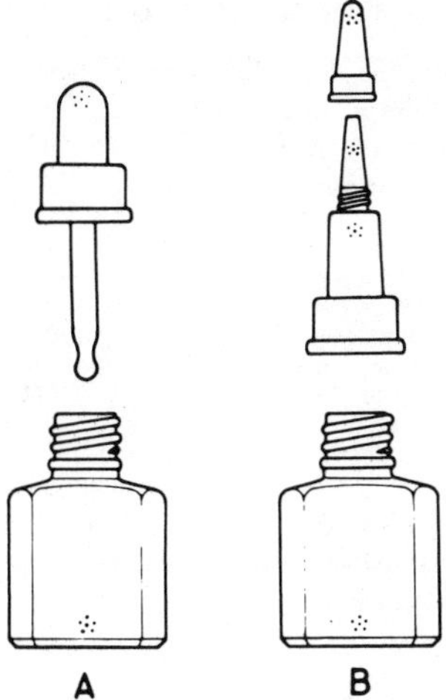

Figure 2. Contaminated dropper bottles taken apart. The dots show the spots of contamination (soil spores). For type A bottles, the bulb does not become sterile by autoclaving without pre-evacuation. For type B bottles, no pre-evacuation of the autoclave is necessary if parts are properly cleaned.

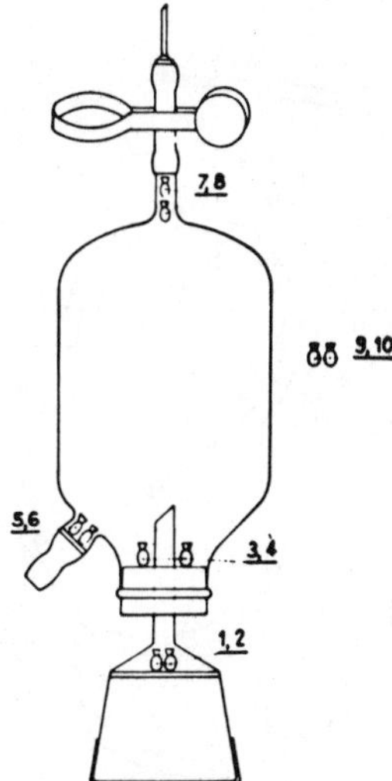

Figure 3. Bacterial filtration apparatus with pouches filled with soil which contained spores (No. 1 to 10). Parchment paper covered suction filter. The spores at contamination positions 3,4,5,6,7, and 8 are not sufficiently reached by the autoclave steam and are not positively destroyed.

the pipette and up into the rubber bulb. Therefore, this type of dopper bottle definitely requires pre-evacuation. Positive sterility for type B bottles can be achieved by autoclaving without pre-evacuation if the individual parts are properly cleaned (Fig. 2).

Hypodermic Syringes

Assembled syringes are so inaccessible to gas permeation that autoclaving without pre-evacuation is only a symbolic action and definitely is not sterilization. Here, the best procedure is still the dry heat method for 2 hours at 160°C or 30 minutes at 180°C which, however, calls for a syringe made of high quality material.

Bacterial Filtration Apparatus

A dry, readily assembled bacterial filtration apparatus (Fig. 3) cannot be sterilized in the autoclave by the ordinary method either with or without pre-evacuation.

Since the saturated steam under pressure reaches only insufficiently the corners and angles inside the container, even if the tube clamp is removed, the vapor has to be *generated* within the vessel. It is sufficient if a little over 0.1 percent of the interior space is filled with water and if the air, which is heavier than the water vapor, is permitted to escape in order to obtain sufficient vapor concentration (one kilogram water yields at 120°C approximately 891 liters of steam). As a simple rule for the antimicrobial treatment of such complicated equipment, the following should be valid: Thorough cleaning of the equipment, leaving inside and outside completely wet, to be followed immediately by autoclaving.

Infusion Sets

The positive successful antimicrobial treatment of infusion sets with heat still represents an unsolved problem. Not only is the lumen of the tubings and needles, etc., too small to allow for free steam flow but also the tubing material is too thermolabile to tolerate effective sterilization temperatures. Unfortunately, even pre-evacuation is not sufficient in cases of heavy contamination.

For these tests, the soil which contained spores was triturated with tragacanth mucilage which was then smeared on a strong thread and dried at 105°C for 2 hours. The thread was then passed into the tubings. The assembled sets were wrapped into commonly used sterilization cloth and exposed to saturated vapor at 120°C for 20 minutes. The contamination spots 1, 2, 3, 8, and 9 as well as the control soil sample 10 were sterilized in each case with and without pre-evacuation. The spores at the central spots 4, 5, 6, and 7 remained viable (Fig. 4).

Since the destruction of microorganisms represents also a quantitative problem, the attempt must be made to keep the number of microorganisms as low as pos-

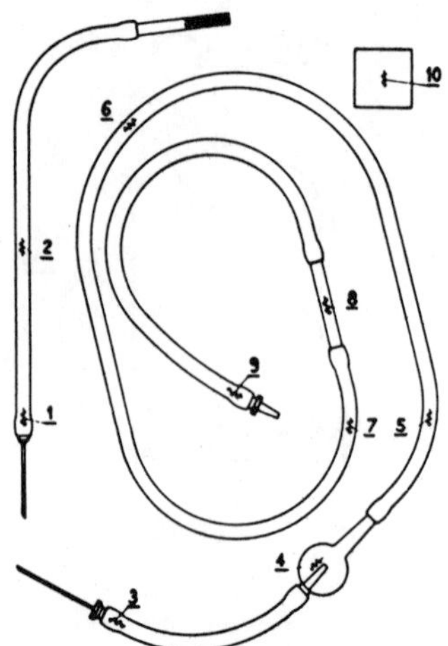

Figure 4. Infusion set, contaminated with soil which contained spores. The spores at contamination spots 4,5,6, and 7 were not killed by autoclaving with or without pre-evacuation.

sible. Therefore, a very important factor is the cleaning of the tubing. The exclusive use of new, disposable plastic tubing is warranted since such tubing is, due to the manufacturing process, practically free of microorganisms. A complete reliability on the germicidal power of steam under pressure at 120°C is not warranted in the case of infusion sets. The heat sensitivity of the plastics prohibits the use of higher temperatures. Likewise, sterility tests on a few sets out of one lot furnish only a limited safety factor.

The infusion sets are the prototype of often-used sterile equipment for which the thermal antimicrobial methods do not offer enough safety.

Antimicrobial Treatment of Glycols and Glycerin

Propylene glycol, polyethylene glycol and glycerin pose numerous problems as regards sterilization techniques. Geist[4] pointed out the danger of explosion when mixtures of glycerin and water are exposed to heat in a drying oven; heating of anhydrous polyalcohols in the autoclave at 120°C for 20 minutes is entirely unsatisfactory for the destruction of soil spores.

Flury[3] determined the following minimum water content for successful antimicrobial treatment in the autoclave at 120°C and 20 minutes:

	PERCENT WATER
Polyethylene glycol 400	10
Polyethylene glycol 4000	10
Propylene glycol	20
Glycerin	80-90

Glycerin seems to act like a protective agent for the spores. If there is little water present, then heating in the drying oven is recommended. The following temperatures and times are needed to destroy the soil spores:

Glycerin, 95-98 percent	150°C for 1 hr.
	or 140°C for 3 hr.
Glycerin, 90 percent	140°C for 2 hr.
Glycerin, 80 percent	130°C for 2 hr.
Propylene glycol, 100 percent	140°C for 2 hr.
Polyethylene glycol 400, 100 percent	140°C for 2 hr.
Polyethylene glycol 4000, 100 percent	150°C for 2 hr.

All these observations indicate that even our best antimicrobial methods have their pitfalls and, consequently, should be judged critically.

Modern Methods of Antimicrobial Treatment

Bacterial Filtration

The advantages and disadvantages of the bacterial filtration are so well known that we can omit their discussion. Only the new filter materials, nickel, bronze, and steel should be mentioned. Unbreakability and the possibility of cleaning such filters by igniting them to red heat distinguishes them from the common glass, porcelain, diatomaceous earth, cellulose ester, and asbestos-cellulose filters. The significance of the metal filters has been reviewed by Agte and Ocetck[5] and Frehn, Hotop and Stempel.[6]

Flury[3] was never able to obtain a microorganism-free filtrate with these filters during his investigations. Their largest pore diameter is given as "below 1 μ".[7] In addition, the use of these metal filters is quite restricted since they tend to release Fe^{+++} and Cu^{++} into the filtrate.

Fluorinated polyethylenes, such as Teflon®, Hostaflon®, Gaflon®, etc., are so hydrophobic that aqueous solutions, which generally have high surface tension, pass through the filters of fine porosity only with great difficulty. Therefore, their use as bacterial filters in the hospital pharmacy will probably continue to be problematical.

The polyvinylchloride filters of the Porvic® type material possess too high a lead content to be used in the manufacture of injectable solutions. Also, in our experience, the pore diameter is not sufficiently uniform as yet.

Antimicrobial Treatment with Ionizing Radiation

Primarily, two types of ionizing radiation are used for the destruction of microorganisms:

1. Electromagnetic oscillations: X-rays or Roentgen rays
   Gamma rays.
2. Accelerated electrons : Beta rays.

Electromagnetic Oscillations

Different wave lengths sections of the electromagnetic spectrum have been used for antimicrobial treatment of articles and substances:

Radio waves
Infrared waves
U.V. radiation
X-rays
Gamma rays

Guillot[8] reported on these methods in 1953 at the General Assembly of the FIP.

Qualitatively, the above mentioned rays all belong to the same family. Quantitatively, however, they differ widely from each other (Table I).

Table I. Electromagnetic Rays

	Frequency γ	Wave Length λ	Energy Quantum E
Radio waves	10^6 Hertz	3.10^4 cm.	$6.62 . 10^{-21}$ erg.
Infrared	10^{14} Hertz	3.10^{-4} cm.	$6.62 . 10^{-13}$ erg.
Ultraviolet	10^{16} Hertz	3.10^{-6} cm.	$6.62 . 10^{-11}$ erg.
X-rays	10^{18} Hertz	3.10^{-8} cm.	$6.62 . 10^{-9}$ erg.
Gamma rays	10^{22} Hertz	3.10^{-12} cm.	$6.62 . 10^{-5}$ erg.

The amount of energy of a quantum is 10^{16} times greater for gamma rays than for radio waves. Gamma and x-rays, therefore, can very profoundly interfere with the structure of substances and can produce irreversible changes even in the simplest substances. This leads us to the field of radiation chemistry, a field of science which, according to Minder,[9] encompasses all chemical changes of any material systems which occur under the influence of "ionizing radiation."

A few definitions will be helpful in giving us a common basis for the following discussion on this subject. The measurement of the *dosage of ionizing radiations* is usually based on the determination of the ionization which this radiation produces in air. The *unit of the radiation dosage* is the Roentgen (r). It is that amount of Roentgen or gamma radiation such that the associated corpuscular emission per 0.001293 Gm. of air (equivalent to the weight of 1 ml. dry air at 760 mm. Hg and 0°C) produces, in air, ions carrying 1 esu of quantity of electricity of either sign.

$$
\begin{aligned}
1 \text{ r (Roentgen)} &= 83.8 \text{ erg/Gm. air}^{(10)} \\
&= 2.00 \times 10^{-9} \text{ Kcal/Gm. air} \\
&= 2.00 \times 10^{-6} \text{ Kcal/Kg. air} \\
&= 2.33 \times 10^{-6} \text{ watt hours/Kg. air}
\end{aligned}
$$

As unit for the *"absorbed radiation doses,"* the *"rad"* is used which corresponds to an energy absorption of 100 erg/Gm. irradiated material.

$$
\begin{aligned}
1 \text{ rad} &= 100 \text{ erg/Gm.} \\
&= 2.39 \times 10^{-9} \text{ Kcal/Gm. tissue} \\
&= 2.39 \times 10^{-6} \text{ Kcal/Kg. tissue} \\
&= 2.78 \times 10^{-6} \text{ watt hours/Kg. tissue}
\end{aligned}
$$

Frequently, the literature mentions the unit *"rep"* (roentgen-equivalent-physical) which is equivalent to 83.8 ergs absorbed per gram of irradiated tissue. Other authors use 93 erg/Gm. instead of 83.8 erg/Gm. Therefore, each time it should be ascertained if rep_{83} or rep_{93} is meant.

$$
\begin{aligned}
1 \text{ rep}_{83} &= 83.8 \text{ erg/Gm. tissue} \\
&= 2.00 \times 10^{-9} \text{ Kcal/Gm. tissue} \\
&= 2.00 \times 10^{-6} \text{ Kcal/Kg. tissue} \\
&= 2.33 \times 10^{-6} \text{ watt hours/Kg. tissue}
\end{aligned}
$$

The *energy capacity of the radiation* is expressed in *electron volts* (eV). 1 eV is defined as the energy which one electron with a charge of 1.602×10^{-19} coulombs gains when rising through a potential difference of one volt.[11]

$$
\begin{aligned}
1 \text{ eV} &= 1.6 \times 10^{-12} \text{ erg} \\
1 \text{ million eV} &= 1\text{MeV} = 1.6 \times 10^{-6} \text{ erg}
\end{aligned}
$$

The effect of energy-rich irradiations is the following: Electrons of an atom are driven out of their shell and continue to move on their own along the path of ionization, in the direction of the beam, until they unite again with ionized molecules to become a more or less excited unstable particle which subsequently can split up again. These fragments consist in part of free radicals which are very reactive.[12] In the case of water there can be formed:
H_2, H_2O_2, $HO_2^{\cdot}$, H_2O^+, H^+, OH^+, H_2^+, O^+, H_3O^+, H^-, O^-, OH^-.
According to Magee and Burton,[13,14] the simplest reactions of water can be given as follows:

$$
\begin{aligned}
H_2O &\rightsquigarrow H_2O^+ + e \\
H_2O^+ + e &\rightsquigarrow H_2O^* \text{ (excited water)} \\
H_2O + e &\longrightarrow {}^{\cdot}H + OH^- .
\end{aligned}
$$

If the OH^- ion meets a positive water ion (H_2O^+) then water and an •OH radical is formed. The free hydrogen atoms unite to form hydrogen molecules, the •OH radicals can form H_2O_2.

If a simple compound, like water, can yield so many reaction products, then it is easy to understand that

Figure 5. Inactivation doses for different microorganisms by cathode rays (after Moriarty[15] cited by Lück[16])

the situation becomes very complicated for high molecular weight substances or mixtures of substances. It has been established that micro- and macroorganisms can be severely injured by ionizing radiation. Such injury causes complete inactivation of most of the microorganisms at 500 Krep to 2 Mrep (Fig. 5). The destruction of the microorganisms follows an exponential death rate, as did the thermal antimicrobial treatment. This is, with prolongation of the irradiation period, the same fraction, *e.g.* 1/2 or 1/5, etc., of the surviving microorganisms is always killed per unit time. Sterility is obtained when less than one microorganism survives.

Spores are more resistant to radiation than many vegetative microorganisms. At the Symposium on Sterilization Problems in London 1961, Trump,[17] one of the most prominent experts in this field, pointed out that viruses are even more resistant to radiation than spores.

How much the active agents will be altered by Roentgen and beta rays has to be examined and decided in each individual case. According to Miller,[18] penicillin appears to tolerate doses of 500 Krad without loss of potency. Insulin, however, becomes inactivated. Lück reported that at a radiation dosis of 2.8 Mrep, vitamin B_1, suffers about a ⅔ loss of potency but that lactoflavin, pantothenic acid, niacin and folic acid remain undamaged, results which Kuprianoff and Lang[19] confirmed and completed with numerical data. According to Schwenker and Vogt,[20] paraffins are only slightly attacked by sterilizing radiation doses. Thus, we find here a situation similar to that of heat sterilization: There are microorganisms and materials which are more resistant to radiation and others which are more sensitive to radiation, properties which can be evaluated only experimentally.

In addition, secondary effects caused by the irradiation have to be considered, *e.g.* the brown discoloration of the ampul glass (Controulis *et al.*[21]), the alteration of the medium, etc. A paradoxical secondary effect should particularly be considered: insufficient radiation doses may stimulate and enhance the growth of molds.

Gamma rays, when compared with beta rays, show a distinctive advantage. The depth of penetration of the gamma rays is relatively great, namely 10 to 15 cm. per MeV. Beta rays of 1 MeV penetrate to a depth of only 0.5 cm. Sources of gamma rays are primarily reactor waste products, *e.g.* Co_{60} and Cs_{137}. These products are now relatively inexpensive. However, the cost of irradiation installation is quite high. Lück and Kühn[11] mentioned for radiation processing of 14 metric tons (1 ton = 1000 Kg.) of potatoes per hour with 10,000 rep, which is about 1/200 of the sterilization dose, an irradiation installation which would cost approximately $500,000.00. The costs of irradiation per ton were estimated at $3.60 to $5.00.

Figure 6. 2 MeV Van de Graff Electron Accelerator for radiation processing (after Trump[17])

Beta Rays

Beta rays consist of a stream of highly accelerated electrons. Rays with 4 to 8 MeV and with output electron beam power of 250 to 500 watts proved to be appropriate. Their effect on microorganisms is similar to the effect of gamma rays. Beta rays are produced in linear, Van de Graff, accelerators (Fig. 6).

As was previously mentioned, beta rays penetrate only 1/20 to 1/30 as deep as the gamma rays. Therefore, antimicrobial treatment with beta rays may be used only for small objects, *e.g.* ampuls.

Beta rays, because of their limited penetrating power, are easier to shield than gamma rays. For this reason they are already used to some extent by industry in the antimicrobial treatment of thermolabile materials, *e.g* the antimicrobial treatment of catgut, bones for trans-

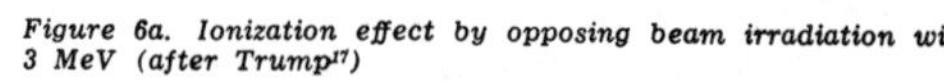

Figure 6a. Ionization effect by opposing beam irradiation with 3 MeV (after Trump[17])

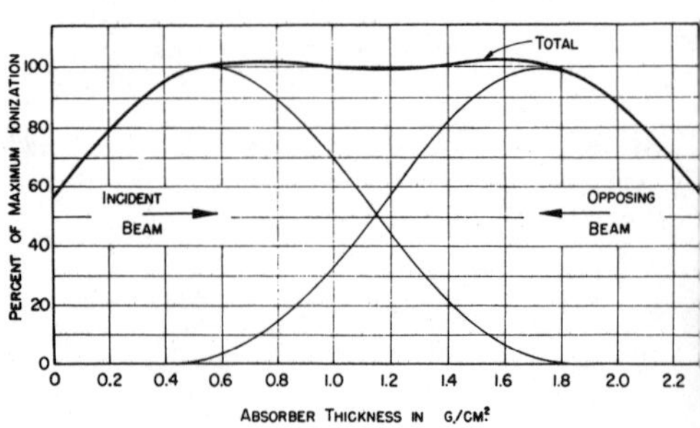

plantations, etc. The necessary radiation dose is 2 Mrad. Miller[18] calculated that 2000 catgut tubes per hour can be irradiated, involving an irradiation expenditure of ¼ d per tube which is easily tolerated by such material.

Evaluation of the Use of Ionizing Radiation

The destructive effect on microorganisms is not more reliable with ordinary radiation sources of 4 to 8 MeV than with the autoclave. Consequently, no gain in safety is to be expected over the autoclaving process. Economically, when based on a reasonable amortization, the radiation equipment does not offer any gain over the autoclaves.

The decisive advantages in employing ionizing rays as the antimicrobial treatment show up in those cases where heat or filters cannot be used. However, in such cases it must also be proved that the irradiation is harmless to the product.

The use of ionizing radiation as antimicrobial treatment is obviously worthwhile only in those instances where, in a continuous operation, very large batches of production in their final packaging, which are sensitive to heat but not affected by irradiation, have to be rendered microorganism-free. In such special cases, the ionizing rays represent probably not only the most appropriate but also the only useful antimicrobial method.

Antimicrobial Treatment with Gases

The principle of inactivating microorganisms by gases was known in ancient times. Burning of herbs containing volatile oils, sulfur, etc., was and is still done for the purpose of disinfection. Formaldehyde belongs to the standard disinfectants. Other, newer antimicrobial agents which can effectively render contaminated material free from microorganisms are the following:

Ethylene Oxide $\begin{matrix} CH_2 \\ | \\ CH_2 \end{matrix}\!\!>\!O$

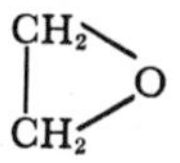

Propylene Oxide $\begin{matrix} CH_3\text{-}CH \\ | \\ CH_2 \end{matrix}\!\!>\!O$

Beta-Propiolactone $\begin{matrix} CH_2 & — & C{=}O \\ | & & | \\ CH_2 & — & O \end{matrix}$

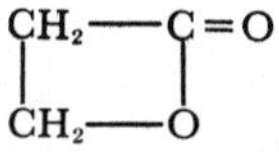

The two most important agents are probably ethylene oxide and beta-propiolactone. Bruhin, Bühlman, Vischer and Lammers,[22] bacteriologists at J. R. Geigy AG., Basle, described extensively the fundamentals and possibilities of application of ethylene oxide. The literature on beta-propiolactone is still quite scattered.

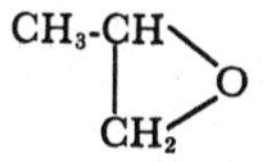

Physico-Chemical Properties

The following table lists the physical properties of ethylene oxide and beta-propiolactone.[23]

	Ethylene Oxide	*Beta-Propiolactone*
Molecular weight	44	72
Boiling point (760 mm. Hg.)	10.7°C	155°C
Melting point		–33.4°C
Freezing point	–111°C	
Vapor pressure	1140 mm. Hg (at 20°C)	3.4 mm. Hg (at 25°C)
Density	0.8694 (at 20°C liquefied)	1.149
Water solubility	Miscible	37.5% Vol.

The effect of ethylene oxide on bacteria cannot, according to Fraenkel-Courat,[24] be attributed to an oxidation of the essential bacterial substances but to alkylation or esterification of acids and to ether- or thioether formation on the proteins. According to these

ETHYLENE OXIDE REACTIONS

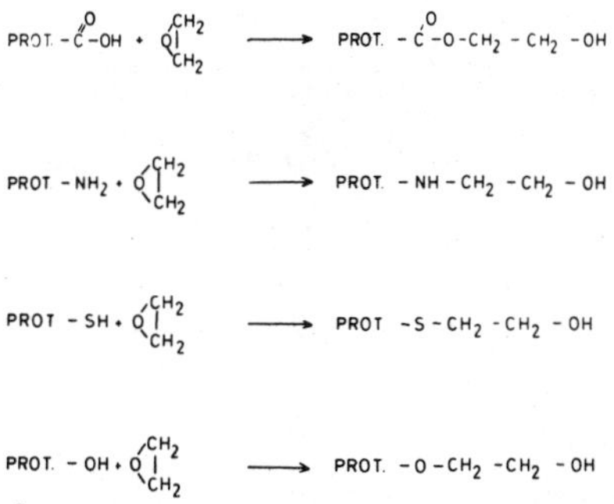

$$PROT.-\overset{O}{C}-OH + \begin{matrix} CH_2 \\ O| \\ CH_2 \end{matrix} \longrightarrow PROT.-\overset{O}{C}-O-CH_2-CH_2-OH$$

$$PROT-NH_2 + \begin{matrix} CH_2 \\ O| \\ CH_2 \end{matrix} \longrightarrow PROT.-NH-CH_2-CH_2-OH$$

$$PROT-SH + \begin{matrix} CH_2 \\ O| \\ CH_2 \end{matrix} \longrightarrow PROT-S-CH_2-CH_2-OH$$

$$PROT.-OH + \begin{matrix} CH_2 \\ O| \\ CH_2 \end{matrix} \longrightarrow PROT.-O-CH_2-CH_2-OH$$

Figure 7

equations, the reactions do not require water. However, the destructive effect of ethylene oxide is significantly enhanced by 10 to 20 percent relative humidity.

Beta-propiolactone also acts not simply as an oxidizing agent but, according to Machell,[25] reactions such as the following take place:

BETA-PROPIOLACTONE REACTIONS

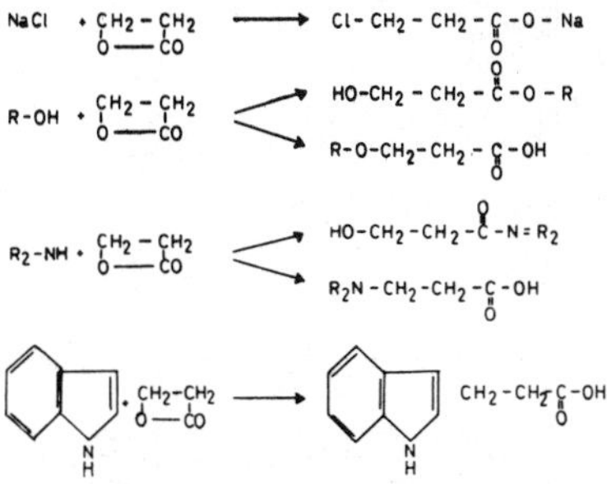

$$NaCl + \begin{matrix} CH_2-CH_2 \\ O — CO \end{matrix} \longrightarrow Cl-CH_2-CH_2-\underset{O}{\overset{\|}{C}}-O-Na$$

$$R-OH + \begin{matrix} CH_2-CH_2 \\ O — CO \end{matrix} \begin{cases} \nearrow HO-CH_2-CH_2-\overset{O}{\overset{\|}{C}}-O-R \\ \searrow R-O-CH_2-CH_2-\underset{O}{\overset{\|}{C}}-OH \end{cases}$$

$$R_2-NH + \begin{matrix} CH_2-CH_2 \\ O — CO \end{matrix} \begin{cases} \nearrow HO-CH_2-CH_2-\overset{O}{\overset{\|}{C}}-N=R_2 \\ \searrow R_2N-CH_2-CH_2-\underset{O}{\overset{\|}{C}}-OH \end{cases}$$

$$\text{(indole, NH)} + \begin{matrix} CH_2-CH_2 \\ O — CO \end{matrix} \longrightarrow \text{(indole, NH)}\ CH_2-CH_2-\underset{O}{\overset{\|}{C}}-OH$$

Figure 8

METHODS OF ANTIMICROBIAL TREATMENT

The decisive property of the two agents is their germicidal effect. Bruhin *et al.*[22] found the concentration of ethylene oxide for suitable antimicrobial treatment as follows: 1200 mg. per liter, at 6 atmosphere gage (CO_2), at a temperature of 55°C and 10 to 20 percent relative humidity. For the complete destruction of soil spores on plastic petri dishes, they recommend a treatment for 45 minutes. Under the conditions cited in figure 8a, 90 percent of the spores were destroyed—

at 1.6 mg. per liter beta-propiolactone after 2 minutes

at 0.1 mg. per liter beta-propiolactone after 42 minutes

The effect of beta-propiolactone is best at 75 to 85 percent relative humidity and diminishes rapidly with

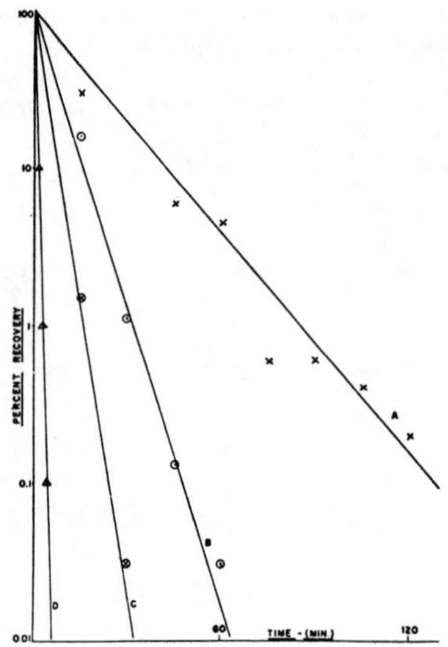

Figure 8a. Effect of beta-propiolactone concentration on death rate of spores of Bacillus subtilis var. niger. Relative humidity, 80 ± 5 percent; temperature 27 ± 2 C. Concentrations (mg. per L.): A, 0.1; B, 0.2; C, 0.4; D, 1.6 (cited from paper of Hoffmann, R. K. and Warshowsky, B.: Appl. Microbiol. 6:358, 1958)

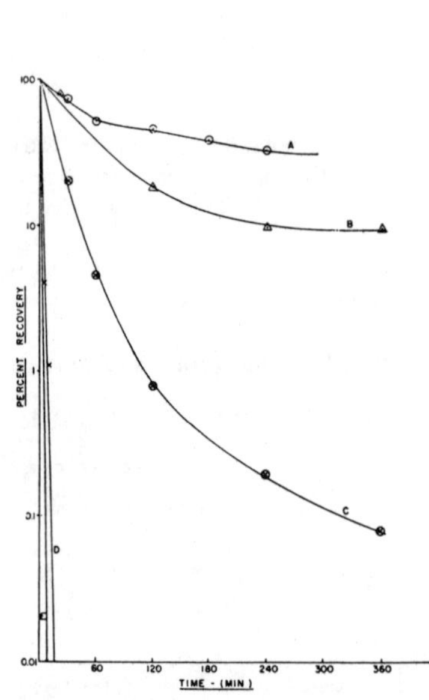

Figure 8b. Effect of relative humidity on death rate of spores of Bacillus subtilis var. niger exposed to beta-propiolactone vapor. Lactone concentration, 1.5 ± 0.3 mg. per L.; temperature, 27 ± 2 C. Relative humidities: A, 45 percent; B, 50 percent; C, 60 percent; D, 75 percent; and E, 85 percent (cited from paper of Hoffmann, R. K. and Warshowsky, B.: Appl. Microbiol. 6:358, 1958)

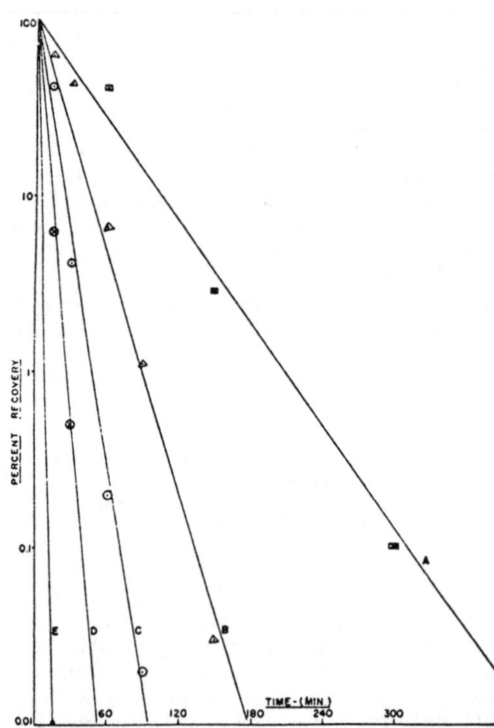

Figure 8c. Effect of temperature on death rate of spores of Bacillus subtilis var. niger exposed to beta-propiolactone vapor. Lactone concentration, 1.5 ± 0.3 mg. per L.; relative humidity 80 ± 5 percent. Temperatures: A, −10°C; B, −2°C; C, +6°C; D, +15 C; and E, +25 C (cited from paper of Hoffmann, R. K. and Warshowsky, B.: Appl. Microbiol. 6:358, 1958)

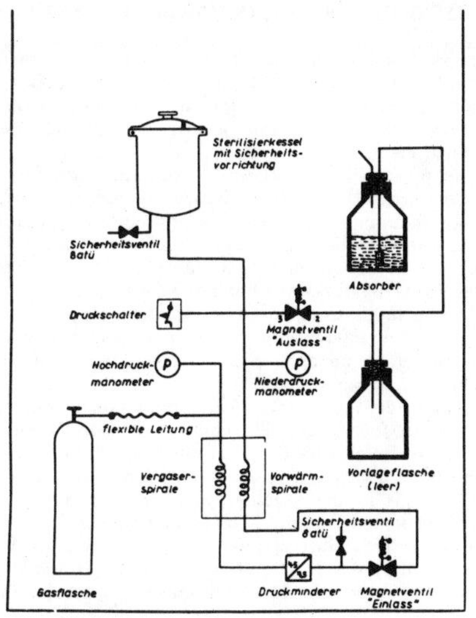

Figure 9a. Scheme of the ethylene oxide autoclave.

TRANSLATION: Absorber—absorber
Druckminderer—pressure reducer
Druckschalter—pressure switch
Flexible Leitung—flexible pipe
Gasflasche—gas cylinder
Hochdruckmanometer—high pressure-gauge
Magnetventil "Auslass"—magnet valve "exhaust"
Magnetventil "Einlass"—magnet valve "inlet"
Niederdruckmanometer—low pressure-gauge
Sicherheitsventil 8 atü—safety valve 8 atü
Sterilisierkessel mit Sicherheitsvorrichtung—sterilization vessel with safety equipment
Vergaserspirale—carburettor coil
Vorwärmspirale—pre-heating coil
Vorlageflasche (leer)—receiving flask (empty)

Figure 9b. Ethylene oxide autoclave, 100 liter capacity DMB-Sterivit-Automatic.

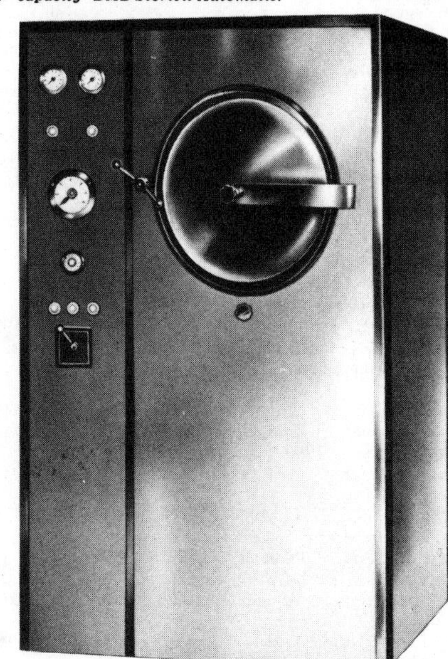

a decrease in the water content of the air. Sixty per cent relative humidity is insufficient for adequate effect (Fig. 8b). On the other hand, the effect remains excellent at temperatures from +15 to +25°C (Fig. 8c).

Application of Ethylene Oxide and Beta-Propiolactone

Application of ethylene oxide in gaseous form takes place in an autoclave-like apparatus which allows for production of vacuum or pressure. Frequently the apparatus possesses instruments to measure and control the relative humidity.

The ethylene oxide is introduced into the apparatus from a steel cylinder in suitable amount and concentration, mixed with carbon dioxide, Freon, or other inert gases. The proportion of ethylene oxide: inert gas is usually 10:90 or 20:80. The admixture of inert gas is an absolutely necessary precaution because even a 3 per cent ethylene oxide-air mixture is explosive. Following its use, the ethylene oxide is rendered harmless by passing it through a gas absorber.

Beta-propiolactone can be applied in any closed area, or in the autoclave, or if necessary, even in a drum with a tightly fitting cover. It is applied in the form of an aerosol which is sprayed into the closed area. It is rather stable in its pure form but hydrolyzes rapidly when diluted with water.[26] Therefore, the aqueous aerosol solution should be prepared just prior to use. Beta-propiolactone is extremely irritating to the eyes and mucosae.

In order to evaluate correctly possible applications of ethylene oxide and beta-propiolactone, the particular properties of the two agents have to be considered carefully. Both agents, in contrast to the thermal methods or the ionizing radiation, exhibit their effect primarily at the surface of the materials to be sterilized. Microorganisms which are enclosed in crystals will not be reached. This especially has to be considered in the antimicrobial treatment of powders. Both agents are also not suitable for the antimicrobial treatment of solutions because the quantitative removal of the antimicrobial agent or of its hydrolysis products from the solution is difficult to accomplish. In general, antimicrobial treatment with ethylene oxide is appropriate for objects and substances which are not damaged when heated to 50 to 60°C and for which low humidity (10 to 20 percent relative humidity) is desirable. It is useful to wrap the objects to be treated in polyethylene film which is permeable to ethylene oxide but impermeable to germs.

Beta-propiolactone is of advantage for the antimicrobial treatment of materials which, under no circumstances, can be exposed to temperatures above room temperature. However, those materials which are sensitive to humidity cannot be treated since effective treatment requires 75 to 85 percent relative humidity.

In each case, the possibility of reaction to the materials to be treated with the antimicrobial agent has to be determined carefully. Furthermore, it should not be overlooked that antimicrobial agents are only effective if they come in contact with the material to be treated. Complete diffusion into all "dead corners and ends" is not entirely guaranteed for very short treatment periods. Therefore, sterility testing always has to follow the treatment.

Summary and Conclusions

Evaluating the pros and cons of the methods, the following conclusions can be drawn.

Certainty of the Destruction of Microorganisms

1. Heating in live steam at 100°C is insufficient even if the treatment is carried out for many hours.

2. Heating in saturated steam at 120°C for 15 to 20 minutes offers complete guarantee of the destruction of all vegetative microorganisms, spores and viruses which are found in correctly prepared pharmaceutical materials, if a sufficient amount of water is present in such preparations and equipment. In any case, care has to be taken that all parts of the equipment come in contact with steam either by allowing for an escape of the air or by filling at least 0.1 percent of the hollow spaces with water.

3. There is probably not a single aqueous solution in a hospital pharmacy for which the autoclaving method at 140°C for 20 minutes is justifiable. Glass, rubber stoppers, active ingredients and additives suffer considerably more at this condition than at 120°C. The gain in safety for these preparations is null.

4. In concentrated glycerin, propylene glycol or polyethylene glycols, however, spores will not positively be destroyed by steam treatment at 120°C for 20 minutes.

5. Ionizing radiations yield, according to our information, positive destruction of microorganisms and spores if the radiation dose absorbed by the material amounts to 2.5 to 3 Mrad.

6. Ethylene oxide and beta-propiolactone yield—at the right concentration, humidity, pressure, temperature, and period of exposure—sufficient safety for the destruction of microorganisms at the surface of materials.

7. For the ethylene oxide method the following was found to be appropriate: 1200 mg. ethylene oxide per liter, 10 to 20 percent relative humidity, 6 atmosphere gage at 55°C for 45 minutes.

8. The beta-propiolactone procedure requires: 1.6 mg. beta-propiolactone per liter for 2 minutes or 0.1 mg. per liter for 42 minutes at 75 to 85 percent relative humidity, atmospheric pressure and room temperature.

Other Considerations

1. Many preparations and materials will, however, be adversely effected under the conditions of the above mentioned reliable methods. Therefore, the suitability of a method has to be determined experimentally for each case.

2. Beta-propiolactone treatment appears to be the most economical method because no installation, with the exception of good ventilation, is necessary. Its use, however, is relatively limited due to its irritant effect.

3. For general applications the autoclave method of 120°C for 15 to 20 minutes is economically unexcelled. If, however, some materials have to be autoclaved at 140°C, *i.e.* at 3.6 atmospheres, and others, at 121°C, this not only increases equipment costs and loss of time but also increases the possibility of errors because of the thermolabile properties of many substances (rubber and plastic, glass, vehicles, active ingredients, etc.).

4. The personnel runs relatively little risk with the autoclave. Beta-propiolactone is an irritant to the eyes and mucosae so that one has to take appropriate precautions. Ethylene oxide without the addition of inert gas is highly explosive; the commercially available 10 to 20 percent ethylene oxide mixtures are not hazardous.

5. The methods using ionizing radiations require a large expenditure for safety protection. Of principal importance here is the shielding against primary and secondary radiations, by lead, concrete, etc.

6. It is evident that the ideal antimicrobial process has not yet been found. It still requires critical, careful consideration to decide which process offers the most advantages and the least disadvantages in a particular case. The more choice there is in the selection of substances and processes and the deeper our insight is into the problems, the greater will be the responsibility of judgement placed on us to make the correct decision. It is and it will be the pride of each pharmacist to meet these constantly increasing responsibilities.

References

1. Kurzweil, H.: *Schweiz. Z. fuer allgem. Pathol. u. Bakteriol. 20*:505, 1957.
2. Dosch, F.: Paper presented at Deutsche Therapiewoche, Karlsruhe, 1961.
3. Flury, F.: Thesis, Swiss Federal Institute of Technology, Zurich 1962 (No. 3202).
4. Geist, G.: *Deut. Apotheker-Ztg. 101*:110, 1961.
5. Agte, C. and Ocetck, K.: *Metal Filters: Their Manufacture, Properties and Uses,* Berlin 1957.
6. Frehn, F., Hotop, W. and Stempel, G.: *Dechema Monograph.,* volume 28.
7. Deutsche Edelstahlwerke brochure on Siperm sinter materials, 1955. (Note: This information is obsolete for the newer Siperm-Filters.)
8. Guillot, M.: General Assembly, Federation Internationale Pharmaceutique, 1953.
9. Minder, W.: *Chimia (Aarau) 12*:17, 1958.
10. Diem, K.: *Documenta Geigy,* 6th edition, 1960, page 187.
11. Lück, H. and Kühn, H.: *Deut. Lebensm. Rundschau 55*:37, 1959.
12. Minder, W.: *Bull. Schweiz. Akad. Med. Wiss. 12*:353, 1956.
13. Magee, J. L. and Burton, M.: *J. Am. Chem. Soc. 72*: 1965, 1950.
14. *Ibid.*: *ibid. 73*:523, 1951.
15. Moriarty, J. H.: *Gt. Brit. Dept. Sci. Ind. Res., Food Invest., Spec. Rep.,* number 61, London, 1955.
16. Lück, H.: *Deut. Lebensm. Rundschau 55*:135, 1959.
17. Trump, J. G.: Sterilization of Surgical Materials, Report of a Symposium, Pharmaceutical Press, London, 1961, page 16 ff.
18. Miller, C. W.: *Brit. Instu. Radio Engrs. 14*:637, 1954.
19. Kuprianoff, J. and Lang, K.: Strahlenkonservierung, Verlag Steinkopff, 1960, page 69.
20. Schwenker G. and Vogt, H.: *Pharm. Ind. 24*:163, 1962.
21. Controulis, J., Lawrence, C. A. and Brownell, L. E.: *J. Am. Pharm. Assoc., Sci. Ed. 43*:65, 1954.
22. Bruhin, H., Bühlmann, X., Vischer, W. A. and Lammers, Th.: *Schweiz. Med. Wochschr. 91*:607, 1961.
23. Hoffmann, R. K. and Warshowsky, B.: *Appl. Microbiol. 6*:358, 1958.
24. Fraenkel-Courat, H.: *J. Biol. Chem. 154*:227, 1944.
25. Machell, G.: *Ind. Chemist 36*:13, 1960.
26. Lo Grippo, G. A., Overhulse, P. R., Szilagyi, D. E. and Hartman, F. W.: *Lab. Invest. 4*:217, 1955.

Editor's Comments on Papers 14 through 22

This series of papers shows the biological properties and the methods of evaluation to determine the efficacy of various categories of antimicrobial agents. The antiviral properties of a number of germicides were reported by Klein and Deforest; Zedler and Beiter chose to show the biological activity of a singular group, the organotins.

Burdon and Whitby, and Adair, Geftic, and Gelzer, showed contamination of disinfectants with *Pseudomonas* sp. and determined the resistance of these microorganisms to quaternary ammonium compounds. Walter and Gump tested the antimicrobial activity of combinations of quaternary ammonium compounds with hexachlorophene and showed some advantages and shortcomings that occurred when these mixtures were tested for antimicrobial activity.

Reprinted from *Soap Chem. Specialties* **39**, 70–72ff. (1963)

14

Antiviral Action of Germicides

By Morton Klein* and Adamadia Deforest,

Temple University
School of Medicine
Philadelphia

THE in vitro inactivation of bacteria by the common germicides has been quite thoroughly documented. Problems of evaluation now more commonly involve effectiveness in a given environmental situation. However, evaluation of the virucidal action of germicides is still poorly documented at the level of in vitro inactivation. There are at least a dozen different classes of germicides, some 150 human viruses and a far larger number of animal viruses. To test all possible combinations is a prohibitive task and any attempt to generalize from the limited number of studies is precarious for, as we will emphasize, viruses are not homogeneous in their susceptibility to a given germicide.

If one attempted even a tentative explanation for differences in resistance of viruses to germicides some 15 years ago one could not even begin to think of the question effectively. A virus was merely a small filterable agent needing living cells to grow and this information offered no basis for understanding patterns of resistance or susceptibility. Within the last 10 years, a body of knowledge has accumulated concerning the morphology and chemical structure of viruses. One can now take a group of viruses about which something is known and attempt to relate the structure and chemical properties of the virus and its susceptibility to germicides. This we have tried to do in our study.

Rather than review the literature in detail, let me make certain generalizations that I think summarize most of the studies:

1. Certain viruses, such as influenza, vaccinia, and Eastern equine encephalomyelitis, are readily killed by a variety of germicides at germicide levels similar to those of vegetative bacteria.

2. Other viruses, including polioviruses and coxsackie viruses, can be inactivated by germicides such as sodium hypochlorite though they have a resistance somewhat greater than that of vegetative bacteria.

3. The most striking deviation from the usual pattern of inactivation is an observation we made some 20 years ago, namely, a cationic detergent, "Zephiran," (Winthrop) was completely inactive against the Lansing Type 2 strain of poliovirus grown in mouse brain. This resistance of poliovirus was confirmed with tissue culture preparations of all three types of virus (1). We thus knew that viruses varied in their resistance to certain germicides and, as new viruses were isolated, the question arose how they would react to a germicide. In this study, we will present a hypothesis for predicting the resistance of some viruses to certain germicides.

Experimental Procedure

We have determined the inactivation of seven viruses by 10 germicides, repeating some studies already reported in the literature in order to present a summary picture. The properties of the seven viruses are shown in Table 1.

We tested three representatives of the some 60 viruses that comprise the enterovirus group, namely poliovirus Type 1, coxsackie B-1 and Echo 6. Adenovirus Type 2 is the representative of the large family of adenoviruses that cause infections in man and animals. Herpes simplex causes, among other things, the common fever blister. Vaccinia is the pox virus used for vaccination of man and is the representative of the family of myxoviruses that include the virus of mumps and the parainfluenza viruses.

Some of the viruses contain ribonucleic acid, others desoxyribonucleic acid. Some of the viruses are small, others large. We have found no correlation in this study

Table 1. Viruses Included in Germicide Study

Virus	Nucleic Acid	Size (mu)	Membrane	Lipid	Ether Sus.	Adsorption by Cholesterol
Polio Type 1	RNA	30				Hydrophilic
Coxsackie B-1	RNA	30				Hydrophilic
Echo 6	RNA	25				Hydrophilic
AdenoType 2	DNA	75				Lipophilic
H. simplex	DNA	130	+	+	+	Lipophilic
Vaccinia	DNA	250	+	+		Lipophilic
Influenza (Asian)	RNA	100	+	+	+	Lipophilic

*Paper presented at 49th midyear meeting, Chemical Specialties Manufacturers Association, Chicago, May 21.

between the size, kind of nucleic acid and susceptibility to germicides.

The three enteroviruses and adenovirus have as their basic structure an inner core of nucleic acid and an outer protein shell, the capsid, which consists of identical subunits of protein, called capsomers. The three other viruses, Herpes simplex, vaccinia and Asian influenza, have an outer envelope containing lipid. The three viruses with the outer envelope are usually susceptible to germicides, no matter whether they are ether resistant or not.

Adenovirus, like the three enteroviruses, has no lipid, no outer membrane and is unusually stable to environmental conditions. We anticipated that its resistance to germicides would be similar to that of the enteroviruses. We found, however, that the adenovirus had a pattern of resistance similar to the viruses having a lipid-containing envelope. In an attempt to find a property of the adenovirus that would explain this pattern of germicidal susceptibility we noted the study of Noll and Youngner (2). They observed that some viruses (Influenza—8 strains) combine with lipids; they called them lipophilic viruses. Viruses which did not combine with lipids they called hydrophilic. Polioviruses (2 types), coxsackie (1 type), and Echo viruses (2 types) were hydrophilic. The virus of infectious canine hepatitis, even though it apparently does not contain lipid, still, like the envelope lipid-containing viruses, was lipophilic because it was absorbed with lipids. We have found that the resistance of the hydrophilic viruses to some germicides is based upon the failure of these viruses to react with germicides having lipophilic properties. Lipophilic viruses on the other hand, are unusually susceptible to the killing action of germicides having lipophilic properties.

Determining Inactivation

Influenza virus was grown in the allantoic cavity of the chick embryo. Tests for infectivity were carried out by inoculating the virus into the allantoic cavity of the chick embryo and testing for viral hemagglutinins in the allantoic fluid. All other viruses were grown in cultures of HeLa cells, except Herpes simplex which was grown in freshly trypsinized rabbit kidney. The maintenance medium in which the viruses were harvested consisted of:

- 2% chick serum
- 20% trypticase soy broth
- 78% Eagle's medium (a mixture of amino acids and vitamins) in Earle's balanced salt solution

This medium, plus some tissue debris that remained after sedimenting the harvested virus preparations at 3,000 RPM for 30 minutes, represents the interfering organic matter. All viral titers were in the range of 10^6 to 10^8 infectious doses per ml.

Viral inactivation was determined by mixing 0.9 ml. of the test germicide (9.9 ml. of germicide was used with ethyl and isopropyl alcohol) with 0.1 ml. of undiluted virus. In some studies, virus was diluted in saline at 1:100. After contact at room temperature for 1, 3, 5 and 10 minutes, viral inactivation was determined by titering the virus and comparing the titer with that of the untreated controls. Germicide carried over in the early dilutions was frequently toxic for tissue culture cells and thus we could not determine complete viral inactivation.

Results

A summary of the results appears in Table 2:

Sodium hypochlorite. We used the commercially available "Clorox" starting with 200 p.p.m. which is approximately the concentration recommended for disinfection. At the level of the organic load in our media 200 p.p.m. inactivated all seven viruses. We have found that this chlorine concentration also inactivates a virus of monkeys, Simian virus #40, that causes tumors in hamsters and was present as a contaminant in early preparations of the Salk vaccine. The chlorine demand of the tissue culture preparations was approximately 40 p.p.m. thus 20 p.p.m. of free available chlorine failed to inactivate the viruses. However, at this concentration adenovirus showed an *increase* of 1-2 logs in viral titer. We have observed this increase in adenovirus titer at concentrations just below the inactivating dilutions with phenol and iodine. This stimulation is somewhat irregular but sufficiently consistent to be a recognizable phenomenon. This phenomenon was not observed with

Specificity of a germicide against certain virus types can be predicted on the basis of its lipophilic or hydrophilic character; antimicrobial activity offers no criterion.

Table 2. Lowest Concentrations of Germicides Inactivating in 10 Minutes

A — Sodium hypochlorite
B — Weladyne
C — Bichloride of mercury
D — Formalin
E — Glutaraldehyde
F — Ethyl alcohol
G — Isopropyl alcohol
H — Phenol
I — O-phenylphenol
J — Zephiran (Winthrop)

	A	B	C	D
Poliovirus Type 1	200 ppm	150 ppm	1:500	8%
Coxsackie B-1	200 ppm	150 ppm	1:500	2%
Echo 6	200 ppm	150 ppm	1:500	2%
Adenovirus Type 2	200 ppm	150 ppm	1:5,000	2%
Herpes simplex	200 ppm	75 ppm	1:5,000	2%
Vaccinia	200 ppm	75 ppm	1:5,000	2%
Asian influenza	200 ppm	75 ppm	1:5,000	2%

	E	F	G	H
Poliovirus Type 1	2%	70%	95% (Neg.)	5%
Coxsackie B-1	1%	60%	95% (Neg.)	5%
Echo 6	1%	50%	90%	5%
Adenovirus Type 2	0.02%	50%	50%	5%
Herpes Simplex	0.02%	30%	20%	1%
Vaccinia	0.02%	40%	30%	2%
Asian influenza	0.02%	30%	30%	2%

	I	J
Poliovirus Type 1	12% (Neg.)	10%-24 hrs. contact (Neg.)
Coxsackie B-1	"	" " " "
Echo 6	"	" " " "
Adenovirus Type 2	0.12%	1:1,000
Herpes simple	0.12%	1:10,000
Vaccinia	0.12%	1:10,000
Asian influenza	0.12%	1:10,000

1.5% HCl inactivated all of the above viruses

any of the other viruses. We have no firm explanation, but it is known that an inhibitor of adenovirus multiplication is released from infected cells and we may suggest that the inhibitor is more susceptible to the germicide than the virus itself. Thus germicidal concentrations that fail to inactivate the virus, inactivate the inhibitor with an increase in viral titer.

Provided the virus was diluted in saline 1:100, concentrations of 2 p.p.m. of free available chlorine inactivated all the viruses. We have found, as have others, Kelly and Sanderson (3), Clark and Kabler (4), that if you dilute your virus still further, until there is no organic load, as little as 0.2-0.3 p.p.m. of free available chlorine will inactivate polioviruses or coxsackie viruses. Sodium hypochlorite is a broadly reactive virucidal agent.

Wladyne. This is iodine complexed with nonionic detergents at a low pH. It was quite similar in activity to sodium hypochlorite inactivating all our test viruses at 150 p.p.m. If one diluted the viral challenge the germicidal concentration needed to inhibit dropped accordingly. One might recall that a mild tincture of 2% iodine contains 20,000 p.p.m. of iodine, over 100 times the concentration needed to inactivate all of our test viruses. Tincture of iodine is obviously a potent virucidal agent.

Bichloride of Mercury. A 1:500 dilution of $HgCl_2$ killed all of our test viruses. Though the inactivation of influenza by $HgCl_2$ can be reversed by reducing agents (5) there is no evidence that reactivation occurs in the animal body.

Formalin. This compound has long been used for the preparation of vaccines since low concentrations (1:4,000) and prolonged inactivation times preserve antigenicity. However, high concentrations (8 per cent) are needed to obtain complete inactivation of all viruses in 10 minutes.

The four germicides that we have considered thus far are highly reactive, small molecular weight compounds that show no unusual affinity for lipophilic viruses. Note that other than formaldehyde none of these compounds has any carbon atoms. However, and this will be our major observation, with the introduction of additional carbons into a germicide the compound becomes more lipophilic and will react more readily with lipophilic viruses. But a germicide may possess such a high ratio of carbon to polar groups that the compound becomes completely nonreactive with hydrophilic viruses.

Glutaraldehyde. Glutaraldehyde activiated by raising the pH with sodium bicarbonate is a recently introduced preparation ("Cidex," Ethicon, Inc.) for the sterilization of hospital equipment. At the recommended 2 per cent use dilution, it inactivated all of the test viruses in one minute. It is a powerful virucidal agent. If we compare the structure of formaldehyde and glutaraldehyde, we see that the latter is a dialdehyde containing five carbons rather than the one, as in formaldehyde. Glutaraldehyde still has its reactive polar groups, hence can inactivate hydrophilic viruses like the enteroviruses but the additional carbons give it a 50-fold greater activity against the lipophilic viruses. Glutaraldehyde is then a germicide in which the additional carbons are associated with an increased activity against the hydrophilic enteroviruses.

Ethyl vs. isopropyl alcohol. Ethyl alcohol is a very potent virucidal agent and within the range of 70-95 per cent all of the viruses were inactivated within one minute. It exhibits a slightly greater activity against the lipophilic viruses.

Isopropyl alcohol has been widely used as a substitute for ethyl alcohol and all available data indicate that it is as active as ethyl alcohol against bacteria. Isopropyl alochol has one more carbon than ethyl alcohol, giving it somewhat greater lipophilic properties. We would predict that isopropyl alcohol should be less active against the hydrophilic enteroviruses but fully active against the lipophilic viruses. As shown in the table, iso-

(*Turn to Page* 95)

Antiviral Germicides

(From Page 72)

propyl alcohol is as active--in fact somewhat more so—against the lipophilic viruses than ethyl alcohol. However, against the enteroviruses there is a dramatic loss in activity. There is no inactivation of any of the three enteroviruses at concentrations of 70-80 per cent isopropyl alcohol. The 95 per cent isopropyl has limited and irregular activity against both the polioviruses and the coxsackie viruses, though Echo 6 is somewhat more susceptible. These results indicate that isopropyl alcohol should not be considered as the germicidal equivalent of ethyl alcohol.

Phenol vs. o-phenylphenol. Phenol at concentrations of 5 per cent inactivated all of the seven viruses. However, the compound is active over a rather narrow range and 1 per cent phenol inactivates only Herpes simplex.

O-phenylphenol is used in commercial germicides. In tests against bacteria, all of which have lipid in their outer membrane, o-phenylphenol has greater activity than phenol. O-phenylphenol, by virtue of the additional carbons in the added phenyl group is a markedly lipophilic compound, quite insoluble in water and usually solubilized with soap. One would predict that, compared to phenol, it would have a greater activity against lipophilic viruses and less activity against the hydrophilic enteroviruses. As shown in the table, o-phenylphenol is approximately ten times as active as phenol against the lipophilic viruses but it has completely lost its activity against the hydrophilic viruses. At 12 per cent concentration, o-phenylphenol fails to inactivate any of the three hydrophilic viruses after 10 minutes contact.

"Zephiran," a cationic detergent. This is a distinctly lipophilic compound due to the long chain alkyl groups in the active portion of the molecule. One would expect activity against the lipophilic viruses and limited activity against the hydrophilic viruses. A 1:100 dilution of "Zephiran" readily inactivated the four lipophilic viruses while a 10 per cent solution of "Zephiran," even after 24 hours contact at room temperature, was completely inert against any of the three enteroviruses. We would expect that an arbor virus like the virus of Eastern equine encephalomyelitis, even though it is an RNA virus within the size range of the enteroiruses, would be susceptible to "Zephiran" because of its high lipid content. This susceptibility to "Zephiran" has been noted by Bucca (6). Finally, as observed by Theiler (7), bile salts destroy influenza virus and the virus of Eastern equine encephalomyelitis but fail to destroy polio and coxsackie viruses. This activity is also predictable based on the affinity of lipophilic compounds for the lipophilic viruses.

Summary

The unusual resistance of enteroviruses to certain germicides is associated with the hydrophilic nature of the virus particle and the lipophilic nature of the germicide. Bacteria are lipophilic and their use in the past for the evaluation of germicides has failed to detect the limited activity of certain germicides against the hydrophilic viruses. Isopropyl alcohol, cationic detergents and certain derivatives of phenol, though highly active against bacteria and liphophilic viruses have been found deficient in their action against hydrophilic viruses.■

Bibliography

1. Klein, M. 1956. The evaluation of the virucidal activity of germicides. *Proc. Chem. Specialties Manufacturers Assoc.*, May, 98-100.
2. Noll, H., and Youngner, J. S. 1959. Virus-lipid Interactions. II. The mechanism of adsorption of lipophilic viruses to water-insoluble polar lipids. *Virology*, 8, 319-343.
3. Kelly, S. and Sanderson, W. W. 1958. The effect of chlorine in water on enteric viruses. *Am. J. Public Health*, 48: 1323-1334.
4. Clark, N. A., and Kabler, P. W. 1954. The inactivation of purified Coxsackie virus in water by chlorine. *Am. J. Hyg.* 59: 119-127.
5. Klein, M., Brewer, J. H., Perez, J. E. and Day, B. 1948. The inactivation of influenza virus by mercurials and their reactivation by sodium thioglycolate and BAL. *J. Immunol.* 59: 135-140.
6. Bucca, M. A. 1956. The effect of various chemical agents on Eastern equine encephalomyelitis virus. *J. Bact.* 71: 491-492.
7. Theiler, M. 1957. Action of sodium desoxycholate on arthropod-borne viruses. *Proc. Soc. Exp. Biol. and Med.* 96: 380-382.

Errata:

Page 190, first column, line -16: "*Wladyne*" should be "*Weladyne.*"
Page 190, second column, line -6: "activiated" should be "activated."

Reprinted from *Soap Chem. Specialties* **40**, 76–80 (1964)

Modified Approach to Laboratory

Evaluation of Disinfectants

15

Modifications in substrate and kill time stipulations of A.O.A.C. Test suggested for more realistic appraisal of hospital hard surface antibacterial preparations

By L. J. Vinson, Ph.D.* and O. M. Dickinson,
Lever Brothers Co.,
Research Center,
Edgewater, N. J.

A GREAT deal has been written in recent years on the need for proper sanitation practices in hospitals and other institutions in controlling staphylococcal infections. One important measure which contributes to staphylococcal control is the regular use of antibacterial agents for treatment of all accessible surfaces in critical areas not only of surgery, obstetrics and nursery but also the wards, corridors, washrooms, laundry and hospital equipment. The need for such treatments has been documented many times and will not be described here. Because of the very large number of antibacterial products available to hospitals and the difficulty encountered in evaluating them correctly on the basis of their germicidal claims, classification of these agents into different activity categories has helped to clarify a confusing situation.

Two types of antibacterial products are covered by this study:

1) Sanitizer — defined by Reddish (1) as an agent that reduces the number of bacterial contaminants to safe levels as may be judged by public health requirements.

2) Disinfectant — defined by Reddish (1) as a chemical agent which destroys disease germs or other harmful microorganisms. An important consideration is that the proper use of a disinfectant is contingent on the purpose for which it is employed or on the type of infectious agent believed to be present. L. S. Stuart states in his chapter on *Methods of Testing Disinfectants* (1) that no single bacteriological test method can be expected to be suitable for determining the efficiency of all germicidal chemicals in all of the disinfecting uses for which they may be recommended. Among other things, a realistic test method should yield data that can be accurately interpreted in terms of practical disinfecting value.

Currently, the A.O.A.C. Use-Dilution Method (2) is employed as a primary evaluation in the regulatory testing of germicides sold specifically for use in disinfecting floors, walls, fixtures and equipment in hospitals. The use-dilution of a disinfectant product is required, under strict and specified conditions, to kill *Staphylococcus aureus* and *Salmonella choleraesuis* on steel cylinders within a period of 10 minutes (3).

This test is satisfactory insofar as it defines a disinfectant as an agent that destroys completely designated infectious organisms on a steel surface in 10 minutes. It does not, however, provide information as to a) what such a disinfectant will do on other surfaces common to the hospital environment and b) the ability of a treated surface to continue to destroy pathogens that may recontaminate the surface. To put it simply, a positive A.O.A.C. Use-Dilution Test indicates that a steel surface treated with an effective disinfectant is free of staphylococci or other pathogens after 10 minutes. There is no assurance, however, that the surface would remain sterile after recontamination, possible in a hospital.

These points, so pertinent in predicting the use performance of a hospital disinfectant, will now be discussed employing data on four commercial liquid disinfectants and a sanitizer:

Disinfectant I — A phenolic based formulation representative of products containing one or more of the phenolic agents—o-phenyl phenol, p-tertiary amyl-phenol, o-benzyl p-chlorophenol;

Disinfectant II — Active ingredients are a phenolic (o-benzyl p-chlorophenol) and a 1:1 mixture of 4',5-dibromosalicylanilide and 3,4',5-tribromosalicylanilide†;

Disinfectant III — A quaternary ammonium halide-based product;

Disinfectant IV — An iodophor-based disinfectant; and

Sanitizer FL—An antibacterial product whose active ingredients are lauryldiethylenetriamine and a 1:1 mixture of 4',5-dibromo-

*Paper presented at 50th annual meeting of Chemical Specialties Manufacturers Assn., Hollywood, Fla., Dec. 10, 1963.

†"Temasept", Fine Organics, Inc.

Table I. Self Sanitizing Performance of Five Hospital Products

Treated Surfaces* Recontaminated with S.aureus** and Incubated in Letheen Broth After Time Lapses

Time held before recontaminated cylinders are placed into Letheen broth	No. of positive tubes out of ten Disinfectants				
	I	II	III	IV	Sanitizer FL
4 hours	10+	6+	10+	10+	5+
6 hours	10+	4+	10+	10+	0
8 hours	10+	0	10+	10+	0
Overnight	10+	0	10+	10+	0

*A.O.A.C. steel cylinders.
**1:100 dilution of 48 hour growth culture.

Table II. Self Sanitizing Performance of Three Hospital Products

Treated Surfaces* Recontaminated with S.aureus**

Viability check following recontamination at times indicated	No. of positive tubes out of ten		
	Disinfectant I	Disinfectant II	Sanitizer FL
1 hour	10+	0	0
1 day	10+	0	0
2 days	10+	0	0
3 days	10+	0	0
6 days	10+	0	6+
7 days	10+	2+	10+
14 days	10+	10+	

*A.O.A.C. steel cylinders.
**1:100 dilution of 48 hour growth culture.

salicylanilide and 3,4',5-tribromo-salicylanilide.

Experimental

The capacity of a treated surface to continue to destroy staphylococci, applied as a repeat contamination, was evaluated. The four designated disinfectants and one sanitizer described above were subjected to the A.O.A.C. Use-Dilution Test procedure up to the point of placing the series of 10 treated steel cylinders into Letheen broth. In our procedure, the cylinders, after the 10 minute exposure to the disinfectant solution, were allowed to drain for 10 minutes on sterile filter paper placed on a Petri plate. They were then recontaminated by dipping into a 1:100 dilution of a 48 hour serial broth culture of *S.aureus*. The carriers were then placed on sterile filter paper in a Petri plate and held for 4, 6, 8 hours and overnight before placing into Letheen broth for 48 hours incubation at 37°C. as called for in the regular A.O.A.C. Use-Dilution procedure. Tubes showing positive growth evidenced by turbidity indicated treatment by the disinfectant to be ineffectual. Clear tubes signified kill of the test organism. Table I indicates that only surfaces treated with Disinfectant II and the Sanitizer have the capacity to continue to kill *S.aureus* applied as a recontamination. The time required to give complete kill under these conditions is between 4-6 hours for the Sanitizer FL and 6-8 hours for Disinfectant II. Of particular significance is the action of Sanitizer FL which did not pass the regular A.O.A.C. Use-Dilution Test only because of the time limitation of 10 minutes to effect kill of the test organism.

In a similiar study, the cylinders treated with the hospital products, according to the A.O.A.C. Use-Dilution Test, were held after removal from the disinfectant solutions for varying periods of time—1 hour, 1 day and longer—before recontamination with a 1:100 dilution of a 48 hour serial broth culture of *S. aureus*. All carriers were then held overnight and placed in Letheen broth for 48 hours at 37°C. Data on Disinfectants I and II and the Sanitizer are given in Table II. Disinfectant I showed no activity against recontamination while Disinfectant II provided a self-sanitizing surface capable of activity up to 6-7 days following treatment. Sanitizer FL also exhibited prolonged activity, with treated surfaces showing self-sanitizing action for at least 3 days.

The effect of relative humidity on the capacity of hospital formulations to impart self-sanitizing activity to treated surfaces was studied. The procedure was the same as previously described: The

Table III. Effect of Relative Humidity on Self Sanitizing Activity of Hard Surfaces Treated With Hospital Products

(Re-Inoculation with S.aureus of Treated A.O.A.C. Steel Cylinders)

Relative humidity	No. of positive tubes per indicated total tubes		
	Disinfectant I	Disinfectant II	Sanitizer FL
Not controlled	30/30	0/30	0/30
0% R.H.	30/30	0/30	3/30
33% R.H.	20/20	0/30	0/20
53% R.H.	20/20	1/30	0/20
75% R.H.	10/10	0/30	0/30
100% R.H.	20/20	0/30	0/30

Table IV. Activity of Three Hospital Products on Different Hard Surfaces Employing Modified A.O.A.C. Use-Dilution Procedure

Surface	No. positive tubes per indicated total tubes samples incubated in Letheen broth		
	Disinfectant I	Disinfectant II	Sanitizer FL
Linoleum—unwaxed	44/50	27/50	—
waxed	10/10	11/30	20/20
Vinyl—unwaxed	50/50	31/50	—
waxed	20/50	20/30	8/10
Rubber—unwaxed	50/50	36/50	—
waxed	10/10	19/30	10/10
Asphalt—unwaxed	50/50	50/50	—
waxed	20/20	24/30	12/20
Steel cylinder	0/30	0/30	10/10
Painted plasterboard	0/20	0/20	10/10
Ceramic tile	0/20	0/20	10/10

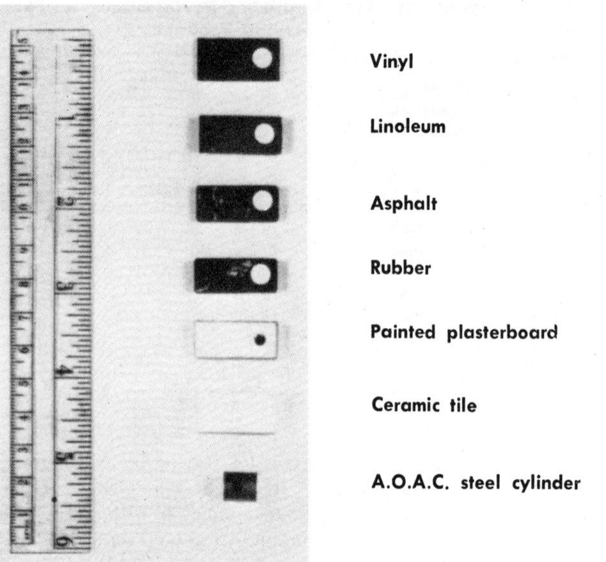

Figure 1. Hard surface materials employed in the disinfectant testing of hospital products.

steel cylinders, after being treated with the disinfectant, were drained for 10 minutes and reinoculated by dipping into a 1:1000 dilution of a 48 hour serial broth culture of *S.aureus* in 0.1% peptone water. One set of treated cylinders was observed without controlled relative humidity and other sets were left overnight in desiccators maintained at the following relative humidities: 0%, 33%, 55%, 75% and 100% R.H. As can be seen in Table III, Disinfectant I is inactive at all relative humidities while Disinfectant II and Sanitizer FL are active at all levels. It should be pointed out that the desiccators were sterilized by ethylene oxide to prevent chance contamination from moisture condensation at high R.H.

Evaluation on Different Surfaces

The antimicrobials were evaluated for disinfectant action on the following realistic surfaces: Linoleum, vinyl, asphalt, rubber, ceramic tile and painted plasterboard. Tiles were cut into 5 x 30 mm. samples and each had a hole punched out at one end to facilitate transfer by a platinum wire or similar device. Figure 1 is a photograph of these samples and in Figure 2 a tile sample is seen being handled by the bacteriologist.

The A.O.A.C. Use-Dilution procedure was modified slightly, since, for the most part, these surfaces could not be treated like steel cylinders because of a) their susceptibility to the high temperature of autoclaving and b) the flooring materials used have thick backing or felt making inoculation by total immersion impractical. The changes made to overcome these difficulties were:

1) All tile samples were sterilized overnight in desiccators filled with ethylene oxide.

2) Inoculation of the surfaces of these tiles was accomplished by platinum loop calibrated to deliver 0.001 ml. This gave an inoculum of approximately 100,000 cells, a number found on steel cylinders inoculated by the conventional A.O.A.C. Use-Dilution technique. After loop inoculation, the tile surfaces were dried for 20 minutes in a 37°C. incubator.

The tile samples, in series of 10 replicates, were immersed in 10 ml. of use-dilution of the test products for exactly 10 minutes. Transfers were then made into each of two subculture media, a) A.O.A.C. Letheen broth and b) A.O.A.C. nutrient broth. All tiles were incubated for 48 hours. Those subcultured into nutrient broth showing no growth were re-subcultured into Letheen broth for an additional 48 hours. Results of the Letheen broth series appear in Table IV. Both Disinfectants I and

Figure 2. Tile sample being handled by bacteriologist.

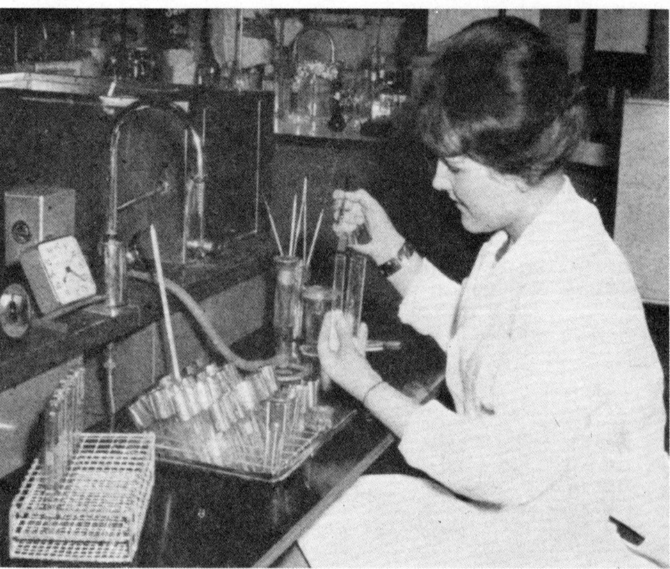

Table V. Activity of Three Products on Contaminated Waxed Asphalt Tile by Modified A.O.A.C. Use-Dilution Procedure

Samples Held Overnight Before Placing in Letheen Broth

	Disinfectant I	Disinfectant II	Sanitizer FL
	No. of positive tubes out of ten		
Treated samples placed directly into Letheen broth after holding overnight	0	0	0
Treated samples recontaminated before holding overnight and placing into Leethen broth	8+	0	0

Table VI. Activity of Three Hospital Products on Different Hard Surfaces Employing Modified A.O.A.C. Use-Dilution Procedure

Surface	Disinfectant I	Disinfectant II	Sanitizer FL
	No. positive tubes per indicated total tubes samples incubated in nutrient broth		
Linoleum—unwaxed	30/30	1/30	
waxed		0/10	
Vinyl—unwaxed	30/30	0/30	
waxed		0/10	1/10
Rubber—unwaxed	30/30	6/30	
waxed		2/30	2/10
Asphalt—unwaxed	30/30	28/30	
waxed	9/10	2/10	0/10
Steel cylinders	0/20	0/20	0/10
Painted plasterboard	0/20	0/20	0/10
Ceramic tile	0/20	0/20	0/10

II were effective on hard surfaces—steel cylinders, painted plasterboard and ceramic tile. However, Disinfectant I was inactive on linoleum, vinyl, rubber and asphalt tiles. Disinfectant II showed partial activity and some evidence that it performs better on waxed surfaces. Sanitizer FL was not effective on any of the surfaces, since the Letheen broth limits the kill time to 10 minutes, a period too short for Sanitizer FL to act.

In a limited study, Disinfectant III, the quaternary-ammonium halide-based product was found to be inactive when checked on waxed asphalt while Disinfectant IV, the iodophor preparation, gave almost complete kill.

To determine whether the treated porous surface (waxed asphalt), if given sufficient time to act, will kill the test organism, the following test was run: Waxed asphalt tiles were contaminated by loop with *S.aureus* and treated with the disinfectant preparation. Before being placed into Letheen broth, the tiles were allowed to stand overnight. After 48 hours' incubation, all tiles treated with Disinfectants I and II, and Sanitizer FL were found free of staphylococci, indicating kill on prolonged contact (Table V). If the treated tiles are recontaminated before being held overnight, the results show tiles treated with Disinfectant II and Sanitizer FL to have the capacity to destroy the second inoculum of *S. aureus*. Disinfectant I fails in this case (Table V). In a separate test, Disinfectants III and IV were observed to fail in the re-inoculation study of treated waxed asphalt.

In the nutrient broth series (Table VI), Disinfectants I and II as well as the Sanitizer FL were effective on the hard surfaces— steel cylinders, painted plasterboard and ceramic tile. However, there were significant differences in activity on the porous tiles. Disinfectant I failed again while Disinfectant II and Sanitizer FL were, for the most part, effective. Of particular interest was the increased activity of Disinfectant II on waxed asphalt compared with unwaxed asphalt.

Discussion, Conclusions

Four hospital disinfectants, different in composition and similar in action in the A.O.A.C. Use-Dilution Test, were found to differ in antibacterial action in other tests simulating use conditions. In fact, Sanitizer FL, which does not qualify as a disinfectant under existing standards, is superior in action in these tests to some disinfectants which do so qualify.

Several of the findings reported have an important bearing on the hospital performance characteristics of disinfectants:

1. Hard surfaces treated with a disinfectant can—for a reasonable period of time—continue to destroy subsequent contamination. Surprisingly, some disinfectants which destroy staphylococci on contact (within 10 minutes) do not render treated surfaces self-sanitizing *viz.*, able to kill new additions of staphylococci.

2. Of the five hospital preparations tested only Disinfectant II and Sanitizer FL demonstrated self-sanitizing activity at all relative humidities checked.

3. The self-sanitizing properties of steel surfaces treated with Disinfectant II last up to 6 days and, in the case of Sanitizer FL, somewhat shorter. Such treated surfaces become an important tool in combating cross-contamination known to exist in hospitals.

4. We employed conditions stipulated in the A.O.A.C. Use-Dilution Test with only minor modifications in sample preparation and inoculation technique. We made the rather disturbing discovery that porous surfaces such as vinyl, linoleum, asbestos, and rubber cannot be disinfected within the required 10 minutes. This applies to all hospital preparations tested. However, if Letheen broth is replaced by nutrient broth which permits continued action by the germicide, Disinfectant II and Sanitizer FL will destroy the staphylococcal inoculum almost completely. Disinfectant I fails in nutrient broth.

In another series of experiments the porous tiles treated once with the disinfectant preparations were allowed to stand overnight before being placed into Letheen broth. They destroyed the test organism completely. Disinfectants I and II and Sanitizer FL were effective under these conditions. However, if the porous tiles are recontaminated immediately with *S.aureus*, before being allowed to stand overnight, Disinfectant I fails, while Disinfectant II and Sanitizer FL provide complete protection.

The importance of these findings lies in the observation that a 10 minute period for kill action, as required in the A.O.A.C. Use-Dilution Test on steel cylinders, is insufficient to kill *S.aureus* on realistic porous surfaces. Apparently, penetration of porous surfaces is a very important consideration in the evaluation of disinfectant action by hospital antibacterials. A summary of results obtained in the various tests described is given in Table VII. All disinfectants tested are similar in action on hard and impervious surfaces like steel, painted plasterboard and ceramic tile. Disinfectants differ in their action on porous surfaces, some showing poor activity. They also differ in their ability to provide self-sanitizing properties to hard surfaces. Interestingly enough, Sanitizer FL, although not active in the Standard A.O.A.C. Use-Dilution Test, is superior to some disinfectants in the modified tests.

The difference in activity of disinfectants tested on porous *vs.* unporous surfaces was pointed out also in an interesting paper by Walter and Foris on "Antibacterial Residuals on Inanimate Surfaces" given at the 49th Annual Meeting of CSMA in Washington, D. C. (4) Phenolic disinfectants were found active on glass slides contaminated with a dry inoculum of the test organism in talc powder, but were not active when tested on similarly contaminated vinyl asbestos. These authors also observed that activity was poor at low relative humidity in contrast to some of the results given in this report. The difference is probably due to the fact that Walter and Foris employ a dry inoculum on a talc carrier making it difficult for the residual disinfectant left on the surface to reach the test organism effectively.

About two years ago, Reddish (5) stressed the importance of performance tests in the evaluation of germicidal preparations for use in hospitals. He suggested that performance tests should be employ[ed] in determining the effectiveness [of] all disinfectants, and label clai[ms] and directions for use be based [on] results from such practical tes[ts]. Because of the many difficulties i[n]volved in conducting actual p[er]formance tests in hospitals, the [al]ternative is to predict use prope[r]ties of disinfectants by laborato[ry] tests that simulate more close[ly] the performance of disinfectants [in] hospitals.

In conclusion, the offici[al] A.O.A.C. Use-Dilution Test is [an] important primary evaluation [in] the regulatory testing of disinfe[c]tants. However, additional pra[c]tical information on disinfectan[ts] and sanitizers can be obtained [by] evaluating their antibacterial acti[v]ities on different hard surfaces ar[nd] determining the activity of treate[d] surfaces exposed to recontamin[a]tion. Results show that hospit[al] preparations, classed as disinfe[c]tants under the conditions of t[he] A.O.A.C. Use-Dilution Test, [may] show differences in disinfecting ar[nd] self-sanitizing activities in tests d[e]scribed in this report.

Table VII. Summary of Antibacterial Activity Ratings* of Hospital Products

Tests	Disinfectants I	II	III	IV	Sanitizer FL
Official A.O.A.C.					
Use-Dilution Test	A	A	A	A	NA
Recontamination control					
Steel cylinders	NA	A	NA	NA	A
Asphalt	NA	A	NA	NA	A
A.O.A.C.-type test					
Vinyl – Letheen	NA	PA			NA
Vinyl – nutrient	NA	A			A
Linoleum – Letheen	NA	PA			NA
Linoleum – nutrient	NA	A			A
Rubber – Letheen	NA	PA			NA
Rubber – nutrient	NA	A			A
Asphalt – Letheen	NA	PA	NA	A	NA
Asphalt – nutrient	NA	A	NA	A	A
Painted plasterboard	A	A			**
Ceramic tile	A	A			**
Steel cylinder	A	A			**

*Ratings: A, active; PA, partly active; NA, not active; ** in nutrient broth only.

Bibliography

1. Antiseptics, Disinfectants, Fungicid[es] and Sterilization; edited by G. Reddish; Lea and Febiger, 2nd ed[i]tion, 1957.
2. Official Method of Analysis, 9th E[d.] Association of Official Agricultur[al] Chemists, Washington, D. C. 196[0] 5.006-5.009.
3. L. F. Ortenzio and L. S. Stua[rt] Adapation of the Use-Dilution Meth[od] to Primary Evaluations of Disinfe[c]tants. *Journal of Official Agricultu[ral] Chemists*, 44, No. 3, 416-421 (1961
4. G. Walter and S. Foris. Antibacteri[al] Residual on Inanimate Surfaces. *So[ap] and Chemical Specialties*, March, 196[2]
5. G. F. Reddish. Sanitation in Ho[s]pitals: The Importance of Perform[m]ance Tests. *Sanitarian*, p. 132-13[?] Nov./Dec., 1961.

—★—

Reprinted from *Soap Chem. Specialties* **45**, 79–80, 84–85 (1969)

Testing Sterilizers, Disinfectants, Sanitizers and Bacteriostats

16

By L. S. Stuart*

IN THE regulation of sterilizers, disinfectants, sanitizers, and bacteriostatic materials recommended for use in the inanimate environment, judgments as to compliance with efficacy requirements of the Federal Insecticide, Fungicide and Rodenticide Act are made largely on the basis of laboratory test data. In the enforcement of the law, samples collected from interstate shipments by official inspectors are tested in the Microbiological Laboratory of the Pesticides Regulation Division (PRD). Where applicable, methods of Association of Official Analytical Chemists are used. However, if no available AOAC method is considered applicable, simulated use methods are employed. Failure in these tests usually provides positive evidence that a product will fail in a given recommended application. However, effective performance in these tests usually falls considerably short of providing adequate assurance that a product will, in fact, give effective performance in the same application. This discrepancy can, in certain respects, be alleviated by increasing the number of samples and replicate determinations on individual samples. Thus, when the test methods employed in the PRD's enforcement program are used by applicants for registration to satisfy the documentary evidence on efficacy now required, it is essential to conduct sufficient testing to establish at the 95 per cent confidence level that the product will be effective as claimed with a representative sample. Also, the manufacturer must insure that he can replicate the preparation and that it will possess sufficient shelf-life to be effective as long as the product is offered for sale.

It is perhaps unfortunate that the amount of replication required to provide a 95 per cent confidence level with biological testing methods is much greater than bacteriologists have been accustomed to do or even admit. Thus, the upgraded documentary requirements for efficacy as outlined by Dr. Harry W. Hays, director of PRD, last December have been labeled by some as harsh and unrealistic. Some reevaluations on this score with the U.S. Department of Agriculture's Biometrical Services have permitted certain modifications, but for the most part the proposed testing schedules will remain as basic requirements for the registration of new products. Manufacturers also will be required to develop equivalent documentary evidence for existing registration files.

A study of our enforcement records with products in this category has clearly revealed a level of violation from an efficacy standpoint greater than the administration is willing to accept and this is the preferred action to correct this situation.

In evaluating sterilizing and sporicidal claims, the PRD's laboratory employs the AOAC sporicidal test. In this method, vacuum dried spores of specified strains of *Bacillus subtilis* and *Clostridium sporogenes* are employed. Two types of surface carriers are provided, porcelain penicylinders and surgical silk suture loops. Thirty replicates with each organism on each carrier are required for the condition of exposure recommended. Thus, a total of 120 carriers is needed for each set of exposure conditions involving time, temperature, and/or pretreatment routines to be evaluated. An exposure temperature of 20° C is a prescribed constant for chemical solutions unless a manufacturer clearly reveals that added heat is a prerequisite for efficacy. The incubation time is 21 days, followed by an additional 72 hours after a stipulated heat shock to eliminate possible error due to the presence of viable dormant spores.

Applicants for the registration of chemicals under labels bearing a sterilizing claim must submit data by this procedure on three different preparations of

Pesticides Regulation Division's testing program requires 95 per cent confidence level in product's efficacy. Manufacturer must insure that shelf life lasts as long as product is offered for sale.

---

* Dr. Stuart is chief staff officer, Disinfectants Evaluation Staff, Pesticides Regulation Division, Agricultural Research Service, United States Department of Agriculture. Paper presented May 20, 1969 during 55th midyear meeting, Chemical Specialties Manufacturers Association, Chicago.

the proposed formula and on duplicate samples of one formula following a 60-day shelf life study. This adds up to a total of 600 tubes. However, the absolute nature of a sterilizing claim is such that this cannot be considered an unreasonable requirement.

The basic feature of this test is that it starts with the vacuum dried spore. This has been found essential for replication of results in processes involving both gaseous and liquid chemical preparations.

With germicides, bactericides, and disinfectants recommended for environmental surfaces, PRD employs results obtained in the AOAC use-dilution method as the primary index to efficacy. The number and nature of the test organisms employed depends upon the claims made and the areas of use recommended.

Minimal Claims

Where minimal claims such as "germicide," "disinfectant," or "bactericide" are all that are involved—and the areas of recommended use are limited to those situations where effectiveness against Gram negative enteric bacteria is of primary importance and lack of efficacy against other species may not be a critical factor—tests using the single organism *Salmonella choleraesuis* are all that is required. In this situation, 60 replicates on three preparations with 30 replicates on duplicate samples of one of these preparations after a 60-day shelf life study have been specified as minimal requirements for registration for the concentration of the product recommended for use. This adds up to a total of 240 carriers.

The basic feature of this test is that a direct evaluation is made on the concentration of the product recommended to disinfect rather than an evaluation of an indirect type such as is provided by the AOAC phenol coefficient method. This is a carrier procedure employing stainless steel rings. The exposure temperature is 20°C, the exposure time is 10 minutes. Both resubculture and subculture media containing neutralizers are prescribed if necessary to overcome false results due to a carry-over of bacteriostatic concentrations of the chemical under test.

"General Disinfection"

With germicides recommended for "general disinfection" or for which representations such as "broad spectrum" are made, applicants for registration are required to submit the data as specified above for products bearing a minimal claim. In addition, data using the same procedure on three preparations employing two other test species, *Staphylococcus aureus* and another organism elected by the applicant, are required. In these cases, 30 replicates for each organism and each preparation will suffice. For this type of product a total of 420 carriers is required.

With germicides recommended for disinfection in hospital clinics, dental offices, veterinary hospitals, and as adjuvants to medical and veterinary medical practice, the primary test organism is *Staphylococcus aureus*. Here, applicants for registration are required to submit data using 60 replicates on three preparations with this test organism and on 30 replicates each on duplicate samples of one of these preparations after a 60-day shelf life study. In addition to this evaluation, tests using both *S. choleraesuis* and *Pseudomonas aeruginosa* also must be submitted on each of the three preparations using 30 replicates each. Thus, as in the case of the "general disinfectants" and "broad spectrum" products, a minimal requirement of 420 carriers is involved.

A product which is not effective against *Pseudomonas aeruginosa* may be accepted for registration bearing hospital, medical, dental, clinical, and veterinary representations. In this case, the label must bear a prominent disclaimer to this effect. If it is only effective against this organism when applied at special concentrations or in a special manner, then th label disclaimer may be replace by the special directions neede to assure efficacy against this o ganism.

If an unqualified phen coefficient claim is made on th labels of any of these product duplicate determinations on on preparation using *Salmonella ty phosa* must also be submitted. should be pointed out that this claim is made, the maximu dilution recommended to disin fect may not exceed that repre sented by one part of product t a number of parts of water, de termined by multiplying th phenol coefficient number by th figure 20, regardless of the ef ficacy found in the AOAC use dilution procedure.

If a claim for efficac against pathogenic fungi is mad for any of these products, dat on duplicate samples of on preparation using the AOAC fungicide test also are required This is an adjusted dilution tub test rather than a carrier pro cedure.

If a claim for effectivenes against the organisms causing tuberculosis is made, tests on on preparation using the AOAC tu berculocidal test also must b submitted.

Germicidal Sprays

With germicidal sprays including pressurized spot dis infectants, the requirements fo sample numbers and replicatio are the same, except that the use dilution method is replaced by the AOAC germicidal spray test The single deviation here is tha evaluations for effectivenes against the spread of pathogeni fungi are made by spraying the test slides, rather than by the AOAC fungicide method.

Added claims for effectiveness against specific organisms other than those involved in the tests specified above, can be accepted only when supported by data on at least one preparation with 30 replicates, using such modifications of the procedures specified as may be necessary to provide eaningful results. With fastidious organisms, special test culture media, enrichment subculture media, etc., are frequently required to provide meaningful results.

Claims for effectiveness against viruses or specific viruses must be supported by data on at least one preparation against the specific viruses named according to accepted virological techniques. Standardized procedures have not been developed in this area to a point where PRD feels justified in making specific recommendations. With the tissue culture procedures now being evaluated, a basic problem for accurate estimations as to the concentration of a product necessary to inactivate a virus irreversibly, or eliminate live virus, is the testing of undiluted or low dilutions of the virus-test chemical-mixtures so that accurate differentiations between the cytotoxic effects of the chemical and the cyto-pathogenic effects of the virus can be made. Preferential adsorption techniques with the exposed virus-chemical mixtures can apparently be employed effectively to resolve this problem but further standardization as to detail is necessary.

With iodophors, mixed halide preparations and organic chlorine-bearing chemical formulations recommended as germicidal rinses for previously cleaned, hard, nonporous surfaces, the PRD continues to rely on the AOAC available chlorine germicidal equivalent concentration procedure. Data showing the concentrations of the formulas equivalent in activity to the reference standards of 50, 100, and 220 ppm of available chlorine as sodium hypochlorite are required for registration. The test organism here is *Salmonella typhosa*. For registration, data on three separate preparations are required. Also, data on duplicate samples of one preparation after a 60-day shelf life study are necessary.

With quaternary ammonium sanitizers and anionic detergent-acid formulations recommended for similar applications, data on the same number of samples by the AOAC germicidal detergent sanitizer method are required. This same method is employed by PRD in evaluating hard water tolerance claims for products of this type. Data on duplicate samples of one preparation must be submitted to support a registration representation in this connection.

In the regulation of swimming pool water disinfectants, the Division employs the AOAC swimming pool water disinfectant method. For registration, data on three preparations with the two test organisms *Escherichia coli* and *Streptococcus faecalis* and 60-day shelf life studies on duplicate samples of one preparation with *E. coli* must be submitted. This is a germicidal equivalent procedure in which the activity of the commercial product is directly compared to a prescribed NaOCl control.

Additional standardized testing methods are needed for use with products recommended for applications in which the procedures identified above are not applicable. Sufficient progress has been made in developing a method for evaluating laundry disinfectants, sanitizers and bacteriostatic agents so that a tentative procedure should be available by early next year. Studies to standardize virucidal methods, air-sanitizing test procedures, and a technique for determining disinfecting and sanitizing efficacy in rug and carpet shampoos have been initiated.

The PRD realizes that the success of both its registration and enforcement programs will hinge largely upon the intelligent selection and application of available testing methods to the specific situations involved. A comprehensive understanding with regards to these selections and applications at the time of registration should materially minimize subsequent enforcement difficulties.

Reprinted from *Soap Chem. Specialties* **38**, 75–78, 101 (1962)

Organotins: Biological Activity, Use

17

Organotins show promise for a wide rang of household and industrial application Among them: bactericides, repellents fo rodents, agricultural foliage fungicide

By Robert J. Zedler and Charles B. Beiter*,
Metal & Thermit Corp.
New York

ORGANOTINS are chemicals in which at least one carbon to tin bond exists. The first of these substances was described by Löwig in 1852. (7) However, interest in this area of chemistry was not great until after 1945. The use of compounds such as dibutyltin oxide and dibutyltin dilaurate as heat and light stabilizers for polyvinyl chloride plastics and the use of tribenzyl and other tins as rubber antioxidants encouraged continued research on these unique compounds. Many patents have now been issued on organotins as oil additives and more recently on their use as catalysts for silicone elastomers and for polymerization of olefins and urethane foam.

This paper will be confined to the biologically active organotins and more specifically to their use as industrial preservatives, although agricultural and rodent repellent properties will be included.

Triorganotins as Antimicrobials: C. J. Faulkner of the Tin Research Institute (5) and G. J. M. van der Kerk and J. G. A. Luijten of the Institute for Organic Chemistry T.N.O. of Holland, under the sponsorship of the Tin Research Institute (8), were among the first to recognize the fungistatic activity of triorganotins. The preliminary study was conducted with ethyltins as indicated in Table I by van der Kerk and Luijten (8).

It should be first noted that tin is not active either in a stannic or stannous ion state. This is unusual behavior because such metals as zinc, mercury, copper and cadmium are known to have fungicidal activity, even though their biological activity increases with certain organic configurations. This is not so with tin. Secondly, it is obvious that the R_3Sn moiety is by far the most active. This same picture prevails with trialkyl tins other than triethyltins. The chain length of each alkyl group should not be longer than five carbons or shorter than two when considering the symmetrical types. For example, tri-n-hexyltins and trimethyltins are only mildly active agai fungi.

Van der Kerk further co ments that the electronegative po tion of the molecule, or X portic of the typical R_3SnX compour does not radically affect its activi against fungi. However, substit tion in the X position can chang chemical and physical properties the compound. This certainly m affect performance under use co ditions.

Up until this point we ha been discussing the work of Faul ner, van der Kerk and Luijten an the biological responses have bee limited to fungi. The trialkylti are excellent bacteriostats but, would be expected, there is vari

TABLE I

INFLUENCE OF THE NUMBER OF ALKYL GROUPS DIRECTLY ATTACHED TO THE TIN ATOM ON THE FUNGICIDAL PROPERTIES OF ETHYL COMPOUNDS

COMPOUND		CONCENTRATION (ppm = mg./l) CAUSING COMPLET INHIBITION OF GROWTH OF THE FUNGI			
NAME	FORMULA	BOTRYTIS ALLII	PENICILLIUM ITALICUM	ASPERGILLUS NIGER	RHIZOPUS NIGRICAN
TETRAETHYLTIN	$(C_2H_5)_4Sn$	50	> 1000	100	100
TRIETHYLTIN CHLORIDE	$(C_2H_5)_3SnCl$	0.5	2	5	2
DIETHYLTIN DICHLORIDE	$(C_2H_5)_2SnCl_2$	100	100	500	200
ETHYLTIN TRICHLORIDE	$C_2H_5SnCl_3$	> 1000	> 1000	> 1000	> 1000
STANNIC CHLORIDE	$SnCl_4$	> 1000	> 1000	> 1000	> 1000
STANNOUS CHLORIDE	$SnCl_2 \cdot 2H_2O$	> 1000	> 1000	> 1000	> 1000

*Paper presented during 48th annual meeting, Chemical Specialties Manufacturers Assn., New York, Dec. 6, 1961.

on in performance depending pon the structure involved. As can e seen in Table II, best control f gram negative bacteria results ith triethyl and tri-n-propyl deivatives. This is important with nany preservation applications, here control of the complete specrum is essential. It is also interesting to note that the trimethyls are elatively ineffective bacteriostats nd fungistats.

Toxicology of Triorganotins: t is unusual that metallic tin and norganic tin salts are considerably ess toxic than many of the organic in compounds. For example, the se of tin for plating food-containng cans is indicative of its safety. "The unofficial maximum permited level in the United Kingdom s 250 ppm," report Barnes & Stoner. (3) The use of stannous hloride as a stabilizer for certain oods and of stannous fluoride in lentifrice further supports this hesis.

Organotins are of varying oxicity. Our discussion will be imited to the trialkyltins since hese are of greatest importance as ntimicrobials. As an indication of order of magnitude, Table III prepared by Barnes & Stoner (2) will be of interest.

As might be expected from their bacteriostatic activity, the lower trialkyls are most toxic. However, the literature does show considerable variation in toxicity and only order of magnitude has been firmly established.

The tributyltins characterized by "bioMeT"* and "TBTO"*, bis (tri-n-butyltin) oxide, have been studied quite thoroughly, however. The acute oral LD_{50} on rats is approximately 200 mg/kg. For comparison, phenylmercuric acetate when applied by the same route has an LD_{50} of 35 mg/kg, according to Ramp and Grier (9). The acute dermal LD_{50} established on albino rabbits for "TBTO" is in the range of 11,700 mg/kg. In its undiluted form (95%), "TBTO" is a primary skin irritant and perhaps a skin sensitizer. However, extensive tests have established that less than 500 ppm on a textile has no adverse effects on the skin.

*Trademarks of Metal & Thermit Corporation

TABLE II

INFLUENCE OF GROUP R ON THE BACTERIOSTATIC PROPERTIES OF TRIORGANOTINS

COMPOUND NAME	COMPOUND FORMULA	CONCENTRATION (ppm = mg./l.) CAUSING COMPLETE INHIBITION OF GROWTH OF THE ORGANISM: P. FUNICULOSUM (FUNGUS)	C. ALBICANS (YEAST-LIKE ORGANISM)	S. AUREUS (GRAM POS. BACTERIA)	P. AERUGINOSA (GRAM NEG. BACTERIA)
TRIMETHYLTIN CHLORIDE	$(CH_3)_3SnCl$	500	500	> 500	250
TRIETHYLTIN CHLORIDE	$(C_2H_5)_3SnCl$	16	16	16	16
TRI-n-PROPYLTIN CHLORIDE	$(C_3H_7)_3SnCl$	1	0.5	8	31
TRI-n-BUTYLTIN CHLORIDE	$(C_4H_9)_3SnCl$	4	< 0.125	2	> 500
TRI-n-AMYLTIN ACETATE	$(C_5H_{11})_3SnOOCCH_3$	250	8	1	> 500
TRI-n-OCTENYLTIN CHLORIDE	$(C_8H_{15})_3SnCl$	> 125	> 125	—	> 500
TRIPHENYLTIN CHLORIDE	$(C_6H_5)_3SnCl$	8.0	< 2	1.0	> 500

Triorganotins Applications

Water Treatment: There are three major areas of industrial water treatment which require the use of biocides for the elimination of slimes caused by bacteria, fungi and algae. These are paper mills, industrial cooling water and water used for secondary recovery of oil. Combinations of "TBTO" and quaternaries have shown particular merit especially for industrial cooling water. The quaternary solubilizes the "TBTO" in water and also broadens its spectrum against bacteria. "TBTO" enhances the control of fungi and algae. Formulations of one part "TBTO" to four or five parts of a quaternary are in common use today.

The laboratory data in Table IV compare this type of formulation with "TBTO" and the quat alone in an enriched pulp slurry. Also, the improved control with bis (tri-n-propyltin) oxide when compared with the tri-n-butyl derivative should be noted.

Wood preservation: Approximate threshold values of "TBTO" for several major wood digesting fungi have been established by G. B. Fahlstrom of the Osmose Wood

TABLE III

THE TOXICITY OF SINGLE DOSES OF TRIALKYLTIN ACETATE

ALKYL GROUP	LD_{50} (MG. ACETATE PER KG. BODY WEIGHT)
METHYL (ACQUEUS SOLUTION)	9.1 (7.0 - 11.8)
ETHYL	4.0 (2.9 - 5.5)
n-PROPYL	118.3 (98.3 - 142.4)
ISO-PROPYL	44.1 (36.1 - 53.9)
n-BUTYL	380.2 (238.1 - 607.3)
n-HEXYL	1000.0
n-OCTYL	> 1000.0

EXCEPT WHERE OTHERWISE SHOWN, THE COMPOUNDS WERE DISSOLVED IN ARACHIS OIL AND GIVEN BY MOUTH TO FEMALE RATS (APPROX. 200 G. BODY WEIGHT). THE GROUPS WERE KEPT FOR AT LEAST 6 AND UP TO 21 WEEKS AFTER ADMINISTRATION AND THE LD_{50} CALCULATED BY WEIL'S (1952) METHOD. THE 95% CONFIDENCE LIMITS ARE SHOWN IN PARENTHESES.

TABLE IV

CONCENTRATION (PPMS = MG./l.) CAUSING INHIBITION OF GROWTH OF THE ORGANISM IN PAPER SLIME EVALUATION

COMPOUND	B. MYCOIDES	A. AEROGENES	P. AERUGINOSA
BIS(TRI-n-BUTYLTIN)OXIDE (bioMeT* TBTO*)	<10	500	> 500
bioMeT TBTO PLUS QUAT.	1	100	100
QUAT.	1	100	500
BIS(TRI-n-PROPYLTIN) OXIDE	1	100	500
TRICHLOROPHENOL	10	100	500
ACROLIEN	< 50	100	50

* TRADEMARK

TESTS WERE CONDUCTED IN AN ENRICHED PAPER PULP SUBSTRATE. BACTERIAL COUNTS WERE ESTIMATED AFTER 24 HOURS USING A STANDARD PLATE COUNT TECHNIQUE.[10]

Preserving Company of America, Inc. In his paper presented at the 1958 meeting of the American Wood Preservers' Association, the data in Table IV A were presented.

The sensitivity of *Lentinus lepideus* (Madison 534) to "TB TO" was so great it was not included in this study. However, subsequent investigation has shown the threshold against this organism to be between 0.007 and 0.010 lbs./cu. ft. This certainly suggests that combinations with creosote might be useful to assist in controlling this important wood destroying organism.

Out door stake tests using "TBTO" alone are now in progress. Until extended service results are available, a retention of 0.03 to 0.05 lbs./cu. ft. is suggested as an impregnation treatment. The effect of these levels on termites is being evaluated as are combinations of "TBTO" with aldrin and dieldrin.

"TBTO" lends itself to water repellent formulations for treatment of millwork and use by home owners. "TBTO" at 0.3% in mineral spirits meets or exceeds the performance requirement of the National Woodwork Manufacturer's Association, Inc., and Federal Specification TT-W-572. Such formulations are colorless and can be painted over without difficulty. An example of these products are the formulations now sold by the Osmose Wood Preserving Company of America, Inc., pictured in Figure I.

Its water insolubility and adsorption to cellulose suggests use of "TBTO" in a marine environment. Tests indicate that successful control of marine borers and *L. noria* can be obtained for over t years when wooden panels are i pregnated with 0.27 lbs. per cu foot (6).

Use techniques for mar wood preservation include dip a brush applications in addition impregnation. A 2% solution suitable solvents applied to a n wooden boat hull will protect even if anti-fouling paint is ac dentally removed. The data p sented in Table V demonstra this type of situation. One bru coat of "TBTO" was applied in solution consisting of nine parts fuel oil to one part of mine spirits at the levels indicated. T coats of anti-fouling paint were a plied after treatment of the wo with this solution and two one-in holidays left.

Anti-Fouling Paints: Pai formulations containing "TBT(have controlled marine organis for as long as high-level cupro oxide paints. "TBTO" rates of a plication are also competitive wi cuprous oxide. Like these coppe based paints, the paint formulatio used had a profound effect "TBTO's" biological activity, an it should be chosen with care. general, rates of 15% "TBT(based on solids content are require for good control of fouling. Figu II is a dosage series which dete mined this effective level. Testing lower rates in combination wit cuprous oxide is encouraged if hy droids or algae are a problem.

The advantages of a "T

Figure I. Examples of water repellent formulations made by Osmose Wood Preserving Co. of America, Inc., for treating millwork, and for home owners' us

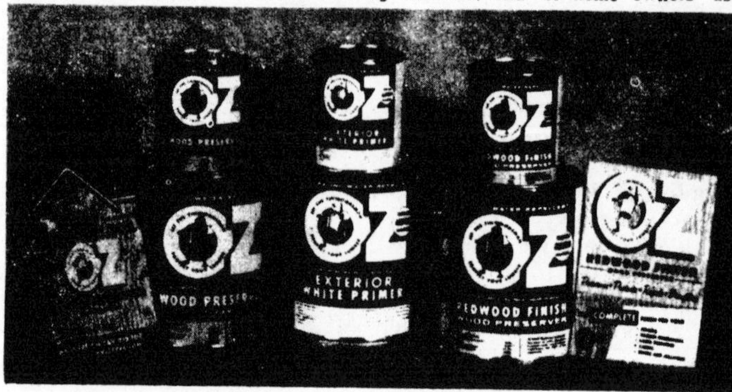

TABLE IV A

TOXIC THRESHOLD USING SOIL BLOCK TECHNIQUE (UNWEATHERED) – bioMeT* TBTO* CONTENT IN LBS./CU. FT.

MADISON 617	MADISON 698
LENZITES TRABEA	PORIA MONTICOLA
0.0138 – 0.0284	0.0055 – 0.0138

* TRADEMARK

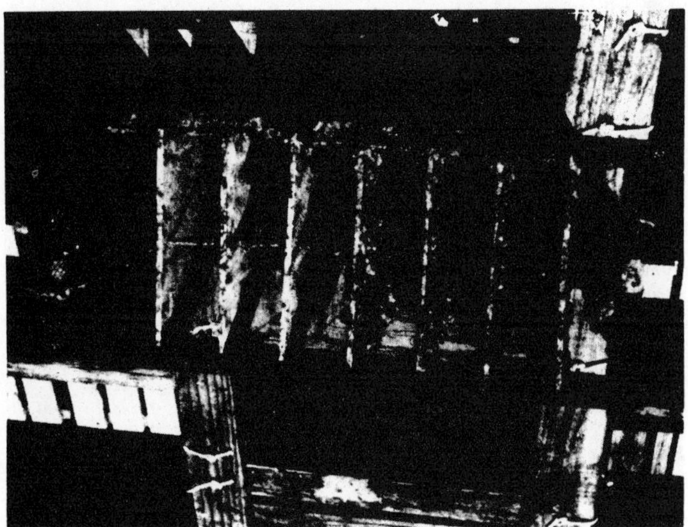

Figure II. Dosage series which determined effective level of 15% "TBTO" based on solids content for good control of fouling in anti-fouling paints.

TO"-based anti-fouling paint are (1) complete freedom of color, (2) ease of manufacture because it is soluble in most organic solvents and no grinding of the anti-fouling ingredient is necessary, (3) "TBTO" is broad in control spectrum, and (4) marine borer control is possible with thinned coats. Relief from corrosion problems is another probable advantage. Detailed tests are in progress on aluminum and steel to further study this aspect of "TBTO" anti-fouling paints.

Mildew Control in Paint: Laboratory tests conducted by Arnold and Clark (1) indicate that 250 ppm of "TBTO" is outstanding for mildew control in a polyvinyl acetate emulsion paint. Our results indicate that higher levels are necessary especially in oil paint. Preliminary laboratory results with bis (tri-n-propyltin) oxide have shown that it is more active than "TBTO" in emulsion paints and is equal to phenylmercuric oleate. These data are presented in Table VI.

Textiles: Chemicals which will prevent odor, germs and mildew on clothing, bedding and similar items have become useful textile sales tools. "TBTO"'s resistance to washing has placed it in a predominant position as a "permanent" bacteriostat and fungistat. Applications can be made as a finish, in the manufacture of a synthetic fiber or in a detergent or textile softener. "TBTO" is not affected by sodium perborate or sodium hpyochlorite bleaches.

In addition to use as a purifying chemical for textiles, there is a large market for rot proofing products for use on awnings and tenting. However, "TBTO" has not performed successfully for this application. We have conducted extensive studies with a large number of triorganotins and have found that the triphenyltins are more promising for this use. Outdoor weathering tests are reported in Table VII.

Home and Institutional Germicides: Staphylococcus aureus 80/81 is very susceptible to "TBTO." In addition, the compound is extremely persistent and resists washing. Because of these advantages, "TBTO" has found a place in formulations especially with quaternaries marketed for hospital treatment. These formulations are used on air filters, in mop water, waxes, laundry washes, and for spot disinfection.

The paper by P. B. Hudson, M.D., *et al*, titled "Effective System of Bactericidal Conditioning for Hospitals" and published in the April 4, 1959, issue of the *Journal of the American Medical Association*, fully describes the system for total environmental control of staph and other bacteria with formulations containing "TBTO." (A similar article appeared in the

(*Turn to Page* 101)

TABLE V

MARINE WOOD PRESERVATION

COMPOUND	DOSAGE	TOTAL NUMBER OF TEREDO AND LIMNORIA ENTRIES (MONTHS)						
		2	4	6	8	10	12	14
bioMeT* TBTO*	1%	0	0	1	1	5	5	21
bioMeT TBTO	1.5%	0	0	1	4	7	5	57
bioMeT TBTO	2.0%	0	0	0	0	2	3	0
UNTREATED CONTROL	—	16	19	18	DESTROYED IN 7 MONTHS			

*TRADEMARK

THE MINOR VARIATION IN THE COUNTS FROM MONTH TO MONTH IS A RESULT OF DIFFICULTY IN POSITIVE DETERMINATION OF ENTRY. THE TEST WAS CONDUCTED AT MIAMI BEACH, FLORIDA.

TABLE VI

PRESERVATION OF P.V.A. EMULSION PAINT

COMPOUND	CONCENTRATION (%) WHICH WILL COMPLETELY INHIBIT FUNGI: PENICILLIUM SP.	PULLULARIA PULLULANS
BIS(TRI-n-BUTYLTIN) OXIDE (bioMeT* TBTO*)	> 0.5	0.05
BIS(TRI-n-PROPYLTIN) OXIDE	0.05	0.05
PHENYLMERCURIC OLEATE	0.05	0.05

*TRADEMARK

TWO COATS OF POLYVINYLACETATE EMULSION PAINT WERE APPLIED TO FILTER PAPER BY BRUSHING. THEY WERE THEN CULTURED ON AGAR FOR A PERIOD OF FOUR WEEKS.[11]

Organotins

(*From Page* 78)

Medical Annals of the District of Columbia, Vol. XXVIII, No. 2, February, 1959.) In general, bactericidal conditioning, as described in this article, reduced the total number of bacteria contaminating the hospital air by 82%. The tests were conducted in the Francis Delafield Hospital, and the figures were obtained after a five-week treatment period.

Agriculture: The agricultural applications of triorganotins in the United States have been limited to the use of dibutyltin dilaurate and dibutyltin maleate as poultry anthelmintics and coccidiostats. However, in recent years there has been interest in triphenyltin acetate as a foliage fungicide. The trialkyltins are in general too phytotoxic for foliage applications. The triphenyls do not have this drawback at least on celery, sugar beets and potatoes. One pound of a 20% wettable powder formulation has been equal to commercial applications of carbamates against such organisms as *Phytophthera*, *Alternaria* and *Cercospora*.

There are also indications that triorganotins are useful as turf and bulb fungicides and as seed treatments.

Rodent Repellents: After screening about 8000 compounds as barrier rodent repellents, the U. S. Fish and Wildlife Service, Department of Interior, reports that tributyltin chloride and triphenyltin chloride are among the most active. These tests were conducted with trapped house mice. (*Mus Musculus*). The organotin compounds were applied at various concentrations by dipping burlap in an acetone solution of the repellent. Bags were then prepared from treated burlap and filled with food. Treated and untreated bags were exposed to individually caged mice. The tests were replicated 50 or more times using 50 or more different animals. The results obtained are found in Table VIII.

Summary

In conclusion, organotins of the R_3SnX type exhibit the most promise as industrial biochemicals. Of these, the tri-n-butyl, tri-n-propyl and perhaps triphenyl derivatives are unique. The tributyls have already found a place in the treatment of water and wood. In addition, bis (tri-n-butyltin) oxide is used as an anti-fouling ingredient in ship bottom paints, as a textile purifier, and as an ingredient in home and institutional germicides. Tributyltin chloride is also a very active rodent repellent.

The tri-n-propyltins exhibit broad spectrum control of bacteria which make them of special interest for water treatment and various preservative applications.

Lastly, the triphenyltins are the most durable on textiles in outdoor weathering and perhaps they will find a place for this use. Interest is already high in this type of compound as an agricultural foliage fungicide. However, testing under field conditions must be conducted for this and its rodent repellent applications, before actual utility can be determined.

References:

1. Arnold, H. M. and Clark, H. J.: *Journal of Oil and Colour Chemists Assoc.*, Vol. 39, (Dec. 1956).
2. Barnes, J. M. and Stoner, H. B.: *British Journal of Industrial Medicine*, Vol. 15 (1958).
3. Barnes, J. M. and Stoner, H. B.: *Pharmacological Reviews*, Vol. II, No. 2 (1959).
4. Fahlstrom, G. B.: Proceedings of American Wood Preservers' Association (1958).
5. Faulkner, C. J.: British Patent #734,119 (1952).
6. Hochman, H. and Roe, T.: Harbor Screening Tests of Marine Borer Inhibitors—III, Y-R005-07-007, Type C., U. S. Naval Civil Engineering Laboratory (1961).
7. Ingham, R. K., Rosenberg, S. D., and Gilman, H.: *Chemical Reviews* (Oct. 1960).
8. Kerk, G. J. M. van der and Luijten, J. G. A.: *Journal of Applied Chemistry*, 4 (1954).
9. Ramp, J. A., and Grier, N.: Proceedings of the Chemical Specialties Manufacturer's Association, Inc. (May, 1961).
10. T.A.P.P.I. Monograph Series, Microbiology of Pulp and Paper, No. 15 (1955).
11. Vickbund, R. E. and Manowitz, M.: Engineer Research Laboratories, Fort Belvoir, Va., Report 1118 (1959).

TABLE VIII

LABORATORY TEST - RODENT REPELLENCY

COMPOUND	CONCENTRATION (mgs. sq. in.)	DAMAGE REDUCTION	LENGTH OF STORAGE
TRIBUTYLTIN CHLORIDE	5.0	96%	INITIAL TEST
TRIBUTYLTIN CHLORIDE	5.0	56%	1 YEAR
TRIBUTYLTIN CHLORIDE	1.25*	88%	INITIAL TEST
TRIBUTYLTIN CHLORIDE	1.25*	90%	1 YEAR
TRIPHENYLTIN ACETATE	5.0	84%	INITIAL TEST
TRIPHENYLTIN ACETATE	5.0	75%	1 YEAR

* POLYVINYLACETATE ADHESIVE USED. NOT TESTED AGAINST BAGS TREATED WITH POLYVINYLACETATE, THEREFORE, A PORTION OF THE REDUCTION MAY BE DUE TO MECHANICAL RESISTANCE RATHER THAN CHEMICAL REPELLENCY.

TABLE VII

MILDEW CONTROL ON CANVAS

% REQUIRED FOR COMPLETE INHIBITION OF CHAETOMIUM GLOBOSUM

COMPOUND	NUMBER OF DAYS WEATHERING 35	85	155	231	263
BIS(TRI-n-BUTYLTIN) OXIDE (bioMeT* TBTO*)	0.5	0.5	1.0	> 1.0	> 1.0
TRIPHENYLTIN CHLORIDE	0.05	0.5	0.5	0.5	1.0
COPPER-8-QUINOLINOLATE	0.05	0.5	0.5	0.5	> 1.0

* TRADEMARK

THE TEXTILES WERE DIPPED IN METHANOL SOLUTIONS OF COMPOUNDS AND EXPOSED AT RAHWAY, N. J. SAMPLES OF THE TEXTILES WERE TAKEN AT INTERVALS AND EVALUATED USING FEDERAL SPECIFICATION CCC-T-191b # 5751.

Reprinted from *J. Pharm. Sci.* **61**, 390–392 (1972)

Interaction of Quaternary Ammonium Bactericides with Biological Materials I: Conductometric Studies with Cephalin

DAVID W. BLOIS* and JAMES SWARBRICK▲

18a

Abstract ☐ Quaternary ammonium surfactants are more active gainst Gram-positive organisms than against Gram-negative acteria. This difference has been attributed to the presence of ephalin in the cell wall of the Gram-negative bacteria. This paper resents a review of previous *in vivo* work reported in the literature. dditionally, as a preliminary step in elucidating the mechanism ehind this difference by studying the molecular interactions beveen these bactericides and bacterial wall constituents by use of an *i vitro* film balance approach, a conductometric study on cephalin nd certain alkylbenzyldimethylammonium chlorides was underken. An interaction in solution was observed, the data indicating at two molecules of cephalin react with one molecule of the quaernary ammonium surfactant.

Keyphrases ☐ Quaternary ammonium bactericides—interaction vith cephalin, *in vivo* literature review, *in vitro* conductometric tudy ☐ Cephalin interaction with quaternary ammonium bacericides—*in vivo* literature review, *in vitro* conductometric study ☐ Conductometric studies—interaction of cephalin with quaternary mmonium bactericides ☐ Bactericidal activity—quaternary amnonium compounds

Since the original observation by Domagk (1) that the lkylbenzyldimethylammonium chlorides were extremely otent antibacterial agents, much work has been devoted o the action of cationic surface-active quaternary ammonium bactericides. Numerous structural modificaions of the original series were carried out in an effort to ncrease the bactericidal activity of the class. In addition, nany studies were conducted to determine the manner n which these compounds exert their action. Howver, the original material, alkylbenzyldimethylmmonium chloride, also known collectively as benzlkonium chloride, is still one of the most widely used gents.

LITERATURE REVIEW

It was observed (2, 3) that the quaternary ammonium compounds re active against Gram-positive and Gram-negative organisms as vell as fungi. However, the Gram-positive organisms show a higher legree of susceptibility to these agents than do the Gram-negative rganisms (2, 3). The resistance of the Gram-negative organism as been ascribed to the phospholipid present in its cell envelope 4), which appears to be of the highly acidic cephalin type. The cell vall of the Gram-positive organism lacks such a phospholipid omponent.

Several observations tend to strengthen this theory. It was observed (5) that prior addition of phospholipids to a media containing Gram-positive cells can prevent the inhibition of metabolism by ationic surfactants. Furthermore, exposure of the cells to cephalin, followed by a washing of the cells, also protected the organisms. Based on these observations, it was postulated that the phospholipid was adsorbed onto the bacterial surface, where it subsequently interacted with the bactericide, rendering it inactive. It also was shown (6) that the prior addition of protamine to a media of Gram-negative organisms markedly increased the susceptibility of these organisms to quaternary ammonium bactericides. The highly basic protamine was shown to form an insoluble precipitate with cephalin (7). Such experimental evidence suggests that the phospholipid portion of the complex cell wall is responsible for the greater degree of protection afforded the Gram-negative bacteria.

Salton (8) proposed that the action of lytic agents on bacteria is as follows: (*a*) adsorption and penetration of the porous wall, (*b*) interaction with lipid–protein membrane, (*c*) leakage of low molecular weight metabolites, (*d*) degradation of proteins and nucleic acids, and (*e*) lysis due to wall-degrading autolytic enzymes. Other studies (4, 9, 10) showed that the cell membrane, rather than the cell wall, is the primary site for the bactericidal action of lytic agents. However, since the cell membranes for the Gram-positive and Gram-negative organisms are in both cases lipoprotein, it would appear that the difference in susceptibility should be ascribed to the difference between the cell walls. Hence, the interaction with the cell wall is of primary importance to the bactericidal action of the compound.

It has been established that the antibacterial action of the quaternary ammonium salts is related to their physical, rather than chemical, properties. The most significant physical property of these compounds is their surface activity. Numerous authors studied the interfacial properties of the antibacterial quaternary ammonium bactericides and attempted to relate these properties to the *in vivo* activity. Zissman (11) compared the minimum effective concentration (MEC) of a series of quaternary ammonium bactericides with surface tension lowering and found that solutions having the same MEC had surface tension values of the same order of magnitude. Others (12, 13) attempted to relate CMC data to the thermodynamic activity of the solution and, in turn, to relate this derived thermodynamic activity to the MEC. As an extension of this work, the Ferguson principle (14) was used to explain the dependence of the MEC on the surface activity.

Ferguson (14) proposed that the chemical potential of a series of substances possessing "physical toxicity" could be used as a toxic index. His theory was based on the fact that at equilibrium the chemical potential and, hence, activity of the substance in the internal and external phases must be equal. In the case of quaternary ammonium bactericides, the external phase is the bulk solution and the internal phase is the cell membrane of the bacteria. Ferguson also showed that the activity at the toxic concentration could be approximated by S_t/S_o, where S_t is the molar concentration of the toxic substance and S_o is its solubility. Thus, if the Ferguson principle holds true, it substantiates the theory that the bactericidal activity is the result of some physical activity rather than its chemical reaction.

Other workers similarly attempted to invoke the Ferguson principle to explain bactericidal activity. Ecanow and Siegel (12) attempted to define the thermodynamic activity as the ratio of the MEC to the CMC. For three quaternary ammonium bactericides of equal alkyl chain length but different polar head groups, Weiner and Zografi (15) defined the activities as the ratio of the Gibbs surface excess at the MEC to that at the CMC. Good agreement was found between the activities of all three quaternary ammonium bactericides when tested against Gram-positive and Gram-negative organisms and fungi. These authors concluded that the mechanism of action of these compounds depends primarily on a physical relationship between the external phase and the internal phase.

In an effort to understand the nature of the interactions that occur between drugs and biological tissues, various authors proposed the use of systems; probably the most useful of these systems is an insoluble monolayer adsorbed at the air/water interface. The first use of insoluble monolayers as models for biological membranes appears to be that of Schulman and Rideal (16). These authors used spread monolayers of gliadin and gliadin–cholesterol as a model of the cell wall of a human red blood corpuscle. They then studied the interaction of hemolytic and agglutinating agents in the subphase on the spread monolayers. The penetration into, as well as association with, an insoluble monolayer by these compounds was monitored as a function of the increase in surface pressure or area and change of surface potential with time. Using criteria established in these studies, a relationship was established (17) between a compound's effect on the erythrocytes and the nature of its interactions with an insoluble monolayer.

The use of monolayers to simulate biological membranes has become greatly expanded since the original work of Schulman and Rideal (16). Since the original investigations into the mechanism of hemolysis, several authors have attempted to correlate monolayer penetration with the activity of other classes of drugs including the sulfas, local anesthetics, tranquilizers, and antibiotics.

Although a great deal is known about the end results of the action of quaternary ammonium compounds on bacteria, *i.e.*, cellular leakage and lysis, and postulates have been presented on the manner in which bacterial death is caused, little is known about the nature of the interactions between the bactericide and the cellular substituents. However, it does appear, as stated by Schulman *et al.* (18), that the greater resistance of Gram-negative over Gram-positive organisms is due to the higher lipid content in the bacterial cell walls of the Gram-negative cell. Many studies using live bacteria have been carried out in an effort to gain insight into the mechanism of action of the cationic bactericides. Under such conditions, it is difficult to determine the nature of the interactions between the bactericide and the cell wall and membrane components that ultimately lead to bacterial cell death.

EXPERIMENTAL

Since the use of insoluble monolayers to simulate cell structures and subsequent study of the action of drugs on these monolayers have been well established in the literature, the purpose of this investigation was to study the interaction that occurs between a quaternary ammonium bactericide and the components of a simulated bacterial cell wall. These studies were carried out through the use of insoluble monomolecular layers and a conductometric analysis of solutions of biological materials.

The model membrane chosen to simulate the Gram-positive cell wall was that of an insoluble monomolecular film of the insoluble protein gliadin spread at the air/water interface. A protein–phospholipid monolayer of gliadin and cephalin was used to simulate the Gram-negative bacterial wall. By studying the interactions that occur between these spread monolayers and the surface active bactericide injected beneath, the role of the components in determining the susceptibility of the organism may be assessed.

In addition, a conductometric study was carried out to establish the presence of an interaction between the bactericide and the cephalin. For this study, both materials were in aqueous solution.

Materials—*Alkylbenzyldimethylammonium Chlorides*—A homologous series of alkylbenzyldimethylammonium chlorides in the monohydrated form (C_{12}–C_{16}) was used[1]. The purity of these compounds was established by the observation that paper chromatography yielded a single spot. This determination was carried out by other workers (using the same batches) and reported previously (2). Certain physical and interfacial properties of this series were presented in an earlier paper (19).

Cephalin—Synthetic L-α-(β,γ-dipalmitoyl)phosphatidylethanolamine[2] was used as received. The cephalin was dissolved in distilled water for the conductometric studies.

Water—The water used was double distilled from an all-glass apparatus[3].

Methods—A conductivity bridge[4] was used to establish the presence of an interaction between cephalin and the C_{14} and C_{16} homologs. Measurements of the specific conductivity *versus:* (*a*) increasing molar concentration of cephalin in the presence and absence of alkylbenzyldimethylammonium chloride and (*b*) increasing molar concentrations of alkylbenzyldimethylammonium chloride in the presence and absence of cephalin were determined. Corrections were applied for the specific conductivity of the distilled water.

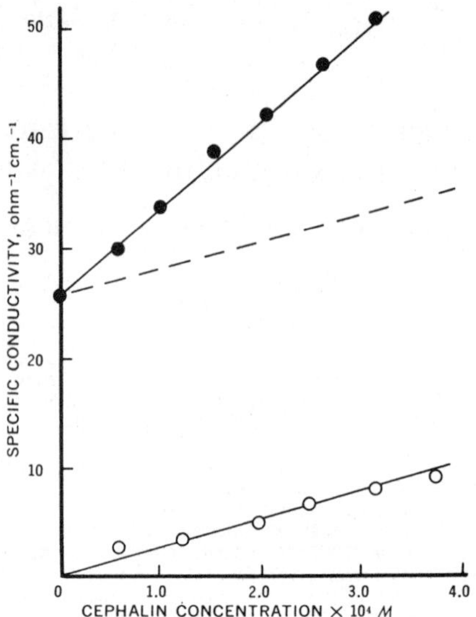

Figure 1—*Conductometric study of increasing concentration of cephalin in the presence and absence of the C_{14} alkylbenzyldimethylammonium chloride. Key:* ○, *no C_{14} alkylbenzyldimethylammonium chloride present; and* ●, *C_{14} alkylbenzyldimethylammonium chloride concentration = 2.51 × 10^{-4}* M. *Dashed line represents the theoretical additive values.*

RESULTS AND DISCUSSION

Due to the instability of cephalin monolayers in the presence of alkylbenzyldimethylammonium chloride injected into the subphase, a quantitative study of the interaction between these two materials could not be carried out using monolayer techniques. Accordingly, a conductometric study was performed to study their interaction

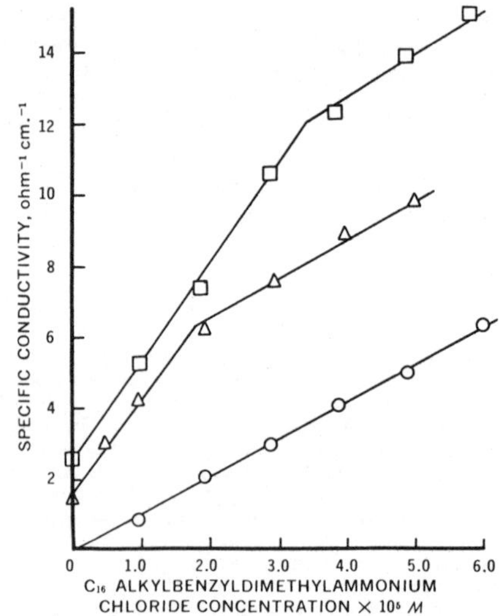

Figure 2—*Conductometric study of increasing concentration of C_{16} alkylbenzyldimethylammonium chloride in the presence and absence of cephalin. Key:* ○, *no cephalin present;* △, *cephalin concentration = 3.43 × 10^{-5}* M; *and* □, *cephalin concentration = 6.86 × 10^{-5}* M.

[1] Supplied by Dr. R. A. Cutler, Sterling-Winthrop Research Institute, Rensselaer, N. Y.
[2] California Corporation for Biochemical Research.
[3] Barnstead Redistiller, EPR-1/2C.
[4] Beckman Instruments, Inc., model RC-19.

Table I—Summary of Conductometric Study of Interaction of Cephalin and Alkylbenzyldimethylammonium Chloride

Homolog	Concentration of Alkylbenzyldimethyl-ammonium Chloride, moles/l.	Concentration of Cephalin, moles/l.	Slope, ohm^{-1} $cm.^{-1}$ $mole^{-1}$ l.	Intersection, moles/l. Alkylbenzyldimethyl-ammonium Chloride
14	0	Varying	2.36×10^{-2}	—
	2.51×10^{-4}	Varying	8.21×10^{-2}	—
14	Varying	0	1.07×10^{-1}	—
	Varying	3.13×10^{-5}	2.14×10^{-1} (Initial region)	1.60×10^{-5}
	Varying	3.13×10^{-5}	1.12×10^{-1} (Second region)	
	Varying	6.25×10^{-5}	2.18×10^{-1} (Initial region)	3.50×10^{-5}
	Varying	6.25×10^{-5}	1.10×10^{-1} (Second region)	
16	Varying	0	1.10×10^{-1}	—
	Varying	3.43×10^{-5}	2.81×10^{-1} (Initial region)	1.60×10^{-5}
	Varying	3.43×10^{-5}	1.20×10^{-1} (Second region)	
	Varying	6.86×10^{-5}	2.69×10^{-1} (Initial region)	3.40×10^{-5}
	Varying	6.86×10^{-5}	1.25×10^{-1} (Second region)	

Typical data are shown in Figs. 1 and 2; a summary is presented in Table I.

Figure 1 shows the specific conductivities resulting from the addition of increasing amounts of cephalin to a constant concentration of the C_{14} alkylbenzyldimethylammonium chloride homolog. Since the slope of the mixed system differs from the sum of the single components in solution, it appears that there is an interaction between them in solution. Thus, the slope of the line in Fig. 1 for cephalin in the presence of C_{14} alkylbenzyldimethylammonium chloride is greater than that for cephalin in the absence of the C_{14} homolog. Similarly, as shown in Fig. 2 for the C_{16} homolog, the initial slopes of the lines in the presence of a constant amount of cephalin are greater than those obtained in its absence. Again, these results indicate that an interaction has occurred between the cephalin and alkylbenzyldimethylammonium chloride, leading to specific conductivity for the solution that is increased over that of the separate parts.

As may be reasoned from Fig. 2, as more alkylbenzyldimethylammonium chloride is added to the cephalin, the latter is used to form the interaction product. When no further cephalin is available, the addition of more alkylbenzyldimethylammonium chloride results in a line whose slope is identical to that for alkylbenzyldimethylammonium chloride in the absence of cephalin. Within the limits of experimental error, this appears to be the case. While the amount of data is not felt to be sufficient to propose a mechanism for the observed increase in conductivity, it is possible to gain an appreciation of the stoichiometry of the reaction. Thus, from the points of intersection in Fig. 2, the ratio of cephalin to C_{14} alkylbenzyldimethylammonium chloride is within the range of 1.8–2.0. With the C_{16} alkylbenzyldimethylammonium chloride homolog, the cephalin–alkylbenzyldimethylammonium chloride ratio is from 2.0 to 2.1.

The significance of this interaction in terms of rationalizing the effect of cephalin on the antibacterial activity of alkylbenzyldimethylammonium chloride will be considered in more detail in a subsequent publication (20).

REFERENCES

(1) G. Domagk, *Deut. Med. Wochenschr.*, **61**, 829(1935); through *Chem. Abstr.*, **29**, 7018(1935).

(2) R. A. Cutler, E. B. Cimijotti, T. J. Okolowich, and W. F. Wetterau, *Soap Chem. Spec.*, **Mar. 1967**, 84.

(3) N. D. Weiner, F. Hart, and G. Zografi, *J. Pharm. Pharmacol.*, **17**, 350(1965).

(4) R. Gilby and A. V. Few, *J. Gen. Microbiol.*, **23**, 19(1960).

(5) Z. Baker, R. W. Harrison, and B. F. Miller, *J. Exp. Med.*, **74**, 621(1941).

(6) B. F. Miller, R. Abrams, A. Dorfman, and A. M. Klein, *Science*, **96**, 428(1942).

(7) R. Chargaff, *J. Biol. Chem.*, **125**, 661(1938).

(8) M. R. J. Salton, *J. Gen. Physiol.*, **52**, 2275(1960).

(9) R. D. Hotchkiss, *Advan. Enzymol.*, **4**, 153(1944).

(10) M. R. J. Salton, *J. Gen. Microbiol.*, **6**, 391(1951).

(11) E. Zissman, *C. R. Acad. Sci.*, **245**, 237(1939).

(12) B. Ecanow and J. Siegel, *J. Pharm. Sci.*, **52**, 812(1963).

(13) J. Cella, D. Eggenberger, D. Noel, L. Harriman, and H. Harwood, *J. Amer. Chem. Soc.*, **74**, 2061(1952).

(14) J. Ferguson, *Proc. Roy. Soc., Ser. B*, **127**, 387(1939).

(15) N. D. Weiner and G. Zografi, *J. Pharm. Sci.*, **54**, 436(1965).

(16) J. H. Schulman and E. K. Rideal, *Proc. Roy. Soc., Ser. B*, **122**, 29(1937).

(17) J. H. Schulman, *Trans. Faraday Soc.*, **33**, 1116(1937).

(18) J. H. Schulman, B. A. Pethica, A. V. Few, and M. R. J. Salton, *Progr. Biophys.*, **5**, 41(1955).

(19) D. W. Blois and J. Swarbrick, *J. Colloid Interface Sci.*, **36**, 226(1971).

(20) D. W. Blois and J. Swarbrick, *J. Pharm. Sci.*, **61**, 393(1972).

ACKNOWLEDGMENTS AND ADDRESSES

Received May 17, 1971, from the *Division of Pharmaceutics, School of Pharmacy, University of Connecticut, Storrs, CT 06268*

Accepted for publication December 10, 1971.

Presented in part to the Basic Pharmaceutics Section, APhA Academy of Pharmaceutical Sciences, San Francisco meeting, March 1971.

Supported in part by Public Health Service Fellowship 5-F01-GM-36,156-02 (to D. W. Blois) and Grant 064 from the University of Connecticut Research Foundation.

* Present address: Sterling-Winthrop Research Institute, Rensselaer, N. Y.

▲ To whom inquiries should be directed.

Reprinted from *J. Pharm. Sci.* **61**, 393–398 (1972)

18b

Interaction of Quaternary Ammonium Bactericides with Biological Materials II: Insoluble Monolayer Studies

DAVID W. BLOIS* and JAMES SWARBRICK▲

Abstract □ The behavior of a series of bactericidal alkylbenzyldimethylammonium chlorides in the presence of various materials spread at the air/water interface was examined, with a view to elucidating the manner these compounds initiate bacteriolysis in Gram-positive and Gram-negative organisms. A monolayer of the protein gliadin was chosen to represent the Gram-positive bacterial wall, while a gliadin–cephalin film was used to simulate the Gram-negative bacterial wall. Interactions between these monolayers and the various alkylbenzyldimethylammonium chloride homologs, alone and in the presence of protamine, were followed by monitoring surface pressure, surface area, and surface potential as a function of time. Recompression studies were also undertaken. The results suggest that with Gram-positive organisms the bactericide first becomes associated with the protein in the cell wall; subsequent penetration leads to disruption of the cell membrane. In the Gram-negative wall, the phospholipid present affords the organism a degree of protection from the bactericide. This effect is removed in the presence of protamine.

Keyphrases □ Quaternary ammonium bactericides—interaction with gliadin and gliadin–cephalin monolayers, presence and absence of protamine □ Gliadin and gliadin–cephalin monolayers—interaction with quaternary ammonium bactericides, presence and absence of protamine □ Cephalin–gliadin and gliadin monolayers—interaction of quaternary ammonium bactericides, presence and absence of protamine □ Protamine—effect on interaction of quaternary ammonium bactericides with gliadin and gliadin–cephalin monolayers □ Bactericidal activity—quaternary ammonium compounds

In another paper (1), the literature concerning the action of the quaternary ammonium bactericides and the methods used to elucidate their mechanisms of action were reviewed. The presence of an interaction between the quaternary ammonium bactericides of the alkylbenzyldimethylammonium chloride series and the phospholipid cephalin also was established *via* a conductometric analysis of aqueous solutions of these materials. This latter experiment was carried out to establish that the bactericide and the phospholipid indigenous to the Gram-negative bacterial cell wall are able to interact with each other.

The present paper concerns itself with the interactions occurring between the bactericide and insoluble monolayers spread at the air/water interface, designed as models for the Gram-positive and Gram-negative bacterial cell walls. A film of the insoluble protein gliadin was used to model the Gram-positive cell wall, while a protein–phospholipid film of gliadin and cephalin was used to mimic the Gram-negative cell wall. The bactericide under study was injected into the aqueous subphase beneath the insoluble monolayer and its interaction was monitored as the time-dependent change in surface pressure or area and surface potential. In addition, an effort was made to elucidate the role played by protamine in altering the susceptibility of Gram-negative organisms to the quaternary ammonium bactericides. These results were then interpreted in view of the ba- teriological activity of this series of compounds c Gram-positive and Gram-negative organisms.

MATERIALS AND METHODS

Alkylbenzyldimethylammonium Chloride—The source, puri and characteristics of the alkylbenzyldimethylammonium chlori series were described previously (1).

Gliadin—The molecular weight of gliadin[1], a protein deriv from wheat, was taken to be 27,000, as determined from monolay properties of the water-insoluble protein (2). Gliadin is report to be soluble in 70% ethanol (3). However, the protein, as pu chased, in 70% ethanol contained insoluble (proteinaceous) mat rial. Therefore, a purification and quantification procedure w used, which involved filtration of the solution containing insolub material followed by a gravimetric analysis for the total protein solution (4).

Cephalin—Synthetic L-α-(β,γ-dipalmitoyl)phosphatidylethan amine[2] was used as received. The cephalin was dissolved in a mixtu of chloroform and ethanol (90:10) for the insoluble monolay studies.

Protamine—Protamine sulfate[3] was used as received. It co tained 67–70% arginine and 24 ± 1.5% nitrogen. A molecu weight of 7000 (5) was used to calculate the molar strength of t aqueous solutions used.

Gliadin–Cephalin Solution—A solution in chloroform–ethanc water (67:24:9) was used in the formation of a mixed protein phospholipid monolayer.

Film Balance Studies—The apparatus, a Wilhelmy-type fil balance, and the calibration procedure used were described in d tail elsewhere (6). The time for equilibration of the film with t barriers set for maximum area was 20 min. The rate of compressi was 2.54 cm. min.$^{-1}$.

Penetration Studies—Since both the gliadin and gliadin–cepha films showed the phenomenon of surface pressure relaxation (the compressed films were allowed to relax to their equilibrium pre sure prior to the start of any penetration studies. This was a complished by compressing the film to a preselected area and th allowing the film to reach equilibrium. The area to which the fil was compressed was such that the equilibrium film pressure, F_e at that area was greater than that pressure generated by the alk benzyldimethylammonium chloride itself at the air/water interfa for the subphase concentration employed in the study. Followi attainment of the equilibrium surface pressure, between 0.5 and ml. of the subphase was removed from behind the barriers a replaced by an equal volume of solution containing the desir amount of alkylbenzyldimethylammonium chloride. The transfer the solution was accomplished by means of a glass syringe fitted wi a 7.62-cm. (3-in.), 18-gauge hypodermic needle. Homogeneity of t subphase was ensured by gently drawing the subphase into t syringe and discharging it several times under the surface. Penet tion into the monolayer was followed as a function of the change surface pressure or surface area and the change of surface potent with time, the initial time being that point when the alkylbenz dimethylammonium chloride was introduced into the subpha Monolayer penetration was monitored until an equilibrium con tion was reached or 90 min. had elapsed, whichever was the soon At that time, the penetrated monolayer was compressed to collapsed area.

[1] Nutritional Biochemical Corp., Cleveland, Ohio.
[2] California Corporation for Biochemical Research.
[3] Salmine, Nutritional Biochemical Corp., Cleveland, Ohio.

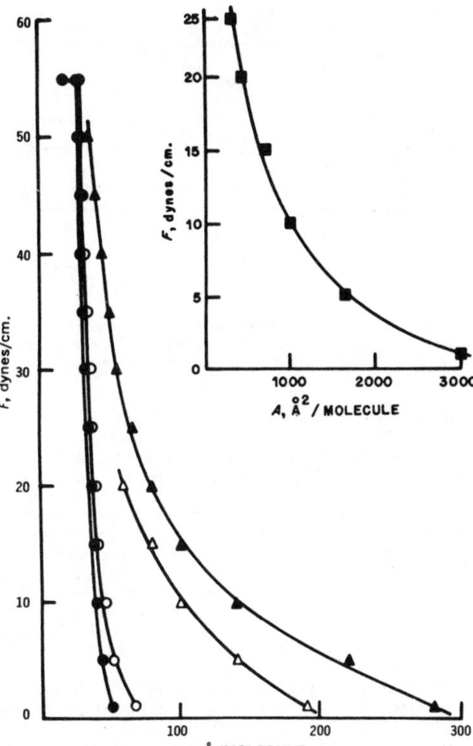

Figure 1—*Surface pressure–area relationships for gliadin* (■), *gliadin–cephalin mixed film* (▲), *gliadin–cephalin derived film* (△), *cephalin* (●), *and cephalin on protamine subphase* (○).

For the studies of monolayer penetration by alkylbenzyldimethylammonium chloride at constant surface pressure, the surface area was increased manually to maintain a constant surface pressure. The distance of separation of the barriers, and, hence, the area per molecule were determined as a function of time.

Surface Potential Measurements—Surface potential measurements were determined by the ionizing electrode method described by Gaines (7). The ionizing electrode consisted of a static eliminator[4] containing 500 μc. of ^{210}Po impregnated in foil. A wire lead was soldered onto the stainless steel back of the unit. The whole electrode was then fastened to an insulated clamp and supported 5 mm. above the water surface in the trough and between the two barriers. The reference electrode was a standard KCl pH electrode[5] immersed in the subphase behind the stationary barrier. The two electrodes were connected by shielded cables to an electrometer[6]. The surface potential, ΔV, was taken as the difference of potential in millivolts between the clean water surface and the film-covered surface. It was not possible to measure the surface potential during the compression phases of the studies due to electrical interference from the electric motor driving the movable barrier.

RESULTS

Definition of Terms—For the purposes of this work, *association* of the penetrant with the insoluble film is defined as the irreversible entry of alkylbenzyldimethylammonium chloride into the film in such a way that it interacts with the film and is not subsequently expelled by compression of the penetrated film. *Penetration* is the general entrance of the alkylbenzyldimethylammonium chloride into the insoluble film and may or may not include association of the penetrant with the film. If the material is not associated, then it can be expelled by compression of the film. Association and penetration are accompanied by a change in both the surface pressure and surface potential.

Anchorage of the alkylbenzyldimethylammonium chloride onto the insoluble film signifies interaction and attachment of the alkylbenzyldimethylammonium chloride in the subphase to the film and involves the attraction between oppositely charged sites on the polar head groups in the subphase. Since this interaction does not occur in the interface but rather immediately below it, it is accompanied by a change in the surface potential with little or no effect on the surface pressure. *Adsorption* onto the film is similar to anchorage but is a more passive, nonspecific process which includes the entrance of the alkyl chain into the interfacial area. Surfactant molecules will be adsorbed at the interface even in the absence of a film. The effect of adsorption on the surface pressure and surface potential is variable.

Table I—Comparison of ΔF and $\Delta(\Delta V)$ for Alkylbenzyldimethylammonium Chloride Homologs 90 min. after Penetration Was Initiated

Homolog	—824 Å²/Molecule— ΔF^a, dynes/cm.	$\Delta(\Delta V)$, mv.	4000 Å²/Molecule, ΔF^b, dynes/cm.	Surface Tension Lowering Produced by 1.6×10^{-5} *M* Alkylbenzyldimethylammonium Chloride, dynes/cm.
12	1.4	+74	1.0	0.2
13	2.0	+93	1.2	0.3
14	3.4	+112	2.3	0.7
15	4.8	+147	3.7	1.2
16	5.5	+157	7.6	—

[a] Surface pressure of film prior to penetration = 6.6 dynes/cm.
[b] Surface pressure of film prior to penetration = 0.8 dyne/cm.

***F–A* Characteristics of Insoluble Films**—*Gliadin*—The surface pressure–area per molecule (*F–A*) isotherm for gliadin is shown in Fig. 1. The surface potential of the spread film was found to be +110 mv. at the maximum area (4000 Å²/molecule) and +328 mv. at the minimum area (324 Å²/molecule). The rate of compression was 503 Å²/molecule/min.

Cephalin—The *F–A* isotherm for cephalin is shown in Fig. 1. The film had a well-defined collapse point at a molecular area of 28.1 Å² and a film pressure of 54 dynes/cm. The extrapolated area per molecule was 39.6 Å²/molecule. The film had a surface potential of +255 mv. at the maximum area (156 Å²/molecule) and +390 mv. at the minimum area. The compression rate was 21.0 Å²/molecule/min.

Gliadin–Cephalin Monolayers—The solution used to produce the mixed monolayer contained a molar ratio of 16:1 cephalin to glia-

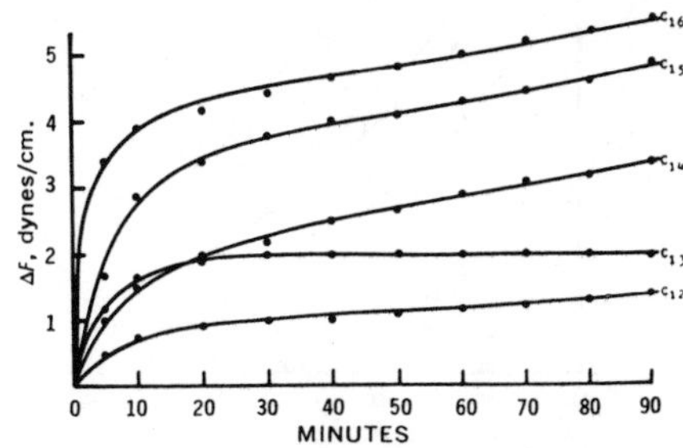

Figure 2—*Increase in surface pressure with time for gliadin monolayers penetrated by alkylbenzyldimethylammonium chloride (subphase concentration* = 1.6×10^{-5} M) *at constant surface area.*

[4] Staticmaster, Will Scientific, catalog No. 24887.
[5] Beckman Instruments, Inc., No. 31970.
[6] Keithley Instruments, model 610B.

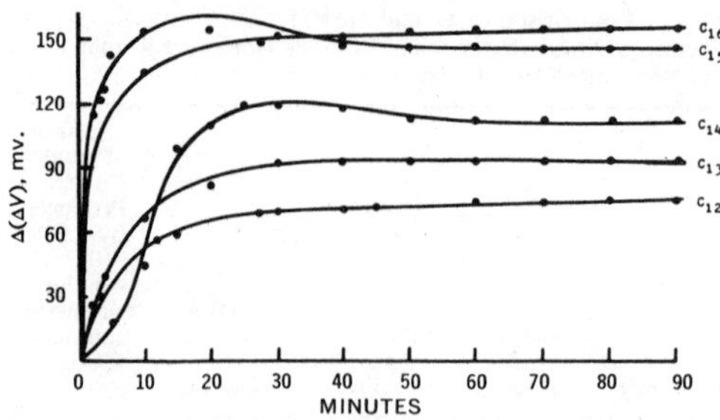

Figure 3—*Increase in surface potential with time for gliadin monolayers penetrated by alkylbenzyldimethylammonium chloride (subphase concentration = 1.6 × 10⁻⁵ M) at constant surface area. Initial surface potential = 264 ± 10 mv.*

din. This ratio is approximately equal to the ratio of 50:20 % w/w for protein to phospholipid commonly found in Gram-negative bacteria (8). The *F–A* isotherm for the mixed gliadin–cephalin film is shown in Fig. 1. The compressed film collapsed at a surface pressure of 50.2 dynes/cm. and an area of 34.9 Å²/molecule and gave an extrapolated area per molecule of 43.5 Å². The surface potential of the spread film was +257 mv. at the maximum area (297 Å²/molecule) and +366 mv. at the minimum area. The compression rate was 39.5 Å²/molecule/min.

Effect of Protamine—To determine if protamine would adsorb onto or penetrate into a spread film, protamine sulfate was injected into the subphase beneath one of the previously mentioned films, and the surface pressure and surface potential were monitored. When the subphase was 3.4×10^{-6} *M* with respect to the protamine, no effect on the surface pressure–area properties of the gliadin or gliadin–cephalin films was observed. A slight expansion was produced in the cephalin film (Fig. 1). With this same concentration of protamine, the surface potential remained constant for the gliadin–cephalin films but increased 38 mv. for the cephalin film.

Penetration Studies—The surface pressure or area increase and the change in surface potential were used to monitor the penetration of the C_{12}–C_{16} alkylbenzyldimethylammonium chloride molecules into the monolayer systems described previously. For the gliadin films, the penetration was followed as: (*a*) the change in the surface pressure, the surface area being held constant, and (*b*) the change in surface area, the surface pressure being held constant.

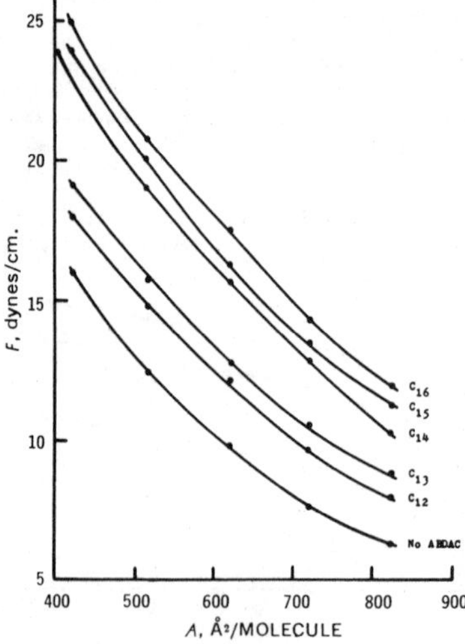

Figure 4—*Recompression of gliadin films previously penetrated at a constant area of 824 Å²/molecule. Subphase concentration of alkylbenzyldimethylammonium chloride = 1.6 × 10⁻⁵ M.*

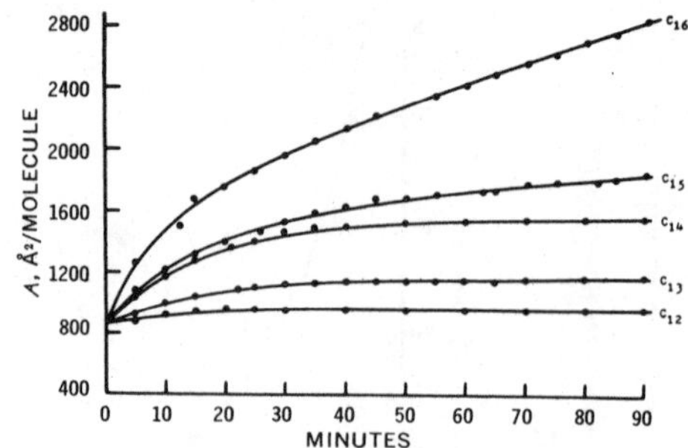

Figure 5—*Increase in surface area with time for gliadin monolayer penetrated by alkylbenzyldimethylammonium chloride (subphas concentration = 1.6 × 10⁻⁵ M) at constant surface pressure of 6. dynes/cm.*

For the gliadin–cephalin mixed film, only Method *a* was employed

Gliadin Monolayers: Penetration at Constant Area—Gliadi films penetrated at constant area showed an initial rapid increase i film pressure and surface potential, followed by a more gradua increase or a leveling off. The penetration was followed for at leas 90 min., at which time there was either no change in the surfac pressure and surface potential or a constant gradual increase that with the higher chain homologs, continued for over 4 hr. withou any apparent plateau being reached. Therefore, the value at the en of 90 min. was taken so that a comparison of the results could b shown (Table I). Plots of ΔF and $\Delta(\Delta V)$ *versus* time are shown i Figs. 2 and 3, respectively. Linear relationships were observed be tween ΔF and alkyl chain length ($r = 0.99$) and $\Delta(\Delta V)$ and alky chain length ($r = 0.99$).

Studies were also carried out using differing initial areas and sur face pressure; the concentration of alkylbenzyldimethylammoniun chloride in the subphase was also varied. It was found that change of the order of ±50 Å²/molecule in the initial area and ±0. dyne/cm. in the initial film pressure did not significantly alter th results shown in Table I. To see a more marked effect, gliadi films occupying an area of 4000 Å²/molecule and having a filn pressure of 0.75 dyne/cm. were penetrated by a concentration c

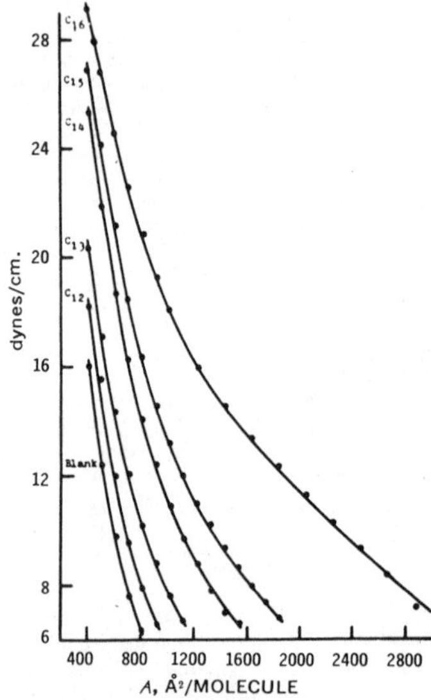

Figure 6—*Recompression of gliadin monolayers previously pene trated at a constant surface pressure of 6.6 dynes/cm. Subphase con centration of alkylbenzyldimethylammonium chloride = 1.6 × 10⁻⁵ M.*

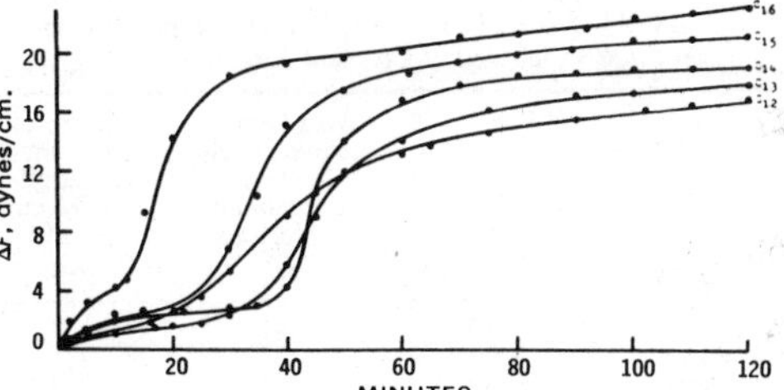

'igure 7—*Change in surface pressure with time for gliadin–cephalin nonolayers penetrated by alkylbenzyldimethylammonium chloride subphase concentration* = *1.6* × *10*$^{-5}$ M) *at a constant area of 139* Å^2*/molecule.*

.6 × 10^{-5} *M* drug in the subphase. Only Δ*F* was monitored in this tudy; the results are shown in Table I. As the concentration of the rug in the subphase increased, the observed change in surface ressure also increased. Following penetration at constant area, the lms were further compressed to their collapse area in order to ifferentiate between adsorbed and associated alkylbenzyldimethyl-mmonium chloride molecules. Typical results are shown in Fig. 4.

Gliadin Monolayers: Penetration at Constant Pressure—The enetration of gliadin films was also studied as a function of changng surface area, the surface pressure being held constant. Matalon) showed that additional quantitative information on the molecular association between a film and penetrating material can be btained by this technique. The change in area, as a function of ime, due to penetration of gliadin by alkylbenzyldimethylamnonium chloride homologs is shown in Fig. 5. Following expansion t constant film pressure, the films were recompressed to their minnum area so as to expel any solute adsorbed by the film. The *F–A* sotherms resulting from this recompression are shown in Fig. 6.

Experiments were also performed to determine the effect of the lm pressure and drug concentration in the subphase on the magniude of the penetration. The equilibrium film pressure prior to enetration was varied from 4.8 to 7.8 dynes/cm., and the concentraon was 1.92 × 10^{-5} *M* alkylbenzyldimethylammonium chloride in he subphase. The results of these experiments indicated that there vas no difference in the value of the extrapolated area per molecule, A_e, within the range of values studied.

Gliadin–Cephalin Mixed Films—The changes in surface pressure nd surface potential were also used to monitor the penetration of he mixed gliadin–cephalin films at constant area. These experinents were carried out with the C_{12}–C_{16} alkylbenzyldimethylamnonium chloride homologs. The penetration of the mixed monoayer showed an initial rapid increase in surface pressure, followed y a plateau (Fig. 7). The plateau pressure (approximately 2–4 ynes/cm. above the initial equilibrium film pressure) was normally eached within 10 min. following the introduction of the alkylbenzyldimethylammonium chloride homolog into the subphase. After a finite period of time, the surface pressure again began to increase rapidly. This second phase of the surface pressure increase was then followed by either a slow increase or a leveling off of the *F–t* plot.

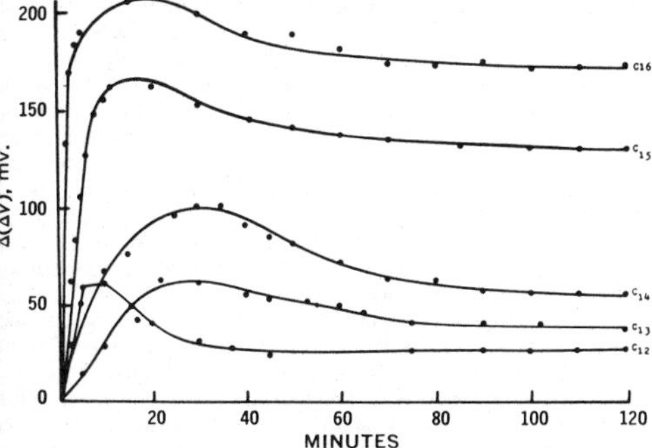

'igure 8—*Change in surface potential with time for gliadin–cephalin nonolayers penetrated by alkylbenzylammonium chloride (subphase oncentration* = *1.6* × *10*$^{-5}$ M) *at a constant area of 139* Å^2*/molecule.*

Table II—Penetration of Cephalin–Gliadin Films[a] by Alkylbenzyldimethylammonium Chloride Homologs

Homolog[b]	Δ$F^{c,d}$, dynes/cm.	Δ(ΔV)[c], mv.
12	17.0	+37
13	18.0	+27
14	19.7	+57
15	21.3	+135
16	23.2	+174

[a] Area = 139 Å^2/molecule. [b] Subphase concentration = 1.6 × 10^{-5} *M*. [c] After 120 min. [d] Initial equilibrium film pressure = 8.3 ± 0.2 dynes/cm.

The surface potential also increased rapidly initially and reached a plateau level at approximately the same time as the surface pressure (Fig. 8). However, as the second phase of surface pressure occurred (Fig. 7), the surface potential began to decrease. The results are summarized in Table II. Linear relationships were also observed between Δ*F* and alkyl chain length (r = 0.99) and Δ(Δ*V*) and alkyl chain length (r = 0.91). Compression curves of the previously penetrated mixed monolayers are shown in Fig. 9.

It was not possible to study the penetration into the mixed film at constant pressure because the film could not be expanded rapidly enough without: (*a*) causing disturbances in the surface, and/or (*b*) maintaining a constant film pressure during the second phase penetration. However, the attempted experiments indicated that the same type of process occurred as with penetration of the mixed film at constant area, *i.e.*, an initial increase and plateau followed by a rapid increase in the surface area.

Penetration of Alkylbenzyldimethylammonium Chloride into Gliadin Films in the Presence of Protamine—The procedure was the same as that used previously, and the penetration was followed as a function of the change in surface pressure and surface potential. Following the introduction of the C_{14} alkylbenzyldimethylammonium chloride homolog into the subphase (1.6 × 10^{-5} *M* concentration), there was an immediate and rapid increase in the surface pressure to a plateau level which was reached within 10 min. This increase was paralleled by a similar increase and plateau in the

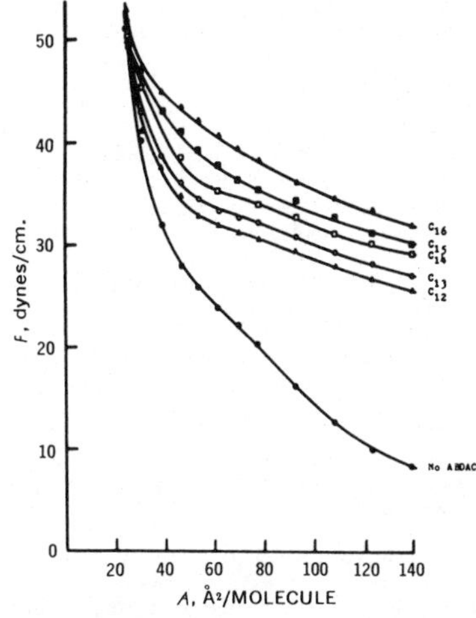

Figure 9—*Compression of gliadin–cephalin monolayers previously penetrated at a constant area of 139* Å^2*/molecule. Subphase concentration of alkylbenzyldimethylammonium chloride* = *1.6* × *10*$^{-5}$ M.

surface potential. A plot of the change in surface pressure and potential as a function of time is shown in Fig. 10*a*.

Penetration of Alkylbenzyldimethylammonium Chloride into Gliadin–Cephalin Films in the Presence of Protamine—The procedure and conditions for this study were those used for the preceding study. The changes in surface pressure and potential *versus* time are shown in Fig. 10*b*.

DISCUSSION

Cutler *et al.* (10) reported that peak bactericidal activity for the alkylbenzyldimethylammonium chloride homologs occurs at an alkyl chain length of 14 carbon atoms when tested against both Gram-positive (*Staphylococcus aureus*) and Gram-negative (*Salmonella typhosa* and *Pseudomonas aeruginosa*) organisms. To gain insight into the mechanism of action of the alkylbenzyldimethylammonium chloride homologs against Gram-positive and Gram-negative organisms, various *in vitro* experiments were performed with the aim of correlating some of the physical properties with the observed bactericidal activity of this series of compounds.

The initial rapid increase in surface pressure shown in Fig. 2, which occurs within 10–15 min., is attributed to the penetration of alkylbenzyldimethylammonium chloride into, and its association with, the gliadin monolayer. The surface potential (Fig. 3) also shows a rapid increase during this time period. However, the rate of increase of the surface potential decreases and then levels off within the first 10–15 min., whereas the surface pressure continues to increase but more gradually. The $\Delta(\Delta V)$ data indicate that the distribution of alkylbenzyldimethylammonium chloride between the interfacial region and the subphase is essentially complete within 15 min. of its introduction into the subphase. However, the subsequent penetration process is slower and continues, although at a slower rate, beyond the first 15 min.

Following anchorage to the gliadin monolayer, it can be postulated that the alkylbenzyldimethylammonium chloride molecule undergoes a reorientation, followed by penetration of the hydrocarbon tail and benzyl ring into the monolayer. This reorientation is necessary because the initial step, prior to actual penetration, presumably involves an interaction between the polar head groups of the gliadin and alkylbenzyldimethylammonium chloride. Following this reorientation, the hydrophobic portion of the alkylbenzyldimethylammonium chloride molecule then associates with the hydrophobic amino acid side chains.

The compression to minimum area of a film previously penetrated at constant area can provide further information on the association complex formed between the materials. That the compressed penetrated films shown in Fig. 4 attained a higher film pressure at the minimum area indicates that the penetrant is not expelled from the interfacial area but is held there by a strong association with the gliadin.

The data presented in Table I indicate that the results observed were not due to simple passive adsorption of the surface-active material at the interface. Thus, the surface pressures generated by the presence of 1.6×10^{-5} *M* alkylbenzyldimethylammonium chloride confirm the observation that the affinity of alkylbenzyldimethylammonium chloride for the insoluble film is greater than the tendency toward simple passive adsorption. Consequently, given sufficient area, alkylbenzyldimethylammonium chloride molecules will penetrate the insoluble film until all the sites where association can take place are filled.

It was shown (9) that data on the formation of the association complex can also be gained from penetration studies conducted at a constant surface pressure and monitored as the change in surface area with time. The curves generated by this technique (Fig. 5) are similar in profile to those for the association between cholesterol and sodium cetyl sulfate and between cholesterol and saponin (9). Recompression (Fig. 6) again shows the presence of a strong association between gliadin and alkylbenzyldimethylammonium chloride.

The expansion curves in Fig. 5 are the result of two simultaneous processes which can be described as follows (9): (*a*) interaction of the solute with the film-forming molecules, the stoichiometry of which is indicated by the value of the area, extrapolated to zero time, and (*b*) solution of the injected solute in the surface structure as demonstrated by the linear expansion.

Extrapolation of the linear gradual increase to zero time will yield the area occupied by the stoichiometric complex formed between the

Table III—Data Derived from Extrapolation of Linear Region of Gliadin Films Penetrated at Constant Pressure

Homolog	A_e, Å²/Molecule	Area Due to Alkylbenzyl-dimethyl-ammonium Chloride, Å²	Ratio of Alkylbenzyl dimethyl-ammonium Chloride to Gliadin
12	970	146	1.7
13	1090	266	3.1
14	1480	656	7.7
15	1520	696	8.2
16	1640	816	9.6

two molecules (9). The values of A_e, the area reached by extrapola tion of the linear portion of the corrected curve to zero time, a given in Table III. From a knowledge of the area occupied by th gliadin molecules and the cross-sectional area of the alkylbenzy dimethylammonium chloride molecule (11), the stoichiometry of th complex can be determined. The molecular ratio of alkylbenzy dimethylammonium chloride to gliadin is also presented in Tab III.

The penetration of alkylbenzyldimethylammonium chloric into gliadin–cephalin mixed films was followed as a function of su face pressure and surface potential *versus* time. Plots of these fun tions are shown in Figs. 7 and 8. Penetration into the gliadin cephalin films is characterized by an initial increase in surface pre sure followed by a plateau. This plateau is reached within 10 mi of the introduction of the alkylbenzyldimethylammonium chloric into the subphase and has a duration of up to 40 min., dependin on the homolog. During this same time interval, the surface po tential rises rapidly to a peak and then starts a gradual declin Comparison of Figs. 7 and 8 during this time period with Figs. and 3 (gliadin monolayer) indicates that this rise in surface pressu and surface potential is due to the penetration of alkylbenzyld methylammonium chloride and its association with the gliad component of the mixed monolayer.

After this plateau region, a second, more drastic, process tak place. During this phase, the surface pressure increases rapidly an then assumes an equilibrium value. At the same time, the surfac potential decreases slightly. This surface pressure increase is a tributed to penetration of the alkylbenzyldimethylammoniu chloride into, and interaction with, the cephalin component of th monolayer, since this second phase process does not occur with th gliadin monolayer. No explanation is advanced at this time for th small, but real, decrease in surface potential.

Figure 9 shows the compression isotherms of the gliadin–ceph lin monolayers previously penetrated at constant area by the alky benzyldimethylammonium chloride homologs. As seen from th figure, the penetrated films collapse at the same area and pressu as the nonpenetrated film. This indicates that during the course compression, the alkylbenzyldimethylammonium chloride is pr gressively forced out of the monolayer, which then behaves ide tically with the two-component gliadin–cephalin film. Previous wo (1) demonstrated a bulk phase ionic interaction between cephal and alkylbenzyldimethylammonium chloride. In addition, it ca be shown that the *F–A* isotherm for the mixed gliadin–cephal film is slightly more expanded than expected on the basis of the is therm derived from the isotherms for the two single-compone systems. This latter phenomenon suggests only a minor interactic between gliadin and cephalin, since a more condensed film wou be expected if a strong interaction existed. On this basis, a ratio alization of the behavior of alkylbenzyldimethylammonium chl ride, in the presence of the gliadin–cephalin mixed monolayer ca be proposed. Thus, the initial stage involves penetration of alky benzyldimethylammonium chloride into and association wi (through London forces) the gliadin component of the mixed mon layer. Subsequently, the alkylbenzyldimethylammonium chlori penetrates and interacts with the cephalin molecules in the mix monolayer; the interaction in this case is ionic in nature. Up compression of the penetrated monolayer, the alkylbenzyldimeth ammonium chloride that is associated with the cephalin is expell from the monolayer but remains anchored in the top layer of t subphase such that the polar head of the alkylbenzyldimethylan monium chloride is adjacent to the negatively charged site on t

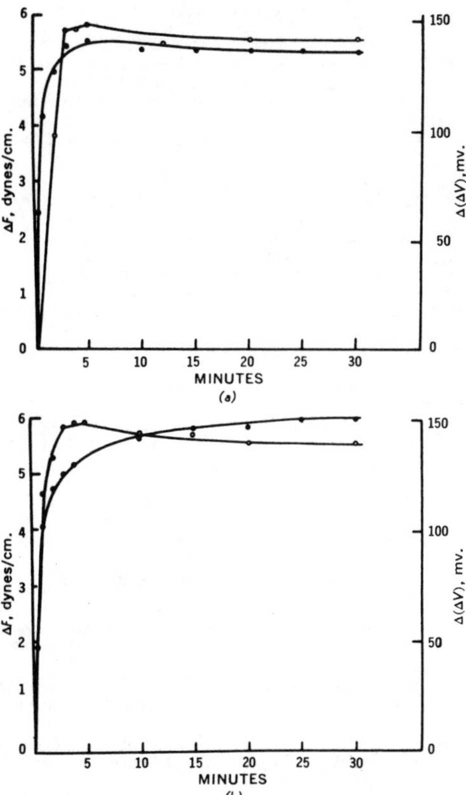

'igure 10—*Penetration of* C_{14} *alkylbenzyldimethylammonium* *hloride into:* (a) *gliadin film in the presence of protamine at a con-* *tant area of 824 Å²/molecule, and* (b) *gliadin–cephalin film at a con-* *tant area of 139 Å²/molecule in the presence of protamine. Key:* ●, *F; and* ○, Δ(ΔV).

ephalin. It is possible that at the relatively high surface pressures btained at maximum compression, the gliadin may also be expelled om the monolayer. Unfortunately, the present data do not permit n unequivocal statement on this possibility. Were this to happen, would presumably also occur in the compression of the simple .*e.*, unpenetrated) mixed gliadin–cephalin monolayer.

The ΔF and $\Delta(\Delta V)$ *versus* time plots for the penetration of alkyl- enzyldimethylammonium chloride into gliadin (Fig. 10*a*) and liadin–cephalin (Fig. 10*b*) monolayers in the presence of protamine dicate that the same penetration process is occurring in both cases. he gliadin content in the two films was essentially the same, the ure monolayer of protamine containing 9.82×10^{14} molecules nd the mixed monolayer containing 7.70×10^{14} molecules of liadin. That the penetration of the two monolayers was nearly iden- ical indicates that the presence of protamine screened the cephalin n the monolayer to the point that it was unable to interact with the lkylbenzyldimethylammonium chloride. Thus, the C_{14} alkylbenzyl- imethylammonium chloride homolog interacted only with the liadin component of the film; since there was approximately an qual amount of gliadin in each monolayer, the surface pressure and urface potential increase was similar.

Protamine is a highly basic protein having an isoelectric point reater than 12 (12). This is due to the high percentage (approxi- nately 70%) of the basic amino acid arginine. It was shown (13) that rotamine forms an insoluble precipitate with cephalin. However, as nentioned previously and as would be expected, the cephalin re- nains in the interface. Certainly, the magnitude of the time-depen- lent rise in ΔF resembles that with gliadin on water (Fig. 2) rather han that with gliadin–cephalin on water (Fig. 7). The results obtained here imply that, as might be expected, the cephalin remains at the interface. It seems likely that the protamine attaches itself by charge neutralization to the negatively charged site on the cephalin molecule. In the absence of protamine this would be the site for attachment of the penetrating alkylbenzyldimethylammonium chloride ion. With the effective elimination (by neutralization) of this charged site from the interface, the alkylbenzyldimethylammonium chloride ion must depend upon the gliadin for its ability to anchor onto and penetrate into the film.

CONCLUSIONS

In view of the experimental results and ensuing discussion derived from the model bacterial cell wall, a general theory can be put forward on the mechanism of action of the homologous series of alkylbenzyldimethylammonium chloride bactericides. It must be realized, however, that the studies discussed here are concerned with only the first event occurring in the sequence of events leading to cell lysis (14), namely, adsorption onto and penetration of the surface of the porous bacterial cell wall. The model does not concern itself with transport through the cell wall and the underlying cell membrane, although it does allow extrapolation of the results obtained to these situations.

The observation that peak activity of the alkylbenzyldimethylammonium chloride series resides with the C_{14} homolog is probably related to more than one physical property of the series. It is unlikely that the C_{14} homolog would possess maximum activity in a series due to its particular intrinsic structure, especially since its action has been theorized to be nonspecific. Rather, it appears that this homolog owes its activity to a combination of effects which determine the relative ease with which the homolog can get to the active site and then exert its action. Thus, the hydrocarbon chain of the molecule is needed so that the material will be adsorbed at the bacterial interface in sufficient quantities. This is related to the fact that the longer the hydrocarbon chain, the greater the tendency to be adsorbed at an interface. Also, it is certain that the onium head group is needed for bactericidal activity. This onium head group also lends aqueous solubility to the molecule; thus, its function should not be overshadowed by the hydrocarbon chain. As such, the magnitude of the bactericidal activity of a particular homolog would be dependent on a balance between two physical properties, the aqueous solubility and the relative surface activity, one of which decreases with increasing chain length and the other of which increases.

A gliadin monolayer was used as the model system for Gram-positive bacteria whose cell walls are principally protein. The penetration studies conducted indicate that the alkylbenzyldimethylammonium chloride molecule was able to penetrate into and become bound to the protein molecules in the insoluble monolayer. Extrapolation of these results to the bacterial cell wall suggests that the alkylbenzyldimethylammonium chloride ion exerts its effect through the development of London forces with the lipophilic side chains of amino acid residues of the protein. As a result of this "solution" within the cell wall, the bactericide is then able to penetrate through the cell wall and disrupt the vital cell membrane. This disruption would then lead to the irreversible permeability change and gross leakage from the cells, which is the first step in bacterial cell death (14).

The observation that Gram-negative organisms are more resistant than Gram-positive organisms to the action of ionic detergents has been ascribed to the difference in lipid content of the cell walls, the Gram-negative membrane having much greater amounts of phospholipid (15). Therefore, a gliadin–cephalin mixed monolayer was used as the model for the Gram-negative cell wall.

As noted previously, large quantities of the alkylbenzyldimethylammonium chloride homologs were able to penetrate into the gliadin–cephalin monolayers in a two-step process. However, following penetration, the alkylbenzyldimethylammonium chloride did not appear to be associated with the film, being expelled from the mixed monolayer on compression. However, it is likely that, because of the ionic interaction between alkylbenzyldimethylammonium chloride and cephalin, the former remains anchored in the subphase immediately below the cephalin. The phospholipid thus serves to protect the cell membrane by reacting ionically with the alkylbenzyldimethylammonium chloride. Only after all ionic sites on the phospholipid have reacted with the alkylbenzyldimethylammonium chloride can the bactericide penetrate through the cell wall and initiate the increase in cell permeability that precedes death. This would account for the fact that higher concentrations of alkylbenzyldimethylammonium chloride are needed to produce the same bactericidal effect in Gram-negative organisms than in Gram-positive organisms.

It was previously observed (16) that the prior addition of small amounts of cephalin to the bulk phase made Gram-positive bacteria more resistant to the action of quaternary ammonium compounds. There are two possible explanations to account for this observation, one or both of which may be operative. One possible explanation is that the phospholipid is adsorbed onto the cell wall and remains there, possibly partially penetrated or merely attached by ionic interactions. When the cationic bactericide is added to the solution and adsorbed onto the cell, it may interact ionically with the cephalin in much the same way as is proposed for the simulated Gram-negative cell wall. In this way, the Gram-positive organisms would be protected. Another possible explanation is that the cephalin in solution interacts with the alkylbenzyldimethylammonium chloride in solution, thereby producing an inactive interaction product. As a result, the effective concentration of the bactericide would be decreased. The conductometric studies (1) confirmed that cephalin and alkylbenzyldimethylammonium chloride reacted with each other in solution, probably through ion-pair formation to form a large complex. Thus, this explanation is also feasible.

It was also observed (17) that addition of protamine to the bulk phase causes Gram-negative bacteria to become more susceptible to the action of quaternary ammonium bactericides. Monolayer studies indicated that protamine is able to interact with the cephalin in the film. This interaction between cephalin and protamine could then nullify the ionic interaction of the phospholipid with the alkylbenzyldimethylammonium chloride. The model may then be considered as having been changed from that representing a Gram-negative bacterial cell wall to that simulating a Gram-positive cell wall. The bactericide would then be free to interact with the protein and freely penetrate the cell wall and cell membrane.

Thus, as a result of studies on a simulated bacterial cell wall, it is felt that the alkylbenzyldimethylammonium chloride series of quaternary ammonium bactericides exert their action by development of London forces with the protein component of the cell wall. This association then leads to penetration of the wall and alteration of the integrity of the cell membrane, with a resulting change in its permeability. This change in permeability allows low molecular weight metabolites to leak out of the cell, followed by complete lysis of the cell by the action of its own autolytic enzymes.

REFERENCES

(1) D. W. Blois and J. Swarbrick, *J. Pharm. Sci.*, **61**, 390(1972).

(2) H. B. Bull, *Advan. Protein Chem.*, **3**, 95(1947).

(3) J. H. Schulman and E. K. Rideal, *Proc. Roy. Soc., Ser. B*, **122**, 29(1937).

(4) D. W. Blois, Ph.D. thesis, University of Connecticut, Storrs, Conn., 1970.

(5) G. R. Tristam, *Nature*, **160**, 137(1947).

(6) J. W. Munden, D. W. Blois, and J. Swarbrick, *J. Pharm. Sci.*, **58**, 1308(1969).

(7) G. L. Gaines, "Insoluble Monolayers at Liquid–Gas Interfaces," Interscience, New York, N. Y., 1966.

(8) M. R. J. Salton, *Biochim. Biophys. Acta*, **8**, 510(1952).

(9) R. Matalon, *J. Colloid Sci.*, **8**, 53(1953).

(10) R. A. Cutler, E. B. Cimijotti, T. J. Okolowich, and W. Wetterau, *Soap Chem. Spec.*, **Mar. 1967**, 84, and **Apr. 1967**, 74.

(11) D. W. Blois and J. Swarbrick, *J. Colloid Interface Sci.*, **36**, 226(1971).

(12) K. Felix, *Advan. Protein Chem.*, **15**, 1(1960).

(13) R. Chargaff, *J. Biol. Chem.*, **125**, 661(1938).

(14) M. R. J. Salton, *Ann. Rev. Microbiol.*, **21**, 417(1967).

(15) R. Gilby and A. V. Few, *J. Gen. Microbiol.*, **23**, 19(1960).

(16) Z. Baker, R. W. Harrison, and B. F. Miller, *J. Exp. Med.*, **74**, 621(1941).

(17) B. F. Miller, R. Abrams, A. Dorfman, and A. M. Kelin, *Science*, **96**, 428(1942).

ACKNOWLEDGMENTS AND ADDRESSES

Received May 17, 1971, from the *Division of Pharmaceutics, School of Pharmacy, University of Connecticut, Storrs, CT 06268*

Accepted for publication December 10, 1971.

Presented in part to the Basic Pharmaceutics Section, APhA Academy of Pharmaceutical Sciences, San Francisco meeting, March 1971.

Supported in part by Public Health Service Fellowship FO1-GM-36156 (to D. W. Blois) and by Grant 064 from the University of Connecticut Research Foundation.

* Present address: Sterling-Winthrop Research Institute, Rensselaer, N. Y.

▲ To whom inquiries should be directed.

Reprinted from *J. Bacteriol.* **86**, 207–211 (1963)

EFFECT OF INORGANIC CATIONS ON BACTERICIDAL ACTIVITY OF ANIONIC SURFACTANTS

19

J. G. VOSS

Miami Valley Laboratories, The Procter & Gamble Co., Cincinnati, Ohio

Received for publication 11 March 1963

Abstract

Voss, J. G. (Procter & Gamble Co., Cincinnati, Ohio). Effect of inorganic cations on bactericidal activity of anionic surfactants. J. Bacteriol. **86:**207–211. 1963.—The bactericidal effectiveness of two alkyl benzene sulfonates and of three other types of anionic surfactants against *Staphylococcus aureus* is increased in the presence of low concentrations of divalent cations, especially alkaline earths and metals of group IIB of the periodic table. The cations may act by decreasing the negative charge at the cell surface and increasing adsorption of the surfactant anions, leading to damage to the cytoplasmic membrane and death of the cell. Increased adsorption of surfactant is also found with *Escherichia coli*, but does not lead to death of the cell.

Synthetic detergents are now widely used for purposes of cleaning and sanitation. The most commonly used synthetic surfactant is the anionic alkyl benzene sulfonate (C_{12}ABS), in which the alkyl is a branched-chain dodecyl group composed of four propylene units. This compound has negligible bactericidal activity against gram-negative bacteria, but appreciable activity against gram-positive species.

In preliminary studies of the bactericidal activity of C_{12}ABS, 0.1 M phosphate buffer was used to control pH. An unexpected increase in bactericidal activity of C_{12}ABS against *Staphylococcus aureus* was observed. Addition of other salts (NaCl, KCl) instead of the buffer showed this to be a nonspecific effect of electrolytes, rather than solely an effect of pH. The work reported here shows that the activity of C_{12}ABS and other anionic surfactants against *S. aureus* may be greatly increased by the addition of some divalent inorganic cations.

Materials and Methods

Five anionic surfactants were studied. The C_{12}ABS was approximately 99% surfactant; C_{15}ABS, with a pentapropylene side chain, was of similar purity. Lauryl glyceryl ether sulfonate was 98.5% surfactant. Lauryl trioxyethylene sulfate was used as a paste containing 55.4% surfactant plus water and a considerable amount of Na_2SO_4. Lauryl sulfate was used as a product containing 90% surfactant and 10% inorganic salts. All three lauryl derivatives were prepared from fatty alcohol produced by reduction of coconut oil fatty acids, and containing predominantly lauryl alcohol. All of the surfactants were used as the sodium salts.

The test organisms, *S. aureus* ATCC 6538 and *Escherichia coli* ATCC 10536, were grown for 24 hr at 37 C in Brain Heart Infusion broth (Difco), centrifuged, washed once in water, and resuspended in water to the original volume. A 2-ml portion of the suspension of washed cells was added to 18 ml of the test solution at 37 C; the final pH was 5.9 to 6.8. The initial population was 100 to 150 million per ml for both organisms, by plate count on Brain Heart Infusion Agar. Plate counts were made in duplicate after 10-min exposure of the cells to the test solution at 37 C.

Electrophoretic measurements on suspensions of *S. aureus* were made by moving-boundary electrophoresis, using a Perkin-Elmer model 38A instrument.

Adsorption of C_{12}ABS by *S. aureus* and *E. coli* was determined with S^{35}-tagged C_{12}ABS, with a specific activity of 10 to 16 mc/g. The adsorption was carried out for 15 min at 37 C in a volume of 10 ml; the cells were then centrifuged, resuspended in water, and sampled for radioassay. Because the adsorption is readily reversible, the cells could not be washed without loss of a large fraction of the adsorbed $C_{12}ABS^{35}$. Calculations of adsorption were corrected for an average 1% carry-over of the supernatant. The samples were assayed for radioactivity by counting in a liquid scintillation counter, using a Packard Tri-Carb spectrometer.

Nitrogen was determined by the micro-Kjeldahl method.

RESULTS

The results of studies on the influence of a number of salts on the bactericidal activity of C_{12}ABS against *S. aureus* are shown in Table 1. Under the conditions of the test, average survival after exposure to 25 ppm of C_{12}ABS alone was 85%. No differences between the effects of sulfates and chlorides were observed; different cations, however, varied markedly in their effect on the bactericidal activity of C_{12}ABS. The most effective were divalent alkaline earth cations, and especially those metals belonging to group IIB of the periodic table. It will be noted that increased bactericidal activity could still be observed at salt concentrations which were lower than the concentration of C_{12}ABS; addition of a quantity of $CaCl_2$ insufficient to convert all of the C_{12}ABS to the calcium salt still permitted only 28% survival of the test organism. With the exception of $HgCl_2$, none of these salts displayed significant bactericidal activity when tested alone at the concentrations shown. Cell stained after death showed no visible alteration and no loss of their gram-positive character.

Other work showed that the effect of $CaCl_2$ i increasing bactericidal activity was not d minished in the presence of a tenfold mola excess of NaCl; no antagonism between th cations was observed.

Since divalent cations had proved effec tive, the effect of a "divalent organic cation was tested. 1,4-Dimethyl-1,4-diazoniabicyclo (2,2,2)-octane diiodide was prepared by reactio of triethylene diamine with excess methyl iodide and was recrystallized from methanol. Thi compound, with two positively charged N atoms was ineffective in increasing the bactericida activity of 25 ppm of C_{12}ABS, when added at concentration of 5×10^{-4} M.

Because the activity of C_{12}ABS had bee studied most extensively in the presence c $CaCl_2$, the behavior of four other anioni surfactants in the presence of this salt was als determined. The data in Table 2 show that th effect of $CaCl_2$ in increasing bactericidal activit

TABLE 1. *Per cent survival of Staphylococcus aureus after 10-min exposure at 37 C to 25 ppm of C_{12}ABS (0.00007 M)[a] plus indicated salts*

Salt	Molar concn of salt									
	0.15	0.05	0.01	0.0025	0.0005	0.0001	0.00005	0.000025	0.00001	0.00000
NaCl	1.4	1.0 (2)[b]	61							
Na_2SO_4		6.1	61	79						
KCl	1.4									
LiCl					>10					
$MgSO_4$		0.034	0.036	3.8						
$MgCl_2$		0.017	0.025	2.5	8.8					
$CaCl_2$		0.017	0.035 (3)	0.055 (2)	5.0 (10)	14 (3)	31 (4)	28	45	
$ZnCl_2$					0.35					
$BaCl_2$					6.0					
$CuSO_4$					3.5					
$MnCl_2$					8.0					
$CdCl_2$					0.086 (2)		6.6		>20	
$HgCl_2$							0.0089[c]		14[d]	25[e]
$SrCl_2$					19					
$FeCl_3$					>25					
$AlCl_3$					>25					
$SnCl_4$					>25					

[a] Used alone, 25 ppm of C_{12}ABS gave 85% survival.
[b] Parenthetical figures indicate number of replicate determinations.
[c] $HgCl_2$ control (no C_{12}ABS): 0.21% survival.
[d] $HgCl_2$ control: 17% survival.
[e] $HgCl_2$ control: 39% survival.

TABLE 2. *Per cent survival of Staphylococcus aureus after 10-min exposure at 37 C to mixtures of anionic surfactants with $CaCl_2$*

Surfactant	Concn	$CaCl_2$	Survival
	ppm	M	%
C_{12}ABS	25 (7 × 10^{-5} M)	—	85 (16)*
	25	5 × 10^{-4}	5.0 (10)
	25	10^{-4}	14 (3)
	25	5 × 10^{-5}	31 (4)
C_{15}ABS	25 (6 × 10^{-5} M)	—	24
	25	5 × 10^{-4}	0.12
	25	10^{-4}	0.15
	25	5 × 10^{-5}	0.26
Lauryl sulfate	25 (8 × 10^{-5} M)	—	56
	25	10^{-3}	25
	25	5 × 10^{-5}	24
	50	—	35
	50	10^{-3}	0.52
	50	5 × 10^{-5}	4.1
Lauryl glyceryl ether sulfonate	25 (6 × 10^{-5} M)	—	89
	25	5 × 10^{-4}	30
	50	—	63
	50	5 × 10^{-4}	2.6
	100	—	28 (2)
	100	5 × 10^{-4}	0.36 (2)
Lauryl trioxyethylene sulfate	50 (12 × 10^{-5} M)	—	25
	50	5 × 10^{-4}	8.6
	100	—	1.8
	100	5 × 10^{-4}	0.55
None	—	5 × 10^{-4}	100

* Parenthetical figures indicate number of replicate determinations.

against *S. aureus* is not limited to C_{12}ABS but is also apparent with other detergent types. The effect was greatest, however, with the two alkyl benzene sulfonates.

It seemed probable that increased kill of *S. aureus* by C_{12}ABS in the presence of added electrolyte was due to increased adsorption of the anionic surfactant by the negatively charged cell. Therefore, the adsorption of reduced concentrations of $C_{12}ABS^{35}$ was determined in the presence and absence of added $CaCl_2$. The influence of $CaCl_2$ on adsorption of $C_{12}ABS^{35}$ by the insusceptible *E. coli* was similarly determined. The results in Table 3 show that the adsorption of $C_{12}ABS^{35}$ by *S. aureus* is indeed increased by $CaCl_2$. Interestingly, although low concentrations of C_{12}ABS have little or no killing action on *E. coli*, the adsorption of $C_{12}ABS^{35}$ by this organism is somewhat greater than that by the susceptible *S. aureus*, and is similarly increased by $CaCl_2$.

Because of its effect on adsorption of C_{12}ABS, a preliminary investigation of the influence of $CaCl_2$ on the electrophoretic behavior of *S. aureus* was carried out. Cells were suspended in 0.01 M $CaCl_2$ or NaCl, and mobility was determined by moving-boundary electrophoresis. Mobilities of the suspended cells, in (μ/sec)/(v/cm), were calculated as 1.18 in $CaCl_2$ and 3.30 in NaCl. Calcium ion is evidently more effective than sodium ion in reducing the net negative charge on the cell, and presumably in increasing adsorption of the C_{12}ABS anion in that manner.

As Hotchkiss (1946) showed, bactericidal activity of surfactants is accompanied by a

TABLE 3. *Adsorption of $C_{12}ABS^{35}$ by bacterial cell suspensions in 15 min at 37 C*

Organism	Added $C_{12}ABS^{35}$	$CaCl_2$	$C_{12}ABS^{35}$ adsorbed by cells
	ppm	M	%
Staphylococcus aureus	8 (2.2×10^{-5} M)	—	2.0
	8	2×10^{-4}	1.9
	8	8×10^{-3}	5.9
	8	8×10^{-2}	10
Escherichia coli	9 (2.9×10^{-5} M)	—	4.3
	9	2.25×10^{-4}	6.9
	9	9×10^{-3}	13
	9	9×10^{-2}	18

TABLE 4. *Release of nitrogen compounds from Staphylococcus aureus after exposure to $C_{12}ABS$ and $CaCl_2$ for 15 min at 37 C*

$C_{12}ABS$	$CaCl_2$	Survival	N in supernatant
ppm	M	%	*μg/ml*
—	—	100	14
25	—	90	29
25	5×10^{-3}	1.3	58

leakage of the constituents of the cell into the environment. Table 4 shows that the increased kill of *S. aureus* by $C_{12}ABS$ in the presence of $CaCl_2$ is accompanied by release of nitrogen compounds into the solution.

Discussion

Relatively little work on the adsorption of electrolytes and surfactants at bacterial surfaces has been reported. Adsorption of cations at the negatively charged cell surface was indicated by the electrophoretic studies of Winslow, Falk, and Caulfield (1923); Ca ions seemed more readily adsorbed than Na ions. McCalla (1940) studied the adsorption of 10^{-3} M and lower concentrations of H ions and of metal, alkali, and alkaline earth cations by *E. coli*, and demonstrated preferential adsorption of Ca, Mg, Ba, Mn, and Hg; more strongly adsorbed ions were able to replace those less strongly adsorbed. The possibility of adsorption at sites other than the surface of the cell wall is indicated by the work of Harris, Eisenstark, and Dragsdorf (1954), who obtained evidence that the site of adsorption of mercuric ions by *E. coli*, *Salmonella pullorum*, and *Azotobacter agile* is inside the cell wall, at the level of the cytoplasmic membrane.

There is also electrophoretic evidence of the adsorption of surfactants on the cell surface. Dyar and Ordal (1946) demonstrated that the negative charge of several species is increased by the anionic surfactant sodium tetradecyl sulfate and decreased by the cationic surfactant cetyl pyridinium chloride. This work, and that of Dyar (1948), implicated the surface lipides of the cell as the constituents primarily responsible for the adsorption of anionic surfactants. In contrast, Loveday and James (1957) found that the electrophoretic mobility of *Aerobacter aerogenes* is decreased at low concentrations of phenol or sodium dodecyl sulfate and increased at higher concentrations; the increased mobility of the cells at the higher concentrations of phenol or dodecyl sulfate was attributed to adsorption of a second layer of ions by van der Waals forces with the polar groups directed outward. The concentration of phenol or surfactant causing 100% kill appeared to be that which gave complete formation of the first layer on the surface of the cell.

If the action of surfactants is not directly on the cell wall, the difference in susceptibility of gram-positive and gram-negative species may be due to an inability of the surfactant ion to penetrate the more complex wall of the gram-negative cell, although adsorption on the cell wall has been shown to occur. The data given here support the assumption that cations are adsorbed on the negatively charged cell wall, or at the cytoplasmic membrane (Harris et al., 1954), and promote the adsorption of surfactant anions. These appear to exert their bactericidal effect by altering the permeability of the cytoplasmic membrane (Hotchkiss, 1946; Newton, 1960). There is direct evidence (Salton, 1957;

Gilby and Few, 1957, 1960) that ionic surfactants can disrupt the cytoplasmic membrane; in this way, they are able to cause the lysis of protoplasts.

There is no *a priori* reason to expect a close correspondence experimentally between bactericidal action and adsorption of the surfactant; e.g., Table 3 shows no increased adsorption by *S. aureus* of 8 ppm of $C_{12}ABS^{35}$ in the presence of 10^{-4} M $CaCl_2$, although $CaCl_2$ concentrations as low as 10^{-5} M cause decreased survival in the presence of 25 ppm of $C_{12}ABS$ (Table 1). Only some fraction of the total surfactant adsorbed need penetrate to the cytoplasmic membrane to cause death of the cell.

The well-known observation that polyvalent cations reduce the antibacterial activity of cationic surfactants may be mentioned here; reduction in activity may be due to exclusion of the surfactant from the bacterial surface.

Thus, the role of the more effective cations in promoting the bactericidal activity of anionic surfactants against *S. aureus* appears to be in increasing adsorption of the surfactant at the cell wall; penetration of the anion to the cytoplasmic membrane then results in disorganization of the membrane, loss of intracellular metabolites, and death of the cell without distinct morphological changes. In this manner, the bactericidal activity of some anionic surfactants may be increased many-fold.

ACKNOWLEDGMENTS

The capable assistance of J. D. Kennedy, H. W. Lampe, and W. L. Gagen in various phases of the work is gratefully acknowledged.

LITERATURE CITED

DYAR, M. T. 1948. Electrokinetical studies on bacterial surfaces. II. Studies on surface lipids, amphoteric material, and some other surface properties. J. Bacteriol. **56**:821–834.

DYAR, M. T., AND E. J. ORDAL. 1946. Electrokinetic studies on bacterial surfaces. I. The effects of surface-active agents on the electrophoretic mobilities of bacteria. J. Bacteriol. **51**:149–167.

GILBY, A. R., AND A. V. FEW. 1957. Reactivity of ionic detergents with *Micrococcus lysodeikticus*. Nature **179**:422–423.

GILBY, A. R., AND A. V. FEW. 1960. Lysis of protoplasts of *Micrococcus lysodeikticus* by ionic detergents. J. Gen. Microbiol. **23**:19–26.

HARRIS, J. O., A. EISENSTARK, AND R. D. DRAGSDORF. 1954. A study of the location of adsorbed mercuric ions in Escherichia coli. J. Bacteriol. **68**:745–748.

HOTCHKISS, R. D. 1946. The nature of the bactericidal action of surface-active agents. Ann. N.Y. Acad. Sci. **46**:479–492.

LOVEDAY, D. E. E., AND A. M. JAMES. 1957. Relationship between the concentration of anionic surface-active agents and the electrophoretic mobility and viability of *Aerobacter aerogenes*. Nature **180**:1121–1122.

MCCALLA, T. M. 1940. Cation adsorption by bacteria. J. Bacteriol. **40**:23–32.

NEWTON, B. A. 1960. The mechanism of the bactericidal action of surface-active compounds: a summary. J. Appl. Bacteriol. **23**:345–349.

SALTON, M. R. J. 1957. The action of lytic agents on the surface structures of the bacterial cell. Proc. Intern. Congr. Surface Activity, 2nd, London **4**:245–253.

WINSLOW, C.-E. A., I. S. FALK, AND M. F. CAULFIELD. 1923. Electrophoresis of bacteria as influenced by hydrogen-ion concentration and the presence of sodium and calcium salts. J. Gen. Physiol. **6**:177–200.

Reprinted from *Brit. Med. J.* **2**, 153–155 (1967)

20

Contamination of Hospital Disinfectants with *Pseudomonas* Species

D. W. BURDON,* M.B., B.S.; J. L. WHITBY,† M.B., M.R.C.P., M.C.PATH.

Brit. med. J., 1967, **2**, 153–155

During the investigation of an outbreak of infection caused by *Proteus mirabilis* in the infants' nursery it was found that solutions of disinfectants in use there were contaminated with viable Gram-negative bacilli. The organisms cultured were not *Proteus* sp., and were quite unconnected with the outbreak. This finding prompted us to examine stocks of disinfectants in the hospital for the presence of living bacteria.

Subsequent investigation showed that aqueous solutions of Hibitane (chlorhexidine) and Savlon (cetrimide-chlorhexidine mixture in the ratio 10:1) issued from the pharmacy and in use throughout the hospital were frequently contaminated with organisms identified as *Pseudomonas* sp. The insidious nature of this contamination and its extensiveness seemed important enough to report, as such contamination may be more widespread than is generally supposed.

Description of Investigation

In the pharmacy batches of chlorhexidine and Savlon are made up in 100- and 90-litre quantities respectively by dilution of stock concentrate and then bottled in litre bottles. We sampled unopened and unused bottles of chlorhexidine 0.05% from one batch, and Savlon 1 in 30 (chlorhexidine 0.05% and cetrimide 0.5%) from three batches. We also sampled residues in bottles returned from the wards from five batches of chlorhexidine 0.05% and five batches of Savlon 1 in 30. All samples were found to be infected with *Pseudomonas* sp. The organisms found were not identical, and three distinct biochemical types were recognized, which we designated in relation to initial positive sample numbers as *Ps.* 10, *Ps.* 60, and *Ps.* 65. *Ps.* 10 was found in all the Savlon batches, and *Ps.* 60 and *Ps.* 65, but not *Ps.* 10, were found in chlorhexidine.

A search was made for the source of these organisms in the pharmacy, as the finding of positive cultures from unopened bottles suggested that contamination was most likely to be occurring there. Samples were taken from bulk stock concentrates of disinfectant, distilled water, measuring-jars, mixing containers, the measuring-stick, polyethylene tubing, bottle-filling apparatus, shelves, benches, sinks, and bottle-washing apparatus. Though many different organisms were found in some of these sites, none having the characteristics of *Ps.* 10, *Ps.* 60 or *Ps.* 65 was recovered. Freshly prepared batches of chlorhexidine and Savlon were also tested immediately before bottling, and were found to be sterile. The bottle-washing apparatus was sampled before a batch of empty Savlon bottles was washed and was free of pseudomonads, but after contaminated bottles had been washed it was found to have become infected. Bottles contaminated with *Ps.* 10 were found to be still contaminated with that organism after washing, and an uncontaminated bottle washed immediately after a contaminated one was found to have become contaminated. We therefore concluded that infection was being maintained by the presence of a residual inoculum of bacteria in the bottles before they were refilled with fresh (sterile) disinfectant. In addition, washing contaminated bottles led to contamination of the washing apparatus, so that infection would subsequently be transfer to clean bottles.

The manufacturers of chlorhexidine and Savlon recomm that bottles should be thoroughly rinsed in tap-water, prefera hot, and then drained before refilling, and that isopropyl alco 4% v/v or ethyl alcohol 6% v/v should be added to the st solutions once or twice a year to eliminate possible conta nating organisms. In our pharmacy the bottle-wash apparatus is connected to the cold-water supply, and bef recommending that a change should be made to hot-wa washing the survival of the *Pseudomonas* strains isolated v tested at higher temperatures. Two strains, *Ps.* 10 and *Ps.* were tested and proved to be remarkably resistant to h temperature, though it was noted that cultures exposed higher temperatures took much longer to grow, and that a h percentage of the initial inoculum was killed. Neverthel exposure to a temperature of 70° C. for five minutes failed sterilize the culture, and this implied that hot water could be relied on to sterilize bottles before refilling.

All three strains were found to survive in chlorhexidine 0.05 freshly prepared in the laboratory, and *Ps.* 60 was also able survive in 0.1% chlorhexidine. When *Ps.* 10 was inocula into Savlon 1 in 30 dilution prepared in the laboratory it fai to survive, though it had been initially isolated from Savlon this concentration. This is at present under further investi tion. None of the strains was found to survive in 0.05 chlorhexidine containing 4% v/v isopropyl alcohol when tes in the laboratory, but recently a strain of *Pseudomonas* havi the biochemical characteristics of *Ps.* 60 has been isolated fr the residues in 3 out of 16 bottles which had been return to the pharmacy after use. These bottles had contained 0.05 chlorhexidine and 4% v/v isopropyl alcohol. This lat finding indicates that continued use of isopropyl alcohol m ultimately select for strains resistant to both isopropyl alco and chlorhexidine, and thus that some other method such autoclaving the returned bottles should be used to break chain of infection, a conclusion reached by Lowbury (1951) relation to bottles of cetrimide. Kelsey and Maurer (196 reported contamination of returned ward stock bottles a freshly filled bottles of a white disinfectant fluid with *Klebsiella* species. They too recommend disinfection of bott before refilling.

Laboratory experiments to determine whether growth of t three strains of *Pseudomonas* would occur in Savlon a chlorhexidine were performed by inoculating 10 ml. of Savl 1 in 30 with *Ps.* 10, and 10 ml. of 0.05% chlorhexidine wi *Ps.* 60 and *Ps.* 65 separately. The dilutions were made fro stock concentrate with sterile distilled water in laboratory glas ware. Inoculation was performed with a straight wire from single colony of the respective organism grown on nutrie agar. Viable colony counts were performed at intervals duri a period of four weeks by spreading 0.1-ml. volumes of appropriate dilution on nutrient agar. Using this method v were able to demonstrate growth of *Ps.* 60 in 0.05% chlo hexidine, but not of *Ps.* 65 in 0.05% chlorhexidine or *Ps.* 10 Savlon 1 in 30. The viable colony count of *Ps.* 60 in 0.05 chlorhexidine showed a 100,000-fold increase during a period three weeks.

* Registrar in Clinical Pathology, United Birmingham Hospitals.
† Consultant Bacteriologist, Queen Elizabeth Hospital, Birmingham 15.

General Characteristics of the Organisms

The three strains of *Pseudomonas, Ps.* 10, *Ps.* 60, and *Ps.* 65, re all motile Gram-negative bacilli, oxidase- and catalase-sitive, and produced nonpigmented colonies on nutrient agar. ucose was utilized by oxidation. Growth on artificial media is characteristically slow, and the initial isolations from dis-ectant solution required five to six days' incubation at room nperature before growth became apparent. Further cultural d biochemical properties are listed in Table I. In the bio-emical and cultural tests we have performed *Ps.* 60 has the aracteristics of *Ps. multivorans,* as described by Stanier, lleroni, and Doudoroff (1966) except that, like three of their strains, it failed to hydrolyse gelatin, and, like one of their ains, it failed to give an egg-yolk reaction. It is interesting at their strain 398, identified as *Ps. multivorans,* also lacked ese two characteristics, and was one of the strains causing inary infection in children described by Mitchell and Hay-rd (1966).

TABLE I.—*Cultural and Biochemical Characteristics*

	Ps. 10	*Ps.* 60	*Ps.* 65
am stain	– bacillus	– bacillus	– bacillus
tility	+	+	+
idase	+	+	+
alase	+	+	+
icose oxidation--fermentation test	Oxidation	Oxidation	Oxidation
owth on MacConkey agar	+	+	+
owth on Cetavlon agar	+	+	+
owth at 42° C.	–	+	–
owth at 5° C.	–	–	–
rate utilization	+	+	+
latin hydrolysis	+	–	+
rch hydrolysis	–	–	–
rate reduction	+	–	–
ease	–	–	+
iconate	+	–	–
ginine dihydrolase	–	–	–
g-yolk reaction	+	–	–

Discussion

The isolation of bacteria from chlorhexidine stock bottles has en recently recognized, and in 1965 the manufacturers (I.C.I.) ued a circular on the subject with recommendations for lucing the incidence of contamination. However, reports contamination of chlorhexidine and of clinical infection used by these contaminants appeared in 1966. Mitchell and ayward (1966) described seven cases of infection of the inary tract in children after cystoscopy. The source of the fection was traced to the chlorhexidine solution used for sinfecting the bladder-irrigation reservoir. The infection was iced back further to the stock bottles of chlorhexidine 1/5,000 use in the hospital, and they concluded that the chlorhexidine ution had deteriorated on storage. Dulake and Kidd (1966) ported finding an organism most nearly identified as *caligenes faecalis* from the urine of 30 gynaecological patients dergoing bladder drainage by indwelling catheter. The same ganism was isolated from the jar used for storage of spigots er these had been sterilized by boiling. The jar contained 1% chlorhexidine.

In other reports of contamination of disinfectants with *eudomonas* species cork closures of bottles have at times en implicated. Lowbury (1951) concluded that contamination bottles was being maintained by showers of bacteria from the rk. Anderson and Keynes (1958) concluded that the ganisms did not actually survive in the disinfectant they were vestigating (cetrimide) but that organisms were released from cork when it was removed and thus passed out of the bottle th the disinfectant. Linton and George (1966) described a bstance, probably a tannin present in cork (and tea), which a very potent inactivator of chlorhexidine. They concluded at the neutralizing action of this substance was responsible the contamination of chlorhexidine solution at Bristol. Cork sures have not been used in our pharmacy for several years, d all bottles tested in the present series had bakelite closures with rubber seals. If a neutralizing substance is involved in the contamination here described we have so far not been able to demonstrate it.

Clinical infections with these organisms have been described elsewhere. In our hospital we have looked for infection caused by *Pseudomonas* sp. other than *Ps. aeruginosa* in all urine and wound swabs received over a period of two months. For this purpose material was inoculated on to cetrimide agar (Lowbury and Collins, 1955) and after overnight incubation at 37° C. keeping the plates at room temperature for a further four days. On no occasion were any of these strains isolated from urine, though *Ps.* 60 and *Ps.* 65 had both been isolated from jars of chlorhexidine used for disinfecting cystoscopes. From wound swabs several other *Pseudomonas* sp. were isolated, but they were all of biochemical types that were distinct from our strains *Ps.* 10, *Ps.* 60, and *Ps.* 65. However, disinfectants may well have been the source of these wound infections, as the disinfectant solution may have become contaminated after issue to the wards. Some support for this view is supplied by the isolation of *Ps. putida* and *Aeromonas* sp. in addition to *Ps.* 10 from a mop and a thermometer standing in Savlon 1 in 30 in the infants' nursery.

Another article better sterilized by other methods but commonly sterilized by chemicals is the cardiac catheter. We investigated two patients undergoing cardiac catheterization where the catheter used had been sterilized in Savlon 1 in 30. *Ps.* 10 was isolated from the Savlon solution employed for sterilization. Blood cultures were taken of venous blood from the right atrium via the catheter and of arterial blood from the brachial artery by means of a stainless-steel cannula that had been sterilized by autoclaving. Six cultures were taken in all, and *Ps.* 10 was isolated from each of them. We have not isolated *Ps.* 10 from blood cultures from suspected cases of bacterial endocarditis, but a serious potential threat obviously exists.

It is perhaps not generally appreciated how widespread contamination of chlorhexidine and Savlon solutions can become, so that ultimately all bottles of the aqueous solutions of these compounds may be contaminated at issue. To illustrate the extent of contamination Tables II and III record the isolations of *Pseudomonas* sp. from chlorhexidine and Savlon bottles issued by the pharmacy. Until the introduction of 4% v/v isopropyl alcohol all samples were contaminated. Since then very few isolations have so far occurred, but it seems possible that continued use of 4% v/v isopropyl alcohol may ultimately result in selection for strains resistant to chlorhexidine and 4% v/v isopropyl alcohol. Later samples of all batches tested have been sterile ; thus the possibility that some organisms may have taken a rather long time to be killed by the low concentration of the alcohol cannot be excluded.

Recently we have had the opportunity of sampling stock solutions of aqueous chlorhexidine and Savlon in four other

TABLE II.—*Organisms Isolated from Different Batches of* 0.05% *Chlorhexidine*

Batch No.	Date of Preparation	Volume Prepared	No. of Bottles Sampled	Source of Sample	Organisms Recovered
5	16/5/66	100 litres	1	Used bottle	*Ps.* 60
8	27/5/66	,,	1	,, ,,	,,
9	1/6/66	,,	1	,, ,,	,,
10	6/6/66	,,	2	,, ,,	*Ps.* 60 (2). *Ps.* 65 (1)
11	9/6/66	,,	2	,, ,,	*Ps.* 60
12	13/6/66	,,	1	Unused bottle	,,
23*	27/7/66	,,	2	Used bottle	None
24*	3/8/66	,,	2	,, ,,	,,
25*	8/8/66	,,	2	,, ,,	,,
26*	9/8/66	,,	3	,, ,,	*Ps.* 60 (2). None (1)
27*	11/8/66	,,	4	,, ,,	*Ps.* 60 (1). None (3)
28*	16/8/66	,,	1	,, ,,	None
29*	22/8/66	,,	2	,, ,,	,,
32*	5/9/66	,,	6	Unused bottle	,,
33*	8/9/66	,,	6	,, ,,	,,
44*	4/11/66	,,	12	,, ,,	,,

* 4% v/v isopropyl alcohol added.

hospitals. In all these hospitals organisms similar to those here reported were found ; 30 out of the 48 samples taken yielded a growth of *Pseudomonas* sp. In one pharmacy the distilled

TABLE III.—*Organisms Isolated from Different Batches of* 1 *in* 30 *Savlon*

Batch No.	Date of Preparation	Volume Prepared	No. of Bottles Sampled	Source of Sample	Organisms Recovered
1	3/5/66	90 litres	1	Used bottle	*Ps.* 10
2	10/5/66	,,	2	,, ,,	,,
3	20/5/66	,,	2	,, ,,	,,
3	—	—	1	Unused bottle	,,
4	31/5/66	90 litres	2	Used bottle	,,
4	—	—	1	Unused bottle	,
5	7/6/66	90 litres	2	Used bottle	,,
14	19/8/66	45 litres	1	Unused bottle	,,
16*	2/9/66	60 litres	6	,, ,,	None
17*	8/9/66	,,	6	,, ,,	,,
23*	31/10/66	,,	4	,, ,,	,,

* 4% v/v isopropyl alcohol added.

water used for dilution was found to be heavily contaminated with the same organism found in samples of disinfectant distributed throughout the hospital.

Storage of distilled water presents a special problem, and we recommend that freshly distilled water, hot from the still, be used. But, this apart, it is important to decide what practicable steps can be taken to prevent contamination assuming significant proportions. If chlorhexidine solutions are sterile at the time of bottling sterilizing the bottles will at least ensure that supplies leave the pharmacy uncontaminated. If in addition 4% v/v isopropyl alcohol is added to aqueous preparations the chance of subsequent contamination on the wards will be very greatly reduced. Though these organisms are not highly pathogenic they are capable of causing human disease under certain circu stances, and unless steps are taken to rid stock solutions of t contamination further case reports can be confidently predict

Summary

Contamination of stocks of chlorhexidine and Savlon w *Pseudomonas* species resistant to the concentrations of chl hexidine and Savlon in clinical use is reported. The contamir tion was maintained by a residual inoculum remaining in bot after washing, and was spread to other bottles in the bot washing apparatus. It is suggested that some wound infectic may be caused by disinfectants contaminated either at is by the pharmacy or during use on the wards. The additi of 4% v/v isopropyl alcohol to aqueous preparations of bc disinfectants was found greatly to reduce the incidence contamination.

We gratefully acknowledge the help of the group pharmacist, M A. E. Marston, and other members of his staff throughout investigation.

REFERENCES

Anderson, K., and Keynes, R. (1958). *Brit. med. J.*, **2**, 274.
Dulake, C., and Kidd, E. (1966). *Lancet*, **1**, 980.
Kelsey, J. C., and Maurer, I. M. (1966). *Mth. Bull. Minist. Hlth L Serv.*, **25**, 180.
Linton, K. B., and George, E. (1966). *Lancet*, **1**, 1353.
Lowbury, E. J. L. (1951). *Brit. J. industr. Med.*, **8**, 22.
—— and Collins, A. (1955). *J. clin. Path.*, **8**, 47.
Mitchell, R. G., and Hayward, A. C. (1966). *Lancet*, **1**, 793.
Stanier, R. Y., Palleroni, N. J., and Doudoroff, M. (1966). *J. g Microbiol.*, **43**, 159.

Reprinted from *Appl. Microbiol.* **18**, 299–302 (1969)

Vol. 18, No. 3
Printed in U.S.A.

Resistance of *Pseudomonas* to Quaternary Ammonium Compounds

21

I. Growth in Benzalkonium Chloride Solution

FRANK W. ADAIR, SAM G. GEFTIC, AND JUSTUS GELZER

Research Department, Ciba Pharmaceutical Company, Summit, New Jersey 0790ı

Received for publication 19 June 1969

Resistant cells of *Pseudomonas aeruginosa* and a waterborne *Pseudomonas* sp. (strain Z-R) were able to multiply in nitrogen-free minimal salts solution containing various concentrations of commercially prepared, ammonium acetate-buffered benzalkonium chloride (CBC), a potent antimicrobial agent. As the CBC concentration increased, growth increased until a point was reached at which the extent of growth leveled off or was completely depressed. Minimal salts solutions of pure benzalkonium chloride (PBC) containing no ammonium acetate did not support bacterial growth. When ammonium acetate was added to PBC solutions in the same concentrations found in CBC solutions, growth patterns developed that were comparable to those found with CBC. Likewise, $(NH_4)_2SO_4$ added to PBC solutions supported growth of both organisms. *P. aeruginosa* was initially resistant to CBC levels of 0.02% and it was adapted to tolerate levels as high as 0.36%. Strain Z-R was naturally resistant to 0.4% CBC. Since ammonium acetate, carried over by the CBC used in drug formulations and disinfectant solutions, has the potential to support the growth of resistant bacteria and thus make possible the risk of serious infection, it is suggested that regulations allowing the presence of ammonium acetate in CBC solution be reconsidered.

Benzalkonium chloride (a mixture of alkyldimethylbenzylammonium chlorides) is a surface-active quaternary ammonium compound. It is widely used as an antimicrobial preservative in pharmaceuticals and in clinical medicine to disinfect thermolabile material. Bacteria resistant to benzalkonium chloride may become a serious health hazard if accidentally introduced during the use of a drug or disinfectant solutions containing this antimicrobial agent. This is especially true if the particular preparation can provide a suitable substrate for growth.

During a comprehensive study on the resistance of bacteria to quaternary ammonium compounds, a strain of *Pseudomonas aeruginosa* and a water-borne *Pseudomonas* sp. were found to not only survive but also to multiply in salt solutions containing commercial benzalkonium chloride (CBC). This study explains this occurrence and discusses its practical importance.

MATERIALS AND METHODS

Organisms. *P. aeruginosa* was ATCC strain 9027. The waterborne organism (hereafter referred to as strain Z-R) was originally isolated from well water; it possessed a single polar flagellum and compared exactly with the description of *P. fluorescens* (1), except that no pigment was produced.

CBC. CBC refers to commercially prepared benzalkonium chloride and ammonium acetate in aqueous solution meeting the requirements of U.S. Pharmacopeia (USP) XVII. Ammonium acetate is allowed as a buffer in such solutions at a level of no more than 40% of the final concentration of CBC. The CBC solutions used in these experiments contained ammonium acetate at a concentration of 38% of the weight of CBC. This type of preparation is registered under various trade names and is commonly used as an antimicrobial preservative in pharmaceutical products and as a disinfectant for medical and surgical materials.

Aqueous solutions of pure benzalkonium chloride (PBC) also met the requirements of USP XVII and differed from CBC solutions only in that they did not contain ammonium acetate.

Media. *P. aeruginosa* and strain Z-R were continually subcultured in a sterile minimal salts-CBC medium composed of the following (per liter of triple distilled water): NaCl, 3.31 g; Na_2HPO_4, 2.58 g; KCl, 2.23 g; KH_2PO_4, 7.42 g; and CBC, 0.1% (v/v). Sterilization was achieved by filtration through a 0.2-μm membrane (Millipore Corp., Bedford, Mass.). If increased growth yields were required, sterile glucose in a final concentration of 0.5% (w/v) was added to the minimal medium along with the following (per liter): $CaCl_2 \cdot 2H_2O$, 0.005 g; $FeSO_4 \cdot 7H_2O$, 0.005 g; $MgSO_4 \cdot 7H_2O$, 0.1 g; and $(NH_4)_2SO_4$, 1.0 g. Using this glucose-expanded salts medium, PBC (0.1%, v/v) could be substituted for CBC.

Growth of cultures. Cultures were grown in 250-ml Erlenmeyer flasks containing 50 ml of medium or in test tubes (13 by 150 mm) containing 10 ml of medium. Incubation was stationary at 30 C. Growth was measured turbidimetrically by use of a Spectronic-20 spectrophotometer (Bausch & Lomb, Inc., Rochester, N.Y.) set at 545 nm.

Preliminary test for the selection of CBC-resistant bacteria. Bacterial isolates (including strain Z-R) that were to be tested for natural resistance to CBC were grown in tryptone soy broth (TSB); they were then centrifuged, washed several times, and suspended in minimal salts medium. The suspensions were adjusted turbidimetrically to contain about 10^8 cells/ml; 1-ml samples were used to inoculate tubes containing 9 ml of a minimal salts-CBC test solution. CBC was present at a final concentration of 0.02%. This concentration was selected on the basis of it being equal to or higher than the level of CBC considered to be highly effective against a wide range of gram-positive and gram-negative bacteria (3, 4, 7). After incubation for 24 hr at 30 C, 1-ml portions were withdrawn from the test solutions and transferred into 9-ml volumes of sterile TSB. If growth occurred in any of these TSB cultures, the organisms present were considered to have a degree of resistance sufficient to make them suitable for further study.

Development of CBC resistance in P. aeruginosa. *P. aeruginosa* was examined for its initial level of resistance to CBC by inoculating 0.1% glucose-expanded salts media containing increasing concentrations of the compound. The organism was found to grow consistently in concentrations of CBC up to 0.02%. Higher levels of resistance were successfully attained by inoculating solutions containing increasing concentrations of CBC in 0.1% glucose-salts medium with cells (at least 10^8/ml) from the highest CBC culture showing growth. The concentration of CBC was increased in increments of 0.0025%. In this manner, the organism acquired a tolerance to 0.36% CBC. Since growth at this CBC concentration tended to be weak, cells to be used in different tests were grown routinely in 0.1% CBC or PBC.

RESULTS

In the preliminary test for resistant isolates, strain Z-R remained viable after 24 hr in the 0.02% CBC-salts test solution, as indicated by growth upon transfer in TSB. It was noted, however, that after 72 hr the test solution itself became turbid. Examination under a phase microscope revealed actively dividing cells, suggesting that the turbidity was due to growth of the organism. Cells from this test solution were centrifuged, washed three times, and suspended in minimal salts solution. Samples of 0.1 ml (about 10^7 cells) were used to inoculate test tubes containing 9.9 ml of minimal salts solution and increasing concentrations of three CBC preparations. Optical density readings were taken after 14 days when increases in turbidity had ceased. As is illustrated in Fig. 1A, the CBC-salts solutions supported the growth of strain Z-R (Fig. 1A), whereas no growth occurred upon replacement of CBC by PBC. However, when ammonium acetate was added to the PBC-salts solutions in the same concentrations

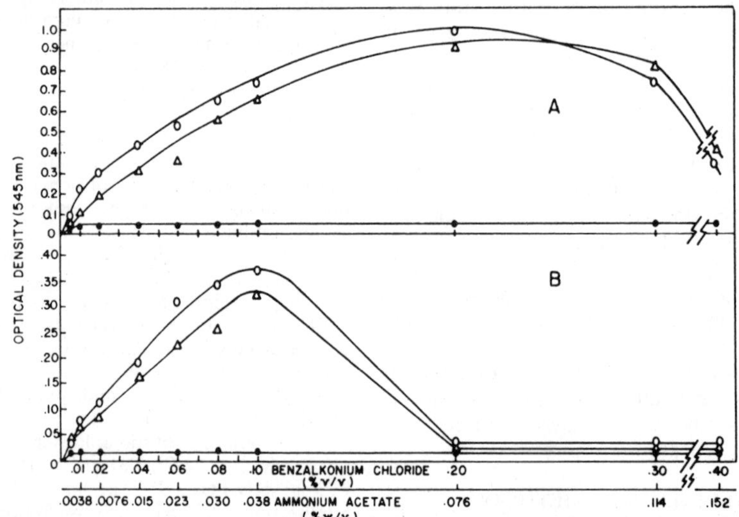

FIG. 1. *Growth of strain Z-R and P. aeruginosa in minimal salts solutions containing increasing concentrations of three types of benzalkonium chloride preparations. Symbols:* ○, *commercial benzalkonium chloride containing ammonium acetate;* ●, *pure benzalkonium chloride (PBC) containing no ammonium acetate;* △, *PBC plus added ammonium acetate. (A) Strain Z-R; (B) P. aeruginosa.*

TABLE 1. *Effect of replacing ammonium acetate with either ammonium sulfate or sodium acetate on the growth of strain Z-R and P. aeruginosa in PBC-minimal salts solution*[a]

Addition to minimal salts solution[b]	Growth[c]	
	Strain Z-R	*P. aeruginosa*
None	−	−
Pure benzalkonium chloride (PBC)	−	−
PBC plus ammonium acetate	+	+
PBC plus ammonium sulfate	+	+
PBC plus sodium acetate	−	−
Ammonium acetate	+	+
Ammonium sulfate	−	−
Sodium acetate	−	−

[a] Minimal salts solution was prepared as described in Materials and Methods.

[b] All additions were present at a final concentration of 0.1% (w/v) except for PBC which was 0.1% (v/v).

[c] Growth was read after 7 days of stationary incubation at 30 C.

found in CBC solutions, strain Z-R resumed a comparable growth pattern.

Cells of *P. aeruginosa* grown in 0.1% glucose-expanded salts solution containing 0.1% PBC were washed three times and suspended in minimal salts solution. These cells had not been adapted to PBC concentrations higher than 0.1%. The suspension (0.1 ml, 10^7 cells) was used to inoculate minimal salts solutions (9.9 ml) containing increasing concentrations of CBC and PBC preparations. Growth was measured after 14 days when the turbidity of the cultures no longer increased. The CBC-salts solutions supported growth of this organism, whereas the PBC-salts solutions did not (Fig. 1B). As in the case of strain Z-R, upon the addition of ammonium acetate to the PBC solutions, growth patterns similar to that obtained with CBC solutions were observed.

In an attempt to gain an initial understanding of the role ammonium acetate played in the nutrition of the two organisms, the experiment shown in Table 1 was devised. It was found that $(NH_4)_2SO_4$, but not sodium acetate, could replace ammonium acetate in the PBC-minimal salts solution and still allow each organism to grow.

DISCUSSION

The data presented indicate that low levels of ammonium acetate found in CBC solutions will support growth of benzalkonium chloride-resistant *P. aeruginosa* and strain Z-R, a water-borne *Pseudomonas* sp., whereas in solutions of PBC containing no ammonium acetate, no growth occurs. The fact that ammonium acetate could be replaced by $(NH_4)_2SO_4$ in PBC solutions suggests that a portion of the benzalkonium chloride molecule was being utilized for carbon and energy, whereas the strongly bonded nitrogen was not attacked. This, in turn, may lead to a chemical modification of the benzalkonium chloride molecule, possibly resulting in an inactivation of its antimicrobial action. Studies are currently underway in this laboratory to determine in detail the nature of these events.

The shape of the CBC growth curves in Fig. 1 may be attributed to several factors. At lower levels of CBC, growth was presumably limited due to the low levels of ammonium acetate introduced with the CBC. Assuming that the organisms can obtain carbon and energy from some part of the CBC molecule in the presence of ammonium acetate, it appears that the ammonium portion of the ammonium acetate molecule, specifically the nitrogen atom, was the sole growth-limiting factor. Thus, an increase in CBC increased the nitrogen level and growth increased proportionally.

In the case of strain Z-R, a point was reached above the 0.2% CBC level where the extent of growth was suppressed regardless of the ammonium acetate concentration. On the other hand, *P. aeruginosa*, which had been adapted to 0.1% benzalkonium chloride, grew optimally at this concentration but did not survive the increase to 0.2% CBC.

In the formulation of a drug, it is mandatory that as few potential microbial substrates as feasible be added. This decreases the chance of growth of resistant bacteria that may be introduced accidentally during normal use of the drug. The antimicrobial preservative should be the least probable source of bacterial substrate. In many drugs in which CBC is used routinely, the addition of ammonium acetate could be a detriment. For example, ophthalmics are usually composed of few organic compounds other than the active agent and the antimicrobial preservative, which in many instances is CBC. Under these conditions, ammonium acetate would at least enhance the growth of a resistant contaminant and could possibly be the sole supporter of growth. Indeed, contamination of ophthalmic solutions by *P. aeruginosa* and other microorganismsas resulted in numerous cases of serious eye infections (2).

The commonplace clinical practice of using CBC solutions as a means of disinfecting needles, swabs, catheters, and surgical instruments precludes survival, much less growth, of bacteria in such solutions. However, many instances of pseudomonal bacteremia, occasionally fatal, have resulted from the use of materials stored in contaminated CBC solutions (5, 6, 7). Furthermore, stored, unused solutions of CBC (0.13%) prepared in a hospital pharmacy have been found to be highly contaminated owing to the growth of resistant bacteria (6). Again, ammonium acetate would only serve to greatly worsen these contamination problems.

Strain Z-R was naturally resistant to CBC concentrations of 0.4%. This level is 20-fold greater than the 0.02% recommended for use in pharmaceuticals (3, 7, 8) and twofold greater than the 0.2% recommended for disinfection of medical materials (9). *P. aeruginosa* was initially resistant to 0.02% CBC and was adapted to tolerate concentrations up to 0.36%. Both organisms serve to illustrate the point that commonly occurring bacteria can multiply in the presence of what is considered high concentrations of CBC if given a carbon and nitrogen source. Thus, the potential capacity of the ammonium acetate contained in CBC solutions to support growth of resistant bacteria with the possibility of serious consequences appears to overshadow any value ammonium acetate may have as a buffering agent under the conditions in which it is used. In view of this, it is important that the U.S.P. regulation allowing its presence in CBC be reconsidered.

LITERATURE CITED

1. Breed, R. S., E. G. D. Murray, and N. R. Smith. 1957. Bergey's manual of determinative bacteriology, p. 105. 7th ed. The Williams & Wilkins Co., Baltimore.
2. Foster, J. H. S. 1965. Preservation of ophthalmic solutions, part I. Mfg. Chemist 36:45–50.
3. Grundy, W. E. 1968. Antimicrobial preservatives in pharmaceuticals, p. 566–574. *In* C. A. Lawrence and S. S. Block (ed.), Disinfection, sterilization and preservation. Lea and Febiger, Philadelphia.
4. Lawrence, C. A. 1968. Quaternary ammonium surface active disinfectants, p. 430–452. *In* C. A. Lawrence and S. S. Block (ed.), Disinfection, sterilization and preservation. Lea and Febiger, Philadelphia.
5. Lee, J. C., and P. J. Kialkow. 1961. Benzalkonium chloride—source of hospital infection with gram-negative bacteria. J. Amer. Med. Ass. 177:708–710.
6. Malezia, W. F., E. J. Gangaros, and A. F. Goley. 1960. Benzalkonium chloride as a source of infection. N. Engl. J. Med. 263:800–802.
7. Plotkin, S. A., and R. Austrian. 1958. Bacteremia caused by *Pseudomonas* sp. following the use of materials stored in solutions of a cationic surface active agent. Amer. J. Med. Sci. 235:621–627.
8. Russel, A. D., J. Jenkins, and I. H. Harrison. 1967. The inclusion of antimicrobial agents in pharmaceutical products, p. 1–38. *In* W. W. Umbreit (ed.), Advances in applied microbiology. Academic Press Inc., New York.
9. Spaulding, E. H. 1968. Chemical disinfection of medical and surgical materials, p. 517–531. *In* C. A. Lawrence and S. S. Block (ed.), Disinfection, sterilization and preservation. Lea and Febiger, Philadelphia.

Reprinted from *J. Pharm. Sci.* **51**, 770–772 (1962)

22

Antibacterial Activity of Mixtures of Quaternary Ammonium Compounds and Hexachlorophene

By G. R. WALTER and W. S. GUMP

Hexachlorophene and several quaternary ammonium compounds in admixture were evaluated for antibacterial activity by *in vitro* techniques commonly employed for the evaluation of lotions, creams, and ointments. It was observed that a maximum decrease in activity occurred as the components of the mixture approached equimolar ratios. The formation of a water-insoluble complex tends to diminish the antibacterial activity of mixtures when tested by broth dilution or agar plate techniques.

NUMEROUS examples of the inactivation of bactericidal cationic substances may be found in the literature and several have been reviewed by Lawrence (1).

The anionic nature of hexachlorophene would also suggest a lesser antibacterial action in the presence of quaternary ammonium compounds. The problem of ascertaining the extent of inactivation, if any, was undertaken because of the possible usage of both hexachlorophene and quaternary ammonium compounds in items such as lotions, powders, and creams. The methods selected for bacteriological evaluation were those commonly associated with the *in vitro* evaluation of these materials; namely, the zone of inhibition type of test and the broth tube serial dilution technique.

Received January 4, 1962, from Sindar Corp., Delawanna, N. J.

Accepted for publication January 26, 1962.

EXPERIMENTAL

Alcoholic stock solutions of benzalkonium chloride (alkylbenzyldimethylammonium chloride) and of hexachlorophene were mixed to give varying ratios of the active materials. In addition to these mixtures, equimolar amounts of hexachlorophene and benzalkonium chloride were brought to reaction in the following manner: To a solution of 8.1 Gm. of hexachlorophene in 100 ml. of acetone was added 15 Gm. of benzalkonium chloride (50% aqueous solution). The mixture was refluxed for 1 hour, the acetone distilled, and the solid removed by filtration, followed by drying at 50° in a 4-mm. vacuum. A slightly sticky material (15.5 Gm.) was obtained. The alkyl group in benzalkonium chloride represents a mixture of the alkyls C_8H_{17} to $C_{18}H_{37}$, the average being about $C_{13}H_{27}$, therefore the molecular weight of benzalkonium chloride approximates 354. The complex obtained from benzalkonium chloride and hexachlorophene would be about 724 (one mole of hydrogen chloride being removed) and its chlorine content 29.4%. The analysis of the product described above gave 29.5% chlorine.

For the bacteriological evaluation, aliquots of the alcoholic mixtures were added to tryptic soy broth (Difco) followed by twofold serial dilution in additional broth. Broth tubes were inoculated with one drop of a 1:100 water dilution of a 24-hour A.O.A.C. broth culture of *Staphylococcus aureus* A.T.C.C. 6538 (2). Tubes were incubated at 34° and growth was recorded by turbidity after 4 days. A slight haze was observed to form when alcoholic aliquots were added to the first tube of the serial dilution series. It was thought that this haze formation might lead to excess variation in the test and obscure any small differences in end points that might occur. For this reason, determinations were replicated seven times, each test being performed on a different day. The log means were analyzed for a significant difference from that of the hexachlorophene mean. It may be noted from Table I that, while both components of the mixture were highly bacteriostatic *per se*, a maximum loss in activity was approached as the ratio of components approached one to one.

An alternate approach for demonstrating the observed loss in activity was performed with the aid of 13-mm. filter paper disks (Schleicher & Schuell No. 740-E) which were impregnated with 0.07 ml. of alcoholic solutions of varying levels of hexachlorophene and benzalkonium chloride. The disks were dried at room temperature to remove solvent and then placed on seeded *S. aureus* plates. Replicate disks were prepared for each solution and placed on assay plates in a random manner. The plates were prepared such that each plate (100 mm. diameter) contained a 20-ml. base layer and a 6-ml. seed layer of agar. Dextrose tryptone extract agar (Difco) was employed for both the base layer and the seed layer. The inoculum consisted of a 1% (v/v) 24-hour A.O.A.C. broth culture of *S. aureus* in agar used for the seed layer. Sharp, well-defined inhibition zones were obtained for both hexachlorophene and benzalkonium chloride by this technique. The loss of zone production by mixtures of the active materials may be noted in Fig. 1. It may be observed that maximum loss of activity was

TABLE I.—BACTERIOSTATIC LEVELS OF MIXTURES OF HEXACHLOROPHENE AND BENZALKONIUM CHLORIDE AGAINST *Staphylococcus aureus*

	Bacteriostatic Levels (mcg./ml.) in Broth of Mixtures of the Following Composition											
% Benzalkonium Chloride	100	90	80	70	60	50	40	30	20	10	0	
% Hexachlorophene	0	10	20	30	40	50	60	70	80	90	100	Complex
Run No. 1	0.39	0.78	0.78	0.78	3.12	3.12	3.12	1.56	1.56	0.78	0.78	3.12
2	0.39	0.78	0.78	1.56	3.12	6.25	6.25	3.12	1.56	0.78	0.39	6.25
3	3.12	0.39	1.56	0.78	1.56	3.12	3.12	0.78	1.56	0.39	0.39	1.56
4	0.78	0.78	0.78	1.56	3.12	6.25	3.12	0.78	1.56	0.78	0.39	6.25
5	3.12	3.12	6.25	12.50	12.50	12.50	1.56	0.78	0.78	0.39	0.78	3.12
6	0.39	0.39	0.39	0.78	1.56	6.25	3.12	3.12	3.12	0.39	1.56	6.25
7	0.39	0.78	1.56	1.56	0.78	1.56	1.56	1.56	1.56	0.78	1.56	12.50
Geometric mean	0.78	0.78	1.16	1.56	2.56	4.60	2.74	1.42	1.56	0.59	0.71	4.65
t^a	...	...	...	1.56	2.75	4.88	4.19	1.85	...	...	...	4.72

a Value of t at the 0.05 level of significance for 12 degrees of freedom is 2.18 (3).

TABLE II.—ZONE PRODUCTION BY EQUIMOLAR MIXTURES OF QUATERNARY AMMONIUM COMPOUNDS AND HEXACHLOROPHENE AGAINST *Staphylococcus aureus*

Quaternary Ammonium Compound	Concentration of Components of Mixture, mcg./ml.		Inhibition Zone,[e] mm.		
	Hexachlorophene	Q.A.C.[d]	Hexa-chlorophene	Q.A.C.	Equimolar Mixture
Hyamine 1622[a]	2500	2750	5.3	1.2	1.7
Hyamine 10-X[b]	2500	2580	5.3	1.1	0.5
Hyamine 2389[c]	2500	2250	5.9	2.0	0.6
Cetylpyridinium chloride	2500	2070	5.8	0.4	0.3

a Hyamine 1622, (Rohm & Haas Co.) (diisobutylphenoxyethoxyethyl)benzyldimethylammonium chloride, monohydrate. *b* Hyamine 10-X (Rohm & Haas Co.) (diisobutylcresoxyethoxyethyl)benzyldimethylammonium chloride, monohydrate. *c* Hyamine 2389 (Rohm & Haas Co.) [alkyl(C9–C15)methylbenzyl]trimethylammonium chloride. *d* Quaternary ammonium compounds. *e* Average zone of three replicates to nearest 0.1 mm.

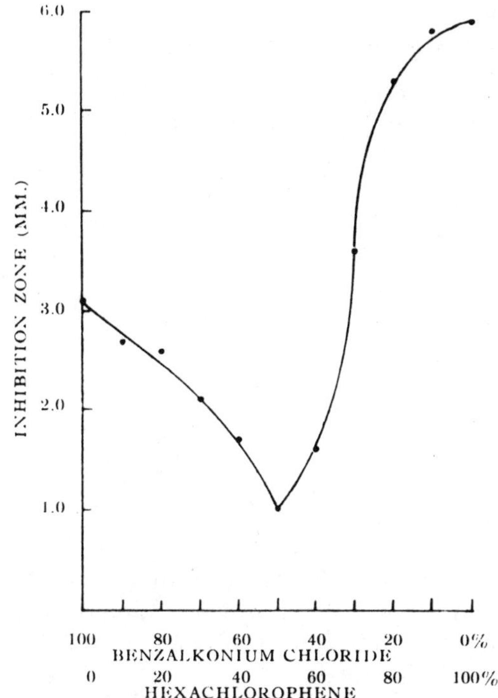

Fig. 1.—Effect of varying ratios of hexachlorophene and benzalkonium chloride on the inhibition zone produced against *S. aureus*. Each point is the mean of three determinations. Solutions were 0.1% with respect to total mixture present.

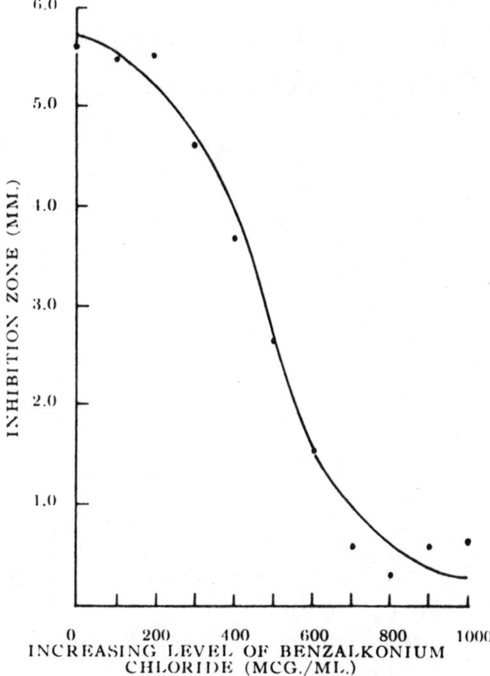

Fig. 2. Diminishing zone production of a 1000 mcg./ml. hexachlorophene solution with increasing levels of benzalkonium chloride.

found at approximately a 1:1 ratio. Alcoholic mixtures of hexachlorophene and benzalkonium chloride, examined by the plate technique, in which the hexachlorophene level was held constant may be seen in Fig. 2. A loss of activity as the mixture approached a 1:1 ratio was observed.

Several quaternary ammonium compounds structurally dissimilar to benzalkonium chloride were examined in equimolar mixtures with hexachlorophene by the plate technique. As may be seen in Table II, zones produced by these mixtures were also considerably smaller than those of the active materials *per se*.

DISCUSSION AND SUMMARY

Bacteriological examination of mixtures of quaternary ammonium compounds and hexachlorophene demonstrated an antagonistic relationship when evaluated by tube dilution and agar plate techniques. The maximum loss of activity was observed at an approximate equimolar concentration of each component of the mixture. The loss of activity by broth dilution was less dramatic than on agar plates. The haze observed in the broth tubes during the conduct of the tests indicates the formation of an insoluble reaction product. This loss of activity was greatly magnified in the plate technique which relies on the ability of materials to diffuse through agar.

Mixtures of hexachlorophene and quaternary ammonium compounds produce a relatively insoluble complex which is less active than the components, *per se*, of the mixture. The activity loss is greatest at an equimolar ratio, and it must be assumed that one is determining the activity of the uncombined excess of one or the other component when ratios other than equimolar are examined.

REFERENCES

(1) Lawrence, C. A., "Surface Active Quaternary Ammonium Germicides," Academic Press, New York, N. Y., 1950, pp. 127, 129.
(2) "Official Methods of Analysis of the Association of Official Agricultural Chemists," 9th ed., Association of Official Agricultural Chemists, Washington, D. C., 1960, p. 63.
(3) Brownlee, K. A., "Industrial Experimentation," 4tn ed., Chemical Publishing Co., Inc., New York, N. Y., 1953.

Editor's Comments on Papers 23 and 24

These two articles deal with evaluation techniques. McGray, Dineen, and Kitzke were able to show that fogging with a quaternary ammonium compound was effective in controlling hospital contaminants—this, in spite of the attitude of some microbiologists, that fogging with disinfectants has limited application.

The Environmental Protection Agency (EPA) (and the USDA before the EPA) has been instrumental in evaluating methods for the efficacy of disinfectants. Chen and Ortenzio present a simple turbidimetric technique used for disinfectant testing. As a consultant to the EPA, I have had the good fortune of collaborating with a number of scientists in this area and have had the opportunity to evaluate some of the methodology for testing antimicrobials.

Reprinted from *Soap Chem. Specialities* **40**, 75–78, 112–114 (1964)

Disinfectant Fogging Techniques

Evaluation of this technique under actual hospital use conditions indicates disinfectant fogging can be an effective adjunct in overall contamination control 23

By R. J. McGray*, P. Dineen, M.D., and E. D. Kitzke*†**

THE possible role of a disinfectant in decontaminating the atmosphere of a room has a growing and interested audience, judging by the recent references in the literature. It is tempting to suspect that the recent availability of mechanical devices designed to monitor microbial populations in the air may have something to do with enlarging research in this area. The relative ease with which precise measurements of air and surfaces can be made certainly encourages exploration of this subject.

Another and coincidental mechanical innovation in the field of disinfection has been the adaptation of insecticide fogging devices to dispersing aqueous germicidal solutions.

During the past year, there has been an increase in the number of hospitals investigating various forms of spraying or fogging machines as a means to distribute a disinfectant vapor. There is evidence that the use of such machines has grown considerably during this period and many hospitals are now relying on fogging periodically as an additional tool for terminal disinfection.

Although most hospitals do not utilize this technique at the present time, several firms have begun selling products specifically intended for use as fogging disinfectants. The new techniques that are becoming available may revolutionize the entire approach to routine terminal disinfection of hospital rooms and greatly improve what has lately become nothing more than a hotel-like housekeeping practice. It is our intention in this paper to present some of the data we have accumulated on disinfectant fogging as related to some of the devices used to disseminate mechanical generated fogs. This research work was started as a reaction to the reports published in the past two years. It was also clear that Federal regulatory and Public Health personnel were dubious about the efficacy of the germicidal fogs described in the reports. This research program was originally intended to confirm the probable inadequacy of the germicidal fogging techniques.

In a paper presented before the 49th annual CSMA meeting in Washington, D. C., in December 1962, Hauser, Crawford, and Clarke (1.) reported on their work in germicidal fogging of sick rooms. They described the use of a Challenger "Fogmaster" and a quaternary ammonium disinfectant as a supplementary disinfection tool for hospitals. Considerable data had been accumulated by these workers and the test method which had been used was one approved by the officials of the USDA. This test method was accepted as a basis for registration of disinfectant fogging formulations.

Figure 1. Challenger "Fogmaster" Tri-Jet sprayer. Capacity: one gallon dispensed in 15 minutes.

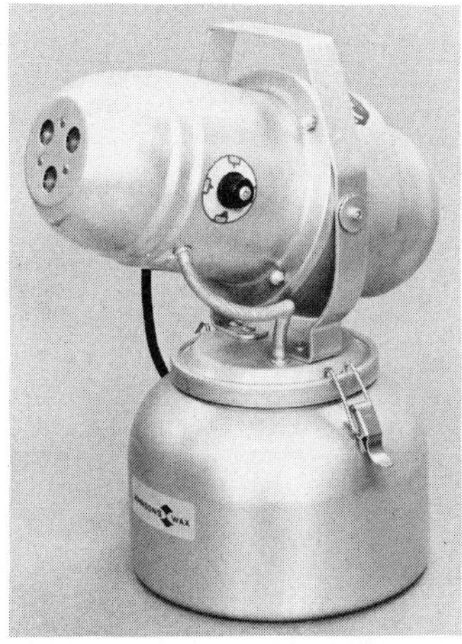

The preliminary work had shown that a stationary Challenger "Fogmaster", distributing 2,000 ppm solution of quaternary ammonium chlorides, resulted in a reduction of contaminants of about 90%. Using a motorized turntable to rotate the fogging machine slowly helped to distribute the fog uniformly throughout a room. This simple mechanical improvement significantly increased the percentage reduction of contaminants. Reductions of between 91 and 100% were obtained on various surfaces at different positions in test rooms. Both hard and porous surfaces were evaluated.

Ostrander and Griffith (2.) at the Veteran's Administration Hospital in Batavia, N. Y., have suggested other test methods.

The Ostrander and Griffith method was developed as an evaluation test for disinfectant fogging under semi-practical use conditions. Practical in-use tests should, of course, be utilized in determin-

†Paper presented at 50th annual meeting, Chemical Specialties Manufacturers Assn., Hollywood, Fla., Dec. 10, 1963.

*Basic research department, S. C. Johnson & Son, Inc., Racine, Wis.

**Department of Surgery, Cornell University Medical College, New York Hospital, New York City.

ing the suitability of products for fogging. However, their method is based on survival recovery by swabbing rather than subculturing the entire test surface.

The use of painted plaster blocks in their method is noteworthy as an attempt to duplicate the wall surface of a hospital. These test surfaces are used only once and must be prepared about two months in advance of the actual tests. Since there are a number of various types of surfaces in the average hospital room, it is difficult to accept a plaster surface as representative of a typical surface. A glass slide, conversely, does not offer any inherent variables and probably is the most inert subtrate on which to compare relative activity of various disinfectant formulations.

In reviewing the methods suggested by these workers and based on our own experience, we feel that the method submitted by Hauser, *et al* has certain advantages.

Of prime importance is the recovery of all possible surviving test organisms with certainty that the germicide involved is completely neutralized in the test system. The use of AOAC Letheen broth for subcultures is essential for tests on quaternary disinfectants. Although most of our data are based on a quaternary germicide, other agents including specially formulated phenolics were used. In the case of phenolics, Letheen broth was also used as a neutralizing medium.

The Hauser test method is a modification of the AOAC test (3.) for pressurized germicides. The percentage reduction is calculated by comparing the number of survivors on fogged inoculated surfaces with the number recovered from non-fogged control surfaces.

Since it is more logical to subculture the entire test surface for survival determinations than attempt to swab a representative test surface, the glass slides were found most adaptable for this purpose. In the Hauser test method, the subculture Letheen medium is plated out for survivor counts, and also incubated to determine whether 100% disinfection occurred on the individual test surfaces. Inoculation of this subculture medium can be done later to determine whether bacteriostasis has occurred from germicide carry-over on the test surface.

Our initial work was done with a stationary Challenger "Fogmaster" sprayer without a turntable. (Figure 1) Our early results coincided with those reported by Hauser, *et al.* To explore a stationary device that could achieve a 360° spray pattern, we experimented with the use of humidifiers which operate on a centrifugal principle and which generate a fine mist. (Figure 2) Using this device, a reduction of only 70-75% was obtained. We then attempted the turntable approach with a Challenger and immediately obtained an increase in effectiveness to 85-95% reduction.

Further experiments indi-

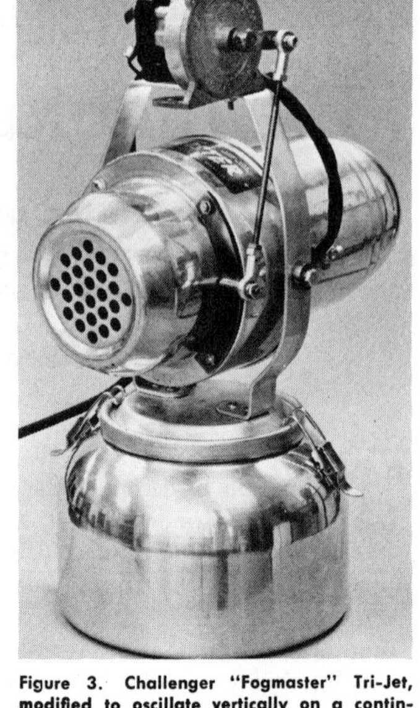

Figure 3. Challenger "Fogmaster" Tri-Jet, modified to oscillate vertically on a continuous basis.

cated that the Challenger "Fogmaster" could be made to perform more efficiently if it were adjusted to deviate from a fixed plane. A standard technique for fogging with the Challenger unit is to incline the direction of spray at a high angle. A mechanical modification of a standard Challenger unit was made which caused it to oscillate slowly and continually in a vertical plane, giving an up and down sweeping motion as the turntable rotated the entire sprayer unit. (Figure 3) The improved performance resulting from this modification was substantial when compared with the use of a standard stationary Challenger on a turntable.

Our final modification of the Challenger being reported at this time consists of a timing mechanism which generally inclines the unit's head from a low angle to the maximum possible inclination for the unit. (Fig. 4, cover) The timing mechanism is graduated in units of five minutes. It is possible, therefore, to adjust the running time to dispense a gallon of disinfectant solution in a range of 15 to 30 minutes. During its operation, the direction of spray is pointed first at

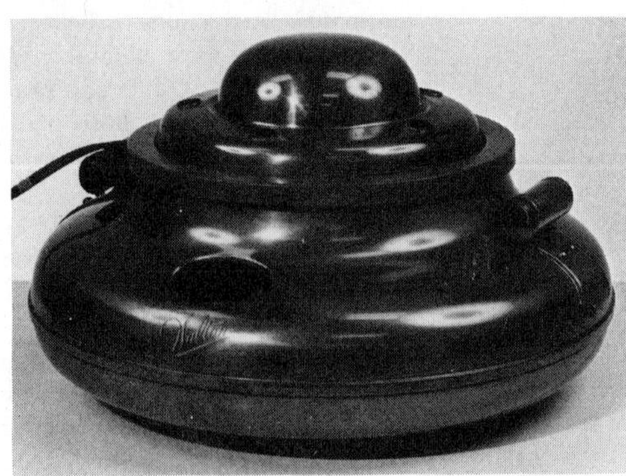

Figure 2. Walton humidifier, centrifugal, "cold steam" generator.

the floor, then at the wall and finally at the ceiling. The net result of this multi-directional spray pattern is a helix or corkscrew-like fogging stream.

Our laboratory data are summarized in Tables I and II. Table I illustrates the gradual increase in effectiveness as the various modifications in fogging techniques were made. It is quite clear that the evolutionary mechanical changes have made significant improvements in performance with the "helix" pattern and providing kill levels of 99.99%. The helix form begins at the floor level, coiling upward toward the ceiling, thus providing a series of 360° sweeps with repeat layers of fog spray fallout to wash and decontaminate the air.

Table II contains data obtained using the self-inclining Challenger-turntable combination. These data in general agree with the results obtained by Hauser, *et al,* as exported at the 1962 annual CSMA meeting. Our data, however, show greater percentage reductions.

Field evaluations to test the efficiency of fogging with the various modified Challenger units were performed at hospitals in Racine, Wisc., and at Cornell University Medical Center—New York Hospital. Operating rooms and patient rooms were treated with the disinfectant fog. The antimicrobial evaluation consisted in using inoculated slides, recovery of surface contaminants before and after fogging, and air sampling with the Reyniers Air Slit Sampler before and after fogging. (see figures 4, 5 and 6).

Surface contaminant recovery was done using both swabs and the special plastic Petri dishes known as Rodac plates (Falcon Plastics). The Rodac plate was described at the 1963 CSMA midyear meeting by Dr. Engley (4.) and is considered by many investigators to give more representative results than swabbing. An impression plate, such as the Rodac, gives an accurate picture of the actual bacterial distribution on a surface as well as a quantitative reading. (Figure 7) The results obtained in our field tests substantiate the

Table I. Relative Effectiveness of Various Fogging Mechanism Combinations Against S. Aureus

Surfaces tested	Average % reduction of inoculum				
	1*	2	3	4	5
Walls	73.2	81.9	95.6	99.64	99.99
Floors	74.3	92.5	89.7	99.99	99.99
Air**	72.9	78.0	85.4	99.88	99.99

(*: 1 - Walton "Herald" centrifugal cold steam generator
2 - Stationary Challenger without turntable
3 - Stationary Challenger with turntable rotating at 3 rpm
4 - Reciprocating Challenger with turntable at 3 rpm
5 - Self-inclining Challenger with turntable at 3 rpm)
(**: Test surfaces suspended from ceiling at different heights in room.)

Table II. Effect of Quaternary Ammonium Formulation (2,000 ppm active concentration)

GRAM POSITIVE (Staphylococcus aureus)

Hard Surface	Avg. % Kill	Soft (Porous) Surface	Avg. % Kill
Walls	99.99	Vertical Surfaces	92.00
Ceiling	98.20	Horizontal Surfaces	99.00
Floors, Tables, etc.	99.99		

GRAM NEGATIVE (Escherichia coli)

Hard Surface	Avg. % Kil'	Soft (Porous) Surface	Avg. % Kill
Walls	99.99	Vertical Surfaces	99.99
Ceiling	99.99	Horizontal Surfaces	99.99
Floors, Tables, etc.	100.00		

GRAM NEGATIVE (Pseudomonas aeruginosa)

Hard Surface	Avg. % Kill	Soft (Porous) Surface	Avg. % Kill
Walls	99.30	Vertical Surfaces	96.85
Floors, Tables, etc.	99.99	Horizontal Surfaces	99.99

Table III. Surface Contaminant Recovery in Rooms Treated with 15 Minute Fog.

Surfaces sampled in Patient Room	Colonies recovered			
	Before fogging		After fogging	
	No. of samples	colonies	No. of samples	colonies
Floor	3	219	4	107
Sink	1	15	1	2
Bedside cart, top	1	7	1	0
Bedrail	1	1	1	0
Wall	2	11	3	12
Locker door	1	5	1	0
	9	258	11	121

Surfaces sampled in Operating Room	Colonies recovered			
	Before fogging		After fogging	
	No. of samples	colonies	No. of samples	colonies
Floor	7	45	4	9
Cart top	4	5	2	1
Door	1	5	1	0
Lamp housing	2	4	2	0
	14	59	9	10

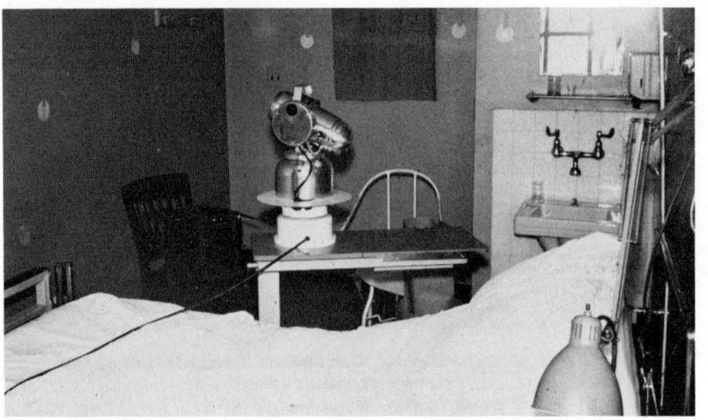

Figure 5. Self-inclining Challenger "Fogmaster" Tri-Jet modification set up for tests on inoculated surfaces (glass slides) in patient's room. White circles are sterile filter paper backings for test surfaces.

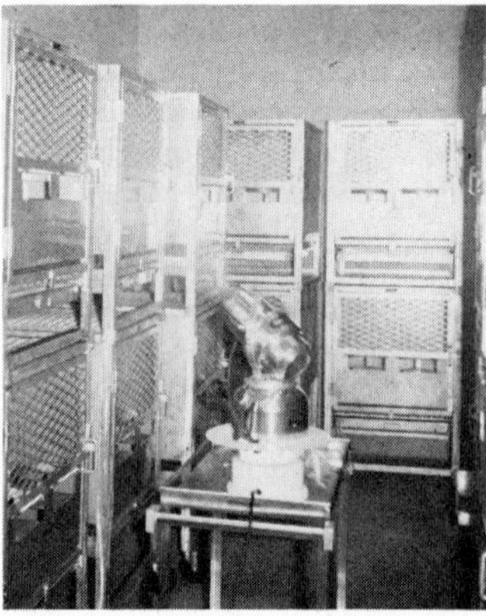

Figure 6. Animal room disinfection using Challenger "Fogmaster" Tri-Jet and turntable.

exploratory evaluations in laboratory test rooms. Using glass slides (1″ x 3″) inoculated with *S. aureus* (FDA 209) the percentage reduction was determined in patient rooms. From 99.8 to 100% reduction was obtained on these simulated hard surfaces.

Subculturing of the slides was done in AOAC Letheen broth to detect possible stasis from the quaternary ammonium disinfectant used. Incubation of the test slides in the recovery medium showed that in a significant number of instances, the slides had been completely disinfected.

During the course of many trials, numerous surfaces in the test area were swabbed or sampled with the Rodac plates before and after fogging of these hospital rooms. With the exception of coagulase determinations on recovered staphylococci, no attempt was made to classify all the types recovered before and after fogging. The quantitative analysis of the effect of fogging can be seen in Table II. Of the 258 colonies isolated before fogging in one patient's room, 35 were staphylococci of which approximately 50% were coagulase positive. Of the 121 colonies isolated after fogging, only three were staphylococci and only one was coagulase positive.

Air samples taken with the Reyniers sampler after fogging show a dramatic reduction in air contaminants. Close to 100% of air borne particles are removed by fogging. Figure 8 shows an air sampler recovery dish with contaminants picked up from a patient's room before fogging. A woolen blanket was shaken at the beginning of the test and the blanket

Figure 7. Rodac plates (Falcon Plastics) containing differential agar, showing "Staphylococcus" colonies. (Mannitol salt agar, "Staphylococcus" Medium #100 (Difco), and A.O.A.C. Letheen agar).

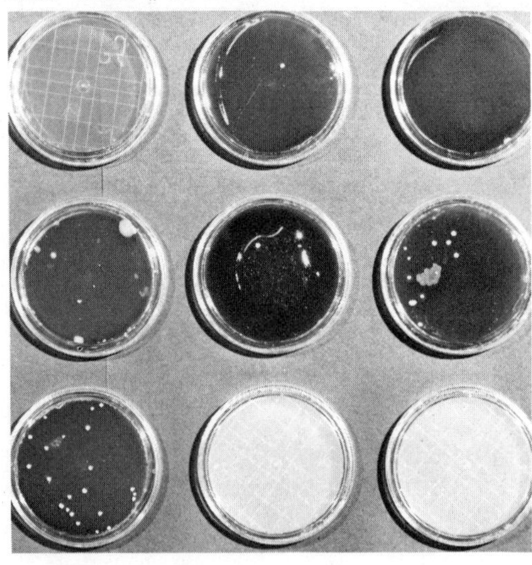

Figure 8. Reyniers Air Slit Sampler plate, showing effects of air sanitizing fog on air borne contaminants. Plate shows bacterial population from 60 cubic feet of air. (See text for details of test.) Read plate clockwise from black line.

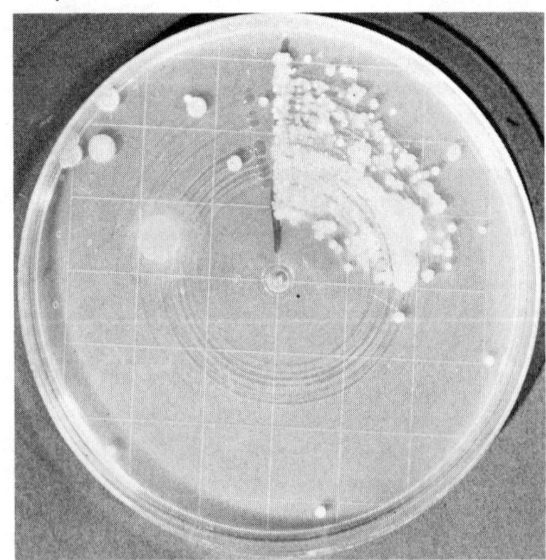

flora was then blown about the room with an air blast. The air sampler ran 15 minutes before it was shut down and covered.

Fogging was then done for 15 minutes. After a 20 minute waiting period, the room was re-entered with minimal activity and the sampler turned back on. Few colonies were recovered during the remaining 45 minute sampling period. We had previously determined that the AOAC Letheen agar medium would neutralize any quaternary carried over into the Reyniers sampler. Other air sampling tests in laboratory test rooms have given equally significant results in air sanitization.

The results we have obtained in lab and field tests indicate that a significant reduction in bacterial contamination occurs when this fog technique is employed to apply a quaternary ammonium formulation at 2,000 ppm active concentration. In controlled studies, 100% reduction is obtained regularly on horizontal surfaces. Reductions of 98 to 99.99% are obtained on walls and other vertical surfaces.

The possible residual effect of germicides deposited by means of a fog has not been evaluated for lack of a significantly reliable test method. With existing methods, no doubt residual antibacterial activity can be demonstrated. However, residual action can perhaps best be shown by a long term evaluation program based on regular and routine use of this fogging technique as a special adjunct to the standard terminal disinfection procedures. Such a program is being prepared for test under actual hospital conditions.

It is evident upon close examination of the cleaning and disinfection procedures in many hospitals that the thoroughness of a given clean-up depends on attitude of individual employees. Effective procedures can be painstakingly devised without real benefit in the hospital where lack of interest or absence of training interferes with the program.

In too many instances today, routine disinfection of a hospital room is construed as a simple clean-up and clean-out. Perhaps several surfaces in the room may hastily be wiped with a disinfectant solution, but time and available labor do not permit effective coverage of all of the surfaces in the room.

Obviously, in contagious disease cases, more emphasis is given to terminal disinfection procedures. The technique of room disinfection by means of an apparatus to dispense a germicidal fog certainly can also apply to such cases. At this time, the question of whether to initiate a program of periodical germicidal fogging of non-isolation rooms must be answered by those responsible for the prevention of cross-contamination in hospitals. It is likely that the lack of a labor-saving procedure for routine disinfection has, until the present time, made it impractical to institute disinfectant procedures for non-contagious areas.

It would appear that fogging with a disinfectant formulation can be a highly effective adjunct or supplementary technique to an overall contamination control program. Used in combination with cleaner-disinfectants, a maximum effort against cross-contamination can be launched with a minimal expenditure in labor costs.

Fogging alone should not, of course, be considered as a complete disinfection treatment. It is not a "cure-all" for infectious epidemic control, but properly used, will prevent the establishment of "room reservoirs" of pathogens. Periodic use of this technique rather than reliance on infrequent or annual general housecleaning would seem to be preferable to avoid maintaining an active "pool" for cross-contamination between rooms.

In theory, most water soluble germicides can be dispensed via fogging to obtain a degree of anti-bacterial activity. However, several considerations must be faced in the choice of the proper agent. To date, quaternary ammonium compounds of a low order of toxicity and irritation at use concentrations (2,000 ppm) have been demonstrated to be effective as disinfectants by this technique. Certain phenolic combinations have been found to possess a marked demonstrable activity, but irritation to the operator and patients has been a primary objection to their use.

Other agents have been suggested for use in fogging applications, but prior experience with them as cleaners limits their use due to excessive chemical deposit and build-up on equipment, floors, and walls.

A certain amount of opposition and natural disbelief in the efficacy of germicidal fogging has arisen which stems from a lack of experience with this technique. Evidence has been accumulating which impressively substantiates a basis for consideration of the technique as a useful tool, not merely as an idea or theory. The disinfectant industry as a whole is aware of the potential in effective anti-microbial procedures represented by disinfectant fogging. The ratio of labor cost to contamination prevention is favorable.

Part of the burden shared by hospital administrators and infection control committees in setting up effective anti-microbial environmental sanitation programs can now be substantially alleviated. Reliance upon the disinfectant industry for effective products can be extended to include new techniques for contamination control. It is the responsibility of disinfectant manufacturers to develop realistic solutions to the problem of environmental contamination.

Summary

In summary, fogging with a quaternary ammonium disinfectant by a procedure using a modified Challenger Fogmaster and turntable has been found to be effective in controlling hospital contaminants. The use of this procedure in combination with other disinfecting clean-up methods will significantly improve the degree of antimicrobial control. Although several disinfectants may be feasible for fogging, quaternaries have been the agents of choice in most fogging applications. The proven effectiveness, low order of toxicity and irritation, and the cost factor involved with quarternaries are prime considerations in this choice. An additional feature is the acute irritation property that forewarns the operator that this fog is a germicide and can be toxic. However, within 15 minutes after fogging, the air no longer is irritating but in fact seems quite refreshing.

Test methods for evaluating the efficacy of fogging are important. They can be performed with a minimum of expense and labor by hospital bacteriologists. The method by Hauser, as mentioned above, is a reasonable approach and may be explored with a variety of test organisms. Disinfectant fogging is considered by those who have evaluated it under actual use conditions to be a valuble too in contamination control program when used for the purposes intend ed in its development.

References

1. "Germicidal Fogging of Sic Rooms," C.S.M.A. 49th Annual Meet ing, Washington, D.C., December 5 1962.

2. "Method for Selecting Disinfec tant Used in Fogging," *Hospital Man agement*, September 1963.

3. *Journal of A.O.A.C.*, Volum 44, No. 1, pp. 137-138, 1961.

4. "Surface Sampling Studies—A Review and Preview," C.S.M.A. 49t Mid-Year Meeting, Chicago, May 2 1963.

Reprinted from *J. Ass. Offic. Anal. Chem.* **55**, 219–223 (1972)

Turbidimetric Evaluation of Bacterial Culture Resistance in Disinfectant Testing

24

By JOHN H. S. CHEN[1] and L. F. ORTENZIO (Pesticides Regulation Division, Environmental Protection Agency, Agricultural Research Center, Beltsville, Md. 20705)

A simple turbidimetric method has been developed for determining the degree of phenol resistance of cultures used for disinfectant testing. Net transmission values are used to assess the degree of resistance; these are based on the measurement of the total amount of light scattered by the bacterial growth in the AOAC broth medium without interfering turbidity of the dissolved ingredients. A decrease in the net transmission value corresponds to a decrease in phenol resistance; the converse is also true. The transmission values obtained in a 10 month study of a total of 77 weekly random samples of AOAC nutrient broth media blanks showed no substantial differences among the broth media tested by the turbidimetric method. Net transmission values were obtained for 71 broth cultures of *Salmonella choleraesuis*, 74 of *Staphylococcus aureus*, and 78 of *Pseudomonas aeruginosa* having the same required resistance against phenol. These values, which fell within a wider range than would be expected, are given. The effect of the number of 10-carrier-soakings on the net transmission value and equivalent phenol resistance of the cultures was determined for 60 broth cultures of the 3 test organisms named above. Soaking wet cylinder carriers in a given volume of test cultures used for the AOAC use-dilution test directly reduced the net transmission value and equivalently decreased the phenol resistance of the cultures. The turbidimetric method has proven experimentally satisfactory in several hundred determinations and in selecting test cultures of uniform quality for disinfectant testing.

Maintaining the resistance of the test culture is of fundamental importance in the testing of sporicides, disinfectants, and sanitizers. The test procedure for evaluating these products must include the control provisions for determining the resistance of the test culture to phenol (with the exception of sporicides) during the test and incorporating this resistance in the final results (1–6).

[1] Present address: Pesticides Regulation Division, Environmental Protection Agency, Washington, D.C. 20250.

The standard culture method for maintaining, propagating, and restandardizing test cultures to the phenol resistance level desired was developed by Ortenzio *et al.* in 1948 (7). Modifications involving the use of specific media, temperature, age of culture, and apparatus for making culture transfers have been introduced by many workers in recent years (7–17). However, considerable interest is still being shown in the cause of the variations resulting when the AOAC use-dilution test is performed under controlled conditions. Indirect evidence indicated that variations were due to changes in growth opacity, which is the quantitative estimation of both number of bacteria and protoplasmic mass. Only indirect evidence was available because a suitable method for measuring the degree of growth opacity was lacking.

In this study, a simple turbidimetric measurement method was developed for determining the degree of phenol resistance of cultures in disinfectant testing; Anatone (Cudahy Laboratories, Omaha, Neb. 68107) is used as the source of peptone. After considerable basic study, the technique described below was tested and the observations on the precision of this method have proven the method to be satisfactory in several hundred determinations.

Experimental

Turbidimetric Measurement

A Lumetron photoelectric colorimeter Model 401 equipped with 14 mm tubes was chosen for this study. A standard set of 6 glass filters is provided which isolates properly spaced narrow spectral bands that are identified by the wavelength of their transmission maxima. This instrument is equipped with a single photocell which provides an inverse logarithmic scale (absorbance) and, in addition, a uniform transmission scale (per cent transmission).

The turbidimetric procedure for determining the degree of growth opacity of AOAC broth cultures corresponding to their resistance against the phenol dilution was based on a measurement of the amount of light scattered by the bacterial growth in the AOAC nutrient broth (2). The interfering turbidity resulting from the dissolved ingredients in the broth was corrected for by subtracting the amount of light scattered by the dissolved ingredients from the amount of light scattered by the bacterial growth in the broth. When a Lumetron photoelectric colorimeter is used, the direct reading in logarithmic form is given as absorbance and the following equations are justified:

$$\begin{aligned} \text{Growth opacity} &= \text{net absorbance value} \\ &= \log_{10} I_o/I_c - \log_{10} I_o/I_b \\ &= \text{net transmission value} \\ &= \%T_b - \%T_c \end{aligned}$$

The equations above represent the light loss by absorption by the bacterial growth in the AOAC nutrient broth, where I_o, I_c, and I_b are the intensity of incident light, light scattered by the bacterial growth, and light scattered by the dissolved ingredients in the broth, respectively, and T_b and T_c are the transmission values of the broth and the culture, respectively. The concentration of bacterial growth, expressed as the degree of growth opacity, is directly proportional to the net absorbance value or net transmission value. For reading convenience, the uniform transmission scale was adopted in this study.

Bacterial Broth Cultures

Salmonella choleraesuis ATCC No. 10708, *Staphylococcus aureus* ATCC No. 6538, and *Pseudomonas aeruginosa* ATCC No. 15442 were used exclusively in this study. The stock cultures of *S. choleraesuis* and *S. aureus* were maintained on nutrient agar slants (2). *Ps. aeruginosa* was maintained on semisolid cystine trypticase agar stabs by monthly transfers (2). Daily transfers of these cultures were carried on AOAC nutrient broth as specified in the method (2). The 48 hr broth cultures were tested for their resistance to dilutions of phenol by the official phenol coefficient test (2) and their corresponding degree of growth opacity by the light transmission measurement method previously described.

Phenol

Pure chemical phenol (USP) that congealed at $\geq 39°C$ was standardized as a 5% solution by the official potassium bromide-bromate titration method (2). The minimum required resistances to phenol of *S. aureus*, *S. choleraesuis*, and *Ps. aeruginosa* are 1–65, 1–95, and 1–90 dilutions, respectively (2).

Compilation of Data

A total of 77 weekly random samples of AOAC nutrient broth media from this laboratory were examined by using the turbidimetric measurement method. The data were collected over a period of 10 months. The results were subjected to statistical analysis (18). The variation of transmission value of broth media was determined by the coefficient of variation, $C = S/\bar{Y}$, where C is the variation expressed as a percentage, S is the standard deviation, and $\bar{Y}$ is the mean transmission value. During the same period, random samples of 71 broth cultures of *S. choleraesuis*, 74 broth cultures of *S. aureus*, and 78 broth cultures of *Ps. aeruginosa* were examined to determine the frequency distribution ranges in terms of net transmission values. An additional 45 samples of representative broth cultures of these test organisms were diluted aseptically with nutrient broth to a level in which the critical value of net transmission at the minimum acceptability could be determined.

An additional 60 broth cultures of these 3 test organisms were tested to determine the effect of the number of 10-carrier-soakings on the net transmission value and equivalent phenol resistance of the cultures. The objective was to establish the prediction equation relating absorbance to carrier-soaking. The best fitting straight lines for the plots of numbers of 10-carrier-soakings vs. net transmission values were determined by the linear regression equation. The mathematical model for this analysis is: $Y = a + bX$ (2), where Y is the net transmission value, X is the number of 10-carrier-soakings, and a and b are the y-intercept and the regression slope of the linear regression line, respectively.

Results and Discussion

The results of a preliminary study of the turbidimetric determination of 77 AOAC nutrient broth blanks on random samples over a period of 10 months are shown in Table 1. Data indicate that there are no substantial differences among the broth media tested and that the laboratory systematic error (coefficient of variation of $\pm 1.42\%$) is considered normal (16). Individual systematic errors in making the broth media could contribute to the variations in the turbidimetric results. On the basis of the evidence obtained (19), the variation caused by interfering turbidity in the AOAC nutrient broth blanks can be minimized.

The mean values of net transmission and the frequency distribution (expressed in percentage units) for the test cultures are presented in Table 2. The net transmission values obtained at the required resistance levels against phenol fall in a much wider range than most microbiologists would have expected. The broth culture of *S. choleraesuis* definitely showed a much lower mean net transmission value of 14.9% and a narrow range of 12–18% net transmission. The broth

Table 1. Transmission values of AOAC nutrient broth blank obtained by using the turbidimetric method

Detn	T, %[a]	$\bar{T} - T$	$(\bar{T} - T)^2$	Detn	T, %[a]	$\bar{T} - T$	$(\bar{T} - T)^2$
1	59.0	1.7	2.89	41	60.0	0.7	0.49
2	59.0	1.7	2.89	42	61.0	0.3	0.09
3	59.0	1.7	2.89	43	62.0	1.3	1.69
4	60.0	0.7	0.49	44	61.0	0.3	0.09
5	60.0	0.7	0.49	45	59.0	1.7	2.89
6	61.5	0.8	0.64	46	59.5	1.2	1.44
7	61.0	0.3	0.09	47	60.0	0.7	0.49
8	59.0	1.7	2.89	48	61.0	0.3	0.09
9	59.0	1.7	2.89	49	62.0	1.3	1.69
10	60.0	0.7	0.49	50	62.0	1.3	1.69
11	60.0	0.7	0.49	51	61.0	0.3	0.09
12	61.0	0.3	0.09	52	60.0	0.7	0.49
13	60.0	0.7	0.49	53	61.0	0.3	0.09
14	60.0	0.7	0.49	54	61.0	0.3	0.09
15	60.0	0.7	0.49	55	61.0	0.3	0.09
16	61.0	0.3	0.09	56	62.0	1.3	1.69
17	60.0	0.7	0.49	57	61.0	0.3	0.09
18	60.5	0.2	0.04	58	61.5	0.8	0.64
19	60.0	0.7	0.49	59	60.0	0.7	0.49
20	61.0	0.3	0.09	60	60.0	0.7	0.49
21	61.0	0.3	0.09	61	62.0	1.3	1.69
22	61.0	0.3	0.09	62	61.5	0.8	0.64
23	61.5	0.8	0.64	63	61.0	0.3	0.09
24	61.0	0.3	0.09	64	62.0	1.3	1.69
25	61.0	0.3	0.09	65	61.0	0.3	0.09
26	60.5	0.2	0.04	66	60.0	0.7	0.49
27	62.0	1.3	1.69	67	61.0	0.3	0.09
28	61.0	0.3	0.09	68	60.0	0.7	0.49
29	61.0	0.3	0.09	69	60.0	0.7	0.49
30	60.0	0.7	0.49	70	61.0	0.3	0.09
31	60.0	0.7	0.49	71	60.0	0.7	0.49
32	60.0	0.7	0.49	72	62.0	1.3	1.69
33	60.0	0.7	0.49	73	61.0	0.3	0.09
34	60.0	0.7	0.49	74	60.0	0.7	0.49
35	60.0	0.7	0.49	75	62.0	1.3	1.69
36	61.0	0.3	0.09	76	62.0	1.3	1.69
37	61.0	0.3	0.09	77	61.0	0.3	0.09
38	62.0	1.3	1.69	Av. ($\bar{T}$)	60.7		
39	61.5	0.8	0.64	Std dev.	±0.86		
40	60.0	0.7	0.49	Coeff. of var., %[b]	±1.42		

[a] Per cent transmission at 530 nm.
[b] In authors' laboratory.

culture of *S. aureus* yielded a higher mean net transmission value of 33.4% with a wider range (20–48%), which is caused by the higher density growing characteristic of this organism. With *Ps. aeruginosa*, the net per cent transmission was between 25 and 51 and had the highest mean value of 40.2%. This suggests that a gentle handling technique should be exercised in separating the pellicle from the broth culture.

The acceptable and unacceptable ranges of the test cultures evaluated by the turbidimetric measurement are summarized in Table 3. The term "unacceptable" as used here is associated with the net per cent transmission which is beyond or below the required resistance level against phenol. A definite relationship exists: As the net transmission value decreases, the phenol resistance decreases in a step-like fashion. The converse is also true.

The acceptable range for the *S. choleraesuis* culture is between 12 and 20% net transmission. This narrow range of growth indicates that the culture is remarkably easy to maintain during daily transfers. Outside of this range (<7 or $>20\%$), the culture tends to be either less or more resistant than required for use in disinfectant testing. The per cent net transmission range between 7 and 12 could be considered as marginal.

The unacceptable broth cultures of *S. aureus* were found to be outside of the range of 20–45% net transmission. The cultures with a per cent net transmission of ≤ 11 were considered to be weaker than the required resistance against phenol. The

Table 2. Frequency distribution of per cent net transmission[a] at 530 nm of AOAC bacterial cultures employed in the use-dilution test

Culture[b]	No. of Samples	Range	Frequency Distribution, %	Mean Net T
S. choleraesuis	71	<12.0	0	14.9
		12.0–13.9	25.35	
		14.0–15.9	43.66	
		16.0–18.0	31.99	
		>18.0	0	
S. aureus	74	<20.0	0	33.4
		20.0–29.9	24.32	
		30.0–39.9	56.76	
		40.0–48.0	18.92	
		>48.0	0	
Ps. aeruginosa	78	<25.0	0	40.2
		25.0–34.9	25.64	
		35.0–44.9	46.15	
		45.0–51.0	28.21	
		>51.0	0	

[a] Per cent net transmission calculated by subtracting the per cent transmission of the culture from the per cent transmission of the broth.

[b] *S. choleraesuis*, *S. aureus*, and *Ps. aeruginosa* cultures were previously assessed for phenol resistance by the official phenol coefficient test and were found to be acceptable at 1–95, 1–65, and 1–90 dilutions, respectively.

wide range of growth indicates that this organism is more susceptible to change during daily transfers.

The results with *Ps. aeruginosa* show that the acceptable range of per cent net transmission falls between 25 and 50 and the unacceptable range is much wider than for the other 2 organisms. This organism appears to be most difficult to handle for maintaining a consistent absorbance.

These 3 test organisms are the most commonly used organisms in the AOAC use-dilution method (2) for determining the maximum safe use-dilution for disinfectants. The sterile metal cylinder carriers are stored in a 0.1% solution of "Bacto" asparagine and when a series of wet carriers are inserted in a given volume of broth culture, they tend to dilute the culture, thereby weakening the cultures' resistance.

Figure 1 shows the plot of the net per cent transmission vs. the number of 10-carrier-soakings applied for these 3 cultures. The slopes (b), possible intercepts (a_1 and a_2) of these lines, and the correlation coefficients (r) are given in Table 4. The correlation coefficient was calculated between the net per cent transmission and the number of times 10-carriers were soaked in each culture. Results indicate that all the sample points are reasonably close to each individual regression

Table 3. Summary of acceptable and unacceptable ranges of net transmission values of AOAC broth cultures evaluated by the turbidimetric method

Culture	Range of Net Transmission Values: Resistance Level Against Phenol Dilution[a] A	B	C
S. choleraesuis	>20	12–20	<7.0
S. aureus	>45	20–45	<11.0
Ps. aeruginosa	>50	25–50	<9.0

[a] The required resistances to phenol of the 3 cultures are specified in Table 2, footnote *b*. A, stronger than required resistance; B, required resistance level; C, weaker than required resistance.

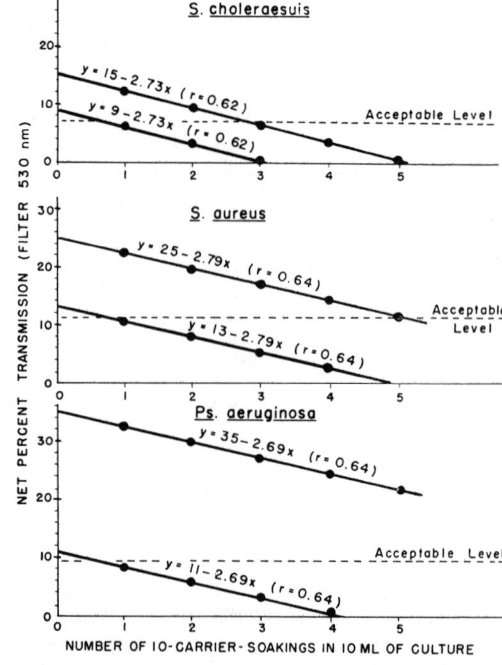

FIG. 1—Regression of the net per cent transmission following 10-carrier-soakings of *S. choleraesuis*, *S. aureus*, and *Ps. aeruginosa*.

line (0.62–0.64). The acceptable net transmission values used significantly affected the phenol resistance data. However, this effect was mostly on the intercepts rather than on the slope of the response line and, if the diluting factor caused by carrier soaking is constant, the slope of the regression line should always be the same for a given culture. Therefore, it is practical to use the same slope of a regression line at various intercepts for predicting the acceptability of a broth

Table 4. Slope (*b*), intercepts (a_1 and a_2), and correlation coefficient (*r*) of determination of linear regression, $Y = a + bX$, predicting the resistance response of the culture at the number of carrier-soakings

Culture	a_1	a_2	b	r
S. choleraesuis	15.0	9.0	−2.73	0.62
S. aureus	25.0	13.0	−2.79	0.64
Ps. aeruginosa	35.0	11.0	−2.69	0.64

[a] a_1, acceptable ranges; a_2, unacceptable ranges.

culture before soaking the 10-carriers. The regression slopes of Y on X were −2.73, −2.79, and −2.69 for *S. choleraesuis*, *S. aureus*, and *Ps. aeruginosa*, respectively. The regression equations, $Y = a - 2.73\ X$, $Y = a - 2.79\ X$, and $Y = a - 2.69\ X$ are shown in Fig. 1. In instances where the culture exhibits a net transmission range which is marginal, it is very likely that the culture will fall below the acceptable level during the first 10-carrier-soaking. This prediction is confirmed by calculations as shown in Fig. 1.

In conclusion, the turbidimetric measurement method is simple and fairly accurate to determine the degree of uniformity of the cultures at the required resistance levels against phenol. The results of this study also suggest that this method may be used as a practical means in selecting test cultures of uniform quality for disinfectant testing. The possibly interfering turbidity of the broth medium is not an evident factor to be considered a limitation of the method.

References

(1) American Public Health Association (1918) Report of Committee on Standard Method of Examining Disinfectants, *Amer. J. Pub. Health* **8**, 506–521

(2) *Official Methods of Analysis* (1970) 11th Ed., AOAC, Washington, D.C., pp. 59–72

(3) Brewer, C. M., & Reddish, G. F. (1929) *J. Bacteriol.* **17**, 44–45

(4) Rideal, S., & Walker, J. T. A. (1903) *J. Roy. Sanit. Inst.* **24**, 424–441

(5) Ruehl, S., & Brewer, C. M. (1931) "United States Food and Drug Administration Methods of Testing Antiseptics and Disinfectants," USDA Circular 198

(6) Wright, J. H. (1917) *J. Bacteriol.* **2**, 315–346

(7) Ortenzio, L. F., Friedl, J. L., & Stuart, L. S. (1949) *JAOAC* **32**, 408–417

(8) Lawrence, C. A., & Black, S. S. (1968) *Disinfection, Sterilization and Preservation*, Lea and Febiger, Philadelphia, pp. 109–178

(9) Ortenzio, L. F., Stuart, L. S., & Friedl, J. L. (1953) *JAOAC* **36**, 480–484

(10) Ortenzio, L. F., Friedl, J. L., & Stuart, L. S. (1955) "The practical disinfecting value of some acids and alkalies as revealed by the AOAC Use-Dilution Test", Paper presented at 41st meeting of the Chemical Specialties Manufacturing Association, May 16–17, 1955, Chicago, Ill.

(11) Ortenzio, L. F., Opalsky, C. D., & Stuart, L. S. (1960) *J. Appl. Microbiol.* **6**, 562–566

(12) Ortenzio, L. F., & Stuart, L. S. (1961) *JAOAC* **44**, 416–421

(13) Ortenzio, L. F. (1968) *JAOAC* **51**, 948–949

(14) Stuart, L. S., Ortenzio, L. F., & Friedl, J. L. (1953) *JAOAC* **36**, 465–478

(15) Stuart, L. S., Ortenzio, L. F., & Friedl, J. L. (1955) *JAOAC* **38**, 465–478

(16) Stuart, L. S., Ortenzio, L. F., & Friedl, J. L. (1958) *Soap Chem. Spec.* **34**, 79–82

(17) Wright, E. S. (1970) *JAOAC* **53**, 857–859

(18) Ostle, B. (1963) *Statistics in Research*, 2nd Ed., Iowa State University Press, Ames, pp. 40–51

(19) Youden, W. J. (1967) *Statistical Techniques for Collaborative Tests*, AOAC, Washington, D.C., pp. 4–6

Received September 14, 1971.

Editor's Comments on Papers 25, 26, and 27

The use of antimicrobial agents in controlling microorganisms is of extreme importance in the hospital. The authors in this section have had vast experience in this area. It should be pointed out that although this text is entitled "Chemical Sterilization," this condition is virtually impossible to achieve where human beings or animals are concerned unless they have been reared in a germ-free environment. Lowbury, Lilly, and Bull show that a high degree of destruction of microorganisms on the skin (99.1 percent) has been achieved using an organic iodine antiseptic solution.

Spaulding has long been active in the control of microorganisms in the hospital, and he and his group at Temple University Medical School have advocated the use of various antimicrobial agents for the elimination of microbes. His paper deals with a number of these agents.

Reprinted from *J. Hosp. Res.* **9**, 5–31 (1972)

CHEMICAL DISINFECTION AND ANTISEPSIS IN THE HOSPITAL

Earle H. Spaulding, Ph.D.

25

Introduction

IN THE LITERAL SENSE, "disinfection" should mean that the risk of infection has been completely eliminated. Instead, this meaning is reserved for the word *sterilization,* which is the total destruction of all microbial forms; a *sterilization procedure* is one which guarantees this absolute end point (sterility).

Thus, *disinfection* is something less than sterilization, and the crucial deficiency in a *disinfection procedure* is that it cannot be relied upon to produce sterility. Whether or not it actually does this in a particular situation will depend upon a number of factors, e.g., the nature of the contaminating microorganisms and especially the presence of highly resistant bacterial spores, the length of time of application, the number of microorganisms in the contamination, amount of organic "soil" present and the temperature. All of these factors influence the rapidity and level of antimicrobial action. Thus, disinfection is a procedure which does reduce the risk of infection but with a range of end results extending from actual sterility to a minimal reduction. It should be apparent by now that the distinction between sterilization and disinfection is an important concept.

That distinction is also of practical significance. A disinfection procedure may destroy all forms of microbial contamination (produce sterility) under certain circumstances, e.g., when only a few nonsporulating microorganisms are present. Likewise, a very strong chemical disinfectant can actually kill spores if it is used long enough. However, the time required in both instances *may be* much longer than is the case with any sterilization procedure such as the autoclave. Thus, for practical purposes disinfection and sterilization represent two distinctly different levels of microbicidal action.

Both sterilization and disinfection, as just defined, are carried out with physical agents, such as heat and irradiation, and with chemicals in either liquid or gaseous form. Heat or ionizing irradiation can sterilize in a matter of minutes or even seconds; whereas chemical methods are slower. Moist heat at 121°C, for example, sterilizes within 10 minutes the same spore-contaminated object which withstands exposure to a strong chemical solution or gas for two hours or longer. The end results may be the same, but the comparatively long time required for chemical sterilization is an unfortunate practical disadvantage.

The distinctions of disinfection and sterilization apply equally well to both physical and chemical procedures. Some heating methods do not guarantee sterility, e.g., immersion of an instrument in boiling water, which is therefore an example of physical disinfection. Immersion in most germicidal solutions is even less likely to result in sterility since their sporicidal capabilities are less than that of boiling water.

Nevertheless, disinfection procedures are of great practical importance in the hospital for they can destroy most – and often all – of the microorganisms contaminating those surfaces and objects which contribute to the spread of nosocomial infections. One of the major achievements of man has been his gradual control of those microorganisms in his environment which in the past devastated whole populations and made admissions to hospitals almost literally death sentences. And the tool for this greatly improved state has been disinfection, physical and chemical. Physical agents, of course, play the principal role, but chemicals have also contributed significantly to this control – and still do.

This review deals with chemical, and not with physical, disinfection. Therefore, from now on the terms "disinfection" and "sterilization" apply only to chemical agents.

Chemical disinfection is generally practiced with solutions, but gases are also used. The latter application is referred to in the vernacular as "gas sterilization," just as disinfection with chemical solutions becomes in common parlance "chemical sterilization." Neither term is appropriate unless the application of the chemical solution or gas guarantees sterility when a substantial number (approximately 1×10^5) of bacterial spores are present. For example, the implication that glutaraldehyde, formaldehyde or ethylene oxide (EtO) always sterilize, no matter how they are used, is misleading, for these sterilizing chemicals are frequently employed in such a way as to fall short of the level needed to guarantee sterility. It would be highly desirable to state when describing such procedures the nature of the chemical agent, the precise method used, as well as contact time. For example, exposure to Pennoxide® (ethylene oxide) in a Cryotherm apparatus for 3 hours at 130°F leaves no doubt. When less potent procedures are employed, sterilization depends even more upon other factors, primarily the types and numbers of contaminating microorganisms and the time of contact or exposure. The point I am emphasizing is that the chemical is only the tool. What result is achieved with it depends first, upon the strength of the chemical; second, upon the way it is used; third, upon several other factors already mentioned, such as nature of the contamination, contact time, temperature, and so on. It is like a hammer (the tool). Whether or not the hammer will crack a nut depends first, upon the weight of the hammer; second, upon how hard you hit the nut, if at all (the procedure); and, third, upon how tough the shell is and how many times you try to hit it. Let me illustrate again by returning to a physical procedure already referred to, i.e., immersion in boiling water which does not guarantee sterility. Yet the application of moist heat at 121°C (autoclave) does guarantee sterility. Moist heat was the tool in both instances, but the first procedure is only disinfection, whereas the second constitutes sterilization because it involves a more intense application of heat. Similarly, some EtO procedures are appropriately termed sterilization; others should be – but are not always – called disinfection.

In the absence of bacterial spores, some chemical disinfection procedures are capable of producing sterility and probably do so frequently; but there are others which only destroy the less resistant of the nonsporulating bacteria. How much these different levels of procedures can accomplish in reducing the risk of infection in the hospital is an important matter which is included in the ensuing discussion. It can be seen at this point that chemicals can be used in such a way as to produce three levels of disinfection: sporicidal, cidal for all nonsporulating types, cidal for some nonsporulating types.

This seems to be a good time to call the reader's attention to two excellent texts on the general subject of disinfection, the first edited by Lawrence and Block[1], the second written by Sykes[2].

Some readers may want to consult other discussions of hospital disinfection by the writer. For example, a comparison of the content of the present review with a 1965 discussion of the same subject[3] reveals the amount of progress which has been made in the past 7 years. Also, there is a chapter in reference 1 dealing in more detail with instrument-equipment disinfection. Quite a different approach was taken in a recent paper on the role of chemical disinfection in the control of nosocomial infections[4].

NATURE OF THE PROBLEM

Hospital disinfection consists of two major types of application. The first is upon inanimate materials such as floors, furniture, equipment and instruments. In order to avoid confusion, chemicals used in this way should be referred to as *disinfectants,* whether they be in the form of a liquid, gas or aerosol mist. The second application is to body surfaces, a practice called *antisepsis,* and chemicals used in this way are *antiseptics.* Antisepsis therefore is a special application of disinfection in which mild and comparatively weak chemicals are applied to skin or mucous membranes. The distinction between application to inanimate objects vs. application to tissues is an important one because these two procedures in general require different kinds and concentrations of chemicals. An exception, incidentally, is alcohol, which in the same concentration is useful both as a disinfectant and antiseptic. *Germicide* is a broader term including both disinfectants and antiseptics.

Disinfection of inanimate objects in the hospital may be conveniently subdivided into *instrument-equipment disinfection* and *housekeeping disinfection.* Furthermore, instrument-equipment disinfection can be understood better and practiced more effectively if it is, in turn, divided into three categories based upon the risk of infection involved in the use of the disinfected materials (Table I). The first of these is *critical items,* so-called because they are introduced beneath the surface of the body or attached to other objects so used, e.g., transfer forceps, scalpel blades, cardiac catheters, plastic components of the heart-lung oxygenator. Consequently, all contaminating microorganisms must be destroyed; in other words, the requirement is for sterility. The risk involved in using disinfected endotracheal and aspirator tubes, thermometers, cystoscopes and inhalation therapy nebulizers is considerably less and these are classified as *semi-critical* items. Although these objects come in contact

TABLE I – HOSPITAL GERMICIDES FOR INANIMATE OBJECTS

Area of Use vs. Level of Cidal Action

	BACTERIA			FUNGI[2]	VIRUSES	
	Vegetative[1]	Tubercle Bacillus	Spores		Lipid and Medium Size	Nonlipid and Small
Disinfection						
Instruments & Equipment						
Critical	+*	+	+	+	+	+
Semi-critical	+	+	+ or –	+	+	+
Noncritical	+	+ or –	–	+	+	+ or –
Housekeeping	+	+ or –	–	+	+	+ or –

* + indicates that the designated level of cidal action occurs within a useful period of time.

(1) Common forms of bacterial cells, e.g., staphylococcus. (2) Includes usual asexual "spores," but not necessarily dried chlamydospores and sexual spores.

with intact mucous membrane, they do not ordinarily penetrate body surfaces. Sterilization is desirable but not essential. A reasonable objective therefore is to employ a procedure which can be expected to destroy viruses, fungal spores, the tubercle bacillus and most viruses. *Noncritical* materials consist of a wide variety of objects and surfaces such as face masks, carafes and humidifiers which do not ordinarily come in contact with mucous membranes and thus carry the least risk.

Housekeeping disinfection pertains to articles of furniture, drapes, linens, walls, floor surfaces, etc. A satisfactory level of disinfection both here and for noncritical materials, is achieved with prompt destruction of the common nonsporulating bacteria. Destruction of the tubercle bacillus is highly desirable but not likely with many procedures in current use. These are also capable of some good virucidal action, but the level which can be expected or is needed remains unclear.

Most *antispetic* procedures, because of restrictions imposed on them by tissue toxicity, are unable to accomplish more than a reduction (largely by physical removal, no doubt) of the less-resistant nonsporulating microorganisms on skin and mucous membranes.

It may seem to the reader that I have complicated the subject unnecessarily by creating so many categories, but these divisions represent significantly different sets of requirements for good disinfection. Furthermore, failure to recognize their significance has contributed to the confusion which exists about this subject and has retarded the rate of improvement in this field.

There is a great difference between the practice of disinfection vs. antisepsis, as well as the types of germicides which are appropriate. The cell walls of bacteria and fungi are much more resistant to chemical injury than are our tissue cells. Therefore, only the keratinized cells of the skin, and to a lesser degree the epithelial lining of mucous membranes, can tolerate the irritating action of germicides. Since antiseptics are applied directly to skin and mucous membranes, the maximum concentration of a germicidal chemical which should be used this way is limited by its toxicity for these tissues. Thus, there are fewer useful antiseptics than disinfectants (Table II). Strong disinfectants

TABLE II – CLASSES OF CHEMICAL COMPOUNDS USEFUL AS

	Disinfectants	Antiseptics
Vegetative Bacteria	Many	Few
Lipid & Medium-sized Viruses	Many	Few
Nonlipid & Small Viruses	Mod. no.	Very few
Tubercle Bacillus	Few	Very few
Bacterial Spores	Very few	None

such as ethylene oxide, formaldehyde and glutaraldehyde are entirely too toxic for tissue, and they lose their germicidal power if they are diluted to the point where they are nontoxic. The class of phenolic germicides also contains examples of good disinfectants which do not qualify as acceptable antiseptics, irrespective of concentration, and for the same reason. An exception is hexachlorophene, a bis-phenol compound with six chlorine atoms attached to the basic molecule. It is a poor disinfectant but enjoys wide acceptance as an antiseptic because it is non-irritating for skin in relatively high concentrations and retains its bacteriostatic properties in the presence of soap. (Recent reports indicate, however, that hexachlorophene is readily absorbed through skin and with continued and heavy use may cause damage to nervous tissue.) A few germicides can be tolerated by our skin in bactericidal concentrations which bring about significant reductions in the microbial population, and it is this select group which constitutes the most useful antiseptics.

Disinfectants, on the other hand, can be employed in much higher concentrations, and some good ones are definitely toxic for skin. The reason is, of course, that they are applied to inanimate objects and not directly to skin. Consequently the limiting factor for determining the highest concentration of a chemical to be used for disinfection is damage to metal, wood, rubber, plastic, etc. But it is well to note that not all bactericidal chemicals are useful disinfectants. For example, strong sulfuric acid destroys spores rapidly but is not a disinfectant because it is corrosive in sporicidal concentrations and almost devoid of antimicrobial properties in noncorrosive concentrations.

The best housekeeping disinfectants are not the best instrument disinfectants. The phenolics, for example, deserve their widespread use on floors, walls and furniture, but they are not good choices for instruments. Conversely, strong glutaraldehyde and formaldehyde solutions are good instrument-equipment germicides but inappropriate for floors. And finally, some instrument-equipment germicides are satisfactory for semi-critical items but do not have sufficient sporicidal activity to qualify them for critical items. An example is 80 to 90% alcohol.

It should be clear by now that there is no such thing as an "all-purpose" disinfectant, just as there is no "all-purpose" antibiotic. If a single germicidal solution is used for all the different applications needed for good hospital asepsis, it will in one or more of these applications fall short of the level available with some other disinfectant. And this point is still valid even though a different concentration of the "all-purpose" product is used for each application. Proper practice of chemical disinfection, therefore, is based on the selection of the best available germicide for each type of application and its use in the most effective way. To do this one must be familiar with the major principles of chemical disinfection and the properties of the available germicides.

PRINCIPLES OF CHEMICAL DISINFECTION

The major principles of chemical disinfection can be stated as follows:

1. Microorganisms differ markedly in their resistance to chemicals.

2. Germicides differ widely in the level of cidal action they produce, and these several levels involve different mechanisms.

3. There are secondary factors which influence the results obtained when a certain type of microorganism is exposed to a particular concentration of germicide; the most important of these are the number of microbial cells present, the time of contact and the amount of organic "soil" present.

How these principles govern the results obtainable with chemical disinfection is the next topic.

Nature of the Microbial Contamination

Because bacteria exhibit a wide range of resistance to chemicals, it follows that the kinds of microorganisms known or presumed to be present as contaminants must be the first consideration when deciding upon the level of disinfection needed.

The four major classes of microorganisms are bacteria, viruses, fungi and animal parasites. For hospital disinfection, the last two classes can be disregarded; thus the problem is how to destroy bacteria and viruses.

The nature of bacteria and viruses, with special reference to germicidal resistance, was the subject of an earlier article by the writer[5]. Most types of bacteria occur as a single form, the vegetative (growing) cell; a few species also produce spores. Bacterial spores are the most resistant form of microbial life, and their resistance to germicides is enormously greater than that of vegetative cells. The tetanus bacillus in its vegetative form, for example, is no more resistant to a disinfectant than the staphylococcus, but its spores can survive exposure to many of the commonly used germicides for days or weeks. Consequently, the statement that a certain germicide "kills spore-formers" is meaningless and misleading.

Once formed within the bacterial cell, the spore remains dormant until the proper growth conditions cause it to germinate into a vegetative cell. Because this dormant period may last for years, viable spores are disseminated so widely in nature that we must assume they are present in many situations involving hospital disinfection. And because they can withstand exposures to very strong germicides for several hours, spores constitute the principal obstacle to chemical sterilization.

In contrast, the differences among the various kinds of vegetative bacteria are relatively minor, with one exception. This is the tubercle bacillus which, because of its waxy envelope, is comparatively resistant to aqueous germicides, and almost completely so to quaternary ammonium ("quats") compounds and hexachlorophene. Among the other vegetative bacteria, staphylococci and enterococci (intestinal streptococci) are somewhat more resistant than other Gram-positives. The Gram-positives as a whole are slightly more resistant to some classes of germicides than Gram-negatives, whereas the Gram-negatives are more resistant to others. In recent years, however, the "nonfermenting Gram-negatives" such as Pseudomonas have become important causes of nosocomial infections[6]. These are bacilli with comparatively high resistance to antibiotics; they are also somewhat more resistant to germicides[7]. Also prominent among these emerging pathogens are enteric bacilli such as Klebsiella, Enterobacter and Serratia species. Another group are the "water bacteria," a collection of types widely distributed in nature and considered in the past as inocuous. However, there are now many reports documenting these organisms as the agents responsible for outbreaks of hospital infection, particularly as contaminants of inhalation therapy equipment[8].

These differences in resistance are of practical significance only when marginal concentrations of low-level germicide are used, for they disappear upon application of a stronger preparation. An important improvement in hospital disinfection could be made today by the widespread use of concentrations of proprietary disinfectants (not antiseptics) twice as strong as those currently recommended by their manufacturers. Incidentally, antibiotic-resistant "hospital" strains of staphylococci are no more resistant to germicides than any other staphylococcus.

Viruses also differ in germicidal resistance, and these differences may be important. Furthermore, the number of human pathogenic viruses is at least as large as the number of pathogenic bacteria and, because they are frequently present on and in our bodies, we must assume that pathogenic viruses are regularly present in the air and surfaces of the hospital environment.

A major concern with respect to viral resistance has to do with the human hepatitis viruses. Because man is the only susceptible species and infection is often life-threatening it has not been possible to carry out the tests needed to determine germicidal resistance. Until this can be done, the correct statement to make about their levels of resistance to chemicals is that we do not yet know the answer. Because, like other viruses, they appear to consist of nucleic acid wrapped in a protein coat, one assumes that their resistance to germicides cannot possibly be of the order of that of bacterial spores. On the other hand, the serious nature of viral hepatitis dictates the necessity of using a sterilization procedure whenever the presence of these viruses is a possibility.

There are also differences in resistance to antimicrobial chemicals among the other viruses. One of these appears to depend upon the presence or absence of lipid. Klein and Deforest[9] noted that the presence of lipid in the protein coat makes viruses so constituted (lipid viruses) susceptible to germicidal solutions which fail to inactivate lipid-free viruses. Among the more resistant, lipid-free picornaviruses is the important enterovirus group containing the poliomyelitis, Coxsackie and Echo viruses, many of which are recognized human pathogens. Also comparatively resistant are the rhinoviruses of the common cold. Therefore, we now recognize the existence of two distinct classes of viruses with respect to resistance to chemicals (Tables I and II).

A consideration of microbial resistance to germicides leads to the realization that all microorganisms fall into three fairly distinct groups. Most vegetative bacteria and fungi, as well as most viruses (designated here as medium-sized and lipid), appear to be comparatively susceptible to the usual applications of germicides. Turbercle bacilli and some – perhaps all – of the small nonlipid viruses, e.g., the picornaviruses, are significantly more resistant. Finally, there are bacterial spores which may be tremendously resistant.

Levels of Germicidal Action

Chemical disinfection in general differs from sterilization by its lack of sporicidal power. The germicides which do have this capability are few, indeed, and constitute that select class known as sporicides. Those which are not sporicidal exhibit significantly different levels of antimicrobial activity. Some kill within a few minutes not only the ordinary vegetative forms of bacteria (i.e., staphylococcus), fungi and lipid-containing viruses, but also the tubercle bacillus and nonlipid viruses. These germicides are intermediate between sporicides and the nonsporicidal ones whose effective cidal range is limited to the less resistant vegetative bacteria and lipid-containing viruses.

Thus, these three levels of germicidal action must be recognized if hospital disinfection is to be carried out properly. The adjectives used to designate them are, respectively: (1) high-level; (2) intermediate-level; (3) low-level (Table III). A tacit but important part of these definitions (and of sterilization, too) is that the cidal effect must occur within a practicable period of time. What is practicable in any given situation is a decision for the operator to make.

High-level Disinfection. Because certain critical items are thermolabile and must be disinfected by chemicals, a question of great practical importance is whether high-level germicides can be depended upon to sterilize medical and surgical materials. In the absence of spores they certainly can, and do so promptly. But one must assume that spores are present in some in-use situations, although the number will probably be small[10]. The sporicidal capacity of these agents, therefore, is a crucial property.

Three high-level germicides are 3 to 8% formaldehyde (7.5 to 20% formalin) in aqueous or alcoholic solution, 2% alkalinized aqueous glutaraldehyde, and gaseous ethylene oxide. Although all of these can kill large numbers of resistant spores under severe test conditions, they may require from 10 to 24 hours to do so[11,12]. On the other hand, sterilization may

TABLE III – LEVELS OF DISINFECTANT ACTION

	BACTERIA			FUNGI[2]	VIRUSES	
	Vege-[1] tative	Tubercle Bacillus	Spores		Lipid and Medium Size	Nonlipid and Small
HIGH	+*	+	+	+	+	+
INTERMEDIATE	+	+	–	+	+	+
LOW	+	–	–	+	+	–

*** + indicates that a cidal effect can be expected when use-concentrations of available disinfectants are properly employed. (1) Common forms of bacterial cells, e.g., staphylococcus. (2) Includes usual asexual "spores," but not necessarily dried chlamydospores and sexual spores.**

occur in 2 hours or less if only a small number of spores are present (Table IV). In summary it

TABLE IV

EFFECT OF NUMBERS ON SPORICIDAL TIME

B. subtilis Spores, Germicide: 8% HCHO-isopropanol + 0.5% G11

Spore Count (per blade)	Test Procedure	RESULTS	
		Positive	Negative
100,000	Dried Blood Blade	2 hrs.	3 hrs.
1,000	"	1 hr.	2 hrs.
10	"	. . .	30 min.

can be said that these agents can be relied upon to produce sterility if they are used properly and the exposure is long enough.

Another interesting question is whether or not high-level germicides (sporicides) should be designated as sterilizing agents. To illustrate, ethylene oxide (EtO) has been widely accepted, and has received official recognition, as a sterilizing agent. But in reality its sterilizing capacity varies widely with the procedure used. The commercial processes of reliable manufacturers ensure sterilization by incorporation of prehumidification, heat, evacuation of the chamber, and by the use of high concentrations of the gas and operating cycles of 16 to 20 hours. However, the EtO "sterilization" methods being carried out in hospitals and medical offices are quite a different matter. In our experiments with a large autoclave-type of EtO apparatus, exposures as long as 12 hours are required for consistent sterilization of test objects heavily contaminated with dry *Clostridium sporogenes* spores (unless they are presoaked in water). Indeed, this apparatus was less rapidly cidal for these spores than the strong formaldehyde and glutaraldehyde solutions mentioned earlier, the latter being intermediate between the two types of EtO apparatus. How many of these high-level germicides should be classified as sterilizing agents is a moot question, particularly in view of the fact that they take so much longer than the autoclave. There are as yet no universally accepted criteria for deciding whether a microbiocidal process (chemical or physical) should be called sterilizing rather than disinfecting.

Stuart, Ortenzio and collaborators in the Pesticides Regulation Division of the U.S. Department of Agriculture (recently moved to the Environmental Protection Agency) developed the A.O.A.C. Sporicidal Test some years ago[11] which has attained in the U.S. the status of an official test. It is a severe one. When the test organism is *Cl. sporogenes*, contaminated porcelain cylinders and suture loop carriers may show spore counts in the range of 10^6 to 10^7. This large number of spores is so much greater than that found on materials[10] that the results are unrealistic with respect to practical situations in the hospital. Because of its severity, the A.O.A.C. Sporicidal Test can serve as a reliable criterion for chemical *sterilization*. The time required for a germicidal solution or gas to pass this test becomes its sterilization time. The A.O.A.C. Test calls for two test organisms, *Cl. sporogenes* and *Bacillus subtilis* on two types of carriers. When there are differences in the end points, the longest time period producing at least 59 negatives from 60 replicates becomes the sterilization time for that disinfectant.

Before leaving this topic it seems worthwhile to put into proper perspective the long exposure periods needed for chemical sterilization. When the dried *Cl. sporogenes*-contaminated porcelain cylinders used as test carriers in the A.O.A.C. Sporicidal Test are autoclaved at 121°C, they are sterilized within 10 minutes; immersion in boiling water requires 2 to 3 hours; a good EtO procedure (without presoak) takes from 1 to 12 hours or longer depending upon the procedure and the dryness of the spore. High-level germicidal solutions require from 3 to 24 hours.

Intermediate-level Disinfection. The tubercle bacillus is significantly more resistant to other vegetative bacteria than aqueous germicides. In some instances, a tuberculocidal effect can be obtained by using a greater concentration than the one commonly employed (e.g., iodophors); whereas this is for all practical purposes beyond the capability of aqueous "quats" at any concentration. Although the risk of transmitting tuberculosis with medical and surgical materials is much less than formerly, it is still a primary consideration in some situations.

Viruses also differ in their resistance to chemicals. In the test system used by Klein and Deforest[9] a number of commonly employed liquid germicides did not destroy the important picornaviruses which contain the enterovirus group (polio, Echo and Coxsackie) and the rhinoviruses of the common cold. Not all germicides with good tuberculocidal activity destroy the small nonlipid viruses used by Klein and Deforest. According to their findings isopropanol is an example of a good tuberculocide which lacks this virucidal power, and there may be some germicides with the reverse properties. On the other hand, 70 to 95% ethanol is rapidly tuberculocidal (Table VIII page 22) and picornavirucidal[9]. Additional studies are needed to determine which of the presently available germicides fulfill both of these criteria of intermediate-level disinfection.

Low-level Disinfection. Some of the germicides in common use today not only lack sporicidal power, but also fail to destroy quickly either the tubercle bacillus or the small nonlipid viruses. These low-level germicides are nonetheless useful in practice because they can rapidly kill the vegetative forms of bacteria and fungi, as well as the medium-sized and lipid-containing viruses.

In some instances the level of cidal activity can be raised from low to intermediate simply by increasing the concentration as, for example, from 75 to 450 ppm with iodophors. But all germicidal chemicals do not have this capacity, for a concentration of a quaternary ammonium compound as high as 10% fails to meet either the tuberculocidal or virucidal criterion for intermediate-level disinfection. In recent years an increase in the use-concentration of "quats" from the 1:1000 to 1:750 has been widely adopted so as, among other reasons, to obtain better cidal activity for the comparatively resistant Pseudomonas organisms. This was a step in the right direction, but it still does not produce second-level disinfection.

How Germicides Kill Microorganisms

A good germicide must be rapidly lethal for microorganisms at its use-concentration. Some strong disinfectants do this the same way heat does, by coagulating the protein of microbial cells, which is the same process as the clotting of casein in milk or the hardening of egg white. The change is irreversible. Thus, formalin (a solution of formaldehyde in water) in high concentrations (8%, for example) kills most vegetative bacteria on contact by coagulating its proteins. But it also kills tissue cells the same way. Indeed, all germicides are protoplasmic poisons, which means that they are toxic for the protoplasm (and outer membranes) of all cells, mammalian as well as microbial. In fact, tissue cells are destroyed sooner than the bacterial cells when exposed to the same germicide because they lack the protection provided by the thick and rigid cell walls of bacteria. Consequently, the application of a germicidal solution to delicate tissues is almost certain to do more harm than good.

More often, however, the germicidal effect is not due to actual coagulation but to a less obvious denaturation of protein. Some of the proteins of microbial cells are enzymes and subject to denaturation by heat or chemicals. Although this process may be slower than gross coagulation, this type of denaturation can also kill the microbial cell if essential enzymes or vital structures are rendered nonfunctional.

There are other bactericidal mechanisms and a single disinfectant may act through several of them. Phenolic and quaternary ammonium compounds in high concentrations, for example, cause rapid lysis of the bacterial cell; whereas leakage of cell constituents without lysis and denaturation of enzymes are the principal modes of cidal action when the concentration is decreased. Obviously, the last-named group of mechanisms is slower than the first one, and so the killing time (time required for total killing of a test microbial population in a given situation) is directly correlated with germicidal concentration.

Still another germicidal mechanism is represented by some of the antiseptics. The maximum concentrations which can be tolerated on skin and mucous membrane are still relatively weak and bring about their cidal effects in subtle ways, such as irreversible oxidation of essential enzymes (iodine), binding of enzymes (mercurials) or by some unknown mechanism (hexachlorophene). Discernible germicidal effects take place slowly, and in the case of mercurials can be reversed if a neutralizing chemical is added before the microorganisms have been irreversibly damaged.

The mechanisms just described pertain to vegetative bacterial cells. Sporicidal action is not well understood, but it is apparent that the thick wall and low water content of spores are important. The mechanism of virucidal action is probably based on denaturation and coagulation of protein, but there may be more to it than that[9].

which must be destroyed grows larger, there is a corresponding increase in the number of resistant cells and therefore in the overall resistance level of that bacterial population. This principle is illustrated in Table IV.

The important relationship between population size and killing time is shown graphically in Fig. 1. It shows the results obtained when a rapidly cidal concentration of disinfectant was added to an aqueous suspension of staphylococci. It can be seen that approximately 90% of the initial population was killed during the first minute of exposure since only 10% of the bacteria present originally were able to grow out when subcultured after one minute. A similar situation exists at 2 minutes vs. one minute, and so on. Looked at in a different way, the data show

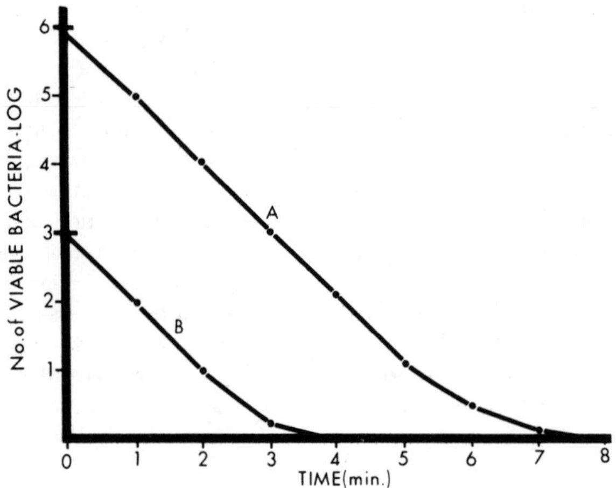

Fig. 1: Influence of the numbers of bacterial cells present when a rapidly cidal concentration of disinfectant was added to a suspension of staphylococci.

Influence of Numbers

The larger the number of bacteria contaminating skin or inanimate objects, the longer it takes for a germicide to destroy them all. The reason is that all the bacterial populations are heterogeneous, even when they consist entirely of a single type of microorganism. This means that individual cells will differ in any one of a number of properties, including resistance to germicides. Thus, as the number of bacteria

that one half of the entire exposure time was needed to destroy one cell in 10,000 in curve A (100 vs. 1,000,000), or one cell in 100 in curve B (10 vs. 1000). The principle this illustrates is that a disproportionate amount of the killing time in chemical disinfection is required to destroy a very small (resistant) portion of any bacterial population.

Upon studying the sporicidal results in Table IV one may ask the question: How long must this germicidal solution be used in actual practice in order to be sure sterility is achieved? It is a good question, and the answer must be based on a judgment decision revolving around another question: What is a reasonable number of spores to include in such a test which make the results relevant to in-use situations? The fact that large numbers of spores are seldom present in actual practice, including surgical instruments used in intestinal surgery[3], suggests that a number much smaller than the 10^6 to 10^7 used in the official A.O.A.C. Sporicidal Test[11] provides an adequate margin of safety.

I discuss the importance of numbers at some length because there seems to be so little awareness of it and especially of its influence on killing times. Also this factor has an important application to instrument disinfection, and this is the necessity for good physical cleansing prior to disinfection. By reducing the number of microorganisms which remain to be destroyed by the chemical, one correspondingly shortens the time required to bring about complete destruction (killing time). This principle applies equally well to all types of chemical disinfection including housekeeping and antisepsis, and to physical agents as well.

Influence of "Soil"

Organic dirt such as blood, plasma, feces and tissue absorbs germicidal molecules and inactivates them, leaving only the excess free chemical to act upon microbial cells. This is, of course, a second – and the major – reason for thorough cleansing of instruments, etc. prior to application of chemical disinfection.

Strong concentrations of some germicides usually retain an effective level of activity in the presence of heavy organic soil, e.g., phenolic disinfectants. Iodophors (iodine-detergent complexes), on the other hand, are much more subject to inactivation by organic soil, and so are the "quats" and chlorine compounds. The adverse effect of organic soil is, of course, much greater with low-level germicides than with high-level ones, particularly in marginal concentrations.

Influence of Germicide Concentration

The killing time can be shortened by increasing the concentration of germicide[13], and this is illustrated in Table V where the

TABLE V – ETHYL ALCOHOL: CONCENTRATION VS. CIDAL ACTION*

Free Suspension – Room Temperature

	STAPHYLOCOCCUS		PSEUDOMONAS	
%/Vol.	Pos.	Neg.	Pos.	Neg.
100	40 sec.	50 sec.	–	10 sec.
95-60	–	10 sec.	–	10 sec.
50	10 sec.	20 sec.	–	10 sec.
40	45 sec.	60 sec.	–	10 sec.
30	45 min.	60 min.	–	10 sec.
20	2 hrs.	3 hrs.	25 min.	30 min.

*Adapted from a paper by Morton (see ref. 13).

number of bacteria and other test conditions remain the same, the only variable being the alcohol concentration. As this increases, additional cidal mechanisms come into play and those already operating become more intense. It is apparent from this table that alcohol is an active germicide only in relatively high concentrations. Other germicides which also show sharp drops in activity upon dilution are formaldehyde, glutaraldehyde and ethylene oxide[1].

The point has already been made, but it is worth repeating, that some low-level germicides become intermediate and even high-level ones if the use-concentration can be increased sufficiently. Thus, aqueous iodophors and certain aqueous phenolics are tuberculocides of practical value at 450 ppm and 3% respectively, whereas they lack this capacity at 75 ppm and 1%. And further increase in concentration may result in some sporicidal action. More importantly, vegetative bacteria – and probably viruses as well – can be destroyed more rapidly by a modest increase in the concentration of some germicides. Bactericidal tests in the writer's laboratory showed that this is true for "quats," iodophors and phenolics. To paraphrase a suggestion made earlier, the rapidity of disinfection can be significantly increased by doubling the concentration of active ingredients in most proprietary disinfectants.

Keeping in mind the various disinfection requirements in the hospital and what the three levels of disinfection are, we are ready to examine the disinfectants and antiseptics which are available, and to see if there are useful criteria for deciding which to use when one is faced with a disinfection problem. Hundreds of proprietary germicides are available in this country. Consequently they need to be arranged in an orderly fashion, and this can be done on the basis of chemical similarities. When we do this we discover that they fall rather neatly into three categories according to the three levels of germicidal action described earlier.

Classification of germicides on the basis of their killing power involves evaluation, and it may be helpful to see how this is done before we look at the germicides themselves.

EVALUATION OF GERMICIDES

Problems

The first problem is commercialism. We, the users, are faced with a plethora of proprietary solutions, hundreds of which are insignificant modifications – if, indeed, they are modifications at all – of well-known products. Many of them are promoted vigorously and backed by exaggerated claims. As early as 1959, there were registered with the United States Department of Agriculture about 450 products specifically recommended for hospital application[14]. Several hundred more have been added since then. Fortunately, this federal agency is doing much to curb the sale of poor germicides by establishing performance standards which must be met if the product enters interstate commerce. These "official" A.O.A.C. tests[1] provide a practical means for eliminating products which do not fulfill the claims made for them.

The second problem is how to evaluate germicides. This is a complex technical subject which is not appropriate for detailed discussion here. However, a few general comments may be helpful.

Testing Methods

These consist of laboratory tests and in-use tests. I will dismiss the former with the remark that the emphasis in most "official" tests is on minimum standards. An exception is the A.O.A.C. Sporicidal Test, which has already been discussed with regard to this point. There is now need for the development and wider use of good in-use tests which evaluate germicides for a specific application by testing them under actual or simulated conditions of use.

In-use tests with critical and semicritical articles involve nurses and Central Service personnel who assist the bacteriologist in determining whether the results of laboratory tests hold up in actual practice. With floor decontamination this means a series of cleaning-disinfection tests which, if properly designed and carried out, will answer the question: How can we get the most efficient decontamination? Good examples of in-use testing of operating rooms and of the floors in hospital wards are those of Kundsin and Walter[15], Adams and Fahlman[16] and Vesley *et al.*[17]. Edmondson and Sanford suggested an in-use method for inhalation equipment in 1966[18], and the same group later did a study under controlled conditions of use[19].

The evaluation of antiseptics *must* be done by in-use testing because *"in vitro"* laboratory tests mean very little. The most comprehensive and reproducible method for doing this is the serial basin procedure of Price[20,21] which, unfortunately, is tedious, inconvenient and time-consuming. Consequently, short-cut methods are generally employed. The three most widely used at the present time have been discussed by Dineen[22].

CLASSES OF GERMICIDES

Liquids vs. Gases

Most germicides are used as aqueous solutions. The water brings the chemical in contact with the microorganisms and constitutes the "water of reaction" without which the disinfection process practically stops. A few germicidal chemicals have vapor pressures low enough to be gases at room temperature, and these compounds can be used as gaseous disinfectants or sterilizing agents.

Tables VI (this page) and VII (on next page) contain summary evaluations and some pertinent properties of the major classes of germicides. These notations are based upon my own experience, published laboratory data and in-use reports. Some of the evaluations and properties, which had to be limited to one or two words in the tables, need clarification and discussion. The liquid germicides will be considered first.

TABLE VI
ACTIVITY LEVELS OF
SELECTED CLASSES GERMICIDES

	Class	Use-Concentrations	Activity Level
GAS			
	Ethylene oxide	450 to 800 mgm/L (1)	High
LIQUID			
	Glutaraldehyde, aq.	2%	High
	Formaldehyde + alcohol	8% + 70%	High
	Formaldehyde, aq.	3 to 8%	High to Intermediate
	Iodine + alcohol	0.5% + 70%	Intermediate
	Alcohols	70 to 90%	Intermediate
	Chlorine cpds.	500 to 5000 ppm. (2)	Intermediate
	Phenolic cpds.	1 to 3% (3)	Intermediate
	Iodine, aq.	1%	Intermediate
	Iodophors	75 to 150 ppm. (4)	Intermediate to Low
	Quaternary ammon. cpds.	1:750 to 1:500	Low
	Hexachlorophene	1%	Low
	Mercurial cpds.	1:1000 to 1:500	Low

(1) In autoclave-type equipment at 55 to 60°C.

(2) Available chlorine.

(3) Dilution of concentrate containing 5% to 10% phenolics.

(4) Available iodine.

TABLE VII – CLASSES OF GERMICIDES

Usefulness and Selected Properties

Class	Usefulness as		Selected Secondary Properties
	Disinfectants	Antiseptics	
GAS			
Ethylene oxide	+2 to +4*	0	Toxic; good penetration; req. R.H. of 30% or more; bactericidal activity varies with apparatus used; absorbed by porous materials. Dry spores highly resistant, moisture must be present and presoak is desirable.
LIQUID			
Glutaraldehyde, aq.	+3	0	Sporicidal; active solution unstable; toxic
Formaldehyde + alcohol	+2	0	Sporicidal; noxious fumes; toxic; volatile
Formaldehyde, aq.	+1 to +2	0	Sporicidal; noxious fumes; toxic
Phenolic cpds.	+3	±	Stable; corrosive; little inactiv. by organ. matter; irritates skin
Chlorine cpds.	+1	±	Flash action; much inactiv. by organ. matter; corrosive; irritates skin
Alcohols	+2	+3	Rapidly cidal; volatile; flammable; dries and irritates skin
Iodine + alcohol	0	+4	Corrosive; very rapidly cidal; causes staining; irritates skin; flammable
Iodophors	+1	+3	Somewhat unstable; rel. bland; staining temporary; corrosive
Iodine, aq.	0	+2	Rapidly cidal; corrosive; stains fabrics; stains and irritates skin
Quaternary ammon. cpds.	+1	+2	Bland; inactiv. by soap and anionics; absorbed by fabrics
Hexachlorophene	0	+2	Bland; isol. in H_2O; sol. in alc.; not inactiv. by soap; weakly cidal
Mercurial cpds.	0	+1	Bland; much inactiv. by organ. matter; weakly cidal

* +4 denotes maximum usefulness; 0 indicates little or no usefulness.

Comment: More detailed information may be obtained from descriptive brochures, journal articles and books[1, 2]. Selection of the most appropriate germicide for a particular situation should be made by the responsible personnel in each hospital and based upon: (1) whether it is to be used as a disinfectant or an antiseptic; (2) estimation of the level of antimicrobial action needed; (3) the hospital's scope of services, physical facilities and personnel.

Instruments, apparatus and other objects should be cleansed to remove gross organic soil prior to the use of chemical disinfectants which coagulate protein in order to get good penetration of crevices and porous material. Instruments, as well as rubber and plastic tubing, must be rinsed or flushed with sterile water before coming into contact with skin and especially mucous membrane in order to avoid irritation. For the same reason, aeration is necessary after exposure to ethylene oxide.

Some of the above material was suggested, modified or contributed by Mr. G. F. Mallison, U.S.P.H.S. Center for Disease Control, who always cooperates fully and helps greatly with efforts such as this.

LIQUID GERMICIDES

Mercurials

Relatively high concentrations are required to achieve significant cidal activity. For this and other reasons the mercurials have no place in modern disinfection. Their value as antiseptics is also limited.

Phenolic Compounds

Phenol or carbolic acid is the oldest of the major classes of germicides. Although the parent chemical is no longer used, hundreds of compounds related to it have been synthesized and proposed as disinfectants. These constitute the class of substituted phenolics (often referred to simply as the phenolics). This class is the most popular one for housekeeping disinfection, and properly so. Not only are the phenolics good bactericides, but they also have the desirable property of stability, meaning that they remain active after mild heating and prolonged drying. Thus, subsequent application of moisture to a dry surface previously treated with a phenolic can redissolve the chemical so that it again becomes bactericidal. In addition, concentrations of the order of 2 to 3% remain quite active when in contact with organic soil; for this reason phenolics are also the disinfectants of choice for dealing with fecal contamination.

On the other hand, unpleasant odor and tissue irritation preclude their useful application on the skin. Indeed, the continued use of phenolics on objects which may come in close and prolonged contact with skin and mucous membranes, e.g., anesthesia equipment, has come under close scrutiny because of reported depigmentation of skin[23].

Quaternary Ammonium Compounds

Synthetic chemists have created hundreds of synthetic chemicals with good cleaning properties, some of them being widely used household products. One group, known as the cationic detergents, contains quaternary ammonium compounds which have definite germicidal activity. Zephiran® is the prototype.

The "quats" have enjoyed wide usage both as disinfectants and antiseptics. They have the important property of being bland and are therefore popular. On the other hand, they have serious limitations. For example, they are selectively absorbed by fabrics so that a 1:1000 solution may become a 1:1500 or 1:2000 if gauze is immersed in such a solution[24,25]. This situation has apparently resulted in severe, and even fatal, infections[26]. Hospital infections from other uses – or misuses – of "quats' were reported and reviewed by Lee and Fialkow[27]. Even the use of hard water for dilution reduces the active concentration of Zephiran® [28]. In general recognition of the fact that the traditional 1:1000 concentration was not enough, it has become common practice in recent years to use 1:750; and in the writer's opinion it should be further increased to 1:500. The "quats" are devoid of tuberculocidal activity[29].

Their value as antiseptics is limited by the fact that, being cationic compounds, they are neutralized by anionic chemicals such as soap. Nevertheless, their blandness for tissue is a favorable property, and it makes them particularly attractive for vaginal "preps" and other mucous membrane applications.

Chlorine Compounds

Inorganic chlorine is valuable for disinfection of water but it has limited use in hospital disinfection. Yet hypochlorite solutions are still among the best and most convenient germicides for spot disinfection of floors. In the concentration generally employed for this purpose (5000 ppm) they are also tuberculocidal.

They have very little use as antiseptics.

Iodine and Iodophors

Iodine is a good bactericide, but it stains fabrics and tissue. The staining can be reduced and made temporary by complexing iodine with a detergent. Such complexes are known as iodophors, and many of them have been placed on the market as germicides. Some of them are unstable in the presence of hard water, heat and organic soil; yet they are reliable general purpose disinfectants if employed in adequate concentration. Instruments are likely to be corroded.

They are good antiseptics because they are relatively nontoxic and produce rapid degerming. The old problem of iodine burns was the result of careless contact with excessively high concentrations and need not be considered any longer. The germicidal action is due mostly or entirely to the release of free iodine and not to the complex itself[30].

The Alcohols

This subject has been reviewed by the author in some detail[31]. Therefore the present discussion is confined to summary comments. Ethyl and isopropyl alcohol are much more useful as antiseptics than as disinfectants. Disinfectants can act only as long as they are in solution, and this means that the alcohols become ineffectual as soon as they evaporate. Although this property has the advantage of leaving no residue on treated surfaces, it often makes repeated applications desirable in order to get adequate exposure.

Nevertheless, the alcohols are rapidly bactericidal[31] and, in the writer's experience, they are the most active germicides against tubercle bacillus (Table VIII). They can be relied upon to destroy other vegetative bacteria promptly, provided little or no organic soil is present and they have not been diluted too much. Since it is convenient to use a single concentration throughout the hospital, one can select 85% by volume as suitable for general use. Because the alcohols rapidly lose their cidal activity when diluted below 50% concentration (see Table V), solutions should be watched closely with this in mind and discarded at frequent intervals. The alcohols dissolve cement mountings of lensed instruments and they blanch the asphalt tiles of floors. On long exposure they harden and swell plastic tubing, including polyethylene.

Ethyl and isopropyl alcohol are clearly the most effective of all antiseptics[20,21]. The cidal action is very rapid and includes all bacterial forms except spores. Ethyl alcohol has less drying action upon skin than isopropyl which is a better fat solvent, and so the former is the preferred degerming agent for skin. Their antiseptic potencies are about the same.

TABLE VIII
TUBERCULOCIDAL ACTIVITY
Simultaneous Mucin-loop Method*

	Disinfection Times
Phenolic I, 3%	**2 to 3 hours**
Phenolic II, 3%	**45 to 60 minutes**
Iodophor, 450 ppm.	**2 to 3 hours**
Isopropanol, 70% vol.	**5 minutes**

*No. of *Myco. tuberculosis* (H37-Rv) per loop — approximately 10^4.

Formalin

Formalin is a solution of approximately 40% formaldehyde in water. Therefore, 8% formaldehyde is 20% formalin. This strong concentration is a high-level germicide and it can be used as a sterilizing agent provided the contact time is as long as 12 hours. Its activity is further increased for the tubercle bacillus by diluting it in alcohol.

The irritating fumes of formaldehyde limit its usefulness and its toxicity for tissue requires that materials treated with it be thoroughly rinsed before use.

Glutaraldehyde

This chemical relative of formaldehyde is more active than the latter in that a 2% aqueous alkaline concentration (Cidex®) has been reported[32] as being the approximate sporicidal equivalent of 8% formaldehyde in alcohol (Bard-Parker Germicide®). It is a high-level disinfectant, and is tuberculocidal within a few minutes. Glutaraldehyde is the liquid disinfectant of choice for lensed instruments, inhalation therapy apparatus and critical items which should be sterile when used. Contact times of 8 to 10 hours guarantee sterility. The fumes are less irritating than those of formaldehyde.

GASEOUS DISINFECTANTS

Formaldehyde and ethylene oxide (EtO) are very reactive chemicals which become gases at room temperatures. If enough moisture is present (50% relative humidity or higher), strong concentrations are sporicidal. Both gases are, of course, toxic for tissues, and articles exposed to them should be aerated to avoid subsequent irritation upon contact with tissue.

Because of its high-level cidal action, disinfection procedures using EtO are often termed "gas sterilization." For reasons explained earlier in this review, many applications of EtO fail to sterilize. Consequently, the term "gas sterilization" should be restricted to those procedures which pass the A.O.A.C. Sporicidal Test[11].

Formaldehyde

This gas has been employed as a fumigant for many years, usually in the traditional – actually, antiquated – formaldehyde chamber. The bactericidal (and especially the sporicidal) effect is disappointing unless much moisture (70% R.H.) is present. This much moisture tends to corrode metal, and its fumes are, of course, very irritating.

Ethylene Oxide

The general subject of ethylene oxide sterilization was discussed in detail in a recent issue of this journal[33]. This compound has a much more rapid sporicidal action than formaldehyde, and its other properties are such that EtO is widely used commercially for the gas sterilization of prepackaged medical and surgical articles. The EtO sterilization procedures in industry can be correctly called gas sterilization. But it is also important to remember, as noted earlier, that they employ relatively high gas concentrations, exposure times of 16 to 20 hours in a controlled and heated environment containing high relative humidity, and often preceded by a period of preconditioning in a moist environment. These specifications are very different from those of much of the equipment recommended for office and hospital use. It is not at all surprising that so-called ethylene oxide "sterilizers" often fail the A.O.A.C. Sporicidal Test.

Indeed, the procedures being used in hospitals should be examined critically. Those which incorporate a heating coil, produce EtO concentrations of at least 450 milligrams per liter (mg/L) and provide adequate relative humidity, can be depended upon to sterilize if the exposure is long enough. The last-mentioned factor is important, for the time required to guarantee sterility may be several hours longer when spores which have become thoroughly dry (vs. moist ones) are present and the contaminated material has not been preconditioned by exposure to moisture or immersion in water. For example, freshly contaminated filter paper strips carrying about 1×10^5 *Cl. sporogenes* spores in one of our tests were sterilized by a Sterivac® apparatus at 130°C within 45 minutes, but the same type of strips after being allowed to dry 3 weeks were not sterilized in 3 hours. Placing additional moisture in the chamber in the form of wet cotton balls shortened the sterilization time by an hour or so, and a presoak in water for one hour reduced it to the same time as the fresh strip.

There seems to be a lack of general recognition that ethylene oxide is subject to the same factors which are operative for other disinfectants, and that in the case of very dry spores the amount of moisture may be a critical factor. Although EtO disinfection is a very useful tool for preventing hospital infections, it has also been subjected to widespread misuse, primarily because of a compulsive emphasis by manufacturers upon the shortest possible exposure times. As a regrettable consequence, subsequent use of materials so treated constitute a hazard with consequences such as reported by Taguchi *et al.*[34].

Because sterility is guaranteed with some EtO procedures (apparatus) but not with others, one must decide in each instance whether or not sterility is essential. If the answer is yes, one needs a heated apparatus which provides increased moisture and at least 450 mg/L of EtO, and it should be run for the period of time which the manufacturer can document will sterilize paper strips containing about 1 x 10^5 *Cl. sporogenes* spores.

EtO disinfection is also useful for articles which do not have to be sterile but should be free of all contamination except bacterial spores. This can usually be accomplished readily with the small, table-top types of apparatus which are dependent upon the ambient temperature and moisture, provided the manufacturer's directions are followed.

Note is made here, however, of the disturbing reports of nonsporulating bacteria highly resistant to EtO. This subject was dealt with at some length by Kereluk and Lloyd[33].

A major difficulty with the use of EtO is the residual toxicity of materials exposed to it. This gas penetrates solid materials extremely well; it also has a high combining affinity for a variety of substances. Consequently, many types of materials, and rubber articles in particular, are likely to cause tissue irritation, hemolysis of blood, etc., unless they are thoroughly aerated after exposure to the gas[33].

Beta Propiolactone

Beta propiolactone is the most rapidly sporicidal of the three gases, but it has too many detrimental properties to be suitable for hospital disinfection.

FOGGING AND SPRAY DISINFECTION

Fogging

Fogging is the process of filling the air of a room with an aerosol disinfectant sprayed from a centrally located revolving dispenser. The common assumption that such aerosols reach all parts of a fogged room is generally unwarranted, for often many surfaces will have only droplets deposited on them. Unless surfaces are completely covered by a layer of germicidal solution, disinfection will be incomplete. Because fogging is quick and saves labor costs it is an attractive substitute for manual surface disinfection, but the mist which is created has a greater psychological than microbicidal effect. As suggested by McGray *et al.*[35], it should be considered a supplementary procedure to thorough cleansing and surface application of disinfectants. In other words, it is not by itself an adequate method for the terminal disinfection of rooms which have contained infected patients.

Finally, there is reason to be concerned about potential harm to the respirary tissue from inhaling droplets of phenolic disinfectant solutions and other protoplasmic poisons suspended in the air.

Spray Disinfection

This means spot disinfection with an aerosol spray from a pressurized can of disinfectant solution held in the hand. Because it is generally applied close to the area being treated, a complete film can be produced easily and this is the equivalent of the usual hand-wipe method of application. Spraying is a convenient way to get disinfectant into crevices and through ventilation gratings. There is the risk of inhaling germicide here, too.

SELECTION OF DISINFECTANTS

Even though the user may have a good working knowledge of the nature of microbial contamination, the principles of disinfection and the comparative value of available germicides, some practical suggestions may be helpful in selecting the best one for a particular purpose.

1. Determine the level of disinfection required. If the application is the disinfection of a critical item such as transfer forceps, select a high-level solution that is capable of producing sterility if resistant forms happen to be present. When there is a risk of exposure to tubercle bacilli, but not

spores, a good tuberculocide is adequate. Thus it is necessary to consider both the types of microorganisms likely to be present and the nature of the application.

2. There are many proprietary germicidal solutions which have not been subjected to in-use testing. Thus, it seems advisable for users who are unable to get a good bacteriological opinion to choose "brand-name" products which are sold in interstate commerce since these come under federal jurisdiction and have probably been approved as meeting accepted standards.

3. When considering an unfamiliar disinfectant ask for comparative data with a standard germicide of the same type, for example, Zephiran®, if it is a "quat," or Wescodyne if it is an iodophor. Ask a bacteriologist to evaluate the data.

4. Consult Table X (on next page).

ANTISEPSIS*

As pointed out earlier, antisepsis is a special application of chemical disinfection in which the maximum usable concentration of antiseptic is sharply limited by the risk of skin and mucous membrane irritation. Consequently, only low-level and a few intermediate level germicides are applicable; yet some of these bring about a marked reduction in the size of the skin population within a few minutes or even seconds.

The literature on antisepsis is enormous and hexachlorophene has been the most popular antiseptic in recent years. A comprehensive discussion in this review would make it inordinately long. Therefore, the reader is referred to Price's article in a recent issue of this journal[21] for a practical and authoritative treatment of the surgical scrub and preoperative preparation of skin. The material included in the present review is primarily intended to complement the Price article.

The skin cannot be sterilized of its normal flora, but the number of living bacteria can be reduced significantly by scrubbing with soap or detergent, and/or application of antiseptic solution. Normal skin flora consists of the superficial, *transient* bacteria which are acquired casually and removed easily, and the *resident* flora consisting of persisters which live and multiply in the skin at the openings of the hair follicles and sebaceous gland ducts. The graph in Fig. 2 was obtained with the Price serial basin method.

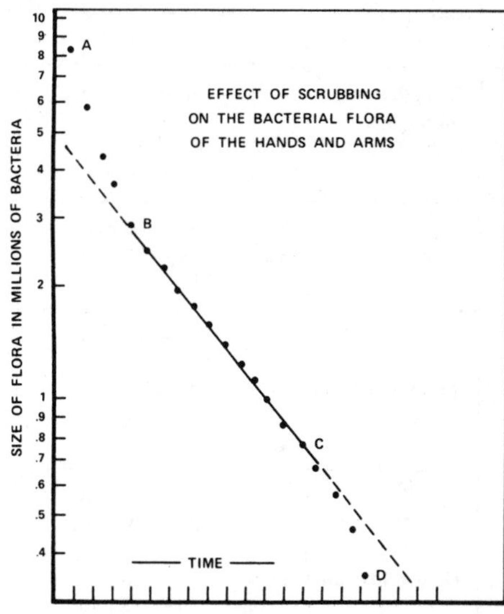

Fig. 2: Graphic indication of the appearance of three divisions of the cutaneous flora – transients, residents, and deep bacteria.

The discovery of hexachlorophene led to the development of the first important germicidal

**Portions of this section are reprinted by permission of the AORN Journal, official publication of the Association of Operating Room Nurses. Figs. 2 to 5 are those of Dr. P. B. Price and they appeared originally in reference 20.*

TABLE IX
RECOMMENDATIONS FOR CHEMICAL DISINFECTION AND STERILIZATION

	Disinfection		Sterilization
Objects	Category A Vegetative bacteria and fungi, influenza viruses.	Category B Category A, plus tubercle bacillus, and enteroviruses.	Categories A & B, plus hepatitis viruses$, bacterial and some fungal spores.
Smooth, hard-surfaced objects	1a – 10 min. 2 – 5 min. 3 – 10 min. 4a – 10 min. 5a – 10 min. 8 – 5 min. 9 – 5 min.	1b – 15 min. 2 – 10 min. 4b – 20 min. 5b – 20 min. 8 – 15 min. 9 – 15 min.	2 – 18 hours 7 – 3 to 12 hours@ 8 – 12 hours 9 – 10 hours
Rubber tubing and catheters#	3 – 10 min. 4a – 10 min. 5a – 5 min.	4b – 20 min. 5b – 20 min. 9 – 15 min.	7 – 3 to 12 hours@
Polyethylene tubing and catheters#	1a – 10 min. 3 – 10 min. 4a – 10 min. 5 – 10 min.	1b – 15 min. 4b – 20 min. 5b – 20 min. 9 – 15 min.	2 – 12 hours 7 – 3 to 12 hours@ 8 – 12 hours 9 – 10 hours
Lensed instruments	3 – 10 min. 4a – 10 min. 5a – 10 min.	8 – 15 min. 9 – 15 min.	7 – 3 to 12 hours@ 8 – 12 hours 9 – 10 hours
Thermometers ‡	1c – 10 min.	1c – 15 min.	2 – 12 hours 7 – 3 to 12 hours@ (cold cycle only) 8 – 12 hours 9 – 10 hours
Hinged instruments %	1a – 15 min. 2 – 10 min. 3 – 20 min. 4a – 20 min. 5a – 15 min. 8 – 10 min. 9 – 10 min.	1b – 20 min. 2 – 15 min. 4b – 30 min. 5b – 30 min. 8 – 20 min. 9 – 20 min.	7 – 3 to 12 hours@ 8 – 12 hours 9 – 10 hours
Inhalation and anesthesia equipment	1a – 15 min. 3 – 20 min. 9 – 5 min.	1b – 20 min. 9 – 20 min.	7 – 3 to 12 hours@ 9 – 10 hours
Floors, furniture, walls, etc.	3 4a 5a 6a	4b 5b 6b	None

See next page for key to agents appearing in Table.

KEY TO AGENTS APPEARING IN TABLE IX ON PREVIOUS PAGE

1a. Ethyl or isopropyl alcohol* (70-90%)
1b. Ethyl alcohol (70-90%)
1c. 1a. + 0.2% iodine
2. Formaldehyde (8%) + alcohol (70%) solution*
3. Quaternary ammonium solutions* (1:500 aq.)
4a. Iodophor – 100 ppm available iodine*
4b. Iodophor – 500 ppm available iodine*
5a. Phenolic solutions (1% aq.)*
5b. Phenolic solutions (2% aq.)*
6a. Sodium hypochlorite, 2000 ppm
6b. Sodium hypochlorite (1%)
7. Ethylene oxide gas
8. Aqueous formalin (20%)
9. Activated glutaraldehyde (2% aq.)

*** 0.2% sodium nitrite should be present in alcohols, formalin, formaldehyde-alcohol, quaternary ammonium, and iodophor solutions to prevent corrosion; and 0.5% sodium bicarbonate should be present in phenolic solutions to prevent corrosion.**

$ Very little direct observation has been possible.

 # Be certain tubing is completely filled.

‡ Thermometers must be thoroughly wiped, preferably with soap and water, before disinfection or sterilization. Alcohol-iodine solutions will remove markings on poor-grade thermometers.

@ Depending upon procedure used, more rapidly cidal for category A and B microorganisms.

% Must first be cleansed grossly free of organic salt.

(G. F. Mallison, U.S.P.H.S. National Center for Disease Control, contributed substantially to the format and detail of this table.)

soap, made possible by two important properties of this chemical. First is retention of germicidal activity in the presence of soap, whereas most germicides are cationic and neutralized by anionic substances such as soap. This is the case with "quats." Secondly, hexachlorophene is insoluble in water; thus its continual use results in an accumulative deposit on the skin which only very slowly washes off with water. Its bactericidal action is due to that amount of hexachlorophene which dissolves in the fatty acids of the skin. After several days of continual use the skin flora may be reduced significantly and kept at a low level by repeated applications.

On the other hand, the rate with which hexachlorophene kills is slow (Fig. 3 [see next page]). Ivory soap has the same effect as a single scrub with hexachlorophene, therefore, hexachlorophene has no virtue for emergency preps[20]. With continuous use, a Gram-negative replacement flora may develop.

Hexachlorophene is completely and immediately soluble in alcohol. Thus the usual hexachlorophene scrub regimen omits alcohol. This is unfortunate because Price has shown repeatedly that alcohol is the most effective degerming agent for skin[20,21]. Also see Fig. 4 (on next page).

The great value of alcohol as a skin degerming agent is beautifully illustrated in Fig. 5 (page 29). The steepness of the slope of the lines indicates the degree of killing (degerming) produced. Note that the alcohol-acetone base alone is more active than the tincture of merthiolate containing the same base. In other words, the degerming action of alcohol (the active component in the tincture base) was actually *reduced* by the addition of the mercurial compound. Note also that this alcohol base was more effective than the aqueous Zephiran®, but also observe the effect

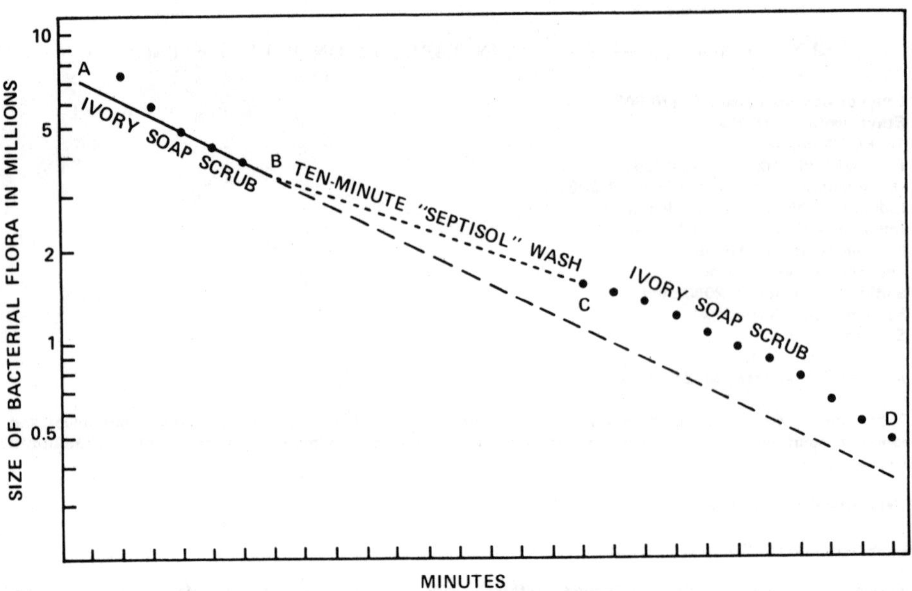

Fig. 3: Absence of immediate degerming effect of 2% hexachlorophene liquid soap; in fact, less action than an equal scrub with an ordinary soap.

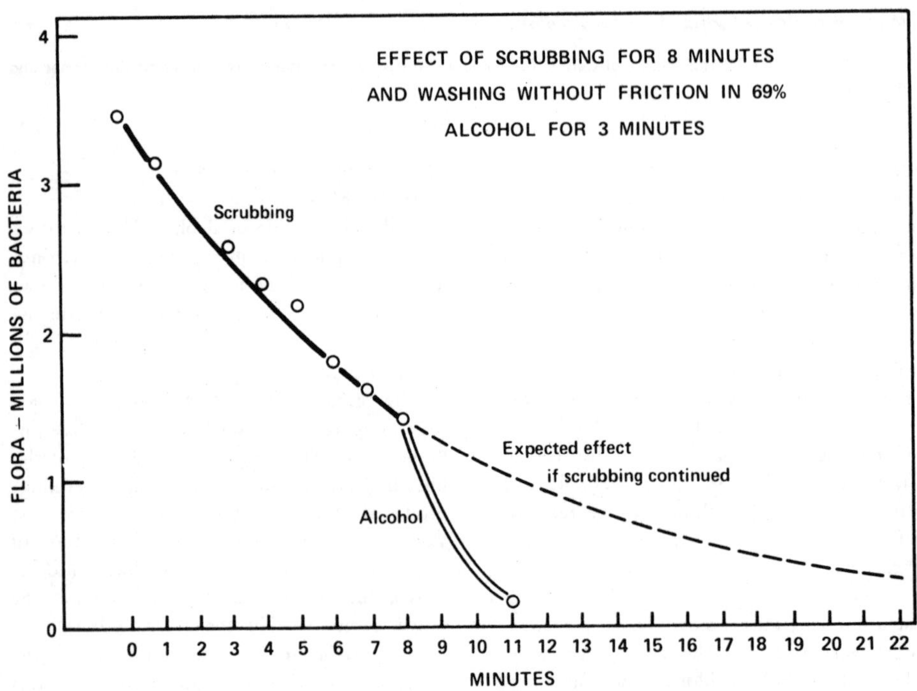

Fig. 4: Degerming effects of scrubbing followed by an alcohol wash.

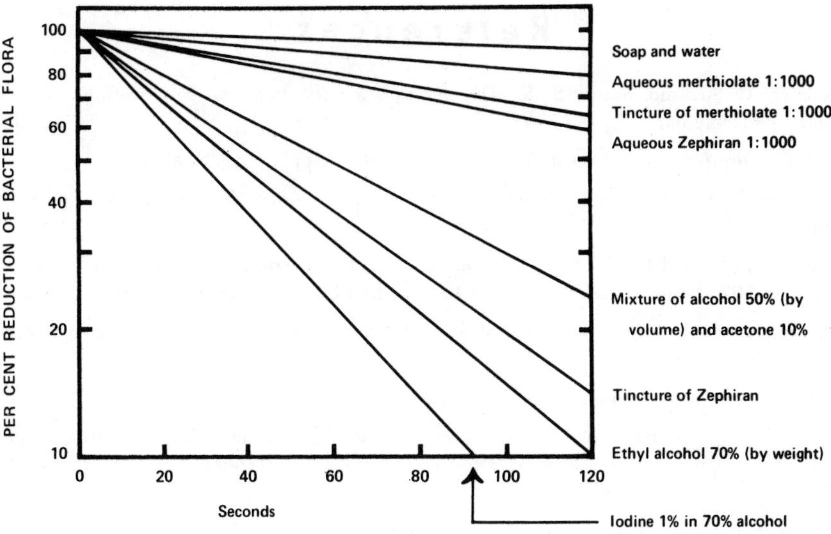

Fig. 5: Comparative effects when hands and arms are washed in various antiseptic solutions, including iodine.

of dissolving Zephiran® in the alcohol-acetone base (Tincture of Zephiran®) instead of water. Other significant information shown here indicates the superiority of 70% alcohol by weight (about 80% by volume) over the pharmaceutical 50-10% base, and also the added activity achieved by adding 1% iodine to 70% alcohol.

Therefore one is entitled to question the wisdom of abandoning entirely this highly efficient antiseptic. In fact, a good standard procedure for hand-arm scrub is Ivory soap and isopropyl alcohol wash, a procedure recommended by Price[36]. The drying effect of alcohol can be reduced by the incorporation of the emollient cetyl alcohol in 0.5% final concentration[37]. At least one manufacturer* recommends dilution of its hexachlorophene in alcohol in order to combine the rapid degerming action of alcohol with the continuous bacteriostasis produced by residual hexachlorophene left on the skin after the alcohol has evaporated. This makes sense, and would deserve wide adoption if it were not for the recent disturbing reports of central nervous system toxicity (in rats) caused by hexachlorophene absorbed through the skin[38].

From the bacteriological viewpoint it is a reasonable step to combine hexachlorophene with alcohol. The usual scrub procedure (Price recommends 7 minutes) may be carried out with plain or hexachlorophene soap, followed by a water rinse and then a wash in a hexachlorophene-isopropanol-cetyl alcohol solution[37] which leaves a hexachlorophene-cetyl alcohol residue on the skin. Continual use of a hexachlorophene soap outside the operating room is also indicated.

The results in Fig. 5 also suggest that the best antiseptic for preoperative preparation of the skin is alcohol and iodine. This does not preclude prior washes with a hexachlorophene soap or, for that matter, any one of a number of different antiseptics. The one essential step is the application of alcohol rubbed in with gauze and allowed to evaporate.

Vestal Laboratories, Div. of W. R. Grace & Co.

References

[1] Lawrence, C. A., and Block, S. S.: *Disinfection, Sterilization and Preservation,* 1968, Lea & Febiger, Philadelphia.

[2] Sykes, G.: *Disinfection and Sterilization,* 2nd ed., 1965, Lippincott, Philadelphia.

[3] Spaulding, E. H.: Chemical Disinfection in the Hospital, *Jour. Hosp. Research, 3* (No. 1):5-25, 1965.

[4] Brachman, P. S., and Eickhoff, T. F.: *Proceedings of the International Conference on Nosocomial Infections,* 1971, Amer. Hospital Assoc., 840 Lake Shore Drive, Chicago, Ill., 60611, pp. 247-254.

[5] Spaulding, E. H.: Principles of Microbiology as Applied to Operating Room Nursing, *AORN Jour., 1*:49-57, 1963.

[6] Knight, Vernon: Instruments and Infection, *Hospital Practice, 2*:82-95, 1967.

[7] Bassett, D. C. J., Stokes, K. J., and Thomas, W. R. G.: Wound Infections with *Pseudomonas multivorans:* A Water-borne Contamination of Disinfectant Solutions, *The Lancet, 2*:1188-1191, 1970.

[8] Rhoades, E.R., *et al.*: Contamination of Ultrasonic Nebulization Equipment with Gram-negative Bacteria, *Arch. Intern. Med., 127*:228-232, 1971.

[9] Klein, M., and Deforest, Adamadia: Antiviral Action of Germicides, *Soap and Chemical Specialties, 39*:70-72, 95-97, 1963.

[10] Spaulding, E. H.: Chemical Sterilization of Surgical Instruments, *Surg., Gynec. & Obstet., 69*:738-744, 1939.

[11] Ortenzio, L. F.: Collaborative Study of Improved Sporicidal Test, *Journ. Assoc. Official Analytical Chemists, 49*:721-726, 1966.

[12] Spaulding, E.H.: Unpublished data.

[13] Morton, H. E.: The Relationship of Concentration and Germicidal Efficiency of Ethyl Alcohol, *Ann. N.Y. Acad. Sc., 53*:191-196, 1950.

[14] Stuart, L. S.: How Effective are Chemical Germicides in Maintaining Hospital Asepsis?, *Hospitals, 33*:46-47, 59, 62, 66, 1959 (May 16).

[15] Kundsin, R. B., and Walter, C. W.: In-use Testing of Bactericidal Agents in Hospitals, *Applied Microb., 9*:167-171, 1961.

[16] Adams, R., and Fahlman, B.: Prevention of Infections in the Operating Room, *Trans. Amer. Acad. Ophth. & Otolaryng, 65:*16-32, 1961.

[17] Vesley, D., *et al.*: A Cooperative Microbiological Evaluation of Floor-cleaning Procedures in Hospital Patient Rooms: A Committee Report. *Health Lab. Science, 1*:256-264, 1970.

[18] Edmondson, E. B., and Sanford, J. P.: Simple Methods of Bacteriologic Sampling of Nebulization Equipment, *Amer. Rev. Resp. Dis., 94*:450-453, 1966.

[19] Pierce, A. K., *et al.*: Long-term Evaluation of Decontamination of Inhalation-Therapy Equipment and the Occurrence of Necrotizing Pneumonia, *New Eng. Jour. Med., 282*:528-531, 1970.

[20] Price, P. B.: Skin Antisepsis, *Becton Dickinson Lectures on Sterilization,* 1957-1959, pp. 79-98. Becton, Dickinson and Company, Rutherford, New Jersey.

[21] Price, P. B.: Surgical Scrubs and Preoperative Skin Disinfection, *Jour. Hosp. Research, 5* (No. 1):7-19, 1967.

[22] Dineen, Peter: The Use of a Polyurethane Sponge in Surgical Scrubbing, *Surg., Gynec. & Obstet., 123*:595-598, 1966.

[23] Kahn, G.: Depigmentation Caused by Phenolic Detergent Germicides, *Arch. Dermat., 102*:177-187, 1970.

[24] Kundsin, R. B., and Walter, C. W.: Investigations on Adsorption of Benzalkonium Chloride USP by Skin, Gloves and Sponges, *Hospital Topics, 36*:108-113, 1958.

[25] Myers, G. E., and Lefebvre, C.: Antibacterial Activity of Benzalkonium Chloride in the Presence of Cotton and Nylon Fibers, *Canad. Pharmaceut. Jour., 94*:55-57, 1961.

[26] Plotkin, S. A., and Austrian, R.: Bacteremia Caused by Pseudomonas sp. Following the Use of Materials Stores in Solutions of a Cationic Surface-active Agent, *Amer. Jour. Med. Sc., 235*:621-627, 1958.

[27] Lee, J. C., and Fialkow, P. J.: Benzalkonium Chloride – Source of Hospital Infection with Gram-negative Bacteria, *Jour. Amer. Med. Assoc., 177*:708-710, 1961.

[28] Babcock, K. B.: Maintaining Standards and Quality Care in the Operating Room, *OR Nursing, 2*:44-86, 1961.

[29] Hirsch, J. G.: The Resistance of Tubercle Bacilli to the Bactericidal Action of Benzalkonium Chloride (Zephiran), *Amer. Rev. Tuberc., 70*:312-319, 1954.

[30] Blatt, Ronald, and Maloney, J. V.: An Evaluation of the Iodophor Compounds as Surgical Germicides, *Surg., Gynec. & Obstet., 113*:699-704, 1961.

[31] Spaulding, E. H.: Alcohol as a Surgical Disinfectant, *AORN Journal, 2* (No. 5):67-71, 1964.

[32] Stonehill, A. A., Krop, S., and Boric, P. M.: Buffered Glutaraldehyde, a New Chemical Sterilizing Solution, *Amer. Jour. Hosp. Pharmacy, 20*:458-465, 1963.

[33] Kereluk, Karl, and Lloyd, R. S.: Ethylene Oxide Sterilization, *Jour. Hosp. Research, 7* (No. 1):5-75, 1969.

[34] Taguchi, J. T., Edmonds, P., and Harmon, G. A.: Serious Limitations of a Portable Ethylene Oxide Sterilizer, *Amer. Jour. Med. Sc., 245*:299-304, 1963.

[35] McGray, R. J., Dineen, P., and Kitske, E. D.: Disinfectant Fogging Techniques, *Soap and Sanitary Chemicals, 40*:75-78, 112-114, 1964.

[36] Price, P.B.: Hand Scrubs and Skin Preparations, *Hosp. Topics, 38*:61-68, 1960.

[37] Blank, I. H., *et al.*: A Study of the Surgical Scrub, *Surg., Gynec. & Obstet., 91*:577-584, 1950.

[38] Wade, Nicholas: Hexachlorophene: FDA Temporizes on Brain-damaging Chemical, *Science, 174*:805-807, 1971 (Nov. 19).

Reprinted from *Brit. Med. J.* **2**, 442–445 (1966)

26 Cleaning and Disinfection of Hospital Floors

G. A. J. AYLIFFE,* M.D., M.C.PATH. ; B. J. COLLINS,* A.I.M.L.T. ; E. J. L. LOWBURY,* D.M., F.C.PATH.

Hospital floors become contaminated by settlement of airborne bacteria, by contact with shoes, trolley wheels, and other solid objects, and occasionally by the spilling of urine, pus, sputum, and other fluids. Pathogens commonly present on the floor include *Staphylococcus aureus* dispersed by patients and staff, and (in much smaller numbers) Gram-negative rods, such as *Pseudomonas aeruginosa.* Spores of *Clostridium tetani* and gas-gangrene bacilli are also present on floors, probably deposited in larger numbers from shoes and trolley wheels than by deposition from the air. Some of the bacteria lie loosely in dust, while others are ingrained into the surface and between cracks.

The removal of this reservoir is one of the normal aims in the control of hospital infection. Dispersal of bacteria into the air has been greatly reduced through the replacement of brooms by vacuum cleaners in wards (Rogers, 1951 ; Bate, 1961 ; Babb, Lilley, and Lowbury, 1963), but vacuum cleaners and also oiled mops do not remove a large proportion of the bacteria from floors (Babb *et al.,* 1963). Scrubbing and disinfection might be expected to have a larger effect, and useful results of disinfection are reported by Foster (1960). Finegold, Sweeney, Gaylor, Brady, and Miller (1962) and Vesley and Michaelsen (1964), on the other hand, have reported no significant difference in the reduction of bacterial counts on floors washed with detergents or with disinfectants.

We describe here a comparison of alternative methods of disinfecting and cleaning ward floors. The prompt recontamination of disinfected areas, and the consequent need to cover test areas during assessments of disinfection, became apparent during the study.

Materials and Methods

Disinfectants

A selection of agents commonly recommended for surface disinfection was investigated. The concentration chosen was 1/100 of concentrate or 1% w/v for most of the disinfectants, but the concentration recommended by the manufacturers was used if this was markedly different.

Aqueous solutions of the following compounds were studied :

1. Phenolic compounds: Sudol 1/100, Hycolin 1/100, Izal 1/100 and 1/160.
2. Chloroxylenol: Dettol 1/100 and 1/40.
3. Quaternary ammonium compounds: Benzalkonium chloride (Roccal) 0.1%, Cetrimide *B.P.* 0.1%.
4. Ampholytic compound: Tego M.H.G. 1/100.
5. Combination of tri-*n*-butyltin, a quaternary ammonium compound (alkyl dimethylchlorobenzyl ammonium chloride) and isopropyl alcohol: Micro Gard with Trimicrotin 1/100.
6. A mixture containing a non-ionic detergent and a quaternary ammonium compound (alkyl dimethylbenzyl ammonium chloride): Shield 1/40.
7. Chlorhexidine (Hibitane) 1/500 and 1/5,000.
8. Iodophors: Idokyl and Wescodyne 1/100 and 1/160.
9. Chlorine compounds: Domestos 1/100 and 1/160 ; chlorine cleaning powders, Diversol BX 1% and Septonite 1%.
10. Ethyl alcohol 70%.

* M.R.C. Hospital Infection Research Laboratory, Summerfield Hospital, Birmingham.

Laboratory Tests

A bactericidal test was used for a preliminary study of t disinfectants. The test organisms were strains of *Staph. aure* and *Ps. aeruginosa* isolated from clinical sources. In the te 0.5 ml. of an 18-hour broth culture of the test organism w added to 4.5 ml. of disinfectant solution at room temperatu Three standard loopfuls were transferred to an agar pla and one loopful to 2 ml. of nutrient broth at intervals 1, 2½, 5, and 10 minutes. The inoculated plates and bro were incubated at 37° C. for 24 hours, and the broths were th subcultured on to agar plates which were incubated at 37° (for 24 hours. The minimum time of exposure after whi no growth was obtained on the agar plate or in the tub of broth was recorded. The tests were repeated with 20 serum added to the disinfectant solutions before addition the organisms. Egg-yolk Tween 80 agar plates, and egg-yo Tween 80 broth (Morris and Darlow, 1959), were used f sampling quaternary ammonium and Tego compound Sodium thiosulphate 0.5% was added to the nutrient bro for sampling iodine and chlorine compounds. To exclu the possibility of carry-over of a bacteriostatic amount disinfectant, tubes of broth showing no growth were inoculate with one drop of a suspension of *Staph. aureus* (approximate 10 organisms) and examined for growth after 18 hours' incub tion at 37° C.

Surface Disinfection Tests

The effect of cleaning a contaminated glass plate and similarly contaminated floor covered with polyvinyl tiles wi a disinfectant or a detergent was investigated. A glass pla 32 by 22 in. (81 by 56 cm.) was divided into 15 square Six randomly selected squares were inoculated with five standar loopfuls of a suspension of organisms in horse serum (5×1 orgs./ml.). Three of these squares were inoculated wi *Staph. aureus,* and the other three squares with *Ps. aerugino* (the same strains as in the last experiment). After drying f one hour one square inoculated with *Staph. aureus,* and anothe with *Ps. aeruginosa,* were sampled with moistened throat swab A pad of cotton-wool (approximately 2 by 2 by 1 in. (5 by by 2.5 cm.) was immersed in disinfectant or detergent, exce fluid was drained off, and the whole surface of the glass plat was thoroughly cleaned with the pad. After drying the oth four contaminated squares were sampled by rubbing over t surface of each with a throat swab moistened with a solutio containing lecithin, Lubrol, and sodium thiosulphate (Lowbu and Lilly, 1960). The swabs were inoculated on to nutrie agar or egg Tween 80 agar and incubated at 37° for 48 hour Similar tests were also made on a floor covered with polyvin tiles.

Ward Study

Sampling Techniques

Floors were sampled with agar impression plates (Foste 1960 ; Babb *et al.,* 1963), each plate covering an area 9.6 sq. in. (62 sq. cm.). Phenolphthalein diphosphate wa added to the agar to obtain presumptive counts of *Staph. aure* (Barber and Kuper, 1951) ; egg yolk and Tween 80 we ded to plates for tests with Tego and quaternary ammonium mpounds. Counts of total organisms and presumptive *ıph. aureus* were made after 24 hours' incubation at 37° C. ests for carry-over of disinfectant were also made by adding ops of a suspension of *Staph. aureus* (approximately 10 ganisms/drop) to impression plates which showed little or growth after sampling a treated floor ; there was no hibition of growth from these inocula.

loor-cleansing

The experiments were performed in a 28-bedded male surgical ard with a terrazzo floor.

Experiment 1.—The ward floor was swept with a broom d mopped with soap and water or disinfectant solution ward cleaners at 7 a.m. according to the usual routine. easured quantities of neat disinfectant were supplied to the eaners in bottles and added to a bucket of hot water to give e required concentration. The floors were sampled one hour ıd nine hours after mopping. Six impression plates were sed for each test, and tests were repeated daily with each isinfectant for three or five days. Tests were made with soap ıd water, Shield, Tego M.H.G., and Sudol.

Experiment 2.—In Experiment I the high total bacterial ounts obtained one hour after cleaning with a disinfectant ıggested either heavy recontamination or ineffective disinfec-on. To solve this problem the following tests were made. our impression plates were taken from an area of floor, hich was then mopped with soap and water or disinfectant y the ward-cleaner. The mop and bucket were rinsed in the olution before use and a fresh solution was used for the floor eatment. A cardboard box (15 by 9 by 9 in. ; 38 by 23 by 3 cm.) open on one side was placed on the treated floor ith the open side downwards to prevent recontamination. fter one hour two impression-plate samples were taken from ıe area covered by the box, and two plates were also taken om an adjacent treated but uncovered area. Two settle plates ere exposed on top of the box during the test period. Tests ere made with soap and water and 10 disinfectants.

Experiment 3.—Further tests were made with the use of the ox to compare the effectiveness of soap and water, Tego, Micro Gard, Hycolin, and Sudol. Mops were used for all ests except the one in which a Cimex Eagle combined scrubbing nd vacuum-drying machine was used with a detergent. Six npression plates were taken from a selected area of floor, hich was then treated as in Experiment 2, and the open ardboard box was inverted over part of the treated floor. fter one hour six impression plates were taken from the area overed by the box. Two tests were performed with each leaning agent in the experiments with mops, and one test with ıe scrubbing-and-drying machine.

Results

acterical Tests

Table I shows the minimum exposure time required to kill single strain each of *Staph. aureus* and *Ps. aeruginosa* with nd without the addition of 20% serum to the disinfectant. he results indicate that in these tests most of the disinfectants ere effective against both organisms in the absence of organic atter. Sudol, Izal, and 0.2% chlorhexidine were effective gainst both organisms in one minute in the presence of 20% erum. Shield was slightly less effective against *Staph. aureus* ı the presence of serum, and the other quaternary ammonium ompounds were less effective against *Ps. aeruginosa* in the resence of serum. Tego and the chlorine compounds were ess effective against *Staph. aureus* than against *Ps. aeruginosa*. The iodophors, the chlorine compounds, Tego, and to a less extent Hycolin showed reduced activity in the presence of serum. An unexpected finding was the greater activity of Dettol against *Ps. aeruginosa* than against *Staph. aureus* ; preliminary tests with another chloroxylenol preparation (D.C.M.X.) had shown that this had poor activity against *Ps. aeruginosa*. Activity of Dettol against both organisms was reduced in the presence of serum. Chlorhexidine at a dilution of 0.02% was less effective against either organism than most of the other disinfectants tested.

TABLE I.—*Time in Minutes Taken to Kill Strains of Staph. aureus and Ps. aeruginosa in Solutions of Disinfectants*

Disinfectant	*Staph. aureus*		*Ps. aeruginosa*	
	No Serum	20% Serum	No Serum	20% Serum
Phenolic compounds:				
Sudol 1/100	1	1	1	1
Izal 1/100	1	1	1	1
Hycolin 1/100 ..	1	2½	1	5
Chloroxylenol:				
Dettol 1/100	5	> 10	1	> 10
Dettol 1/40	2½	10	1	5
Chlorhexidine:				
Hibitane 0·2% ..	1	1	1	1
Hibitane 0·02% ..	5	> 10	5	> 10
Quaternary ammonium compounds:				
Benzalkonium chloride (Roccal) 0·1% ..	1	1	1	10
Cetrimide *B.P.* 0·1%	1	1	1	10
Tri-*n*-butyltin + quaternary ammonium compounds:				
Micro Gard 1/100 ..	1	1	2½	> 10
Quaternary ammonium compound + detergent:				
Shield 1/40	1	2½	1	1
Ampholytic compound:				
Tego 1/100	10	> 10	1	> 10
Iodophors:				
Idokyl 1/100	1	> 10	2½	> 10
Wescodyne 1/100 ..	1	> 10	5	> 10
Chlorine compounds:				
Domestos 1/100 ..	2½	> 10	1	> 10
Diversol BX 1% ..	> 10	> 10	2½	> 10
Septonite 1% ..	> 10	> 10	2½	> 10

Surface Disinfection Tests

Ps. aeruginosa was not isolated from the glass plate after cleaning with any of the disinfectants or with a non-ionic detergent alone. Sudol 1/100, Izal 1/100, Hycolin 1/100, Dettol 1/40, Roccal 0.1%, cetrimide 0.1%, Micro Gard 1/100, Shield 1/40, Tego 1/100, Domestos 1/100, Idokyl 1/100, ethyl alcohol 70%, chlorhexidine 0.2%, and Diversol BX 1% were all effective against *Staph. aureus*, and no growth was obtained from the plate after treatment with these disinfectants. *Staph. aureus* was still isolated in large numbers from all squares following the use of 0.02% chlorhexidine and of a non-ionic detergent. Similar results were obtained with polyvinyl tiles as with the glass plate. The results indicate that cleaning with detergent alone, followed by drying, was sufficient to kill or remove *Ps. aeruginosa*, and that similar treatment with all but one of the disinfectants, even if their activity is reduced by serum, was also effective against *Staph. aureus*. Cleaning with detergent alone was not sufficient to remove or kill *Staph. aureus* present in dried serum.

Ward Tests

The results obtained from Experiment 1 are shown in Table II. The total counts of impression plates taken one hour

TABLE II.—*Mean Bacterial Counts on Impression Plates from Ward Floors*

Treatment	1 hour After Cleaning			9 hours After Cleaning		
	Total	*Staph. aureus*	No. of Plates	Total	*Staph. aureus*	No. of Plates
Soap and water	423	4·6	30	661	9·1	30
Shield 1/40 ..	470	7·7	30	532	20·2	30
Tego 1/100 ..	921	17	18	644	3·6	18
Sudol 1/100 ..	859	2·7	18	863	4·5	18

after cleaning were very high, and indicate rapid and heavy recontamination. With Sudol the mean total counts at nine hours were the same as at one hour ; they were slightly higher with soap and water and with Shield, and lower with Tego. When recontamination was prevented by protecting an area of floor with a box, as in Experiment 2, a considerable reduction in total bacterial counts and a reduction in the numbers of *Staph. aureus* was found one hour after all methods of cleaning. Table III shows a reduction of 89.7% in bacterial counts with soap and water, and reduction of 93.7 to 99.9% following the use of disinfectants. The counts of samples taken from a treated area outside the box were much higher, indicating recontamination and an absence of continuing disinfection after drying. The counts from the uncovered area were variable, and lower than those obtained in Experiment 1, as the tests in Experiment 2 were performed at a time of less ward activity. Settle plates exposed on the box during the test (one hour) showed an average of 59 colonies/plate.

TABLE III.—*Effects of Cleaning and Disinfection on Exposed and Covered Areas of Ward Floor*

Treatment	Mean Bacterial Counts						% Reduction (Total Organisms) After Treatment: Covered Areas
	Before Treatment		After Treatment				
			Floor Exposed		Floor Covered		
	Total	*Staph. aureus*	Total	*Staph. aureus*	Total	*Staph. aureus*	
Sudol 1/100 ..	190	4·5	75	0	2·5	0	98·7
Izal 1/160 ..	945	4·5	179	3	9	0·5	99·1
Dettol 1/40 ..	445	1·2	144	1	5·5	0	98·8
Hycolin 1/100 ..	261	2·8	221	2·5	16·5	0·5	93·7
Micro Gard 1/100	788	24	261	0·5	1	0	99·9
Shield 1/40 ..	210	0·3	142	1	2·5	0	98·8
Tego 1/100 ..	400	0	684	0	24	0	94
Idokyl 1/160 ..	267	0	79	0	6	0	97·8
Domestos 1/160	162	2·5	120	6	5	0	96·9
Diversol BX 1%	830	8·5	243	2·5	18·5	0·5	97·8
Soap and water..	397	13	460	3	41	0	89·7

The results of Experiment 3 are shown in Table IV. They confirm with a larger series of observations the results obtained in Experiment 2 with soap and water, Sudol, Micro Gard, Hycolin, and Tego. A significant reduction in the mean of total organisms was obtained after cleaning the floor with soap and water ($t=9.16$, $P<0.001$). The mean bacterial counts obtained after using disinfectants were significantly lower than those obtained with soap and water (Sudol: $t=10.7$, $P<0.001$; Micro Gard: $t=11.6$, $P<0.001$; Hycolin: $t=8.6$, $P<0.001$; Tego: $t=8.3$, $P<0.001$).

The mean bacterial counts from the floor after cleaning with Sudol and with Micro Gard were significantly lower than that obtained with Tego (Sudol: $t=3.6$, $P<0.01$; Micro Gard: $t=4.8$, $P<0.001$).

In the experiment with a Cimex Eagle combined scrubbing and vacuum-drying machine the mean reduction by use of detergent was 80.7% (approximately the same as that obtained with a mop and soap and water).

Discussion

The bacteria in an area of terrazzo hospital-ward floor protected from recontamination were greatly reduced in numbers after each of the methods of cleaning and disinfection tested. In contrast with the 40–50% reduction in floor bacteria obtained by using dry methods (a vacuum cleaner or oi mops) (Babb *et al.*, 1963), washing with soap and water a detergent, either with a mop or with a combined scrubbi and vacuum-drying machine, caused a reduction of about 80 and much larger effects were obtained with disinfectants. T most active agents tested caused a reduction of over 99 and all the disinfectants included in our study had an app ciably greater effect than soap and water. The value disinfectants in removing bacteria from a floor corresponded most cases with their performance in killing *Staph. aureus* tube tests and on a glass plate—for example, Sudol and Mi Gard were highly active, and the halogens (hypochlorite a iodophor solutions), which are rapidly inactivated by orga matter, were less effective in both laboratory and field tes Hycolin and Tego had an intermediate position in laborato tests, but were the least successful in field tests. Thou *Staph. aureus* was present in the laboratory test after f minutes' exposure to Tego, exposures of one, two and a ha and five minutes showed a considerable reduction in th numbers.

Organic tin compounds have been claimed to exert continuing antibacterial action after use, as a result of wh surfaces can be kept relatively free from contamination (Huds Sanger, and Sproul, 1959). The claim was not supported studies by Finegold *et al.* (1962), or Kingston and Noble (196 or in our studies, which showed as much recontamination unprotected areas of floor treated with Micro Gard as unprotected areas treated with other disinfectants or with so

The benefit of removing bacteria from ward floors is larg annulled by the rapid recontamination of these surfaces. T has also been shown by Vesley and Michaelsen (1964), thou the rate of recontamination in their experiment was less th in the present study. Because of the apparent failure disinfectants to disinfect, some authorities hold that it probably not worth while using them for the cleaning of flo except when there is severe contamination (Report, 1965). B since the level of bacteria in any environment is determined a balance of accretion and elimination, the use of disinfecta must have some value, even if it is not apparent in places whe the rate of recontamination is high ; this condition obvious occurs in certain wards, especially during and after cleani rounds, when there is maximum activity and movement of be

Our results emphasize the need to prevent recontaminati of floors from the air, and from contact with shoes and oth objects. Oiling of bedclothes was shown by van den Ende a Spooner (1941) to reduce the dispersal of bacteria. With change from woollen to boilable cotton blankets, and the intr duction of vacuum cleaners in wards, the practice of oili blankets and floors was quietly abandoned. Experience on t value of dust-laying in preventing cross-infection has vari (Wright, Cruickshank, and Gunn, 1944 ; Clarke, Dalgleis Parry, and Gillespie, 1954). A reassessment of methods whi prevent the dispersal of bacteria from bedclothes, includi cotton cellular blankets, would be useful. Other sources m be still more important, especially the dispersal of epithel scales (Davies and Noble, 1962) ; a more widespread use antiseptic soaps by staff and patients might be expected reduce this source of contamination.

There is uncertainty about the role of floor bacteria as source of hospital infection, but it is rational, when practicab to prevent the establishment of reservoirs of pathogenic bacte

TABLE IV.—*Effects of Cleaning and Disinfection on Covered Areas of Ward Floor : Mean Bacterial Counts*

Treatment	Before Treatment			1 hour After Treatment, Floor Covered			% Reducti Total Organism
	Total	*Staph. aureus*	No. of Plates	Total	*Staph. aureus*	No. of Plates	
Soap and water	699·8 ± 60·4	1·7	12	137 ± 10·7	1·4	12	80·4
Sudol 1/100	1,242 ± 144·1	1·7	12	12·6 ± 4·3	0	12	99·0
Hycolin 1/100	364·2 ± 34·9	7·4	12	21·6 ± 6·5	0·3	12	94·1
Micro Gard 1/100 with Trimicrotin ..	905·7 ± 136·0	22·6	12	8·5 ± 2·6	0·17	12	99·0
Tego 1/100	880·8 ± 121·0	10·1	12	37·5 ± 5·4	3·1	12	95·7

nd to remove such reservoirs. The majority of disinfectants tested at the chosen concentration appeared to be highly effective n this respect. The tests were carried out by using one concentration of disinfectant on terrazzo flooring in one ward, and t is possible that different results might be obtained under other conditions. In the selection of a disinfectant for floor treatment its activity against the range of pathogens in the reservoir, its safety, acceptability in use, aesthetic results, and cost must be considered ; the type of flooring is also relevant, because materials used for flooring may be damaged by some compounds. Some disinfectants which were highly active against *Staph. aureus* but less active against *Ps. aeruginosa* in laboratory tests were effective in field tests, and our experiments suggest that *Ps. aeruginosa* could be successfully removed from surfaces by cleaning with these agents ; as a result of their high death rate on drying, these organisms, when present in floor dust, are very scanty and are probably further depleted by the evaporation of solutions used for disinfecting the floor. Chlorine compounds, though better than soap and water, were less effective than the best of the disinfectants. Phenolic compounds varied in their effectiveness ; the best of these, however, showed highly satisfactory results both in laboratory and in field tests.

Toxicity will also affect the choice of a disinfectant ; many phenolic compounds—for example, Lysol and to a less extent Sudol—and tri-*n*-butyltin compounds may be corrosive, particularly in high concentration, and should be handled with care.

In testing the effectiveness of a new method of disinfection it is perhaps reasonable to require that it shall reduce the total floor bacteria on areas protected from recontamination by about 95–99%, or to fewer than 15 bacterial colonies and less than one colony of *Staph. aureus* per impression plate.

Summary

After preliminary assessments of bactericidal action by 14 disinfectants, the ability of selected agents to remove bacteria from hospital-ward floors was studied and compared. The disinfectants included phenolic, quaternary ammonium, and ampholytic compounds, a tri-*n*-butyltin compound, a chloroxylenol, chlorhexidine, iodophors, chlorine compounds and cleaning powders, and 70% ethyl alcohol.

Impression-plate samples showed little or no reduction in total bacteria or in *Staph. aureus* on exposed floors after washing or disinfection ; but when an area of floor was protected from recontamination by inverting an open box over the area, large reductions in total bacterial counts were found, and *Staph. aureus* was reduced or eliminated after such treatment. Soap and water caused a mean reduction of 80% and disinfectants caused a mean reduction of 93–99% in bacterial counts on areas protected from recontamination. These effects were highly significant, as were the differences between detergent washing and disinfection ; significant differences between certain disinfectants were also found. All of these treatments caused a much larger reduction in bacteria than had been found in earlier studies with dry methods (vacuum cleaners and oiled mops).

Since the benefits of disinfection are frustrated by recontamination, it is necessary also to reduce the access of bacteria by air and by contact if floors are to be kept bacteriologically clean.

We wish to thank Miss Sandra Louis and Mr. M. Wilkins for technical assistance, the Matron and Domestic Supervisor of Dudley Road Hospital for their co-operation, and the manufacturers for supplies of disinfectants.

References

Babb, J. R., Lilly, H. A., and Lowbury, E. J. L. (1963). *J. Hyg. (Lond.)*, **61**, 393.
Barber, M., and Kuper, S. W. A. (1951). *J. Path. Bact.*, **63**, 65.
Bate, J. G. (1961). *Lancet*, **1**, 159.
Clarke, S. K. R., Dalgleish, P. G., Parry, E. W., and Gillespie, W. A. (1954). Ibid., **2**, 211.
Davies, R. R., and Noble, W. C. (1962). Ibid., **2**, 1295.
Finegold, S. M., Sweeney, E. E., Gaylor, D. W., Brady, D., and Miller, L. G. (1962). *Antimicrobial Agents and Chemotherapy*, p. 250.
Foster, W. D. (1960). *Lancet*, **1**, 670.
Hudson, P. B., Sanger, G., and Sproul, E. E. (1959). *J. Amer. med. Ass.*, **169**, 1549.
Kingston, D., and Noble, W. C. (1964). *J. Hyg. (Lond.)*, **62**, 519.
Lowbury, E. J. L., and Lilly, H. A. (1960). *Brit. med. J.*, **1**, 1445.
Morris, E. J., and Darlow, H. M. (1959). *J. appl. Bact.*, **22**, 64.
Report: Public Health Laboratory Service Committee on Testing and Evaluation of Disinfectants (1965). *Brit. med. J.*, **1**, 408.
Rogers, K. B. (1951). *J. Hyg. (Lond.)*, **49**, 497.
van den Ende, M., and Spooner, E. T. C. (1941). *Lancet*, **1**, 751.
Vesley, D., and Michaelsen, G. S. (1964). *Hlth Lab. Sci.*, **1**, 107.
Wright, Joyce, Cruickshank, R., and Gunn, W. (1944). *Brit. med. J.*, **1**, 611.

Reprinted from *Brit. Med. J.* **2**, 531–536 (1964)

Methods for Disinfection of Hands and Operation Sites

27

E. J. L. LOWBURY,* D.M. ; H. A. LILLY,* F.I.M.L.T. ; J. P. BULL,* M.D.

In previous studies we compared the relative value of alternative methods for disinfecting the hands of nurses and surgeons and the skin of operation sites, but a number of relevant questions were not considered. For disinfection of the operation site alcoholic solutions of chlorhexidine (0.5%) and iodine (1%) were found to be equally effective and superior to a number of other agents (Lowbury, Lilly, and Bull, 1960), but we did not include laurolinium acetate, which was later reported by Verdon (1961) to be more effective than nine other antiseptic preparations, including 1% iodine in alcohol ; nor did we examine the removal of spore-bearing organisms. In studies on the disinfection of hands we confirmed the cumulative effect of repeated use of hexachlorophane detergent preparations, obtaining the best results with a liquid soap, and found some alternative methods which had comparable effects in reducing the hand flora and in preventing the emergence of bacteria through holes in rubber gloves (Lowbury and Lilly, 1960 ; Lowbury, Lilly, and Bull, 1963) ; we also assessed the value of ablution and disinfection in removal of transient flora (Lowbury, Lilly, and Bull, 1964). We did not examine the effects of varying the time of disinfection, of repeated treatments with antiseptics other than hexachlorophane, of varying the medium in which the antiseptic was mixed and the method by which it was applied.

Experiments to fill some of these gaps are described below. In the light of these and previous experiments the choice of methods of skin disinfection suitable for various purposes in hospital and elsewhere are discussed.

Comparison of Laurolinium with Other Methods for Disinfection of Operation or Injection Sites

In the following experiment we compared the effectiveness of three preparations of laurolinium acetate (4-aminoquinaldinium-1-lauryl acetate monohydrate), of an iodophor (povidoneiodine), and of 0.5% alcoholic chlorhexidine digluconate in the removal of bacteria from the skin.

Materials and Methods

Antiseptic Preparations.—The following preparations were tested: (1) providone-iodine (" betadine ") antiseptic solution ; (2) chlorhexidine (" hibitane ") digluconate, 0.5%, in 70% ethyl alcohol ; (3) laurolinium acetate (" laurodine "), 5%, in 70 ethyl alcohol ; (4) 5% aqueous laurolinium acetate solution (5) laurolinium skin spray, an aerosol dispersed from a pressu pack containing laurolinium acetate (5% w/v) in industri spirit (50 g.) with propellants (50 g.) ; and (6) contr treatment: no antiseptic preparation.

Application of Antiseptics.—Preparations 1, 2, 3, and 4 we applied with a gauze swab to the whole surface of both hand and reapplied when necessary so that the skin was kept moi for approximately two minutes. In using laurolinium ski spray the whole surface of both hands was sprayed with t aerosol and kept moist for two minutes by repeated spraying.

Testing the Antiseptic Preparations.—The effectivenss of ski disinfection was assessed by a method described in detail els where (Lowbury *et al.*, 1960). Viable counts of bacteria we obtained from standard hand-washings taken before and aga after the application of the antiseptic. A Latin-square desig was used for the experiment, each of the five preparations an a control treatment (rinsing briefly under a tap) being tested c each of six subjects ; the six replicate testings were made c one day in alternate weeks to allow the skin flora to return t its normal level between tests. Both sampling fluid (Ringer solution) and culture medium (pour-plates of nutrient aga contained neutralizers—" lubrol W " (1%), lecithin (0.5% " tween 80 " (1%), and sodium thiosulphate (1%)—and tes were made in each experiment for transfer of inhibitory amoun of antiseptic. The effect of treatment was assessed by a com parison of viable bacterial counts from the first and secon samplings ; the bacterial counts were made after 48 hour incubation of the pour-plates at 37° C.

Results

The reduction in bacterial counts of hand-washings take after various forms of treatment expressed as a percentage c the initial (pretreatment) counts is shown in Table I, an analysis of variance in the experiment is shown in Table I There was a marginally significant variance due to differenc

* From the Medical Research Council Industrial Injuries and Burns Research Unit, Birmingham Accident Hospital.

TABLE II.—*Disinfection of Operation Site : Analysis of Variance*

	Sum of Squares	Degrees of Freedom	Mean Square	Significance
Experiments	1,640	5	328	P < 0·05 > 0·01
Persons	1,852	5	370	P < 0·05 > 0·01
Treatment ..	25,555	5	5,111	P < 0·001
Residual	2,373	20	119	

TABLE I.—*Disinfection of Operation Site : Reduction in Bacterial Counts from Hand-washings Expressed as Percentage of Initial Count*

	Replicate Experiments, Each on One Day						Totals	Mean % Reduction
	1	2	3	4	5	6		
Povidone-iodine	J.L. 44·1	R.J. 83·8	J.D. 74·0	B.C. 59·0	M.K. 52·0	J.O. 61·0	373·9	62·3
Chlorhexidine (0·5%) in 70% alcohol	M.K. 82·4	J.L. 81·1	B.C. 82·2	J.D. 88·6	J.O. 86·2	R.J. 89·2	509·7	84·9
Laurolinium (5%) in 70% alcohol ..	R.J. 82·6	B.C. 84·9	J.O. 86·9	J.L. 86·9	J.D. 88·9	M.K. 76·3	506·5	84·4
Laurolinium (5%) in water	B.C. 88·1	M.K. 86·4	R.J. 80·2	J.O. 72·5	J.L. 80·6	J.D. 79·4	487·2	81·2
Laurolinium spray	J.D. 76·7	J.O. 73·7	M.K. 44·1	R.J. 49·5	B.C. 34·1	J.L. 71·3	349·4	58·2
Control	J.O. 24·6	J.D. 50·0	J.L. −0·4	M.K. −10·3	R.J. −2·1	B.C. −10·5	51·3	8·5
Total	398·5	459·9	367·0	346·2	339·7	366·7		

Initials indicate experimental subjects.

:tween days and individuals, apparently caused by the large duction in bacterial counts after the control treatment in one ıbject (J. D.). In the comparison between different methods treatment, chlorhexidine in alcohol, laurolinium in alcohol, ıd aqueous laurolinium were not significantly different from ch other, but all were significantly better than povidone-dine, laurolinium spray, and control treatment. Povidone-dine and laurolinium spray were not significantly different om each other in their skin-disinfecting action, but both were gnificantly better than the control treatment.

The mean reduction of skin flora by alcoholic chlorhexidine this study (84.9%) was similar to that (81.3%) found in our revious study (Lowbury *et al.*, 1960) ; the mean reduction by coholic laurolinium was in the same range (84.4%), and queous laurolinium was found to be approximately as effective alcoholic laurolinium (mean reduction of skin flora=81.2%).

Disinfection by Alcoholic Chlorhexidine after Repeated Ablutions with Hexachlorophane Detergent Cream

Repeated ablution with hexachlorophane detergent cream or ap has been shown to cause a large progressive reduction in in flora, but appreciable numbers of bacteria can usually be olated from hand-washings even after two or three days' con-stent use of such agents—for example, Lowbury *et al.* (1963). pre-operative preparation with alcoholic chlorhexidine or urolinium were shown to have as great a proportionate effect n skin treated repeatedly with hexachlorophane as on untreated in, it should be possible to reduce the resident flora to a egligible level. The following experiment was made.

Materials and Methods.—Nine subjects were provided with exachlorophane detergent cream ("phisohex"), with which ıey washed their hands in a standard manner for two minutes, ur times on each of two successive days and once on the third ay. Before and after the first ablution and again after the inth ablution bacteriological samples were taken from the ands by a standard hand-washing technique in a bowl of sterile inger's solution containing neutralizers, from which pour-late cultures were inoculated (see Lowbury *et al.*, 1963). After ıe third sampling the skin of both hands was disinfected, as or an operation, by application of chlorhexidine gluconate .5%) in 70% alcohol on a gauze swab, the skin being kept ıoist with the antiseptic for two minutes. It was then allowed dry, and a further bacteriological sample was taken. Tests or transfer of inhibitory concentrations of antiseptic to rinsing uids and to culture plates were made by duplicate inoculation f a culture of *Staphylococcus aureus* on these media and on ontrol media.

Results.—The individual and the mean percentage survival f bacteria after these forms of treatment are summarized in Table III. As in previous studies, the immediate effect of one pplication of the hexachlorophane preparation was negligible, ut repeated use led to a large fall in bacterial counts. The further mean reduction in skin flora after the additional treatment with alcoholic chlorhexidine (96.5%) was no less than that obtained by disinfecting unprepared skin with chlorhexidine in alcohol (see Table I): from four of the nine subjects in the experiment no bacteria were found in 10-ml. amounts of bacteriological hand-washings taken after the last treatment.

TABLE III.—*Effect of Repeated Disinfection of Hands with Hexachlorophane Detergent Cream Followed by Treatment with Alcoholic Chlorhexidine Solution*

Subject	Percentage Survival of Skin Flora after		
	(1.) One Ablution with Phisohex	(2.) 9 Ablutions with Phisohex	(3.) No. 2 followed by 2 Minutes' Treatment with Alcoholic Chlorhexidine
A.J.	92·4	0·29	0·063
M.W.	47·6	0·05	0
H.L.	65·0	0·81	0·030
J.O.	79·2	0·40	0·013
M.S.	70·4	0·03	0
A.K.	45·2	0·85	0·005
V.B.	21·2	0·18	0
G.B.	36·3	0·69	0
M.F.	86·1	0·31	0·015
Mean	60·4	0·40	0·014
S.D. mean	8·9	0·101	0·007

Effect of Varying Time of Exposure to Skin Antiseptics

Material and Methods.—Tests were made with the following agents: (1) chlorhexidine gluconate (0.5%) in 70% alcohol (replicate tests on eight subjects) ; (2) chlorhexidine diacetate (0.5%) in water (replicate tests on eight subjects) ; (3) laurolinium (5%) in 70% alcohol ; and (4) laurolinium (5%) in water (replicate tests on two subjects). Both hands were disinfected by rinsing in 100 ml. of antiseptic solution ; a standard procedure was used, including a constant number of strokes with palm to palm, palm over dorsum, and with fingers interlaced. After 30 seconds, 60 seconds, 90 seconds, and 120 seconds of this disinfecting procedure the bacterial flora of the hands was sampled by a standard hand-washing technique (Lowbury *et al.*, 1963) in Ringer's solution containing neutralizers ; after each sampling the hands were rinsed under running water. Pour-plates were prepared from the hand-washings (with nutrient agar containing neutralizers), and viable counts were made after 42 hours' incubation at 37°C. Tests for carry-over of antiseptics to sampling fluid and to culture medium were made. In the tests with preparation 3 there was considerable inhibition of growth by transfer of antiseptic to culture medium, and no further study was made with this material.

Results.—The results of tests with preparations 1 and 2 are shown in Table IV. In most of the tests the major part of the skin disinfection had been attained after 30 seconds' treatment, but longer treatment removed more organisms. Alcoholic chlorhexidine showed slightly but not significantly less activity than aqueous chlorhexidine in 30 seconds, but after longer intervals results were approximately the same with both agents, and none of the observed differences was significant. In a more limited experiment aqueous laurolinium showed slightly less activity than the chlorhexidine solutions at 30 seconds and at 2 minutes. An unexpected finding was the larger reduction in skin flora when the antiseptic solution was applied by the standard rinsing method than when it was applied, as on an operation site, with a gauze swab (see Lowbury *et al.*, 1960, and above), or than when it was applied in a timed but unstandardized rinse (see Table VI).

TABLE IV.—*Period of Disinfection and Removal of Skin Flora*

Treatment	Sub-jects	Mean Percentage Reduction in Bacterial Counts of Hand Washings after Disinfection for			
		30 Seconds	60 Seconds	90 Seconds	120 Seconds
Alcoholic chlorhexidine (0·5%)	8	84·8 ± 12·3	95·1 ± 6·5	97·8 ± 1·9	99·0 ± 1·4
Aqueous chlorhexidine (0·5%)	8	90·0 ± 7·2	94·0 ± 5·3	95·7 ± 3·9	98·2 ± 10·4

Comparison of Antiseptic Rinses and Creams

In previous experiments (Lowbury *et al.*, 1963) we found that two antiseptics, chlorhexidine and "hycolin," were ineffective in removing resident organisms when applied repeatedly in a cream to the dry skin ; experiments made with hycolin liquid soap showed that this caused a significant reduction in skin flora. A further comparison of cream and aqueous solution as vehicles for antiseptics was therefore made.

Materials and Methods.—The following preparations were studied: (1) chlorhexidine (1%) hand cream ; (2) a solution of chlorhexidine diacetate (0.5%) in water ; (3) a cream containing hexachlorophane (0.5%) ; (4) a cream containing no antiseptic ; and (5) control treatment—no antiseptic. In using the creams the hands were washed with ordinary bar soap and water, and dried on a sterile towel. A small amount (about 1 in. (2.5 cm.) from a tube) of the cream was rubbed thoroughly into the whole surface of both hands until they felt comfortably dry. Chlorhexidine solution was used for a 30-second rinsing (free style) of both hands, followed by rinsing under a tap and drying on a sterile towel. Before each treatment and also in the controls the hands were washed briefly with ordinary bar soap and water. A Latin-square design was used for the experiment, five subjects receiving each treatment. In each of the five replicates of the experiment the subjects' hands were washed and sampled in the manner described elsewhere (Lowbury *et al.*, 1963) for viable counts of skin flora on a Monday ; on Tuesday and again on Wednesday the hands were treated six times with the selected preparation ; on Thursday a second sampling for viable skin flora was made. Experiments were made in alternate weeks to allow a restoration of normal skin flora between tests on the same individuals.

Results.—Table V shows the mean viable counts of bacteria from hand-washings and the analysis of variance of log counts in the experiment. The repeated rinses with chlorhexidine were very significantly effective, but the creams containing chlorhexidine and hexachlorophane were not significantly more effective than the control cream or the untreated control.

TABLE V.—*Effect of Vehicle on Skin Disinfection by Chlorhexidine and Hexachlorophane (Viable Count of Bacteria from 0.1 ml. of Hand-washings)*

	Day	Preparations Used for Hand Treatment				
		Chlor-hexidine Cream	Hexa-chlorophane Cream	Chlor-hexidine Rinse	Control Cream	Control
Mean counts of 5 experiments	1	163	154	475	183	195
	4	164	129	5	271	319

Analysis of Variance (Log Counts)

	Degrees of Freedom	Sum of Squares	Mean Squares	Significance
Experiment ..	4	1·1815	0·2954	NS
Person ..	4	0·7433	0·1858	,,
Treatment ..	4	18·3569	4·5892	Significant
Residual ..	12	2·2988	0·1916	

Continued Action of Antiseptics after Ablution

A hexachlorophane detergent ablution has been shown to have little immediate effect, but when rubber gloves are worn for an hour after a single ablution with such an agent the skin flora is shown to be considerably reduced (Lowbury *et al.*, 1963). This effect has been attributed to the persistence of residues of the slow-acting antiseptic on the skin (Fahlberg, Swan, and Seastone, 1948).

The following experiment was made to determine whether povidone-iodine, which has a similar cumulative skin-disinfecting action to that of hexachlorophane (Lowbury *et al.*, 1963), owes this property to the continued action by residues of the antiseptic left on the skin after ablution.

Method.—The viable counts of bacteria on the hands of six subjects were assessed by the method described previously (Lowbury *et al.*, 1963) (*a*) before treatment, (*b*) immediately after a standard two minutes' hand-wash with povidone-iodine and water, and (*c*) (in a separate experiment) after wearing rubber gloves for one hour after the ablution with povidone-iodine.

Result.—The mean percentage reduction in bacterial counts of skin samples immediately after the treatment with povidone-iodine was 74.3% ; after wearing gloves for one hour following treatment with povidone-iodine, the mean percentage reduction in bacterial counts compared with those obtained before treatment was 80.3%. No important further action by povidone-iodine on skin flora after the ablution could therefore [be] detected.

Effect of Single and of Repeated Rinses with Chlorhexidine Solution

To test the possibility of cumulative or progressive sk[in] disinfection by repeated rinses with chlorhexidine solution [we] made the following experiment.

Materials and Methods.—Four subjects were chosen for [the] experiment. After a quick " social " hand-wash the hands w[ere] sampled by a standard hand-washing test for viable counts [of] bacteria. The hands were then rinsed in an aqueous soluti[on] of chlorhexidine diacetate for 30 seconds ("free style " rinsin[g]) and sampled again for viable counts of bacteria. In the ne[xt] two days the four subjects rinsed their hands 12 times (six tim[es] a day) in the same manner with chlorhexidine solution. [On] the morning after the last chlorhexidine rinse a third series [of] samples for viable counts was taken from the hands of the fo[ur] subjects.

Results.—The percentage reduction of bacterial counts in t[his] experiment is shown in Table VI. There was a large varian[ce]

TABLE VI.—*Effect of Repeated Rinsing of Hands with Aqueous Chl[or]hexidine Solution*

Subject	Percentage Survival of Skin Flora (i.e., Viable Count[s] of Washings after Treatment as % Viable Counts befor[e] Treatment)	
	After First Rinse with Chlorhexidine	After 12th Rinse with Chlorhexidine
P.K.	5·2	1·7
K.P.	66·1	0·75
A.J.	32·1	4·0
B.D.	18·5	0·47
Mean	30·5 ± 13·1	1·73 ± 0·08

in the residual flora after one treatment, but a consistent lar[ge] further reduction in the mean viable counts of hand-washin[gs] to less than 2% of the initial mean counts after a series [of] treatments with chlorhexidine solution.

Effect of Repeated Rinsing on Activity of Chlorhexidine Solution

To assess the possible depletion of antiseptic activity fro[m] bowls of chlorhexidine solution used by nurses for hand-rinsi[ng] we made the following experiment.

Method.—A bowl containing 2 litres of 0.5% aqueous chlo[r]hexidine diacetate solution was used for rinsing the hands [of] laboratory staff. Before rinsing in the antiseptic solution t[he] hands were washed with soap and water and rinsed under [a] running tap, but not dried. The minimal inhibitory concentr[a]tion of the rinsing water was tested with a strain of *Stap[h.] aureus* before use, after 15 rinses, and again after 30 rinses.

Result.—The rinsing fluid became turbid, but there was n[o] reduction in its activity. No bacterial growth was obtained o[n] subculture of the fluid to a large volume of medium containi[ng] neutralizers.

Removal of Bacterial Spores from the Skin of Operation Sit[es]

Because of their resistance to most antiseptics, the spores [of] *Clostridium tetani* and other sporing pathogens are usual[ly] considered insusceptible to skin disinfection, and reliance [is] placed entirely on physical ablution with soap or detergent an[d] water. Iodine is more active against spores than other ant[i]septics used for skin disinfection, but in the form of a tinctu[re] or an aqueous solution with potassium iodide it is too irritant [to] left moist on the skin for more than a very short period ; the complexes of iodine with solubilizers, known as iodophors -for example, povidone-iodine—iodine retains its bactericidal ɑd sporicidal activity, but does not stain the skin, and is aimed to be free from sensitizing or irritant properties Gershenfeld, 1957, 1962 ; Joress, 1962 ; Davis, 1962).

The following experiments were made to determine how uch sporicidal action could be obtained by the application of ovidone-iodine to the skin.

Sporicidal Action of Povidone-iodine Applied to the Skin

Materials and Methods.—A strain of *Bacillus subtilis* var. *obigii* (BSG 63/1) was grown in nutrient broth at 37° C. fter overnight incubation the culture was washed and resusended in sterile distilled water, and heated at 56° C. for one our. Examination of a stained film of the suspension showed ores in 70 to 80% of the bacilli. Viable counts of suspension eated at 56° C. for one hour and at 80° C. for 10 minutes were pproximately the same. On measured circular areas of the skin the forearm of volunteers, 0.02 ml. (1 drop) of the suspension *B. subtilis* var. *globigii* was inoculated with a calibrated ropping-pipette and spread over the whole area with a wire oop. When dry these areas were covered with compresses of nt soaked and kept moist with povidone-iodine antiseptic olution for periods of 15, 30, 60, 90, and 120 minutes. Control eas of skin were covered with compresses soaked and kept wet ith distilled water. From these areas samples were taken for iable counts by rubbing in a standard way for 15 seconds with glass spreader under 5 ml. of sterile Ringer's solution conaining neutralizers (including sodium thiosulphate), the soluon being kept in place by a truncated glass cylinder (Story, 952 ; Lowbury *et al.*, 1960).

Results.—Povidone-iodine compresses were found to reduce e numbers of viable sporing bacilli on the skin by 99.85% in 0 minutes (Table VII) ; the absence of any such reduction after pplication of water compresses showed that this effect was due most entirely to the action of the antiseptic, not to mechanical moval by the compress.

ABLE VII.—*Removal of B. subtilis var. globigii Spores from Skin by Povidone-iodine (P.V.I.)*

Minutes of Exposure to P.V.I. or Control Compresses	Viable Counts of *B. subtilis* in Washings from Skin as % Counts of Initial Washings taken when no Compress had been Applied					
	Experiment 1		Experiment 2		Experiment 3	Experiment 4
	P.V.I.	Control	P.V.I.	Control	(P.V.I.)	(P.V.I.)
15	0·26	30	1·13	68	0·60	1·56
30	0·15	40	0·47	76	0·47	2·17
60	0·05	—	0·32	—	0·33	1·17
90	0·06	—	0·21	—	0·15	0·42
120	0·05	—	0·02	—	0·13	0·14

Comparison of Sporicidal Action by Povidone-iodine on B. Subtilis Var. Globigii and on Cl. Welchii

To assess the probable usefulness of povidone-iodine in emoving a pathogenic sporing organism we compared the urvival of *B. subtilis* var. *globigii*, our test organism in the tudy on skin disinfection, with a sporing culture of *Cl. welchii* 53/2).

Materials and Methods.—A broth culture of *B. subtilis* var. *lobigii* and a sporing culture of *Cl. welchii*, produced by rowing a strain of the organism in Ellner's (1956) medium, were washed and resuspended in distilled water. On microcopical examination, approximately 70 to 80% of the *B. ubtilis* var. *globigii* and 80% of the *Cl. welchii* cells contained pores. Viable counts of the suspensions were made by the method of Miles, Misra, and Irwin (1938) on the untreated uspensions, and on mixtures of 0.1 ml. of the bacterial suspenion with 5 ml. of povidone-iodine antiseptic solution which had been allowed to stand, after mixing, for periods from 5 to 150 minutes.

Results.—Table VIII shows that the spores of *Cl. welchii* were at least as sensitive to the killing action of the iodophor as those of *B. subtilis* var. *globigii*. Neither strain showed any evidence of a sporicidal effect after five minutes' exposure to the antiseptic, but after 15 minutes the counts of both organisms were reduced to less than 0.1%.

TABLE VIII.—*Survival of Spores of Cl. welchii and of B. subtilis var. globigii in Presence of Povidone-iodine*

Time of Exposure (Minutes)	Viable Counts per ml. of Spore Suspensions after Exposure to Povidone-iodine	
	Cl. welchii	*B. subtilis* var. *globigii*
0	4,800,000	3,600,000
5	3,800,000	3,700,000
15	1,000	3,100
30	57	2,200
60	38	480
90	29	23
120	18	5
150	0	3

Discussion

The experiments described above are relevant both to surgeons' and nurses' hands and to the patient's operation site. In the comparison of alternative methods for disinfecting the operation site, for example, it was shown that alcoholic chlorhexidine, alcoholic laurolinium, and aqueous laurolinium were of approximately equal value, but a laurolinium spray was less effective. This confirmed the view that rubbing an antiseptic on to the skin enhances its value (cf. Price, 1957). The same conclusion is suggested by the finding that chlorhexidine in alcohol applied on a swab (see Table I ; also Lowbury *et al.*, 1960) caused a smaller reduction of the skin flora than rinsing the hands with a standard procedure of rubbing palm to palm, palm over dorsum, and with fingers interlaced (see Table IV). The precise technique of rinsing also appears to affect the results, as shown in the greater reduction of skin flora by aqueous chlorhexidine solution when the hands were rinsed for 30 seconds in a standard manner described above than when they were rinsed for the same time but in a random manner (see Table VI).

Practical periods of disinfection vary with clinical circumstances ; for example, periods of disinfection shorter than two minutes are usual before injection or venepuncture, and our study on the relation of disinfecting-time to removal of skin flora showed that treatment with alcoholic chlorhexidine or laurolinium for 30 seconds was slightly less effective than for two minutes. The difference between the effects of treatment in shorter or longer periods of application was smaller with aqueous chlorhexidine, which had almost as good an effect at 30 seconds as it had at two minutes. In an earlier experiment the effect of three successive two-minute rinses with 70% alcohol was studied (Lowbury *et al.*, 1960) ; the second rinse caused an appreciable further reduction in hand flora, but the third treatment caused little or no reduction beyond that reached in the second rinse. It would seem from these studies that all the accessible organisms are removed in a fairly short period of disinfection. The cumulative effects of repeated disinfection at longer intervals with hexachlorophane soap or chlorhexidine rinses, or (still better) with a combination of these methods, suggests that some of the resident organisms which are inaccessible immediately after skin disinfection become accessible to antiseptics after a while, and before the flora has had a chance to proliferate to its previous level.

The cumulative action of povidone-iodine surgical scrub (Lowbury *et al.*, 1963) and of rinsing with chlorhexidine (as described above) shows that this is not a peculiar property of hexachlorophane, and in the former examples it is not dependent on the attachment of antiseptic to the skin (with action continuing after the hands are rinsed and dried). The peculiar ature of hexachlorophane is a slow disinfecting action ; rinsing the hands in alcohol or in an alcoholic solution of chlorhexidine immediately after ablution—for example, to achieve the maximum disinfecting action described above—would remove the hexachlorophane before it had a chance to exert any disinfecting action, and its *regular* use in this way would invalidate the use of hexachlorophane ; but the same objection cannot be raised against repeated use of alcoholic solutions after the use of providone-iodine or chlorhexidine solution, since these agents achieve their full disinfecting action at the time of application.

Spores of *Cl. tetani, Cl. welchii,* and other pathogens are relatively insensitive to most antiseptics, and reliance is usually placed on repeated ablution with detergents to remove these transient organisms from operation sites. This is difficult to achieve in horny skin with much ingrained dirt. Of the antiseptics used for skin disinfection, iodine has a fairly good sporicidal effect *in vitro,* but its action is too slow to be of much use in the routine two minutes' pre-operative skin disinfection, and longer application of the tincture or of Lugol's solution is irritant and potentially toxic. The iodophors, however, can be applied for long periods, leaving no stain and apparently causing no irritation. Our tests showed that the application of an iodophor (povidone-iodine) to skin contaminated with a suspension of *B. subtilis* var. *globigii* spores led to the removal by disinfectant action of a large proportion of these organisms.

In these studies we have distinguished resident from transient organisms as those which are more difficult to remove by ablution or disinfection. *Staph. aureus* sometimes answers to this description. Hare and Ridley (1958) have shown that *Staph. aureus* can multiply on the skin of the perineal area, but it is uncertain to what extent this can occur on the hands. Colonization of the skin by *Staph. aureus* is surprising in the light of experiments which showed that these organisms are killed by unsaturated fatty acids of the skin (Ricketts, Squire, and Topley, 1951). It is possible that individuals vary in respect of the amount of unsaturated fatty acid produced by the skin, or in the presence of factors that inactivate this self-disinfecting mehanism ; these variations may be associated with differences in the ability of the skin to become colonized by *Staph. aureus.*

Choice of Methods

From the studies reported here and in our previous papers it is possible to draw some tentative conclusions about the types of skin disinfection appropriate for different purposes.

1. *Operation Sites.*—When it is necessary to obtain maximum skin disinfection in a single application, as before an emergency operation, chlorhexidine (0.5%), iodine (1%), or laurolinium (5%) in 70% ethyl alcohol applied for two minutes have about the same activity ; laurolinium has rather a high toxic action on skin cells in tissue culture (J. C. Lawrence, personal communication, 1963) and iodine is known to cause sensitization in some individuals, so alcoholic chlorhexidine is probably a good choice. For shorter periods of disinfection—for example, 30 seconds—aqueous chlorhexidine diacetate (0.5%) seems at least as good as the alcoholic solution. Antiseptics should be rubbed in with gauze, not sprayed on.

In "cold" surgery, and particularly when a very high degree of asepsis is required, the cumulative effect of antiseptics applied repeatedly over a period of two to three days is desirable—for example, ablution with hexachlorophane liquid soap or povidone-iodine surgical scrub, three or four times a day for two days—followed by a full pre-operative disinfection with alcoholic chlorhexidine. When the skin contains ingrained soil or road dirt, a compress of povidone-iodine antiseptic solution can be expected to kill a large proportion of the spores of tetanus and gas-gangrene bacilli ; repeated ablution, followed by the application of a compress of povidone-iodine for abo 30 minutes is a desirable procedure in the removal of spor from the skin of such patients when operation can be delaye for two or three days.

Before injection or venepuncture 70% alcohol is general considered acceptable, but a better disinfection can probab be obtained with chlorhexidine or laurolinium solutions (eith alcoholic or aqueous) ; since the time of disinfection is unlike to exceed 30 seconds, an aqueous solution is possibly better tha an alcoholic solution.

2. *Hands.*—The resident flora of surgeons' and nurses' han can be maintained at a low level by repeated use—for examp six times a day—of a liquid soap or a detergent cream contai ing hexacholorophane, or with povidone-iodine surgical scru Regular rinsing with aqueous chlorhexidine solution has similar cumulative effect.

Where the control of cross-infection with Gram-negati bacilli is important—for example, in infants' wards during ou breaks of gastroenteritis, or in burns wards—an antiseptic th is active against these organisms is recommended—for examp rinsing with chlorhexidine solution—but the removal desquamated epithelium by thorough physical ablution is pro ably the most important part of the discipline for removal such transient organisms as pseudomonas, escherichia, ar salmonella.

Summary

In a comparison of five methods for disinfecting the operatic site, approximately the same reduction in resident skin flo (81–85%) was obtained by two minutes' application of chlo hexidine digluconate (0.5%) in 70% alcohol, and of aqueous alcoholic solutions of laurolinium acetate (5%). Treating t skin for two minutes with an aerosol of laurolinum acetate with povidone-iodine antiseptic solution was less effective.

Hands which had been cleared of a large proportion of t skin flora by repeated washing with a hexachlorophane dete gent cream showed a further mean reduction of 96.5% aft two minutes' application of alcoholic chlorhexidine (0.5% after this double treatment four out of nine subjects showed detectable bacteria in washings of the skin, and the me estimated reduction in skin flora was 99.98%.

A comparison of different times for rinsing the hands wi antiseptics showed nearly as large a reduction of flora after seconds' as after two minutes' treatment.

Antiseptic rinsing with a standard number of strokes to cov all surfaces of the hands was more effective than a free-sty method of rinsing.

The application of creams containing hexachloropha (0.5%) and chlorhexidine (1%) repeatedly to the dry hands d not lead to any reduction of the skin flora.

Repeated rinses with aqueous chlorhexidine diacetate solutic (0.5%) caused a progressive reduction in the skin flora ; t mean percentage of surviving bacteria on the skin after a sing rinse was 30.5% but after 12 rinses it was 1.73%.

In contrast with hexachlorophane preparations, which ha no immediate effect but act slowly on the skin after the han have been dried, povidone-iodine was shown to have virtual all its disinfecting action at the time of application.

Sporing bacilli (*B. subtilis* var. *globigii*) were removed fro the skin by a compress of povidone-iodine antiseptic solutior when the compress was kept moist for 15 minutes a me reduction of 99.1% of sporing bacilli was obtained.

The choice of antiseptic preparations for disinfection hands and operation or injection sites is discussed.

We are grateful to Mr. M. D. Wilkins for valuable technic assistance ; to the staff of the M.R.C. Unit for their co-operatior

Berk Pharmaceuticals Ltd. for supplies of povidone-iodine ; and Messrs. Allen & Hanburys for supplies of laurolinium acetate.

REFERENCES

is, J. G. (1962). *J. appl. Bact.*, **25**, 195.
er, P. D. (1956). *J. Bact.*, **71**, 495.
lberg, W. J., Swan, J. C., and Seastone, C. V. (1948). Ibid., **56**, 323.
shenfeld, L. (1957). *Amer. J. Surg.*, **94**, 938.
– (1962). *Amer. J. Pharm.*, **134**, 78.
c, R., and Ridley, M. (1958). *Brit. med. J.*, **1**, 69.
Joress, S. M. (1962). *Ann. Surg.*, **155**, 296.
Lowbury, E. J. L., and Lilly, H. A. (1960). *Brit. med. J.*, **1**, 1445.
—— —— and Bull, J. P. (1960). Ibid., **2**, 1039.
—— —— —— (1963). Ibid., **1**, 1251.
—— —— —— (1964). Ibid. In press.
Miles, A. A., Misra, S. S., and Irwin, J. O. (1938). *J. Hyg. (Camb.)*, **38**, 732.
Price, P. B. (1957). In *Antiseptics, Disinfectants, Fungicides, and Chemical and Physical Sterilization*, edited by G. F. Reddish, 2nd ed., p. 409. Kimpton, London.
Ricketts, C. R., Squire, J. R., and Topley, E. (1951). *Clin. Sci.*, **10**, 89.
Story, P. (1952). *Brit. med. J.*, **2**, 1128.
Verdon, P. E. (1961). *J. clin. Path.*, **14**, 91.

Editor's Comments on Papers 28 and 29

These two articles show the effects of antimicrobial agents on inanimate as well as animate surfaces. Since more potent chemical agents can be employed in the former than in the latter case, it may be virtually impossible to achieve chemical sterilization on the skin. A number of chemical agents have been evaluated by Crisley and Foter, and in their article here they present the use of hand sanitation in the prevention of transmission of pathogenic microorganisms.

Reprinted from *Soap Chem. Specialties* **39**,77–79, 101 (1963)

A technique for evaluating the activity of

Antibacterial Residuals on Inanimate Surfaces

A relatively simple technique for obtaining uniformly contaminated surfaces to compare efficacy of some antibacterial residuals.

28

By G. Walter and S. Foris*,
Givaudan Corporation,
Delawanna, N. J.

THE incidence of staphylococcal infections in hospitals and other institutions during the past decade has resulted in renewed emphasis on environmental sanitation. Antibacterial claims on several product labels have been extended into the area of residual activity. These claims imply that the residual chemical remaining on a surface following treatment exerts bactericidal action against organisms coming into contact with the surface under normal environmental conditions of temperature and relative humidity.

There are a number of publications dealing with the residual activity of surfaces, the majority of which concerns fabrics (1-6). It is interesting to note that many propose a technique utilizing a wet inoculum. It is also interesting to note that several publications make mention of no antibacterial activity of fabrics, such as blankets, when in actual use, implying inactivity with dry microorganisms (4, 5). There are relatively fewer publications dealing directly with hard surfaces and residual activity. Dunklin and Lester demonstrated the important role of relative humidity and presented evidence which suggested that such claims might be possible for hard surfaces (7-9). Other than Dunklin's work and that of Hoffman (10), who dealt primarily with sporicidal coatings, very little direct experimental evidence is available to justify the self-disinfection claims of chemical residuals. There are a variety of inanimate surfaces for which residual claims would be beneficial if they could be substantiated, particularly in view of the work by Rubbo, who demonstrated the rapid spread of a marked Staphylococcus from a dry fabric (11).

The purpose of this investigation has been to develop a technique which would simulate dust-borne Staphylococci falling upon surfaces and to evaluate residual activity against dry bacterial cells. It has been presumed that criteria for a satisfactory technique should include at least the following points: (1) dry bacterial cells on a dry surface, (2) an adequate number of uniformly inoculated replicate test surfaces within a given experiment, (3) complete removal of bacterial cells from the surface for the enumeration of survivors and (4) ease of inoculation regardless of the type of surface, be it hard surfaces or a fabric.

Experimental

The technique of inoculation consisted of dispersing a dried U.S.P. Talc- *S. aureus* powder into the top of an 11 foot, 20 inch diameter, cylindrical tower via an air line connected to a filter flask containing dry powder. The fallout was collected at the base of the tower on the surfaces containing chemical residual. The time of powder spray and fall-out collection may be adjusted to suit the type of experiment. The base of the tower contained a tray-template unit which permitted the time of collection to be constant. The aerosolized "dust" was allowed to equilibrate for one minute to permit rapid settling of larger particles and to allow quiescence of the air currents within the tower. A sliding shield was then removed from the tray unit to permit collection of the dust onto the test surfaces and again inserted into the tray unit at the end of 10 minutes to prevent further fall-out. The entire tray assembly, containing 54 uniformly inoculated surfaces,

Fig. 1. Base of tower assembly with tray-template unit containing samples. (A) sliding shield (B) template (C) tray opening into base of tower (D) ultra-violet tubes (E) 9 foot cylindrical tower.

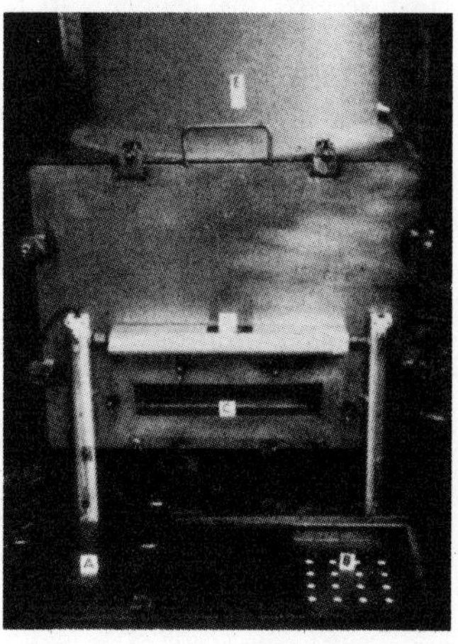

*Paper presented by Dr. Walter during 49th annual meeting, Chemical Specialties Manufacturers Association, Washington, D. C., Dec. 4, 1962.

was then withdrawn from the base and the samples were removed aseptically to humidity chambers. Humidity chambers consisted of tightly closed plastic boxes (7"x-10"x4") fitted with a ¼" mesh stainless steel screen to hold the test surfaces. Each humidity chamber contained 100 ml. of saturated aqueous salt solution to give the desired humidity (12). Saturated calcium chloride and ammonium sulfate were used to give humidities of 30% and 80%, respectively.

Preliminary attempts at obtaining dry inoculum with household dust were unsuccessful; after drying liquid inoculated housedust, we were unable to reproduce a dust fine enough for aerosolization. A finely dispersible powder was formed by the addition of U.S.P. Talc to a 10 ml. 24 hour A.O.A.C. broth culture of *Staphylococcus aureus* A.T.C.C. 6538. The resultant paste was ground after having been dried overnight at 35°C in an air incubator. Excellent viability of the test organism was observed after aerosolization of the dry powder, therefore no further attempt to use household dust was made. It was presumed that this preparation would represent dry *S. aureus* cells on a dry carrier simulating dust-borne organisms.

The area of inoculation was held constant by a metal template under which the test surfaces were fixed in place. It was found necessary to position the surface firmly, particularly glass which tended to slide, by means of wingnut bolts that secured the template to the tray bottom. The test surfaces, sandwiched between the tray bottom and the template, were thus securely held in place.

The interior and exterior areas adjacent to the tray opening were surrounded by 15-watt ultraviolet tubes to minimize airborne contamination of the laboratory. Surprisingly enough, liquid impinger air samplers demonstrated that the laboratory air was of relatively low count during the operation of the unit; small numbers of Staphylococci, however, were recovered from the air of the laboratory which indicate the equipment was not as safe as would be desired.

Table I. Survival of S. aureus on glass surface treated with the use-dilution of four different phenolic disinfectants.

		Bacterial Count per ml Rinse Solution										
		30% relative humidity					80% relative humidity					0 hr.
		A*	B	C	D	E	A*	B	C	D	E	cour
6 hrs.		668	464	364	280	224	636	2	1	7	17	796
		712	484	348	332	308	604	0	1	10	0	696
	$\bar{X}$	690	474	356	306	266	620	1	1	9	9	746
24 hrs.		644	212	176	83	77	572	0	0	0	0	
		596	192	188	172	108	616	0	0	0	0	
	$\bar{X}$	620	202	182	128	93	594	0	0	0	0	

*untreated control

Bacterial counts of the surfaces were determined by hand shaking the test surface in a wide mouth, two ounce, screw cap, glass jar containing 20 ml. of antidote rinse solution. Antidote solution consisted of an aqueous solution of 0.5% "Tween" 80 and 0.07% lecithin. Counts of the rinse solution were determined employing an Astell Roll Tube apparatus* and dextrose tryptone extract agar.

For the evaluation of the residual effect of a given material on dry cells, surfaces were first irradiated with ultraviolet light and then treated with 0.04 ml/inch^2 of the use-dilution of the product as suggested by Klarmann (13). The disinfectant was allowed to dry thoroughly overnight; then the surfaces were inoculated by the aforementioned technique.

*Consolidated Laboratories, Inc., Chicago, Ill.

In order to remove com pletely dust adhering to the sur faces, it was found necessary to em ploy approximately 20, five mm glass beads in the rinse solution This effect was determined by com paring the counts from hard su faces with those from specially pre pared glass surfaces. These specia ly prepared glass surfaces containe a polyvinylpyrrolidone coatin which dissolved readily when pla ed into rinse solution, thereby re leasing the adhering dust film. Re covery tests using glass beads, con sistently demonstrated no signifi ant difference in mean counts be tween the coated glass surfaces an a number of hard surfaces an fabrics.

Results

The residual effect of fou phenolic disinfectants applied a a dilution 20 times the label phenc coefficient, the use-dilution, ma be seen in Table I. A marked bac tericidal action was observed a 80% relative humidity (R.H.); thi greatly diminished when the su

Table II. Survival of dry S. aureus on surfaces previously treate with the use-dilution of a phenolic disinfectant.

	Bacterial Count per ml Rinse Solution								
	0 hr.			6 hr. — 80% R. H. — 25° C.					
	Treated			Untreated			Treated		
			$\bar{X}$			$\bar{X}$			$\bar{X}$
Rubber tile	5000	4550	4775	5650	4750	5200	5170	4180	467
Vinyl tile	4430	4750	4590	5330	5900	5665	2460	1150	180
Vinyl asbestos tile	4950	5330	5140	4850	5000	4925	1470	1970	172
Wood	5300	5100	5200	4600	4430	4515	1970	1310	164
Unglazed ceramic tile	4680	4700	4690	4430	4930	4680	2300	2700	250
Glazed ceramic tile	5500	5000	5275	4930	4680	4805	62	184	12
Stainless steel	4850	5200	5025	5080	5680	5355	113	99	10
Plastic tile	4750	4750	4750	5500	6000	5750	91	84	8
Glass	5400	5660	5530	5830	4350	5090	46	35	4

Table III. The effect of relative humidity and type of surface on the residual antibacterial activity of the use-dilution of a phenolic disinfectant.

		30% Relative Humidity				80% Relative Humidity			
		Glass		Vinyl Asbestos		Glass		Vinyl Asbestos	
		Treated	Control	Treated	Control	Treated	Control	Treated	Control
0 hr.		2460	2340	2090					
		2260	2300	2790					
	$\bar{X}$	2360	2320	2440					
3 hr.		2910	3200	2460	2260	23	3200	2340	2620
		2990	2740	2130	2740	31	2420	2090	2620
	$\bar{X}$	2950	2970	2795	2500	27	2810	2215	2620
6 hr.		2300	2870	2790	2340	8	2300	2170	2540
		2090	2420	2210	2580	0	2500	2260	2740
	$\bar{X}$	2195	2645	2500	2460	4	2400	2215	2640
24 hr.		2070	2190	1620	1040	3	2520	1000	2480
		2320	2320	1530	1240	6	3230	1360	1380
	$\bar{X}$	2195	2255	1575	1140	5	2875	1180	1930

faces were exposed at 30% R.H. This table illustrates the actual survival of the test organism on treated smooth glass surface under differing humidity conditions at room temperature. The viability of the test organism at either of the humidities over the 24 hour period may be noted by column A which is the untreated control glass surface.

That the nature of the surface may be a significant factor in establishing residual claims may be seen in Table II. It may be noted that the surfaces treated with the use-dilution of column E of Table I, which exhibit reasonably good bactericidal action, fall under the smooth group. A very common flooring material, vinyl asbestos tile, was selected for a more detailed comparison with glass. The effect of humidity and the nature of the surface may be seen in Table III in which only the glass surface demonstrated a significant bactericidal action. Repeated applications of the use-dilution of the phenolic disinfectant to vinyl asbestos tile were of little value as may be seen in Table IV. Up to four applications of the disinfectant were without residual effect. Bacteriostasis was encountered with eight applications and was detected by the addition of known numbers of cells to rinse solution containing an equivalent level of disinfectant rinsed from the treated surface. Bacteriostatic effects would necessarily invalidate the counts as representing survivors of the residual treatment.

Table IV. Repeated applications of the use-dilution of a phenolic disinfectant on vinyl asbestos tile and subsequent residual activity against S. aureus after 6 hrs. at room temperature.

		Bacterial Count per ml Rinse Solution					
		Number of Applications					
		0	1	2	4	6	8
30% R.H.		8100	8770	7870	7630	428	200
		8940	7380	8280	8530	648	264
		8940	9910	7550	7950	724	424
		7630	7950	8360	8900	356	268
	$\bar{X}$	8403	8503	8015	7953	539	289
80% R.H.		9670	7870	8360	8100	120	31
		9190	8200	8050	8530	144	17
		8450	9600	8700	3440	444	9
		8600	9270	8770	8050	424	3
	$\bar{X}$	8978	8735	8470	7030	278	15
		2630	2910	2870	2580	3120	0
		2990	2950	2710	2870	2910	0
				stasis detection			
	$\bar{X}$	2810	2930	2790	2725	3015	0

Summary

In conclusion, we have attempted to develop a relatively simple technique of obtaining uniformly contaminated surfaces in order that comparisons for determining the efficacy of certain antibacterial residuals might be made. The data presented were shown to illustrate that any residual claims must take into consideration not only relative humidity but also the nature of the surface itself as both of these factors are critical. In view of the relative inactivity at low humidity and inactivity at high humidity with certain types of surfaces, one should carefully examine claims which imply activity against dust-borne microorganisms which fall upon dry surfaces.

Bibliography

1. Quinn, H., *Appl. Microbiol.*, *10*: 74 (1962).
2. Rountree, P. M., *Med. J. Austr.*, *1*: 539 (1946).
3. Majors, P., *Am. Dyestuff Rep.*, *48*: (3), 91 (1959).
4. Newcastle Regional Hospital Board, *J. Hyg.*, *60*: 85 (1962).
5. Rubbo, S. D., Stratford, B. C., and Dixson, S., *Med. J. Austr.*, *2*: 330 (1960).
6. "Technical Manual of the Am. Assoc. Textile Chemists Colorists," Howes Publishing Co., New York, N. Y. pg. B-131.
7. Dunklin, E. W., and Lester, W., *Soap & San. Chem.*, *27*: (7), 127 (1951).
8. Dunklin, E. W., and Lester, W., *J. Infectious Diseases*, *104*: 41 (1959).
9. Lester, W., and Dunklin, E. W., *J. Infectious Diseases*, *96*: 40 (1955).
10. Hoffman, R. K., Yeager, S. B., and Kaye, S., Proc. 41st Midyear Meeting, Chem. Spec. Mfr. Assoc., Inc., New York, 1955, pgs. 76-81.
11. Rubbo, S. D., Stratford, B. C., and Dixson, S., *Brit. Med. J.*, No. 5300, 282 (1962).
12. "Handbook of Chemistry and Physics," 36th Ed., Chemical Rubber Publishing Co., Cleveland, Ohio.
13. Klarmann, E. G., Wright, E. S., and Shternov, V. A., *Appl. Microbiol.*, 1: 19 (1953).

Reprinted from *J. Milk Food Technol.* **28**, 278–284 (1965)

THE USE OF ANTIMICROBIAL SOAPS AND DETERGENTS FOR HAND WASHING IN FOOD SERVICE ESTABLISHMENTS[1]

FRANCIS D. CRISLEY AND MILTON J. FOTER[2]

Robert A. Taft Sanitary Engineering Center
U. S. Department of Health, Education, and Welfare, Cincinnati, Ohio

29

Considerable interest has been generated in the use of the newer formulations that contain skin sanitizing agents for hand washing in food processing and service establishments. In some areas of the country, the degerming agents have been suggested so often by public health officials that the use of antimicrobial soaps has approached the status of a recommendation. It is the purpose of this paper to briefly review this situation and some of the problems involved in choosing between some of the most common chemical agents that have been suggested for this purpose.

Sanitization of the skin involves a limiting surface that Lane and Blank *(22)* have described generally as a continuous, relatively smooth layer of dead, flattened, keratinized cells made somewhat irregular by various ridges and furrows, by orifices of sweat glands, and by hair follicles and outgrowths of hair. The cutaneous glands secrete a film over these cells, and this film constitutes the absolute limiting boundary between man and his environment. In this film are included salt, urea, and other substances left behind by evaporation of sweat; sebum, which covers all areas except the palms and soles; and a uniform layer of fat. The cells contain proteins, lipids, and water. The protein is largely keratin, which is insoluble in weak acids, weak alkalies, and salt solutions. If the outer layers of the cells of the epidermis are brought into equilibrium with a solution that has a pH to either side of pH 3.70, the isoelectric point of keratin, swelling of the cells will occur. The skin reacts more strongly to alkalies than to acids. Numerous measurements have shown the pH of the skin to range from 3.5 to 7.0.

Although the relative amounts and kinds of the substances of the skin may vary among individuals and from time to time in each individual (as a result of changes in physiological conditions), the structure and composition of the skin generally provide a good environment for bacterial growth. Foci for the establishment of bacterial flora exist in hair follicles, the sweat and subaceous glands, and the numerous ridges and furrows. Price *(29)* has classified the bacteria found on the human skin into two groups, the transient and the resident. The transient types are acquired by contact with other persons or objects in the environment. The resident flora comprise organisms that have established themselves and live in dynamic balance as parasites or saprophytes in the skin.

From the standpoint of sanitation in the food establishment, the ideal situation would be sterilization of the skin on the hands of food handlers; however, it is generally agreed that it is impossible to render skin sterile without destroying it. Transient bacteria are readily removed with ordinary soap and water. The resident organisms, however, are more difficult to remove; and scrubbing in hand-washing procedures is a recognition of this fact. In many persons, staphylococci make up a significant part of the resident flora. Because of the pathogenicity of some staphylococci and their ability to produce enterotoxin, major stress has been placed on the destruction, removal, and control of these organisms by hand-washing procedures. Although there is a paucity of reports on the efficacy of germicidal agents for hand washing in food service establishments, much valuable information can be gleaned from the voluminous literature on preoperative or surgical procedures and, to a lesser degree, from studies of the control of bacteria that produce body odor.

Even if surface bacteria are removed, the bacterial population is easily re-established by the emergence of resident organisms from the deeper structures and the addition of transient types acquired by continual contact with objects in the external environment. Price *(29)* has shown that under normal conditions the skin flora is fully re-established within a week after degerming of the skin. For this reason, the advantages of the deposition of a germicidal residue on the skin after hand washing to exert a continuous antibacterial action on the emerging organisms has been studied. The reliability of data on the efficacy of chemical agents known to be strongly retained on the skin surface is questionable when one moves from the study of operating-room hand-washing procedures (in which most of the rigorous testing has been done), through the simple

[1]The contents of this paper are derived from the available literature and the opinions of the authors and should not be construed to represent the views of the Public Health Service.

[2]Present address: Division of Environmental Engineering and Food Protection, Public Health Service, U. S. Department of Health, Education, and Welfare, Washington, D. C.

control of body odor, to the hands of the food handler. Optimum control of skin bacteria by antibacterial agents in soaps and hand-washing detergents may depend on continuous use of the antibacterial preparation at work and at home, since washing with ordinary soap might tend to remove residual antibacterial agents quickly. Also, the food handler must usually wash utensils in strong cleansing detergents at least intermittently during the day, which causes swelling of the epidermal layer and disruption of the film of active agent deposited by germicidal soaps. To add to these factors, many of the germicidal agents presently in use are soluble in soap fats and fat solvents, and much of the germicide could be lost from the hands by contact with animal and vegetable oils in foods such as salads, meats, etc. Since optimal reduction of skin bacteria by some antibacterial agents has been reported to be based upon continuous use of the agent for as long as 7 days, these limitations must be considered when such agents are proposed for food-handling operations.

Another factor that has not been adequately considered is the ability of certain transient organisms to change their status and become more or less permanent residents. Price *(29)* has given the term "colonization" to this mechanism. While many transient types tend to disappear spontaneously from the skin, apparently because the conditions are not suited to their survival or colonization, Price *(29)* has reported that colon bacilli placed on the hands do not so disappear. He found that prolonged presence of unusual contaminants from wounds, such as *Staphylococcus aureus*, streptococci, *Escherichia coli, Bacillus pyocyaneous* (*Pseudomonas aeruginosa*), resulted in their colonization on the hands as part of the resident flora. Price *(29)* also noted the appearance and persistence for over a year of a nonpathogenic *Trichophyton* on the skin of his hands and arms, although this organism had not been encountered previously and was not present in the air of the laboratory. To what extent the colonization mechanism may operate in food handlers exposed to salmonellae in poultry, or to bacteria in abscesses or other pockets of infection in meat carcasses, has not been adequately studied, to the author's knowledge; this perhaps should be considered in the choice of antibacterial hand-washing compounds.

The degree to which mechanical cleansing alone is responsible for removal of skin bacteria is important *(29)* in the consideration of hand-washing procedures and provides a standard by which the degerming efficiency of antibacterial hand-washing agents can be measured. Price *(29)* concluded that the amount of friction produced at the skin surface by scrubbing appeared to be the most important variable factor in dislodging the resident flora. More firmly imbedded than the transient bacteria that are only lightly attached to the skin by extraneous grease or oils, the resident organisms cannot be removed by soap and water or simple rinsing without the use of friction. Price *(29)* showed that rubbing the hands together was more effective than rinsing, but less effective than scrubbing with a soft brush. A soft brush was less efficient than a stiff one. Brushing the skin without soap reduced the resident flora more rapidly than when soap was used, because soap served as a friction-reducing lubricant for brush bristles. Soap, however, increased the efficiency of removal of grease, dirt, and transient bacteria. Price *(29)* also found brushing with soap in hard water to be more effective than in soft water for removing the basic flora, because hard water precipitated the soap. This finding naturally leads to the possibility that modern detergents, which are not so readily precipitated by hard water, may interfere somewhat with the mechanical cleansing process.

An understanding of these complexities of skin sanitation is needed before an attempt can be made to discuss some of the major types of antibacterial agents that are presently being considered for hand soaps and detergents in food service establishments. Many of the same agents have been proposed for use in lotions or creams. This type of application may be objectionable because of the possibility that the resident bacteria can multiply in the deeper skin layers beneath the preparation *(24)* and also because of the enhanced possibilities for introduction of the agent into foods.

THE BISPHENOLS

Essentially diphenols, the bisphenols are compounds that contain two hydroxyl (OH) groups, only one of which is neutralized by alkalies in soaps and detergents. The second hydroxyl group on the molecule remains free and is completely active against bacteria. In this characteristic the bisphenols are superior to the older phenolics, in which the single hydroxyl groups are easily inactivated by soaps. Of the many bisphenols that have been synthesized, two are most commonly associated with hand soaps. They are hexachlorophene and bithionol. Both are bacteriostatic agents that act by inhibiting the growth of bacteria rather than by killing the organisms.

Hexachlorophene (also known as G-11, AT-7, Gamophen, Hexosan, Exofine, Phisohex, Surgicen, and Surofene[3] is 2, 2'–Dihydroxy–3, 3', 5, 5', 6, 6'–hexachlorodiphenylmethane or bis–(3, 5, 6–trichloro-2-hydroxyphenyl) methane *(26)*. It is usually

[3]Mention of commercial products does not infer endorsement by the Public Health Service.

employed in a concentration of 1 to 3% in liquid or solid soaps, lotions, or emulsions *(26)*. Some skin sensitivity reactions have been known to occur in some individuals *(26)*.

Reduction of skin bacteria has been reported to be considerably greater by hexachlorophene soaps than by ordinary soap *(14, 24)*. No significant reduction occurs immediately after application of the agent *(14, 24)*; and, when used as a single scrub, hexachlorophene soaps are not much more effective than ordinary soaps *(5, 19, 31)*. Routine use for 5 to 10 days, however, has been reported *(2, 4)* to result in a reduction of bacteria as high as 85 to 95% from the original numbers. Only 4% of the food handlers regularly washing with hexachlorophene formulation for a period of over a year harbored coagulase-positive staphylococci, as opposed to a 16% coagulase-positive rate among workers using hexachlorophene-free soap *(7)*. These findings may indicate that some residual antibacterial effect may be present even on individuals who use regular soap away from work. Shemano and Nickerson *(33)*, using hexachlorophene labelled with C-14, found that some of the agent remained on the skin for a considerable time, although some was lost, especially during the first day, by washing with ordinary soap and water. Whether residual agent that remains adsorbed to the skin is as fully active against bacteria as free hexachlorophene is not clear. Some loss of the agent by washing with ordinary soaps between hexachlorophene ablutions is commonly accepted *(16)*.

Following degerming with hexachlorophene and the attainment of a low bacterial level, the normal count returns about 7 days after the use of the agent is stopped. This delay, however, may not be solely due to a residual adsorbed on the skin, since regeneration times of 1 to 7 days occur after disinfection by other means *(29)*, depending on the thoroughness of treatment.

The activity of hexachlorophene is greatly reduced by organic matter such as body fluids, pus, serum, albumin, milk, etc., and non-ionic detergents and emulsifying agents *(31)*. Although there is no evidence that hexachlorophene-resistant bacteria develop as a result of exposure to the agent *(31)*, Price *(28)* pointed out that the microbial flora on the hands of different people vary in susceptibility to the agent with some individuals harboring a resistant flora. This finding introduces some uncertainty as to the reliability of hexachlorophene soaps that is probably more serious in the operating room than in food service establishments; nevertheless it must be considered.

In general, the Gram-positive bacteria are most susceptible to hexachlorophene, and Gram-negatives such as *E. coli* and *Salmonella* are not greatly affected *(31)*. Many Gram-negative types are represented among the transient species encountered in food by the food handler. Post and Balzer *(27)* have reported that hexachlorophene appeared to have some effect on the transient as well as the resident bacterial flora on the hands of four culinary workers. The effect on the Gram-negative organisms was erratic. The authors admitted that the results were inconclusive and in need of further clarification. Furthermore the small number of workers studied and the diversity of their culinary duties suggest that additional studies should be carried out on a greater number of subjects and more attention given to the type of culinary operation performed and the extent to which workers contracts with dishwater and food influence the reduction of bacterial flora by hexachlorophene.

Bithionol (also known as XL-7, Actamer, Lorothiodol, and TBP) is termed 2, 2′-thiobis (4, 6-dichlorophenol) or bis (2-hydroxy-3, 5-dichlorophenyl) *(26)*. It is usually employed in concentrations of 1 to 3% in liquid or solid soap formulations for surgical scrub or other skin disinfection. Lower concentrations may be used, one brand containing only 0.4%.

Soap containing 1 to 2% bithionol is reported to be at least as active as soap with hexachlorophene. It is also more active against the Gram-positive than the Gram-negative bacteria *(1)* and is reported to be fungistatic *(1, 31)*. After 10 to 12 days of continuous use, the bacterial load on hands is said to be reduced by 89 to 97.4% and levels off with no further reduction *(1)*. It is said to be nonirritating when used in soap.

Bithionol, like hexachlorophene, is claimed to resist removal by soap and water *(1)*. It is said to be strongly absorbed by animal tissues such as skin and hair and works best in the acidic range of pH 5.0 to 6.5 *(1)*. Apparently an active residual is maintained *(1)* in the presence of alkali in soaps or detergents, but more study is needed on this aspect of both bithionol and hexachlorophene.

The Iodine Compounds

Free Iodine

Elemental iodine is one of the most effective antimicrobial agents known *(31)*. It is essentially bactericidal, dilutions possessing bacteriostatic and bactericidal action being practically identical *(18)*. Under a variety of exaggerated test conditions, iodine in the proper concentrations is uniformly active against a broad spectrum of pathogenic organisms, including the tubercle bacillus, pathogenic fungi, viruses, and even bacterial and fungal spores. Although effective for antiseptic washes and for irrigation purposes over a wide pH range *(17)*, the activity of iodine solutions is markedly enhanced under acid conditions.

Reddish *(32)* points out that the well-recognized efficacy of iodine is partly due to the margin of safety under which it has been employed. It is used as a skin antiseptic in hospitals in a concentration of 2%, although a level of 0.02% in solution is germicidal within one minute to a variety of pathogenic organisms, including S. *aureus*. Tinctures of iodine have low surface tensions, and the solvent action of the alcohol dissolves skin oils and facilitates penetration into the epidermal layer, thus destroying both the transient and the resident bacterial flora. Aqueous solutions of iodine have also been used successfully and possess certain advantages as preoperative skin disinfectants, and disinfectants for surgical instruments, clinical thermometers, drinking water, and eating and drinking utensils.

The iodophors are chemical complexes of diatomic iodine and solubilizing agents or carriers, usually synthetic nonionic surfactants. A portion of the iodine becomes firmly bound in the complex and is unrecoverable, but the remainder is "available" and is believed to be responsible for the germicidal activity. The iodophors have been reported to be effective sanitizers, good disinfectants *in vitro*, nonallergenic, relatively nontoxic, and noncorrosive.

The activity of the iodophors is directly related to the amount of titratable iodine present in solution. Titratable iodine content is very pertinent in evaluating commercial iodophors *(10)*. Blatt and Maloney *(10)* compared three commercial iodophors with aqueous or alcoholic solutions of elemental iodine on the basis of equivalent amounts of titratable iodine and found no significant differences in germicidal effectiveness. These results indicate that germicidal activity is contributed solely by titratable iodine, and any enhancement of germicidal activity is at least partially due to the wetting action of the detergent compound. Blatt and Maloney *(10)* also found that, once all of the titratable iodine was removed from the compound and after the compound had been allowed to stand, no further iodine could be demonstrated by titration. In the analysis of iodine preparations, it is pertinent that the amount of titratable iodine does not always represent the actual amount of active iodine to be expected under actual conditions of use, because the amount dissociating from the complex at any time is dependent upon the dissociation constant, which is influenced by pH and temperature *(12)*. This amount may be only a fraction of the amount recoverable by titration.

Solutions of elemental iodine, phosphoric acid buffered iodine-I_2 and solutions of certain iodophors with a low pH (even after the addition of test bacteria) are believed to be among the best sanitizing agents *(31)*. Many of the marketed liquid iodophors contain phosphoric acid. A cationic iodophor that possesses an alkaline pH and contains 3.2% elemental iodine has been recommended for disinfection of the skin, for operative procedures, and for disinfection of thermometers and surgical instruments *(31)*. It has been reported *(21)* to be responsible for a reduction in major postoperative wound infection from 14.8% to 6.8%, although minor infections were not significantly reduced.

Comparisons have been made of the effectiveness of free iodine preparations, iodophors, and hexachlorophene. Goldenberg, *et al. (19)*, by culturing washings of the insides of surgeons gloves, found that iodine-detergent surgical scrub was almost three times as effective after 4 minutes of scrubbing (23.5% positive cultures) as a 3% hexachlorophene detergent was after 10 minutes of washing (66.7% positive culture). Recently, King and Price *(20)*, employing the widely used method of Price *(29)*, compared the degerming activity of solutions of several iodophor formulations with simple alcoholic and aqueous solutions that have approximately the same iodine content, and with a scrub with ordinary face soap. Although the iodophors were less effective in reducing bacteria on the skin than were the iodine solutions, they were more effective than ordinary soap. A 2-minute exposure to a tincture of 1% iodine in 70% ethyl alcohol reduced the bacterial flora to less than 20% of the pre-exposure levels (equivalent to 13 minutes of soap and brush scrubbing). The same exposure to the most efficient iodophor reduced the flora to only 54%, equivalent to the efficiency attained in 4 minutes of scrubbing with white soap and brush, or to 35 seconds of exposure to 1% iodine in 70% alcohol. The authors believed that about the only advantage of an iodophor surgical scrub over one incorporating tincture of iodine is that the former is more pleasant and less irritating.

Experimental detergent-iodine cakes containing about 0.7 to 1.0% available iodine have been produced and patented *(15)*, but, to our knowledge, are not yet available commercially *(15)*. The exact details of their composition are not known, and an evaluation should be made when more information is available.

As skin degerming agents for the surgical scrub, the iodophors appear to be generally less efficacious than elemental iodine, but this may be a result of the paucity of information about the amount of titratable and dissociated iodine present in the various compounds under actual conditions of use. The available information does not reveal the presence of true residual activity as occurs with hexachlorophene. The iodophors are attractive to potential users because of the claim that detergency and disinfection can be accomplished simultaneously with the same agent.

The Chlorocarbanilides

TCC is a 3, 4, 4, trichlorocarbanilide *(6)*. Available information from the manufacturer *(6)* indicates bacteriostatic activity against staphylococci in dilutions of 1:5 million to 1:10 million, with some fungistatic action against skin fungi. TCC is used in soaps in concentrations ranging from 0.5 to 2.0% and is claimed to be unaffected by either nonionic or anionic detergent. Data for Gram-positive bacteria only are included *(6)*. Handwashing tests with TCC were strictly controlled to eliminate the use of other handwashing agents, so no skin retention data are available.

Bacteriostat CH3479 (Irgasan CF-3) is 3-trifluoromethyl 4, 4′ dichlorocarbanilide *(3)*. It is used in concentrations of 1% in deodorant soaps or shampoos and in detergents in 0.2 to 0.4% for residual bacteriostatic effect on cotton fabrics. Although ineffective against Gram-negative bacteria, it is claimed by the manufacturer *(3)* to be more effective than TCC against Gram-positive bacteria.

Although extensive evaluations of TCC and CH3479 are not yet available, these compounds seem to require their exclusive use by the food handler in order to be fully effective.

The Quaternary Ammonium Compounds

The quaternary ammonium germicides ("quats") are another class of synthetic chemical disinfectants which are synthesized to form amines in which the nitrogen in the molecule has a covalence of 5. With the quats, however, the hydrogen atoms are replaced by one or more alkyl groups (CH_3, C_2, H_5, etc.), or a phenyl radical, and one or more alkyl groups containing C_8 to C_{18} carbon chain lengths *(31)*. The quats are characterized further by their ability to depress greatly the surface tension of water. This property places them in a class of chemicals frequently described as wetting or surface active agents, detergents, or dispersing agents. Surface active agents are grouped further between "anionic" detergent (natural soaps and many synthetic soap substatutes); "non-ionic" detergents (sudsing agents); and the quats which are "cationic" detergents (substituted ammonia compounds). Only the quats or cationics are discussed in this review.

The antimicrobial properties of quats are attributed to their chemical reactivity and the ease with which they are adsorbed. Likewise, these properties account for their occasional failure. The quats are inactivated by soap, hard waters, lecithin, and other phospholipids, and are adsorbed by charcoal, bentonite, and agar. They combine readily with proteins and thus are less efficient in the presence of serum, milk, and other food soils *(30)*. By 1954, the quats had been demonstrated to be incompatible with thirty-six chemical agents, among which were iodine, lanolin, pine oil, silicates, polyphosphates, and anionic detergents *(23)*. The number of chemical agents with which the quaternaries are incompatible is about equal to the number of agents with which they are compatible. Thus it is critical that the ingredients of a formulation be compatible with the quaternary used.

The literature is replete with studies on the antimicrobial properties of quats alone and in preparations formulated for a variety of uses. *In vitro* they appear to be equally effective against many Gram-positive and Gram-negative bacteria, according to one source *(31)*. Other workers found that quaternary ammonium compounds were slightly less effective against the Gram-negative organisms tested *(8)*. Mallman *(25)* summarized these discrepancies, stating, "By selecting the proper laboratory technic, we can show that the cationics are either poor or unusually good disinfectants."

The most widely used quat is benzalkonium chloride, which is a mixture of alkyldimethylbenzyl ammonium chlorides *(26)* and marketed under a variety of trade names. It has been widely used in hospitals for disinfection in surgery, and in sanitizing utensils, floors, walls, soiled linen, and in other applications. Since benzalkonium chloride *(26)* is incompatible with anionic detergents, such as soap, and the mineral content of hard waters interferes with the bactericidal action of the quats *(11)*, it would not be suitable in hand-washing procedures for food handlers whose hands are in constant contact with soaps, detergents, waters of varying degrees of hardness, and food.

Discussion and Conclusions

Because of the paucity of studies on food handlers *per se*, it is difficult to make an absolute judgment of the type of antibacterial agent that ought to be incorporated into hand-washing agents for use by food handlers, or whether one should be used at all. Most of the studies on the efficacy of hand washing compounds have been directed to the evaluation of cosmetic applications or hospital procedures. The standards of efficacy in the former are not sufficiently critical for adoption in the food-service environment, and those for the latter may well be too stringent. At present, the choice of an antibacterial agent for the food handler must be made without full knowledge of the extent to which food pathogens may colonize on the skin of the worker, although allowance for such an eventuality should probably be made.

In the existing literature, the development of an antibacterial residue on the skin, such as occurs with the bithionols, is stressed. In itself, the maintenance of a continuing low level of bacteria on the hands may not be sufficient evidence for the presence of an active residue with all agents, since Price *(29)* has demonstrated that full establishment of the normal skin flora after the skin has been thoroughly degermed may require as much as 1 week, regardless of the method used. Nevertheless, the apparent residual antibacterial activity of the bithionols requires consideration of this aspect in the study of hand sanitizing agents.

The aim of hand sanitation is to prevent the transmission of possible pathogenic organisms from the hands through food or from food to food via the hands of the food handler. Since it is obviously not practicable to depend on the continual and exclusive use of antibacterial hand soaps outside of working hours, optimal control of skin bacteria during the hours in which food is being handled is the best that can be achieved. The maintenance of an efficient antibacterial residual on the skin can then probably be subordinated to other considerations. The antibacterial agent should not be chosen on the basis of activity against staphylococci and the Gram-positive bacteria alone. Food handlers may also harbor many Gram-negative bacteria of significance, such as *Salmonellae* and pathogenic *E. coli,* as well as *Entamoeba histolytica* or other pathogens, either as transient flora or possibly as established residents acquired through contact. The control of transient organisms by a more positive method than simple removal by soap and water may be desirable, since transfer from one food to another should be minimized. Also, the consistent use of a broadspectrum antibacterial agent during the working day would help to prevent possible colonization on the skin of bacteria acquired from foods.

If all of these points are considered together, a good hand-washing agent for food service establishments probably should: (*a*) kill a wide variety of possible pathogens (inhibition is not sufficient because a single viable one transferred to a food may, under optimal conditions, multiply once the agent is diluted by the food); *(b)* be present, if possible, in sufficient residual concentration from one ablution to another to effect control during the day; and *(c)* be non-irritating to skin.

Iodine is the only agent reviewed in this report that appears to satisfy the above criteria in most respects. It is bactericidal and active against a wide variety of both Gram-positive and Gram-negative bacteria and other organisms. Although Blatt and Maloney *(10)* state that skin flora recovers more rapidly after iodophor treatment than after the application of hexachlorophene treatment, this point requires further study, in view of Price's findings *(29)* on regeneration of the bacterial population of the skin. Any iodine preparation selected for study should have a high free-iodine content, whether it be a solid soap or a detergent-iodine complex. It should meet all of the general criteria accepted as necessary for performance of germicidal agents where-ever sanitation is important *(13).* Its penetration into skin and its residual effect during the working day should be determined, as well as the degree to which it is removed by contact with food substances. Emollient additives must be incorporated, and their effect on the germicidal efficiency of the preparation must be definitely established.

The need continues for simple and more reliable and reproducible techniques for measuring changes in the skin flora. Particularly, a method should be devised for the study of frequent changes in levels of skin bacteria that occur during the working day as a result of exposure of the food handler to different foods. Such a method could conceivably shed light on the extent to which hazardous bacteria may be transmitted between ablutions as well as the degree to which a sudden contact with heavily contaminated food staples may overwhelm the capacity of a residual bactericide on the skin to control the spread of these organisms.

From the present consideration of the status and efficacy of the available hand sanitizing agents, one may conclude that frequent and thorough use of ordinary hand soaps, with the aid of a good brush during the working day, is, for practical purposes, about as efficient in controlling skin bacteria as the commonly available germicidal soaps. Practical experience has shown that the frequency of hand-washing by food service personnel may be greatly increased by installing hand washing facilities in the working area, because of the tendency for personnel to correct one another's lapses in hand sanitation as they occur. This simple expedient tends to greatly enhance the efficacy of the simple soap and brush procedure.

A recent study *(9)* was reported on the efficiency of bar soaps, without antibacterial additives. The results show that bar soaps do not transfer bacteria among individuals in normal use, nor do they support bacterial growth.

Undoubtedly, some additional benefit will accrue from the use of residual germicidal soaps if they are considered as a supplement to, rather than a replacement for, thorough and frequent scrubbing. While deposition of residual germicide on the skin may be real, it may be nullified by the narrow microbial spectrum affected, possible neutralization by kitchen detergents and food constituents, and the tendency of some germicides to produce sensitivity reactions in some persons.

The use of formulations containing agents with a

broad antibacterial spectrum, such as iodine, presents attractive possibilities which, however, require much further testing in the food service environment.

REFERENCES

1. Anonymous. Actamer Bithionol U.S.P. Technol. Bull. No. FC-5, Monsanto Chemical Company, St. Louis, Missouri. 1958.

2. Anonymous. Annotated bibliography on G-11 (Hexachlorophene, U.S.P.) Technol. Bull. No. H-1, Sindar Corp., New York, N. Y. 1962.

3. Anonymous. Bacteriostat CH 3479 (Irgasan CF-3) Technol. Bull., Geigy Chemical Corp., Ordsley, N. Y. January, 1961.

4. Anonymous. G-11 (Brand of Hexachlorophene). Bacteriological properties. Technol. Bull. No. H-4, Sindar Corp., New York, N. Y. 1952.

5. Anonymous. Skin antiseptics. The Lancet 2:1164. 1958.

6. Anonymous. TCC, 3, 4, 4' Trichlorocarbanilide. Technical Bull. No. FC4A, Monsanto Chemical Company. 1963.

7. Bailey, J. and Foster, D. W. Reducing the bacterial danger in food handling. The Sanitarian 70:379-385. 1962.

8. Baker, Z., Harrison, R. W., and Miller, B. F. The bactericidal action of synthetic detergents. J. Exptl. Med. 74: 611-621. 1941.

9. Bannon, E. A. and Judge, L. F. Bacteriological studies relating to handwashing. I. The inability of soap bars to transmit bacteria. Am. J. Public Health. 55:915-922. 1965.

10. Blatt, R. and Maloney, J. V. An evaluation of the iodophor compounds and surgical germicides. Surg. Gynecol. Obstet. 113:699-704. 1961.

11. Chambers, C. W., Kabler, P. W., Bryant, A. R., Chambers, L. A., and Ettinger, M. B. Bactericidal efficiency of Q. A. C. in different waters. Public Health Reports. 70: 545-553. 1955.

12. Chang, S. L. The use of active iodine as a water disinfectant. J. Am. Pharmaceutical Assoc., Scientific Ed. 47:417-423. 1958.

13. Committee on antimicrobial agents (disinfectants). Am. Public Health Assoc. Criteria for the selection of germicides. Am. J. Public Health. 51:1054-1060. 1961.

14. Committee on Cosmetics, Am. Med. Assoc., Status Report on Deodorant Soaps. J. Am. Med. Assoc. 142:814. 1950.

15. Cordle, H. J. Personal communication from the Chilean Iodine Educational Bureau, 120 Broadway, New York, N. Y. 1963.

16. Council on Drugs, American Medical Association. New and Nonofficial Drugs, J. B. Lippincott Company, p. 205, 1962.

17. Gershenfeld, L. and Witlin, B. Evaluation of the antibacterial efficiency of dilute solutions of free halogens. J. Am. Pharm. Assoc., Sci. Ed. 38:411-414. 1949.

18. Gershenfeld, L. and Witlin B. Free halogens: A comparative study of their efficiencies as bactericidal agents. Am. J. Pharm. 121:95-106. 1949.

19. Goldenberg, I. S., Haley, L. D., and Higashi, G. I. An evaluation of an iodine preoperative scrub detergent. Surg. Gynecol. Obstet. 14:329-332. 1962.

20. King, T. C., and Price, P. B. An evaluation of iodophors as skin antiseptics. Surg. Gynecol. Obstet. 116:361-365. 1963.

21. Krippaehne, W., and Frisch, A. W. Clinical trial of a new cationic iodophore as a topical germicide. Western J. Surg. Obstet. and Gynecol. 67:114-117. 1959.

22. Lane, C. G. and Blank, I. H. Cutaneous detergents. J. Am. Med. Assoc. 118:804-817. 1942.

23. Lawrence, C. A. Quaternary ammonium surface-active germicides. Soap, Perfumery, and Cosmetics. 27:369-376. 1954.

24. Lowbury, E. J. L., Lilly, H. A., and Bull, J. P. Disinfection of hands: Removal of resident bacteria. British Med. J. No. 5340:1251-1256. 1963.

25. Mallman, W. L., Kivela, E. W., and Turner, G. Sanitizing dishes. Soap and Sanitary Chemicals. 22:130-133, 161, 163. 1946.

26. Merck Index of Chemicals and Drugs, 7th Ed. Merck and Company, Inc., Rahway, New Jersey. 1960.

27. Post, F. J. and Balzer, J. L. Effect of a hexachlorophene detergent on the microbial population of the hands of food handlers. J. Milk and Food Technol. 26:142-147. 1963.

28. Price, P. B. Fallacy of a current surgical fad—the 3-minute scrub with hexachlorophene soap. Ann. Surg. 134: 476-485. 1951.

29. Price, P. B. The bacteriology of normal skin: A new quantitative test applied to a study of the bacterial flora and the disinfectant action of mechanical cleansing. J. Infectious Diseases. 63:301-318. 1938.

30. Rahn, O. and Van Eseltine, W. P. Quaternary ammonium compounds. Ann. Rev. Microbiol. 173-192. 1947.

31. Reddish, G. F. Antiseptics, disinfectants, fungicides, and chemical and physical sterilization. 2nd Ed., Lea and Febiger. 1957.

32. Reddish, G. F. Antiseptics in the hospital pharmacy. Bulletin Am. Soc. Hosp. Pharmacists. 13:545-556. 1956.

33. Shemano, I. and Nickerson, M. Cutaneous accumulation and retention of hexachlorophene—C14 (G-11). Federation Proc. 13: (Part I) 404. 1954.

Editor's Comments on Paper 30

30 Davis: *Fundamentals of Microbiology in Relation to Cleansing in the Cosmetics Industry*

This is an excellent review of the factors necessary to cleanse and sterilize equipment in the preparation of cosmetics. In the section on sterilization by chemicals, some of the antimicrobial agents required to perform the task are discussed. In addition, bacteriological control methods and factors that can influence the results of antimicrobial testing are presented.

Reprinted from *J. Soc. Cosmetic Chemists* **23**, 45–71 (1972)

30

Fundamentals of microbiology in relation to cleansing in the cosmetics industry

J. G. DAVIS*

Presented on 18th November 1970 at the Symposium on 'Cleansing' organised by the Society of Cosmetic Chemists of Great Britain in Bournemouth, Hants.

Synopsis—The fundamental MICROBIOLOGICAL aspects of modern methods of CLEANING and STERILIZING equipment with special reference to the HAZARDS of COSMETIC PREPARATIONS.

Introduction

Almost every operation involving handling of foods and other materials which can be contaminated by organisms of human or other animal origin is in theory a hazard to health. In practice it is fortunately only a few which are known to be a serious hazard, for example contact with a person suffering from a certain disease, rewarming of processed meat dishes, etc. From the hygienic point of view therefore the degree of risk has to be assessed in relation to the cost of preventive measures. Not only the chances of contamination and infection, but the growth-permitting properties of the commodity, the conditions of storage and its intrinsic nature from the microbiological point of view are equally important. The more favourable the conditions for growth of micro-organisms in the product, the more effective should be the preventive measures adopted in the factory.

For the present purpose we may define hygiene as a system of precautions to maintain safety and keeping quality (KQ) in cosmetic products.

*Consultant Microbiologist, 9 Gerrard Street, London, W1V 7LJ.

The causative agents in this problem are micro-organisms, so that scientifically it becomes a question of how we should kill them or control their growth. Basically the same principles and methods apply to both pathogens and fault-producing organisms (FPO).

The trend of technology today is clearly towards aseptic packaging of liquid products, and more efficient use of refrigeration to maintain keeping quality. From the bacteriological point of view these two methods imply an increasing importance for heat-resistant spores, psychro-philic (-trophic) organisms and environmental sanitation.

Hitherto industries employing sub-sterilization heat treatments have been particularly concerned with the numbers of thermoduric organisms in their raw materials but with the gradual change to UHT heat treatment methods these types will become of less importance.

The status of hygiene in industry

One of the greatest difficulties with which the new thinkers in industry have had to contend has been the long established general tradition that cleaning of any sort is a menial occupation and of no importance, so that the poorest types of labour were usually employed. This was a fallacy of the first magnitude, a fact which is now realized. No aspect of processing is more important than the cleaning and sterilizing of equipment.

Significance of bacteria in cosmetics

Safety and commercial or keeping quality

The safety (freedom from any pathogens) and KQ of any product are quite distinct properties and must never be confused. A commodity may be safe but of poor KQ and it can be dangerous but commercially satisfactory.

Laboratory control tests must therefore cover both aspects. A product may have such physical and chemical properties that one or both types of test are unnecessary. Dryness and acidity are in practice the dominant conditions in this respect, dryness for all micro-organisms and acidity for all pathogens and most bacteria. Acidity is no deterrent for yeasts and moulds, and in fact often favours them.

In general it may be said that cosmetic preparations, like foods, should either be free from micro-organisms capable of damaging the product, or should contain a bacteriostatic substance (or condition) capable of preventing their growth.

For pathogens the requirement is different and more exact. Either the product must be free from pathogens or it must contain a substance (or condition) that kills them. This is because a surviving pathogen may not be able to grow in the preparation itself but may be able to proliferate when applied to the skin or mucous membranes, or when inhaled or ingested.

The expression 'free from pathogens' needs definition, and as a standard we suggest failure to recover recognized pathogens, particularly *Staph. aureus, Ps. aeruginosa* and *Salmonella* from 100 g using the common standard methods. Coliforms constitute a convenient index group as a measure of quality of raw materials, plant sanitation and hygiene in handling, processing and packaging.

The unpredictability of micro-organisms

The classical textbooks divided bacteria into pathogens and harmless organisms, but unfortunately the true position cannot be so lightly dismissed. During the last 25 years many bacteria previously regarded as harmless commensals or possibly as useful indicator organisms, such as *E. coli,* have been shown to possess pathogenic powers and be capable of causing illness and even death.

Whether this is due to the frequent uncritical and perhaps irresponsible use of antibiotics since 1945 by the medical and veterinary professions must be a matter of opinion, but even some members of these professions are beginning to have doubts about the wisdom of the present day widespread use of antibiotics (1).

Whatever the reason, today organisms such as *Pseudomonas aeruginosa, E. coli, Aerobacter, Flavobacterium, Serratia* have been responsible for killing diseases, sometimes in epidemic form. These are all Gram-negative, resistant to disinfectants and antibiotics, and flourish under watery conditions. The irresponsible use of disinfectants, preservatives and antibiotics may even favour the establishment of these types by repressing the Gram-positive organisms, against which they are very effective.

Another aspect of the greatest importance is the considerable degree of variability in any genus, and even in any one species of micro-organism. Textbooks may define the conditions permitting growth and thermal death points, etc., but there will always be exceptions, or in other words, freak organisms. Such atypical strains are often responsible for disease and defects in products such as cosmetics, pharmaceutical preparations and foods. It follows that assumptions must never be made, risks must never be taken, and a substantial margin of safety always allowed in specifying any heat-treatment, conditions of using a disinfectant and concentration for any preservative until certainty of result has been clearly established by a large number of tests.

The chemist and bacteriological phenomena

The chemist who has not received any biological training often has difficulty in appreciating the wide range of variation in biological behaviour, and the relatively enormous and unavoidable errors in micro-biological testing. For example, the ordinary 'total count', generally the most commonly performed test, has a large error, especially when made on solid materials. In solid and semi-solid materials micro-organisms occur in colonies containing possibly millions of cells. Maceration of the product breaks up the colonies with unpredictable scattering, leading to a large error in the resultant count or very poor reproducibility. Chemical analysis can usually give repeated results agreeing within about 0.1%, but in such tests as the total count it is better to think in terms of logarithmic values, e.g. to allow a difference of $\times$ 10 before asserting that one result is really different from another, or that one sample is better than another. Assuming reliable sampling, two chemical laboratories can usually get reasonable agreement with their analyses. In bacteriological work wide differences may be found, because the method of sampling, handling of the sample, temperature of transport and storage, and technique differences between laboratories may be of tremendous significance. The chemical condition of a substance is usually static whereas the microbiological condition may be quite mobile.

Factors controlling bacterial growth

The most important conditions controlling micro-organisms are (1) availability of food for growth and as a source of energy, (2) warmth or a certain range of temperature, (3) moisture, water activity or relative humidity, and (4) absence of lethal factors.

Food

Micro-organisms can flourish with such minute amounts of food that scrupulous cleansing is necessary to free any item of equipment from these food traces. Protein of animal origin may be described as the favoured food for human pathogens, and skin secretions, mucus, etc. afford excellent nutrients for bacteria, assuming conditions are favourable.

Temperature

Broadly speaking, pathogens flourish best at about blood heat, but most can grow over the range 16–45°C. Where conditions are unavoidably favourable for bacterial growth, e.g. a nutrient liquid at pH 7, the best, simplest and least objectionable way to prevent or delay growth is to hold the product at a low temperature, e.g. about 0°C. Cold does not kill bacteria *per se*, but if organisms cannot grow they tend to die out.

It is impossible to generalize about temperature conditions in respect of organisms producing defects; they may vary from psychrophils (psychrotrophs) growing well at –5 to +5°C to the obligate thermophils which grow only above 37°C and flourish happily at 55-63°C. Cosmetic preparations are often, or attempt to be, antiseptic in character, i.e. they contain one or more ingredients possessing some disinfectant power. Unfortunately these may have little efficacy against *Pseudomonas*, etc., so that low temperature storage of cosmetics cannot be relied upon to prevent growth of these types. All *pseudomonads* and many Gram-negative bacteria, yeasts and moulds can grow down to low temperatures, some moulds down to –23°C. Even extreme cold, e.g. —100°C, cannot be relied upon to kill micro-organisms, although they usually die off slowly.

Moisture

A certain 'moisture' or water activity (a_w) is one of the major conditions for bacterial proliferation. On surfaces it is customary to speak in terms of relative humidity, but the essential feature is the water activity (osmotic pressure) of the medium in which the micro-organisms are contained. This may be a protein-fat film of minute thickness, perhaps only a few microns.

The simplest way of restraining growth of all micro-organisms is to keep the product or equipment dry. Thus in powders, even foods, micro-organisms will die out if the moisture content is low, e.g. below 5%, and they will also die out in tanks, fillers, pipelines, homogenizers, containers, etc., if these are kept dry. The one requisite is that they must be absolutely clean i.e. entirely devoid of organic matter. If they are not, then organisms will survive but not grow, and so sterilization becomes ineffective.

There is one important point to bear in mind in this connection. Bacteria are classified in two broad groups on the basis of the gram stain. gram-positive organisms, such as *Streptococcus*, *Staphylococcus*, *Corynebacterium*, are more susceptible to disinfectants and antibiotics than the gram-negative (*Pseudomonas*, *Salmonella*, *Shigella*, coliforms) but are more resistant to drying, especially if protected by traces of organic matter. Thus the *streptococci* of scarlet fever, basically very delicate bacteria, can survive for years in particles of skin shed by patients, be hidden in such places as bed equipment, and cause an infection years later.

The hygiene 'probability equation'

Developing the theme of the factors controlling bacterial growth we may express the situation in highly condensed form as:

P_t = probable bacterial count at time t

= f (N_o, T, a_w (or RH), F_{qn}, F_n, L^{-1}, t)

where N_o = initial number

T = temperature

a_w = water activity in product

RH = relative humidity in equipment

F_{qn} = amount of nutrients available (e.g. soil in equipment)

F_n = nature or type of product

L = lethality factor (e.g. uv, sunlight, acidity, high osmotic pressure)

t = time of observation after production

This means simply that the probable count in a product or in a piece of equipment after time t will be a function of the factors discussed above.

If all factors except two, e.g. T and t, are standardized it may be possible to estimate P_t with a fair degree of accuracy, using data previously obtained.

Acidity

In general, micro-organisms flourish best in the pH range 5–8.5. Pathogens are usually more sensitive to extreme values and many grow well only between pH 5.5 and 8. Any product, including even foods, which is below pH 4.5 can be regarded as safe because no ordinary pathogens can grow, and any present will die out. Yeasts and moulds are a significant exception, and the few pathogenic species (e.g. *Candida albicans*) are much more resistant to acids than bacteria. Thus *C. albicans* grows best over the range 5.1–6.4 and can grow over a wide pH range (2).

This acidity factor is of special interest to cosmetic chemists because the secretions of the skin are acid, being usually about pH 5.4. Moreover the free fatty acids may exercise a germicidal effect *per se*. This natural protective effect probably plays an important role in protecting the skin against invading organisms. These can do little harm against the intact skin but may invade if the skin is damaged. In extreme cases the pH of the skin may be as low as 4, and this secretory mechanism has been called the 'acid mantle' of the skin. It follows that frequent washing with a strongly alkaline soap is not to be recommended, and prolonged soaking in hot baths is also inadvisable for the same reason. Scientifically the skin should be cleansed with a preparation at about pH 5.4 rather than with an alkaline material. Basically it is always sounder to assist and stimulate the body's natural protective mechanism rather than try and kill bacteria by 'disinfectants' and other means. There will always be the occasion when a virulent organism will get through. To be really effective an antiseptic must have strong biocidal properties, and unfortunately there is usually a good correlation between biocidal power and traumatic effect on animal tissue.

Contemporary medical thought is veering in this direction. For example, it is now the practice not to remove the natural protective material (*vernix caseosa*) on the new born infant and wash it by orthodox means (alkaline soap) immediately after birth. The warm water and soap cleansing is left over for a few days, thus allowing the natural mechanisms of the skin to protect the infant against any fortuitous contamination in early extra-uterine existence.

The other major example of a natural acid protective mechanism is the acidity of the stomach. In healthy adults the pH of the active gastric secretion is about 2, at which no ordinary pathogens can survive. Sub-acid secretions (pH 2–5) allow acid-resistant types such as *Str. salivarius* to pass through into the bowel, and in cases of gross acid deficiency (pH $>$ 5) most pathogens can survive easily. This is the main reason why young infants and very old people are much more susceptible to food poisoning or infective enteritis than healthy adults. In general young infants and old people are much more susceptible to infections of any type. The young have not acquired much immunity and in old people there is a lowered efficiency of all biochemical mechanisms in the body.

The quantitative approach–the 'communal phenomenon'

All studies and control tests in bacteriology should be quantitative; in other words an attempt should always be made to estimate the number involved, although the error may be large. The reason is that the onset of an infection, or the development of a microbiological defect in any product, is dependent on the initial number of organisms concerned. Apart from a few exceptions, it is doubtful whether a single bacterial cell ever did anyone any harm. It appears to be necessary for at least a few organisms to establish themselves and adapt their environment for growth (the 'communal effect'). This is clearly illustrated by figures for the *minimum infective dose* for well recognized diseases (*Table I*). It follows that any reduction in numbers of micro-organisms is worthwhile, even if a complete kill is impossible for practical reasons.

Table I.
Minimum infective doses (approx.) for pathogens in human beings

Disease	Number of cells
Typhoid fever	3
Tuberculosis	100
Cutaneous moniliasis	100 000
Salmonelloses (other than typhoid fevers)	100 000 to 1 000 000

Pseudomonas aeruginosa

This organism, also called *Ps. pyocyanea* and the 'green pus organism', has assumed considerable importance in medicine, surgery, pharmaceutics and cosmetic preparations in recent years. Not only is it capable of being a virulent pathogen but it is so resistant to commonly used disinfectants and antiseptic preparations that it can often be isolated from them in startlingly large numbers.

It is now being found in almost all watery environments in hospitals, nurseries, kitchens and other places where food is prepared and human beings work.

Many interesting and disturbing examples are continually coming to light. Quite recently severe cases of mastitis in a valuable dairy herd were found to be caused by a *Pseudomonas aeruginosa* contamination of the water used for washing the cows' udder. This was ultimately traced to a dead rat in a water tank. The water had been assumed to be pure because it came from the mains.

Type of product and potential contamination

Each type of product is liable to its own specific kind of contamination and microbiological growth according to

(i) chemical nature (protein, fat, carbohydrate and mixtures of these);
(ii) pH value;
(iii) oxygen tension;
(iv) surface tension;
(v) other biocidal factors operating;
(vi) presence of biocidal substances.

In practice one organism (e.g. *Pseudomonas*, yeast, mould) may so establish itself that it 'gets away' and the material becomes virtually a pure culture. If this organism is dangerous or affects the life of the product, disaster is inevitable.

PRACTICAL ASPECTS: PROCEDURES IN THE FACTORY

Control of raw materials

All materials used in cosmetics should be checked for quality visually, chemically and where appropriate microbiologically. Specifications to buyers should include microbiological standards where necessary. It may be possible to blend, improve or 'top up' the chemical or functional quality of a crude ingredient, but it is often not possible or practicable to improve the microbiological quality without damaging the product. A defect of this nature can persist right through the processing and packaging to retail sale and use.

Formulation and preservation

In general it is always better to prevent microbiological growth by formulation rather than by relying on preservatives. These, like antioxidants, are rarely completely satisfactory for a prolonged period, especially with warm ambient temperatures, whereas control by formulation (i.e. by physical and chemical means) lasts indefinitely. No organism can grow without nutrients but almost anything organic can act as a nutrient for some organisms. Physical factors are highly specific for particular types of organism, e.g. acidity for most bacteria but not for yeasts or moulds, absence of oxygen for obligate aerobes, aerobic conditions for anaerobes. A useful measure of control can be exercised by designing formulation, processing and cleansing methods with particular reference to the type of infection to which the product is most vulnerable.

Temperature control

Temperature is in practice the most important factor controlling the growth of bacteria, and so the safety and keeping quality of the product, assuming satisfactory hygiene. Two of the biggest mistakes made in factory practice are to assume that dial thermometers and recorders are always accurate, and that calculations made in respect of heat transfer under ordinary conditions also apply in hot weather. Both these fallacious assumptions have led to major catastrophes in more than one industry.

All working (dial) thermometers should be checked against a known accurate thermometer *in the laboratory*. Mercury in glass thermometers should never be used in the factory.

All cooling systems should be calculated allowing for an atmospheric temperature of 27°C and a mains water temperature of 20°C, or alternatively provision made for additional cooling capacity in hot weather.

Design of equipment

In the food industries it took a whole generation to convince engineers that micro-organisms existed and could spoil a product. Early types of equipment were often a paradise for bacteria with their multiplicity of dead ends, crevices, unhygienic joints, indiscriminate use of absorbent materials, etc. and the impossibility of cleaning and sterilizing them.

In early educational work we laid down as a basic principle that all equipment for materials of biological perishability had to be dismantled daily and each item individually cleaned before sterilization. There was even equipment on the market for this purpose which could not be dismantled.

Fortunately engineers have now received the message and equipment in this field today is practically all well designed and hygienically constructed.

Sterilization of equipment by heat

Heat is usually applied as hot water, steam at atmospheric pressure (e.g. in a steam chest) or under pressure (e.g. in an autoclave) usually at 15 lb/sq in.

Hot air requires 160°C for 3 h or 170°C for 2 h to ensure sterility of equipment or powders in thin layers.

Although heat, especially autoclaving, is still the preferred method in medical work, it is often inconvenient or impractical in industry for one or more of the following reasons:

(i) it is expensive;
(ii) it causes deterioration of materials (e.g. plastics and delicate fabrics);
(iii) it causes distortion in equipment (e.g. pipelines and gaskets);
(iv) considerable time is taken to heat and to cool;
(v) residues may be baked on unless the equipment is thoroughly cleaned;
(vi) inefficient heating may result in the incubation of micro-organisms in inaccessible parts of the equipment.

In general, it may be asserted that heating a liquid for a few seconds at 75°C will destroy non-thermoduric vegetative cells, at 90°C all vegetative cells, and at 130-140°C all cells including spores. When considering surfaces, even of such easily cleansed materials as glass and polished stainless steel, a more drastic treatment is necessary, mainly because of the possible presence of very thin, invisible films of soiling matter which are often present although the utensil or equipment appears to be clean. Rubber and similar materials are extremely difficult to clean and sterilize. Thus Anderson, Sage and Spaulding (3) showed that it is necessary to hold contaminated rubber nipples in boiling water for 5 min to destroy *C. albicans*, although a few seconds at 100°C is sufficient to destroy it in milk (4).

Sterilization by chemicals

Broadly speaking there are four ways of chemically sterilizing equipment:

(i) cleaning by a detergent (e.g. alkali) and then sterilization by a sterilant (e.g. hypochlorite) or a quaternary ammonium compound (QAC),
(ii) cleaning by a stronger concentration of a detergent-sterilant followed by sterilization by a weaker concentration (e.g. iodophors)
(iii) cleaning and sterilizing by a detergent-sterilant (e.g. QAC+alkali) followed by a 'sterile rinse' (e.g. QAC or hypochlorite).

(iv) using a single substance which has powerful cleaning and sterilizing properties (e.g. sodium hydroxide or nitric acid) followed by a sterile rinse.

Inter-relationship between detergents and sterilants

In practice it is impossible to dissociate the action of a detergent from that of a sterilant. All detergents have some killing power in addition to their ability to remove most of the micro-organisms from a surface by cleaning which effects mechanical removal. Some sterilants exert a detergent action by chemically attacking a constituent of the soil, e.g. hypochlorites accelerate the degradation of proteins, and dilute acids can dissolve the calcium salts in heated milk deposits and hard water scale and so disintegrate a strongly adhering film.

The action of a detergent is complex. The main aspects are chemical hydrolysis of fat and protein, wetting of the equipment surface, solution of certain constituents, and, when an oxidizing agent such as chlorine, iodine, nitric acid, percarbonate or hydrogen peroxide is present, destruction of substances by oxidation. The combined effect of these activities is to disintegrate and loosen the soil so that it can be washed away.

Bactericidal action of detergents

Many detergents have marked germicidal properties although they are used primarily as detergents, and this may be the only claim made by manufacturers of proprietary products. Hot water at 60-80 °C will kill most or all vegetative cells but few spores. A detergent will always enhance the killing effect of heat. Probably the best example is sodium hydroxide. A treatment of 63 °C for 30 min in water will kill all bacteria except thermoduric ones and spores, but a 1–3% NaOH solution under these conditions will kill all thermoduric cells and a considerable proportion of spores.

Detergents are almost invariably used hot and so act by enhancing the bactericidal effect of heat. This effect is especially valuable against spores in those industrial applications, e.g. bottle-washing followed by cold filling, where excessive temperatures have to be avoided.

Detergent-sterilants are particularly useful where high temperatures cannot be used, as in manual dishwashing or because of delicacy of the material.

According to Monori and Varga (5) even apparently innocuous detergents such as the anionics, non-ionics and trisodium phosphate can exert a powerful killing effect against most pathogens but not against tubercle bacilli or spores.

The effectiveness of alkaline detergents can be improved by incorporation of anionic wetting agents if foaming problems are not likely to arise. The alkyl-aryl sulphonates may improve not only wetting, emulsifying and deflocculating but also the bactericidal action (6).

It is generally accepted that there is no reliable method of testing efficiency of detergent action suitable for application under all conditions or relevant to all problems, although standard test methods for *detergents* as such can be devised.

Comparison of sterilants

All sterilants have their characteristic advantages and disadvantages, and it is quite unsound to attempt to compare them unless consideration is given to the conditions of use.

The following factors should be taken into consideration when deciding on the best method for sterilizing equipment:

(a) Material of construction. Stainless steel and glass are best from the hygiene point of view (7).

(b) Adequacy of supply of steam and/or hot water (85-90°C).

(c) Time available for cleaning and sterilizing. A quick turnover (e.g. for a tanker) may make the use of steam impossible.

(d) Type of equipment, e.g. large tank, long pipeline, equipment susceptible to heat distortion.

The advantages and disadvantages of heat and chemical sterilizing methods are summarized in *Table II* (8).

Recommendations for choice of sterilant are given in *Table III* (8).

Chlorine compounds are particularly indicated where a quick drastic action is required.

The QAC are not recommended where serious gram-negative contamination is possible, or where rinsing is difficult, e.g. where surfaces are rough or absorbent. One danger with QAC preparations is that they may be used as detergents although they are sold only as a sterilant.

Table II.
Sterilizing agents—advantages and disadvantages

	Steam	Hot water (90°C)	Chlorine-releasing compounds	Quaternary ammonium compounds	Iodophors
Cost	Varies	Varies	Low	High	Intermediate
Convenience	Depends on lay-out	Recirculatory system necessary	Very convenient	Very convenient	Very convenient
Penetration	Good if adequate supply	Good	Clean plant essential	Clean plant essential	Has detergent action
Heating effect	Tanks, etc. may require hours to cool. Undesirable stresses may be set up	Less than steam	None	According to temperature	None
Suitability	Very suitable for enclosed systems and small articles in chests	Very suitable for pipelines	All purposes	All purposes	All purposes
Persistence	Not persistent	Not persistent	Not persistent	Persistent	Not persistent
Corrosion	None	None	Very corrosive unless maintained at pH 9 or above	None	Not corrosive if thoroughly rinsed away
Odour	None	None	Marked	None	None below 50°C
Rinsing	Unnecessary	Unnecessary	Good rinsing essential	Good rinsing essential	Good rinsing essential

All chemical sterilants can be corrosive if improperly used, e.g. at too high a concentration, at too high a temperature, for too long, and/or not adequately rinsed away.

Table III.
Recommendations on types of sterilant

Sterilant	Circumstances where indicated	Circumstances where inadvisable
Hypochlorites, chlorocyanuric acids and sodium phosphate hypochlorite.	Where drastic action required. Where low cost is important. Where all types of micro-organisms are likely to be encountered. Where alkaline detergent required	Where odour inadvisable. Where corrosion likely

Continued page 59

TABLE III.—*Continued*

Sterilant	Circumstances where indicated	Circumstances where inadvisable
Quaternary ammonium compounds	Where odour, taste and toxicity to be avoided. Where safety in use important. Where gram-positive organisms chief danger. Where alkaline detergent desired.	Where low cost important. Where gram-negative organisms a likely danger. Where rinsing difficult (e.g. rough surfaces)
Iodophors	Where calcium scale a problem	With galvanized iron
Ortho-phenyl-phenol	For equipment not coming into contact with food	
Nitric acid	Where calcium scale a problem	Where equipment not all stainless steel. Where strong acid dangerous. Where fat-protein films a special problem
Hexachlorophene	Where contact with hands, etc. possible. In toilet preparations, etc.	Not for food equipment
Chlorhexidine	As 'antiseptic'.	Where cost important
Amphoterics	Where neutral conditions required	"

Detergent-sterilants and their use

A detergent-sterilant is required to carry out the following operations:

(i) Remove all soil.

(ii) Remove or kill all pathogens and potential pathogens.

(iii) Remove or kill all fault-producing organisms (FPO).

(iv) Reduce bacteria to 1 per sq cm surface area or per ml cubic capacity.

The main fields of application for detergent-sterilants are given in *Table IV*.

Table IV.

Applications of detergent-sterilants for sanitizing equipment

1. In general for all cleansing purposes where heat cannot be used, e.g. walls, floors, wooden and plastic table tops, refrigerators, cold stores, etc.
2. The food industries, particularly for equipment for perishable foods such as milk and the more vulnerable foods such as meat, poultry, fish and eggs.
3. Medical and surgical activities: hospitals, clinics, surgeries, etc.
4. Sanitary aspects of communal activities: schools, colleges, catering, swimming and shower baths, public lavatories, public transport and all equipment communally used.
5. Institution maintenance cleaning.
6. Domestic: dishwashing, babies' and children's items particularly in nurseries, etc.
7. Cleaning or washing operations where heat cannot be employed: manual operations, delicate fabrics, plastics, etc.
8. Agriculture: particularly dairy farms, animal pens and all equipment wherever animals are involved.
9. Sanitation generally: wherever potentially dangerous material is handled as in slaughter houses, disposal of offal and refuse, etc.
10. Sewage disposal and all operations involving obnoxious material.

In general, detergent-sterilants, like chemical sterilants, are particularly useful where for any reason heat cannot be used, or is expensive or inconvenient.

The value of changing methods and sterilants

Particular methods, and particular chemical formulations are often specially good for certain purposes and against particular types of organism. The consistent use of one method and/or one formulation may lead to a weakness in the overall system because of a slow film build-up (too slight to be noticed) or acclimatization by a particular organism, e.g. coli, spore-former or yeast.

The types of organism surviving on equipment depend on the nature of the soil and the sanitizing method used. It is therefore strongly recommended that at intervals, say once weekly, a different method should be used. For in-place cleaning systems it may not be convenient or economic to change the system drastically, e.g. use steam or hot water instead of hypochlorite, but it is usually possible to change the type of detergent and/or sterilant.

In-place or circulation cleaning

The scale of operations in factories today and the shortage and cost of manpower have revolutionized our attitude to cleaning and sterilizing. The classical idealist methods would be impossible today, and all relevant industries have gone, or are rapidly going over to in-place cleaning. Provided *all* the equipment is suitably designed for this purpose, the method can be entirely successful. The usual system is a closed circuit with spray devices for tanks. A minimum velocity to give turbulent flow in pipelines, and properly formulated detergents and sterilants are essential. Permanent tanks for these solutions, regular laboratory control and automation allow such systems to operate with very little man-power although capital cost may be high.

The problem of emulsions

In addition to the purely physical and chemical problems associated with the formulation of emulsions there will often be microbiological problems. Three phases may be involved—the continuous phase (usually aqueous), the discontinuous phase (usually fatty) and possibly an adsorbed layer phase which may have considerable significance for organisms. This third phase may act as a powerfully adsorbing film for bacterial nutrients and a focus for bacterial clumps or colonies.

Homogenization may lead to biological troubles because clusters of micro-organisms are broken up and the cells dispersed throughout the medium. Homogenizers are also difficult to clean and sterilize.

Emulsions of water in oil are much more stable microbiologically than the reverse, as the organisms are confined to their own water globule. If these globules are very small (a few microns) growth appears to be halted rapidly and the organisms die out.

Unsuspected reservoirs of contamination

When all reasonable precautions have been taken but there still occur sporadic and serious outbreaks of infection the cause is probably an unsuspected reservoir of contamination. The following explanations have been found in factory practice:

(i) poor communication between management and staff;
(ii) poor supervision, especially early in the morning;
(iii) bad hygienic design of equipment or lay-out;
(iv) changes in cleaning/sterilizing procedure to reduce costs;
(v) rapid staff turnover;
(vi) making assumptions without laboratory tests to check them.

Filtration and clarification

When a liquid product has to be cleared of suspended particles, filtration is usually adopted because clarification is expensive and may be impossible. It should be realized however that, if the product is of poor microbiological stability, filtration may do nothing to improve this, and may even worsen it because all the material is forced through a layer of suspended matter which may be building up a substantial bacterial population. Filter cloths or pads should be renewed frequently for this reason, and double alternating filters preceded by fine mesh strainers are to be recommended where the nature of the product makes this desirable.

The size of micro-organisms

One difficulty in teaching hygiene to operatives, and even to factory floor management, is to convince people of the size of bacteria. To talk about microns is meaningless to them. A simple analogy is to point out that if a bacterium were magnified to the size of a man, then the man would have to be magnified to the size of Great Britain to maintain the proportion. No system of filtration practicable for large volumes of liquids can be relied on to remove all bacteria, although yeasts and moulds, being about 10 times the size (diameter) can usually be removed to a considerable extent.

Factory water supplies

The bacteriological purity of water is generally judged on the basis of the Ministry of Health Memo No. 71 which assesses potability by the presumptive and faecal coli tests, supported by total colony counts at 22 and 37°C. Many years' experience has proved the validity of this method, but potability is not the same as quality for a particular industrial purpose. Defects in cosmetic and other preparations may be caused by *Pseudomonas* and similar Gram-negative bacteria, yeasts, moulds and other types of no public health significance. The hazards for water, which is drunk, and for cosmetics, which are applied to *and remain on the skin*, are quite different. The latter include *Staphylococcus aureus, Pseudomonas aeruginosa*, and various skin pathogens which are usually completely ignored in public health water bacteriology. A further fallacy is the assumption that water as used *in* the factory is as pure as water supplied *to* the factory. Storage in tanks and passage through pipelines, pumps, filters, softeners, etc. may easily result in gross contamination. Unless constant testing shows that the water is of adequate purity, mild chlorination (2-5 ppm) is recommended. For a survey of problems and control methods see Davis (9).

Hands as a source of infection

Apart from obviously bad air conditions, contamination or infection of a product is always caused by contact. Of all the ways in which this can occur, there is little doubt that in practice the hands are the commonest means whereby a product becomes contaminated by a pathogenic organism. Skin is impossible to sterilize and the bacterial load may vary from a few thousands to a few millions. *Staphylococci* and enterobacteria are nearly always found (10).

Biological control of pathogens and fault-producing organisms

Considerable success has been achieved in agriculture and in some branches of medicine by using biological control to eliminate pests. The usual method is to liberate one type of living organism that is predatory on the pest. Little has been done in this direction in industry, although it is well known that by the use of 'starters', e.g. in cheesemaking, undesirable organisms can usually be suppressed. It has been observed in some fields of work that there may be an inverse relationship between the numbers of a harmful and of an innocuous organism. Thus we have observed this type of inverse relationship between *Staph. aureus* and *Staph. albus* in foods, and such a relationship may also be found on the skin. This type of approach to problems of infection is largely an unexplored field.

Hygienic packaging

The glass bottle is still the favoured container in the cosmetics, milk and other industries, and likely to remain so for some time. Glass is the most hygienic (i.e. most easily cleansed) of all common materials (7) although it is heavy, fragile and susceptible to neglect and sabotage. It has the advantages of transparency, cheapness (if re-used) and does not have to be imported.

Blow-moulded plastics bottles are gaining favour in the soft drinks and other industries. They are very light, cheap, strong, non-fragile, reasonably rigid and initially sterile by virtue of their method of manufacture which involves a temperature of *ca.* 180 °C. Their use is certain to increase.

The plastics sachet is the lightest and cheapest of all single service containers, but is experiencing some consumer resistance, as of course do all new ventures. It is likely to be the container of the future for many liquid and solid products.

Some progress has been made in the use of sterilizable plastics sachets (11).

General precautions in hygiene, etc.

The most efficient cleansing of equipment is easily invalidated if unhygienic methods are practised subsequently.

The following points should be observed:

(i) Check the quality of all raw materials.

(ii) Unpack raw materials in a separate building, especially if embedded in sawdust, cotton waste, straw, etc.

(iii) Apply a biocidal treatment where necessary if this is practicable. Controlled heat-treatment is usually the simplest and most reliable.

(iv) Control the quality of water *as used in the factory.*
(v) Check the bacterial purity of the air near fillers, etc.
(vi) Check the hygienic condition of all containers.
(vii) Remove all residues, broken or split containers, etc., as soon as possible.
(viii) Do not use cloths for mopping up spillages unless these are maintained in a clean condition. Such cloths can be a menace. Paper towels are much better (12).
(ix) Thoroughly clean equipment *immediately after* use.
(x) Sterilize or cleanse all equipment, as may be necessary, *immediately before* use.

Common fallacies in hygiene

Some common fallacies experienced in commercial life are the assumptions that:
(i) splashing disinfectant over floors, etc. solves the hygiene problem,
(ii) forcing steam through a circuit with the production of great clouds of 'steam' and considerable noise necessarily sterilizes the equipment,
(iii) if equipment looks clean, then it must be clean. This is not true microbiologically,
(iv) 'Window dressing devices' such as making people wear white coats and caps, UV lamps, use of disinfectant aerosols, may serve some useful purpose and undoubtedly exert a psychological influence, but in terms of real worth are not quantitatively very important. Thorough cleaning of all equipment and prevention of contact contamination constitute 99% of factory hygiene.

Air

Most quality controllers in factories have their views as to how the purity of air should be maintained, both for the staff and the product. An air conditioning system which controls temperature, humidity and removes micro-organisms by filtration and/or electrostatic means is by far the best, but is quite expensive.

For the product, as distinct from the staff, an aerosol or fog treatment is the simplest and cheapest, but the choice of biocide is a tricky problem. Chlorine (as hypochlorite) is cheap and effective, but very corrosive.

Formaldehyde is also cheap and effective but very unpleasant for the staff, and somewhat corrosive. It causes eye, nose and throat reactions at 2-3 ppm. Up to 5 ppm can be tolerated for a few minutes, but at 10 ppm it becomes almost unbearable (13).

Fogs of QAC solutions appear to be both effective, cheap and without objection. Little or nothing is known of the effect of repeated inhalation of minute concentrations of QAC (e.g. 1 ppm) but in general they can be regarded as non-toxic. There has been some scare in medical circles about the use of benzene compounds in hygienic measures on account of possible carcinogenic effects, but there appears to be no real evidence for this. For example, the toxicity of benzoic acid is low. It there is any apprehension over the benzyl QAC a twin chain (C_8 or C_{10}) compound may be equally or even more effective.

Walls, roofs and air in factories

These problems are inter-related because whatever organisms may occur on one will be found on the others. Clearly the factory air cannot be free from contamination which occurs on walls and roofs, or is present in air outside the factory.

Moulds, yeasts and algae grow readily on any surface if the RH is over 70% and the merest trace of nutrients is present. The first precaution is therefore to maintain adequate ventilation and at all cost to prevent condensation at any time. Such condensate can be teeming with gram-negative bacteria including coliforms and *Pseudomonas*. The simplest and best treatment for soiled walls and other surfaces is to wet them and 1 h later to apply a penetrative, non-foaming, alkaline detergent by a spray or other suitable means. This will clean the surfaces and exercise a substantial killing effect, but in order to obtain an effective kill a suitable bactericide-fungicide must be incorporated in the detergent. If the wall, etc., has been allowed to get into bad condition, repeated treatments will be necessary.

Needless to say, all walls, etc. in a cosmetics factory should have a smooth, impervious and washable surface.

Methodology in hygiene

Practical recommendations for cleaning, sterilizing and hygiene in public health and various industries are given in (14–19).

One of the most serious problems in the teaching of the principles of hygiene and their application is that there is no glamour, no excitement and no romance in such a subject.

Heart transplants, human organ banks, the fertilization of the human ovum outside the uterus and similar topics hit the headlines, but at the most these advances save an occasional life or prolong a few lives for a few months. On the other hand hygiene has saved millions of lives and prevented many millions of cases of disease. The dramatic rise in the expectation of life during the past 100 years is mainly due to the application of hygienic principles. No branch of medicine or science has contributed more to human health and happiness.

Laboratory control

Laboratory control of cleaning and sterilizing

The choice of a particular method is less important than regular testing. The ultimate criterion must always be the keeping quality and safety of the product, and it is usually easy to link the hygiene aspects in the factory with the quality of the products. The 'first product through' test, swabbings, rinsings or any other sound method is adequate for both staff training and protecting the quality of the product (16).

An important feature in hygiene control is that tests should be surprise tests; the staff should never know when a particular piece of equipment is going to be checked. A rigid and known time-table for plant control defeats its own object.

Laboratory tests are useless unless they are acted upon. I have known of a case where the head of the laboratory put his reports on the manager's desk daily, but it was not until the poor quality of the product was revealed later that the manager studied the reports.

The testing of disinfectants, antiseptics and preservatives

The high degree of competitiveness in this field results in many far-reaching claims being made by manufacturers and salesmen. Unfortunately it is not possible to assess the validity of these claims without a careful examination by an expert with adequate bacteriological facilities, a process which is time-consuming and expensive. There is no single, reliable test which can be applied to any of these preparations. Results vary considerably according to the technique used, and the cynic might with some reason assert that one can get almost any result one likes by selection of the conditions of testing. The only ultimate criterion which is of any value to the user is whether the substance fulfils the claims made for it under the condition of use. Any laboratory test used should therefore simulate as closely as possible these conditions.

Choice of end-point

It should be realized that there is nothing definite about disinfectant studies; everything is arbitrary. Such terms as 'complete kill' or '99.99 per per cent kill' are quite arbitrary and can only be defined in terms of the particular technique used.

There are many factors capable of affecting the result of any disinfectant test, irrespective of its nature (*Table V*). In a laboratory test, these can at least be standardized but under conditions of use such factors may

Table V.

Factors influencing the result of any disinfectant test

1. Type of organism (e.g. *Staph. aureus*)
2. Particular strain used
3. Physiological condition—long term (e.g. how long in artificial culture)
4. Physiological condition—short term (e.g. 24 h at 37°C)
5. Composition of medium used for growth (e.g. nutrient broth)
6. Physical state of medium used for growth (e.g. agar medium)
7. Temperature, humidity, etc. of growth
8. Concentration of disinfectant
9. Stability of disinfectant to moisture, oxygen, etc.
10. Temperature of test
11. Time of contact
12. pH value
13. Osmotic pressure
14. Synergistic effects with other substances, e.g. acids, surfactants, salts.
15. Concomitant substances (e.g. in hard water); compatibility with other substances present
16. Physical nature of suspending fluid, e.g. emulsion
17. Surface tension of suspending liquid (e.g. Teepol)
18. Nature of solvent (e.g. part isopropyl alcohol)
19. Method of mixing disinfectant and cells
20. Type, physical nature and concentration of soiling matter
21. Choice and concentration of inactivator (e.g. Lubrol W)
22. Medium for growing survivors
23. Incubation temperature for plates

Surface film tests

24. Soiling material used (e.g. whole milk)
25. Method of fixing to surface (e.g. drying at 37°C)
26. Chemical nature of surface used (e.g. stainless steel)
27. Condition of surface (e.g. highly polished)

vary considerably, e.g. temperature, time of contact, nature and amount of soilage, hardness of water.

Reports of microbiological examinations

In my opinion many reports and claims for disinfectant power, etc. by manufacturers, are unscientific and even sloppy. Such statements as 'kills typhoid in 2 min', 'coli absent', etc., are meaningless, and in fact may even be misleading. The conditions of testing should always be stated, and reports should state results in a form such as 'coli not detected in 1 ml', etc.

Some recommended microbiological control methods for cosmetic products are given in *Table VI*.

Table VI.
Recommended bacteriological control methods for cosmetic products

Organism	Medium		Temperature °C
Total (public health)	Blood agar		37
Total (general)	Glucose tryptone agar		27
Staphylococcus aureus	Mannitol salt (21)		37
	Egg yolk (22)		37
	Phenol phthalein phosphate (23)		37
Pseudomonas aeruginosa	Acetamide agar (24)		37 (42)
	Cetrimide agar (39)		37
Presumptive coliforms	MacConkey broth		30
	Eosin methylene blue agar (25)	*Escherichia* and *Aerobacter* can be differentiated on these media	30
	Violet red bile agar (26)		30
Faecal coli (follow-up tests)	MacConkey broth	(both must be used)	44
	Peptone water		44
Candida albicans, yeasts and moulds	Malt agar pH 5.4		27
Yeasts and moulds	Malt or buffered beerwort agar pH 3.5 (27)		27
	Buffered citric acid agar pH 3.5 (28)		27
Streptococcus faecalis	Crystal violet azide blood agar (29)		37
Salmonella	Selenite broth (for enrichment) (30)		37 (43)
	Desoxycholate (31)		
	Brilliant green (32) or		
	Bismuth sulphite agar (33)		37
	Kligler iron agar (32), (35)) or		37
	Kohn-Gillies broths (36), (37)		
	Final serological confirmation		
Clostridium spores	Meat broth		37
	Reinforced clostridial medium (38)		37

Oxoid or Difco media (see Manuals issued by these firms)

Microbiological standards

There is now considerable interest in microbiological standards for foods and some other products. This is a subject into which which no-one should enter without experience of the product as well as a knowledge of microbiology. It is very easy to lay down standards which are impracticable, unnecessary or even just ridiculous. The basic requirements are

(i) careful standardization of all aspects of sampling, transporting and storage of the sample,
(ii) standardization of laboratory testing,
(iii) consideration of age of product,
(iv) allowance for error of test,
(v) selection of appropriate tests,
(vi) proper interpretation of results.

Standards should only be advisory, and are mainly a matter between buyer and seller. They can be particularly useful for purchasers of basic materials. For general quality control purposes standards set for production in the factory must be related to the microbiological behaviour of the product between production and final use.

Some suggested standards are given in *Table VII*.

In U.S.A. the F.D.A. have become very concerned with the problem of microbiological contamination of cosmetics, especially in relation to *Ps. aeruginosa*. It can be anticipated that they will shortly issue standards for this purpose, which will obviously be of the greatest importance for the British export trade.

Table VII.
Tentative microbiological standards for cosmetic preparations g^{-1} or ml^{-1}

	Satisfactory	Doubtful	Unsatisfactory
Total colony count*	<1 000	1 000-10 000	> 10 000
Presumptive coliforms*	< 10	10- 100	> 100
Faecal coli	< 1	1- 10	> 10
*Staph. aureus**	< 1	1- 10	> 10
*Ps. aeruginosa**	< 1	1- 10	> 10
Salmonella		Not detectable in 100 g	
Fault producing organisms		Impossible to generalise	

* = first priority in laboratory control work.

Tests and standards for the efficiency of cleansing

Cleansing consists of two treatments—physical cleaning and sterilization or disinfection. There is a steady trend towards combining these.

Cleaning or detergency

There is usually no need to assess this alone, or to set standards.

If required, an assessment of residual organic matter can be obtained by allowing contact with a reactive chemical, e.g. chlorine, for a given time and then determining the loss in available chlorine.

A simple 'spot test' is to take advantage of the fact that iodine, as in iodophors, stains organic matter a yellowish colour. Iodophors do *not* stain clean glass, stainless steel, etc., although allegations have been made to this effect. Any staining indicates a greasy or protein film, hard water scale, etc.

Residual bacteria or 'sterility'

If equipment has been properly cleaned and 'sterilized' the number of bacteria left will not exceed 1 per cm^2 area by a swab test or 1 per ml capacity by a rinse test (14). These tests are therefore quite adequate to assess the efficiency of cleansing in a general sense. It can be assumed under ordinary working conditions that if these results are satisfactory (i.e. less than 1 colony per cm^2 or ml) then all pathogens will have been killed or removed. It is also unlikely that FPO will have survived in sufficient numbers to cause trouble, but as a safeguard 1 000 cm^2 may be swabbed and the 20 ml Ringer solution added to a suitable enrichment medium (*Table VI*) for the cultivation of specific pathogens or FPO.

Alternatively 5 ml could be added to

(i) mannitol salt broth (for *Staphylococcus*),

(ii) selenite broth (for *Salmonella*),

(iii) acetamide broth (for *Pseudomonas aeruginosa*),

(iv) buffered citric acid broth pH 3.5 (for yeasts and moulds),

(the appropriate confirmatory tests must be made) but such a refinement is only necessary when a relevant problem arises.

(Received: 4th September 1970)

REFERENCES

(1) Infantile gastroenteritis. *Brit. Med. J.* **3** 2 (1970).

(2) Johnson, S. A. M., Guzman, M. G. and Aguilera, C. T. Candida (Monilia) albicans. Effect of amino acids, glucose, pH, chlortetracycline, dibasic sodium and calcium phosphates and anaerobic and aerobic conditions on its growth. *Arch. Dermatol. Syphilol. Chicago* **70** 49 (1954).

(3) Anderson, N. A., Sage, D. N. and Spaulding, E. H. Oral moniliasis in newborn infants. *Am. J. Dis. Child.* **67** 450 (1944).

(4) Ludlam, G. B. and Henderson, J. L. Neonatal thrush in a maternity hospital. *Lancet*, **i**, 64 (1942).

(5) Monori, S. and Varga, E. Antimicrobial effect of some cleaning materials used in the food industry. *Budapesti Muszaki Egyet. Elm. Kem. Tansz., D S.A.* **26**, 2211 (1962).

(6) Knafelman, P. Improving the effectiveness of detergents. *Mol. Prom.*, **24** 29 (1963). D.S.A. **26** 684.

(7) Davis, J. G. The cleansability of various materials. *Medical Officer*, **110** 299 (1963).

(8) Davis, J. G. "Chemical sterilization" in *Prog. Industr. Microbiol.* ed. Hockenhull **8** 141 (1968). (Churchill, London).

(9) Davis, J. G. The microbiological control of water in dairies and food factories. *Proc. Soc. Water Treat. Exam.* **8** 31 (1959)
(10) Davis, J. G., Blake, J. R. and Woodall, C. M. The types and numbers of bacteria left on hands after normal washing and drying by various common methods. *Medical Officer*, **122** 235 (1969).
(11) Davis, J. G. Packaging of foodstuffs in sterilisable plastics. *Food Processing Industry*, **47** (September 1970).
(12) Davis, J. G., Blake, J. R. and Woodall, C. M. A survey of the hygienic conditions of dishcloths and tea-towels. *Medical Officer*, **120** 29 (1968).
(13) Fassett, D. W. and Irish, D. D. (ed.). *Patty's Industrial Hygiene and Toxicology* 2nd edn. **2** (1970).
(14) Berger, H. and Illingworth, R. S. (ed.). *Infant hygiene*, (1971). Thema-Verlag, Stuttgart.
(15) Davis, J. G. *A dictionary of dairying* (1955, 1965). (International Textbook, London).
(16) Davis, J. G. *Laboratory control of dairy plant* (1956). (Dairy Industries, London).
(17) Fox, A. (ed.) *Hygiene in the food industry* (1971). (Churchill, London).
(18) Hobbs, B. C. Health problems in quality control in *Quality control in the food industry* (ed. Herschdoerfer) (1967). (Academic Press, London).
(19) Hobbs, B. C. *Food poisoning and food hygiene* (1968). (Arnold, London).
(20) BS. 3286 1960: Method for laboratory evaluation of disinfectant activity of quaternary ammonium compounds. *Brit. Stand. Inst., London.*
(21) Chapman, G. H. The significance of sodium chloride in studies of staphylococci. *J. Bacteriol.* **50** 201 (1945).
(22) Baird-Parker, A. C. An improved diagnostic and selective medium for isolating coagulase-positive staphylococci. *J. Appl. Bacteriol.* **25** 12, 441 (1962).
(23) Barber, M. and Kuper, S W. A. Identification of Staphylococcus pyogenes by the phosphatase reaction. *J. Path. Bacteriol.* **63** 65 (1951).
(24) Hedberg, M. Acetamide agar medium selective for Pseudomonas aeruginosa. *Appl. Microbiol.* **17** 481 (1969).
(25) Levine, M. Differentiation of B. coli and B. aerogenes on a simplified eosin methylene blue agar. *J. Infect. Dis.* **23** 43 (1918).
(26) Druce, R. G., Bebbington, N. B., Elson, K., Harcombe, J. M. and Thomas, S. B. The determination of the coli-aerogenes content of milk and dairy equipment by plating on violet red bile agar incubated at 30°C. *J. Appl. Bacteriol.* **20** 1 (1957).
(27) Davis, J. G. Standardisation of media in the acid ranges with special reference to the use of citric acid and buffer mixtures for yeast and mould media. *J. Dairy Res.* **3** 133 (1931).
(28) Davis, J. G. A convenient, semi-synthetic medium for yeast and mould counts. *Laboratory Practice*, **7** 30 (1958).
(29) Packer, R. A. The use of sodium azide and crystal violet in a selective medium for streptococci and Erysipelothrix rhusiopathiae. *J. Bacteriol.* **46** 343 (1943).
(30) Leifson, E. A new selenite enrichment medium for the isolation of typhoid and paratyphoid (Salmonella) bacilli. *Am. J. Hyg.* **24** 423 (1936).
(31) Hynes, M. The isolation of intestinal pathogens by selective media. *J. Path. Bacteriol.* **54** 193 (1942).
(32) Kaufman, F. Further experiences with combined enrichment methods for salmonella bacteria. *Z. Hyg.* **117** 26 (1935).
(33) Cook, G. T. Comparison of two modifications of bismuth sulphite agar for the isolation and growth of Salmonella typhi and Salmonella typhimurium. *J. Path. Bacteriol.* **64** 559 (1952).
(34) Kligler, I. J. A simple medium for the differentiation of members of the typhoid-paratyphoid group. *Am. J. Public Health*, **7** 1042 (1917).
(35) Kligler, I. J. Modifications of culture media used in the isolation and differentiation of typhoid, dysentery and allied bacilli. *J. Exptl. Med.* **28** 319 (1918).
(36) Kohn, J. A two-tube technique for the identification of organisms of the Enterobacteriaceae group. *J. Path. Bacteriol.* **67** 286 (1954).
(37) Gillies, R. R. An evaluation of two composite media for preliminary identification of Shigella and Salmonella. *J. Clin. Pathol.* **9** 368 (1956).
(38) Hirsch, A. and Grinstead, E. Methods for the growth and enumeration of anaerobic spore-formers from cheese, with observations on the effect of nisin. *J. Dairy Res.* **21** 101 (1954).
(39) Drake, C. H. Evaluation of culture media for the isolation and enumeration of Pseudomonas aeruginosa. *Health Lab. Sci.* **3** 10 (1966).

Editor's Comments on Paper 31

In this article the authors discuss the high degree of resistance of bacterial spores and attempt to show some of the difficulties one may encounter in chemical sterilization where they are present. The chemical and physical characteristics of spores are discussed and methods are presented for evaluating the effectiveness of sporicidal agents as chemosterilizers.

31

4

THE SPORE PROBLEM

PAUL M. BORICK, Ph.D.
ETHICON, INC.
SOMERVILLE, NEW JERSEY

ROLLIN E. PEPPER, Ph.D.
ELIZABETHTOWN COLLEGE
ELIZABETHTOWN, PENNSYLVANIA

I. INTRODUCTION

Spores are highly resistant to present methods of sterilization, i.e., heat, irradiation, or chemicals and their elimination presents a major problem to the microbiologist. Writers of textbooks in microbiology hasten to point out that although vegetative bacterial and fungal cells may be rapidly destroyed by either physical or chemical means, many conditions must be satisfied to assure sporicidal activity. Oginsky and Umbreit(*37*) stated that spore formation, a fortress type of defense, is a restricted mechanism. The capacity of certain microbial cells to form spores gives them a selective status and poses a real problem in disinfection.

Borick(*8*) has shown that although numerous antimicrobial agents are available for use, only a few, e.g., formaldehyde, glutaraldehyde and ethylene oxide, among others, are truly sporicidal and, thus, can be used as chemosterilizers. Alcohol, although frequently used as an antimicrobial agent is not sporicidal; it is frequently employed to maintain spore suspensions. Certain chemical compounds inhibit bacterial growth but are not able to kill microbial spores. To cite an example, methyl-2-cyanoacrylate, a chemical adhesive, was reported by Awe et al.(*4*) to be both bacteriostatic and bactericidal, but Page and Borick(*39*) were able to recover both aerobic and anaerobic spores from the polymer when the material was aseptically transferred to appropriate culture media.

The resistance of spores differs within the microbial population and species variation is common. Some strains of *Bacillus subtilis* spores are rapidly destroyed by heat, whereas others may withstand boiling temperatures for prolonged periods of time. This is also true for chemicals or irradiation used in spore destruction. It has been our experience that spores of *Bacillus globigii* were readily destroyed by chemical agents whereas *B. subtilis* or *B. stearothermophilus* spores were more difficult to destroy. In studying the effects of cathode rays on a wide variety of spores, Pepper et al.(*40*) showed that *Clostridium tetani and B. pumilus* were destroyed by only the highest doses. When spores from the progeny of radiation-resistant isolates were subsequently exposed to cathode-ray doses identical to those received by the parent, the survival curves were similar to those of the parent. Although the progeny were destroyed at high dosages, sublethal doses can produce mutants which show higher survival rates than the parent strain. In spite of the fact that the mechanism of spore resistance is unknown, many factors associated with this phenomenon have been determined. Records of extreme longevity were provided by Sussmann and Halvorson(*56*) who showed that certain spores survived over 40 years either dry or in alcohol. Murrell and Scott(*36*) concluded from their investigations that spores have a low water content. This, too, will make spores more resistant to destruction for the drier the spore, the higher the resistance. Moisture is required for ethylene oxide or other sporicidal gases and vapors to exert their maximum effective action. Low salt concentrations in spores, however, may decrease their resistance, whereas an increase in lipoidal substances in spores increases their heat resistance. The combined use of heat and smoke may not have a detrimental effect on spores, as reported by Christiansen et al.(*20*) who recovered spores of *Cl. botulunum* from fish, smoked to an internal temperature of 180° F for 30 min. The age of the spore is another important consideration. Curran(*23*) did not achieve maximum resistance from bacterial spores until a period of maturation was completed. Heat resistance in spores appears to be associated with the presence of dipicolinic acid (DPA). Powell(*44*) showed that 5–15% of the dry weight of spores was DPA. When spore germination took place, DPA was released with a lowering of heat resistance. Russell(*50*), in attempting to describe the resistance of bacterial spores to various chemical and physical agents, concluded that spores which are highly resistant to one process are not necessarily insensitive to another process. Although this may be so, it should be pointed out that sensitivity to the process varies, and it may be necessary to experimentally determine destruction of the spore, the conditions of destruction, and the microbial types before sterility is achieved. It is the intent of this chapter to discuss some of the major problems encountered with spores, as well as to review the many factors concerned with sporicidal activity.

II. CHEMICAL AND PHYSICAL CHARACTERISTICS OF SPORES

Bacterial spores are much more resistant to adverse effects of heat and chemicals than their corresponding vegetative cells. This resistance has been extensively studied and many publications have appeared over the years on this subject. In spite of these invistigations, the nature of the spore and the cause of its resistance to adverse environmental conditions are not fully known. Consequently this subject continues to be of interest and work in this area continues to be actively pursued. There are, however, certain quantitative and qualitative chemical, as well as physical, differences between vegetative cells and spores which are well documented. In combination, it is highly probable that they are responsible for spore survival. It is not our purpose to review all the chemical and physical factors in detail; this has been done by others [Robinow(*47*), Halvorson(*27*), and Sussmann and Halvorson(*56*)]. Rather we plan to list those which seem to be most important vis-a-vis spore survival after exposure to antimicrobial agents.

First of all, the cytoplasm of the vegetative cell is surrounded by a membrane which limits exchange with the environment through active transport and the cell wall which maintains the integrity and rigidity of the cell. The wall offers only limited protection compared with the spore envelope and penetration, as well as osmotic pressures, can render the cell quite susceptible to detrimental agents. The core of the spore, however, is surrounded by a multilayered covering. Next to the core is the wall surrounded by the cortex, and as many as three spore coats. Finally there is the exosporium, enveloping all the others [Sussmann and Halvorson(*56*)]. Electron micrographs have richly demonstrated these layers; their usefulness in maintaining rigidity is amply shown by the difficulty encountered in obtaining the spore contents for study.

The presence of lipids in the spore may add to its resistance by stabilizing enzymes and by rendering it somewhat hydrophobic. Black and Gerhardt(*7*) found that the spore core is surrounded by a lipid-like substance. Accordingly lipid insoluble agents may be limited to the degree in which they can penetrate the spore. Sugiyama(*55*) reported that fatty acids added to sporulating media increase the heat resistance of spores. He suggested that the fatty acids may aid in protein stabilization since it has been shown that denaturation of protein (serum albumin) is retarded by the presence of fatty acids.

Resistant spores contain high levels of divalent metals, particularly calcium [Sugiyama(*55*)]. Additionally, spores which are produced on a calcium deficient medium are heat sensitive [Slepecky and Foster (*52*)]. Calcium may prevent the denaturation of proteins by linking negatively charged groups, thus keeping the protein chains from unfolding. As previously stated, resistant spores contain DPA, a unique substance, since it has not been reported as common in other biological forms. Above a certain temperature level, thermal resistance is directly proportional to the DPA concentration [Church and Halvorson(*21*) and Collier and Nakata(*22*)]. This can amount to approximately 10% of the dry weight of the spore. DPA chelates strongly with calcium and DPA synthesis can be correlated with calcium uptake [Powell and Strange(*45*)]. The appearance of DPA can also be correlated with the appearance of resistance and its depletion also coincides with the loss of resistance as spores germinate. It has been hypothesized [Sussmann and Halvorson(*56*)] that DPA may protect spores through a DPA-calcium-amino acid complex which could act to stabilize folded peptide chains.

Friedman and Henry(*26*), using freezing point measurements, proposed the theory that spores contain bound water as opposed to the free water in vegetative cells and their resistance to heat might be due to this difference. Using refraction indices as evidence, Ross and Billing(*48*) suggested that spores simply contain less water than vegetative cells. Black and Gerhardt(*7*) found that free water is distributed throughout the spore but that the core contains the least amount. They also suggested a new hypothesis for thermostability, postulating that there is an "occurrence of an insolubly gelled core with cross linking between macromolecules through stable but reversible bonds so as to form a high polymer matrix with entrapped free water." Although Black and Gerhardt(*7*) limited their explanation of resistance to heat, their hypothesis could just as well be extended to resistance to chemicals which attack exposed susceptible chemical groups extending from peptide chains.

Active enzymes are less common in the spore than in the vegetative cell. Using *Bacillus myocoides*, Hardwick and Foster(*28*) assayed 17 enzymes in vegetative cells, pre-spores, and spores. They reported negative results for spores although enzyme activities were quite evident in the other two forms. Stedman(*54*) reported that enzymic action did not take place in mature spores. Doi, Halvorson, and Church (*24*) found that spores of *Bacillus cereus var. terminalis* do not have hexokinase or glucokinase enzymes. However, they found that these spores were able to use a direct oxidative pathway with dissimilation occurring through the pentose shunt. Bach and Sadoff(*5*) demonstrated a heat-resistant glucose dehydrogenase in spores of *B. cereus*. Marr(*34*) listed a heat-resistant ribosidase in the spore coat, a heat-resistant alanine racemase and an adenosine deaminase, presumably outside the spore coat, and a pyrophosphatase and a heat-sensitive catalase within the spore coat. The latter two enzymes are heat resistant only when contained within the spore and since they do not act on substrates outside the spore, it is presumed that they are located within the spore coat.

Antimocrobial agents attack microorganisms in various ways. Some exert osmotic pressure, others may act as general oxidizing agents, and still others may attack specific chemical groups on peptide chains. Alcohol has been used as a general disinfectant for vegetative cells. As stated earlier, alcohol is useless as a sporicidal agent. Considering alcohol as a dehydrating agent, it can readily be seen that hydrated, actively metabolizing vegetative cells would be quite susceptible to alcohol whereas the dormant spore covered with several layers, including a lipid layer, would be resistant. Phillips (*42*) reported that spores are 10^3 to 10^4 times more resistant than vegetative cells to such agents as hypochlorites, heavy metals, phenol, and quaternaries. Such disinfectants may act at the surface or have another limited mode of action. Cationics, such as the quaternaries, adsorb onto the cell wall and disrupt the cell [Moore and Hardwick (*35*)], but this mode of action would be unlikely to affect the viability of spores. Heavy metals such as silver and mercurials react with sulfhydryl groups and, again, this may also be a surface phenomenon. Hypochlorites are oxidizing agents and, although penetration may be limited, exert a sporicidal influence. Iodine has been recognized as having sproicidal properties and has been found to react with many protein groups such as indol, imidazole, phenol, disulfide, and sulfhydryl groups [Carroll, et al. (*18*)]. The general class of alkylating agents appear to be among the strongest sporicidal agents. Phillips (*42*) reports that spores are only 2–15 times more resistant than vegetative cells to these agents as compared to a much higher resistance where other types of disinfectants are concerned. Alkylating agents include ethylene oxide, β-propiolactone, formaldehyde, and glutaraldehyde, as well as other aldehydes. Their points of attack are the sulfhydryl, hydroxyl, amino, and carboxy groups. Since many such groups would be present in spore proteins as well as in vegetative cells proteins, it is not surprising that spores are susceptible to these agents and that their resistance is only a few times greater than vegetative cells. Phillips (*42*) represented alkylation of these protein groups by ethylene oxide in the following manner:

$$\mathrm{P}\!-\!\left\{\begin{array}{l} \mathrm{-C(=O)-OH} \\ \mathrm{-NH_2} \\ \mathrm{-C_6H_4OH} \\ \mathrm{-SH} \end{array}\right. + 4\,\underset{\diagdown\ \mathrm{O}\ \diagup}{\overset{\mathrm{H\,H}}{\mathrm{HC{-}{-}{-}CH}}} \longrightarrow \mathrm{P}\!-\!\left\{\begin{array}{l} \mathrm{-C(=O)-O-CH_2-CH_2-OH} \\ \mathrm{-NH-CH_2-CH_2-OH} \\ \mathrm{-C_6H_4-O-CH_2-CH_2-OH} \\ \mathrm{-S-CH_2-CH_2-OH} \end{array}\right.$$

III. SPORICIDAL TESTS AND THEIR EVALUATION

A. Evaluation

A properly executed test for sporicidal activity should indicate whether a test agent kills a specified number of spores of pre-determined resistance in a specified time at a specific temperature. The resistance of spores is sometimes determined by exposure to constant boiling hydrochloric acid [Horwitz (*29*)]. Another method of determining resistance is via heat shocking of a sample, with subsequent dilution or concentration of the contaminating spore suspension as determined by plate counts [Pepper and Chandler (*41*)].

The exposure period should be exact. Unfortunately, many methods naturally allow the transfer of the test agent to the recovery media, thereby either extending the exposure time of a dilution of the test agent or initiating a condition of sporistasis that impedes the germination and growth of spores which may survive the specified contact period. Since it is the purpose of recovery media to promote growth of any surviving spores, every effort must be made to transfer as little of the agent to the medium as possible. Known neutralizers for test agents can be used to prevent sporistasis. A reasonable incubation period should be allowed and followed by testing for sporistasis by the inoculation of a minimal number of spores of the same species used. It would also be advisable to determine initially the sporicidal activity of agents without the use of carriers. Agents showing activity in such a test can be further tested by using a spore carrier which relates to the eventual use of the sporicide. Appropriate species should be employed depending upon the ultimate use of the sporicide. For example, *Clostridium tetani* and *Cl. welchii* could be used to test materials intended for hospital use.

One of the oldest test methods for determining antimicrobial activity is the phenol coefficient test, with its many variations. Essentially, this method involves inoculating both phenol and a test disinfectant with a known number of microorganisms and the subsequent transfer of loopfuls of this mixture into recovery media at specified time intervals. The transfer of microorganisms into recovery media also necessitates the transfer of chemicals which may be inhibitory to the growth of the injured spores. So-called microbial stasis tests usually involve the inoculation of tubes showing no growth with fresh spores of the same strain used in the test. This inoculation is likely to be larger in number than the viable survivor sample. It is also quite possible that the quantity of antimicrobial agent transferred to the medium may be static to the viable survivors, but not to the unexposed organisms used to determine whether the medium will support growth. Thus a test of this type may give false sporicidal values and stasis may not be indicated on the basis of growth support tests. Furthermore, in the event that actual sporicidal activity is present, the number of survivors diminishes with time and the possibility of picking up survivors in a standard loopful becomes increasingly less. If the sample size is increased to compensate for the decrease in viable survivors, this automatically increases the liklihood of sporistasis.

B. A.O.A.C. Method and Modifications

In another method [Ortenzio et al.(*38*)], silk suture loops were contaminated with acid-resistant spores, dried, and placed in test agents under standardized conditions to test their sporicidal effectiveness. Chemicals with microbiostatic properties tended to appear more effective than they actually were because of the amount of the antimicrobial agent adhering to the loop. It is also possible that chemosterilizers, which might not penetrate all parts of the loop, would appear ineffective in such a test even though these agents kill spores either in or on smooth surfaces. This test was designed to be rigorous in that it required a penetration of textile material, as well as sporicidal activity. Unfortunately, the introduction of static material into culture media is its chief weakness.

Recognizing the sporistatic properties of antimicrobial agents, Klarmann(*31*) modified the suture-loop method by suggesting the transfer of the loop from the original tube of medium into a second tube of medium containing 10% horse serum. This modification was a definite advance in assessing the effectiveness of sporicidal activity, since *Cl. sporogenes* spores, thought to be killed in two hours (as indicated by the original method), were found to survive eight hours. These results also point out defects in the usual tests for sporistasis. Such tests involve the introduction of a small number of unexposed spores (to the disinfectant) into the sporicidal menstruum showing no growth after the specified incubation period. If the spores germinate and grow, it is concluded that stasis does not exist. Although no stasis was found in tests of the suture-loop type without modification, it is obvious from Klarmann's findings that stasis actually did exist, but went undetected by the usual method. A further criticism of this test, is that it would not be applicable to hard surface objects. It should be noted that sutures themselves present a wide variability, depending on the choice of materials and how they are treated. Silk sutures may be silicone treated or have waxy outer coats which would contribute to great differences in results obtained in the test method. These can float on the surface and be incompletely exposed to the test solution.

Quisno et al.(*46*) used 0.07% lecithin and 0.5% Tween-80 in recovery media to elimate bacteriostatic effects caused by quaternary ammonium compounds, and Lawrence and Erlandson(*33*) used 1% Tween-80 to eliminate sporostasis. These media additives have been recognized by the Association of Official Agricultural Chemists [Horwitz(*29*)], although this same publication allows only the suture loop and the porcelain penicylinder to be used as spore carriers in sporicidal tests. This, too, places a limitation on the test as rubber, plastics, stainless steel, or other materials may be better spore carriers depending on the ultimate use for the test agent.

C. Membrane Filter Method

One of the simplest and most effective methods of evaluating sporicidal activity is the membrane filter method. Originally described by Portner et al.(*43*), and employed by Chandler et al.(*19*), and Pepper and Chandler(*41*), with modifications, this method involves the direct mixing of spores and chemosterilizer and the subsequent filtering of samples at various time intervals. The filter pads are washed with the chemosterilizer diluent (or solvent) to eliminate any trace of the chemical agent left on the filter pad. The filter pad containing the spores originally suspended in the test agent is then transferred to the growth medium. The advantages of this test method are the testing of known numbers of spores for viability and the complete elimination of the antimicrobial agent from the culture medium as a source of stasis.

Once an agent shows activity with the membrane filter test method, it can, then, be evaluated by some type of in-use test. It seems logical to use some object or carrier made of the same material as the object to be sterilized. Since surgical instruments are often the objects to be sterilized, it seems reasonable to use a stainless steel carrier for such a test. Thus, the tests employing suture loops and porcelain penicylinders are not adequate. Pepper and Chandler(*41*) used stainless steel penicylinders (8 × 10 mm) as carriers. Both aerobic (*B. subtilis* and *B. pumilus*) and anaerobic (*Cl. tetani* and *Cl. sporogenes*) heat-resistant (80°C for 15 minutes) spores were employed. Carriers were contaminated with various concentrations of spores and the numbers were determined by washing the cylinders and plating heat-shocked samples.

A solution of 8% formaldehyde and 0.5% hexachlorophene, in 70% isopropyl alcohol, was compared with an alkaline solution of 1% glutaraldehyde, in 70% isopropyl alcohol, for sporicidal activity in this method. It can be seen in Table 1 that the glutaraldehyde solution was the more effective agent. Test results also showed that with carriers contaminated with various concentrations of spores, the spores survived 5 and 6 hours in formaldehyde solution. However, when the formaldehyde solution was tested by the suture loop method, results indicated that sterility was achieved after two hours. As formaldehyde and hexachlorophene are considered sporistatic, this may account for the difference in results.

IV. FACTORS INVOLVED IN THE RESISTANCE AND DESTRUCTION OF SPORES

A. Heat

Heat is undoubtedly one of the most important factors employed in the destruction of spores. Both moist and dry heat are readily utilized for sporicidal action, with the former being the more effective agent for destroying both bacterial and fungal spores. Resistance of spores varies from species to species and within strains. According to Wilson and Miles(*60*), some strains of *B. subtilis* are rapidly destroyed, whereas others may withstand boiling for several hours. Anaerobic spores demonstrate a similar degree of resistance. Microbiologists are well aware that spores of *Cl. botulinum* can withstand boiling for several hours, whereas others, e.g., *Cl. welchii* may be destroyed in minutes. Although both methods are effective in spore destruction, Russell(*50*) has reported that there is not necessarily a correlation between resistance to moist and dry heat; *B. stearothermophilus*, for example, is highly resistant to moist heat, but not especially resistant to dry heat.

TABLE I

Sporicidal Activities of a Glutaraldehyde Solution[a]

Contaminated penicylinders[b]			Exposure, hr[c]													
			0		1		2		3		4		5		6	
Group[d,e]	Aerobes	Anaerobes	E	T	E	T	E	T	E	T	E	T	E	T	E	T
Glutaraldehyde solution																
I	380,000	210,000	+	+					−	−	−	+	−	−	+	−
II	2,100	3,000	+	+					+	+	−	−	−	−	−	−
III	570	510	+	+	−	+	+	+	−	−	−	−	−	−	−	−
IV	100	100	+	+	−	+	−	+	−	−	−	−	−	−	−	−
V	10–100	10–100	+	+	−	+	−	−	−	−	−	−	−	−	−	−
Formaldehyde (8%) solution																
I	380,000	210,000	+	+					+	+	+	+	+	+	+	+
II	2,100	3,000	+	+					+	+	+	+	+	+	+	+
III	570	510	+	+					+	+	+	+	−	+	−	+
IV	100	100	+	+					+	+	−	+	−	+	−	−
V	10–100	10–100	+	+					−	+	−	+	−	−	−	−

[a]1% glutaraldehyde, 0.3% $NaHCO_3$, 70% isopropanol) and an 8% formaldehyde solution (70% isopropyl alcohol and 0.5%hexachlorophene). Reprinted from Ref. *41*. courtesy of the American Society for Microbiology.

[b]Spore counts were estimated from heat-shocked samples and are shown as number of spores/cylinder.

[c]Symbols: + = growth; − = no growth; E = Eugonbroth; T = fluid thioglycollate medium.

[d]Groups I to V represent successive dilutions of spores (four species).

[e]Viable numbers of aerobic and anaerobic spores present ascertained by heat shock are shown in appropriate columns.

Bowie(*13*), in discussing the problems involved in heat sterilization, states that in order to kill the microorganisms which contaminate equipment it is essential to have adequate contact between the microorganisms and steam or aqueous solution, at the selected temperature. To achieve sterility, Shotton(*51*) claimed that proper packing of containers in the autoclave is necessary and the location of vent holes or the use of porous materials as wrappers are of paramount importance. The adequacy and reliability of heat sterilization may be further reduced by an overloading of the sterilizing units, the lack of adequate controls, defects in the equipment, or improper operation of the units. This is not to say that heat as a method of sterilization is inadequate, but rather to caution that various conditions must be satisfied before sterilization can be accomplished.

Just as moisture is an important factor in the destruction of spores, the opposite situation may prevail where a low moisture content may aid in their survival. Bullock and Keepe(*16*), in examining bacterial survival in low moisture systems, showed that *B. subtilis* spores remained viable in oils, fats, and liquid paraffin for over 2 years. Bullock and Tallentire(*17*), in studying the relationship of moisture and heat resistance, found that below a designated moisture content spores remained viable and heat resistant, whereas the spores lost their heat resistance and retained their viability above a certain range of moisture uptake. Spores contained in dry products, such as peptone powder, remained viable and heat resistant for long periods of time. Bruch et al. (*15*), in determining the effects of chemical and physical factors on dry heat sterilization, showed that neither a vacuum nor the entrapment of spores in nonaqueous liquids increased the time required for sterilization. The entrapment of spores in certain solids did, however, increase this time. These factors must, then, be studied in detail to assure spore destruction.

B. Irradiation

In a series of studies to determine the effects of radiation on microorganisms conducted by various investigators [Koh et al.(*32*), Bridges et al.(*14*), and Pepper et al.(*40*)], bacterial spores were shown to be most resistant to cathode rays. These findings were in agreement with Bellamy and Lawton(*6*), who also demonstrated the high degree of resistance of bacterial spores. In spite of this, sterilization can be accomplished when sufficient dosages are employed.

The two main sources of irradiation in use today are the microwave linear accelerator and cobalt 60. Artandi and Van Winkle(*3*) discussed the efficacy of the electron beam as a means of sterilization of surgical products, whereas Van Winkle, Borick, and Fogarty(*57*) showed the destructive effects of cobalt 60 irradiation on resistant microorganisms on sutures.

In the destruction of spores by irradiation, as in destruction by heat sterilization, various factors must be considered. Edwards et al.(*25*) found that neither pH nor salt concentration had any effect on the lethality of rays in sterilization. The same author reported that the temperature of the suspending medium had a marked influence on the per cent of spores surviving radiation; exposure to rays at elevated temperatures decreased the kill, at low temperatures it increased the kill. Woese(*61*) reported that higher temperatures enhanced the rate of bacterial inactivation. A logarithmic relationship was shown to exist between the numbers of microorganisms present and the dosage required to achieve complete kill.

The presence of protein provides some protection to the spores and will contribute to their survival. Borick and Fogarty(*12*) reported that *B. pumilus* spores, irradiated in a growth-promoting medium, survived a dose of 2.5 Mr, whereas no survivors were obtained under similar conditions when cellulose materials were employed. Vintner(*58*) contends that certain substances may act as protective agents. He found that an increase in resistance to radiation during sporulation of *B. cereus* parallels an increase of cystine-rich compounds, which offer protection to irradiation.

Apparently, the interruption of radiation cycles does not influence sterilization if growth-promoting properties are not present. Interrupted dosimetry tests, performed with different type materials in our laboratories, showed that various spore types were destroyed when radiation doses were given in two separate exposures, with differing periods of interruption. It should be noted that the presence of suitable conditions for growth could make sterilization more difficult or, perhaps, impossible to achieve.

The resistance of different species of bacterial spores to irradiation will vary as will resistance within a species. A strain of *B. pumilus* is used routinely by us in irradiation work because it shows a high degree of resistance. A less resistant strain of *B. pumilus* is also employed for experimental work. To date, sporeformers resistant to complete destruction by irradiation have not been reported. Whether mutants which are completely radiation resistant can occur is questionable. It would appear that increased doses of radiation would result in destruction of even the most highly resistant species.

Although radiation is now employed throughout the world in medical and food areas, Jefferson (*30*), in comparing heat and radiation sterilization, recommends that the user recognize the inactivation factors which are currently obtained with autoclaving procedures before deciding on an inactivation factor for radiation sterilization. This would assure safer processes and help overcome limitations inherent in presently employed routine sterility tests.

Artandi (*2*), in comparing the advantages of radiation sterilization over autoclaving or gaseous sterilization, pointed out that materials sterilized by irradiation can be run in a continuous process past the irradiating source, whereas other methods require a batch-type operation. For all three methods the type of kill was characterized as a first-order reaction; the effect needed for a tenfold reduction of the concentration of microorganisms was the same regardless of initial concentration. The process selected is dependent on the type of operation to be performed. All three processes are effective in sterilization, but all have their limitations in such areas as inaccessibility of the material to be sterilized, excessive drying, protective coatings, or other factors which influence spore destruction.

C. Chemicals

A good deal of controversy prevails regarding the use of chemosterilizers, and there are many problems inherant in the method. Some of the older workers in this field do not accept the widespread use of chemical agents as sterilizers and advocate their use only as disinfectants. In defining criteria for compounds to be used in this area, Borick (*9*) declared that, in addition to a wide microbiological spectrum, an antimicrobial agent must show sporicidal activity before it can qualify as a chemosterilizer. Granted, that sterilization can be effected by many agents where only vegetative cells are present, a sporicidal agent must be employed where the microbial population is unknown, if sterilization is to be assured.

The general use of chemicals in the United States as chemosterilizers lies within the jurisdiction of the United States Department of Agriculture and all products which make germicidal label claims are covered under the Federal Insecticide, Fungicide, and Rodenticide Act. To date, this agency has restricted this usage to a gaseous agent, ethylene oxide and a liquid aqueous solution, glutaraldehyde. Although now widely used for sterilization, they are relative newcomers to the field and criteria for their employment are still being defined. As noted earlier, many factors must be considered when spore destruction is to be achieved by chemical means. These include temperature, pressure, humidity, gas concentration, the nature and type of product, the variety of spore, and concentration. These problems have been reviewed by Borick(*10*). The action and selection of other sporicidal agents cannot be considered without a regard for other criteria, for here, too, action is dependent on a knowledge of the chemical agent and its intended use. No single method is available to define the selection of a test agent for general use. It is, then, necessary to consider the intent and to evaluate the sporicidal agent in terms which may be extrapolated to an actual in-use situation.

Time and concentration are two major factors involved in sterilization by chemicals. However, if an antimicrobial agent does not have sporicidal activity, neither a high concentration nor an extended period of time will result in spore destruction. Although pH is not a factor in radiation sterilization, and has little effect on heat sterilization, it is an extremely important criterion in the employment of chemical agents. Borick and Dondershine(*11*) showed that glutaraldehyde was a more effective sporicide when used in alkaline solution, and Rubbo and Gardner(*49*) showed that, in addition to the above, this chemosterilizer was effective over a wide range of pH.

Formaldehyde is, according to Willard and Alexander(*59*), one of the oldest chemosterilizers employed for the destruction of spores, and, although 1% to 2% solutions have been used, a relatively long period of time (24 hours) is required to destroy *B. subtilis var. niger*, spores. A much shorter time for destruction of spore was indicated by Spaulding(*53*) with a concentration as high as 8% formaldehyde. Lower concentrations of glutaraldehyde solutions are required for sporicidal activity as compared to formaldehyde solutions; however, formaldehyde vapor is more effective for germicidal activity than glutaraldehyde vapor. The novice, in selecting an agent for destruction of spores cannot conclude that biological activity in one physical state is the same as in another.

Chemicals which have a long and effective history as disinfectants for vegetative cells, may not be sporicidal. Alcohol, phenolics, and quaternaries, for example, are widely used as germicides, but they are not effective against spores unless they are used in conjunction with heat and/or other chemicals. Alcohol is widely used as a solvent for other antimicrobials and, when utilized with formaldehyde, glutaraldehyde, or iodine will exhibit sporicidal activity. Activity here is based on the antimicrobial agent, and not on the alcohol, although the solvent obviously aids in chemical transport to the spore site. Quaternaries, too, when used in conjunction with other antimicrobials, act by lowering the surface tension and their wetting action enhances the activity of the disinfecting chemical. Potent chemical agents, may not destroy spores. The use of strong acids or alkalis would be expected to result in rapid destruction of most biological specimens. Spores, however, were reported by Borick(*10*) to survive a 1-hr exposure to either 2.5 *N* HCl or NaOH. From the foregoing, the high degree of resistance which one may encounter in either aerobic or anaerobic bacterial spores is readily seen.

As might be expected, spores embedded in a crystalline matrix, or some other protective material, would be more dificult to destroy by chemical means than by either heat or irradiation. This is not to imply that the end result would not be the same, but rather that one must realize, in choosing this method of killing spores, that the obstacles may be difficult or practically impossible to overcome. A protective barrier in the form of an overwrap may be impermeable to either liquid or gaseous material, thus, the agent could never reach the spore site. Other methods of sterilization may have limitations, too. Allen and Soike(*1*), advocated the use of the electrohydraulic treatment for the sterilization of various materials and showed that this process was restricted to liquid solutions. Chemical alteration of the spore was necessary, in a combined liquid-physical treatment, to effect sterilization.

Although an attempt has been made to warn of the difficulties which may be encountered in spore destruction by the use of chemosterilizers, this is not to imply that sterilization by chemical means is not without merit. As a matter of fact, our personal experience in the field of sterilization would indicate that this method can be just as effective as other available means, when sufficient knowledge regarding its use is at hand. There are occasions when it can be used more readily, or it may be the only method available for the desired result. The individual must be aware of the circumstances involving its use and must decide which method best suits the situation.

REFERENCES

1. M. Allen and K. Soike, *Science*, **154**, 155 (1966).
2. C. Artandi, *Proc. Conf. on Disposable Sterile Medical Products, Health Indust. Assoc. and USFDA*, 1967 pp. 55–62.
3. C. Artandi and W. Van Winkle, *Nucleonics*, **17**, 86 (1959).
4. W. C. Awe, W. Roberts, and N. S. Braunwald, *Surgery*, **54**, 322 (1963).
5. J. A. Bach and H. L. Sadoff, *J. Bacteriol.*, **83**, 699 (1962).
6. W. C. Bellamy and E. J. Lawton, *Nucleonics*, **12**, 54 (1954).
7. S. H. Black and P. Gerhardt, *J. Bacteriol.*, **83**, 960 (1962).
8. P. M. Borick, *Biotechnol. Bioeng.*, **7**, 435 (1965).
9. P. M. Borick, Division of Microbial Chemistry and Technology, 148th Meeting, American Chemical Society, Chicago, Ill., 1964.
10. P. M. Borick, *Advan. Appl. Microbiol.*, (1968) **10**, 291.
11. P. M. Borick and F. H. Dondershine, *J. Pharm. Sci.*, **53**, 1223 (1964).
12. P. M. Borick and M. G. Fogarty, *Appl. Microbiol.*, **15**, 785 (1967).
13. J. H. Bowie *Symposium on Recent Developments in the Sterilization of Surgical Materials*, Pharmaceutical Press, London, 1961. pp. 109–142.
14. A. E. Bridges, J. P. Olivo, and V. L. Chandler, *Appl. Microbiol.*, **4**, 147 (1956).
15. C. W. Bruch, M. G. Koesterer, and M. K. Bruch, *Develop. Ind. Microbiol.*, **4**, 334 (1963).
16. K. Bullock and W. G. Keepe, *J. Pharm. Pharmacol.*, **3**, 717 (1951).
17. K. Bullock and A. Tallentire, *J. Pharm. Pharmacol.*, **4**, 917 (1952).
18. B. Carroll, J. Keosian, and I. O. Steinman, *J. Newark Beth Israel Hosp.*, **6**, 1 (1955).
19. V. L. Chandler, R. E. Pepper, and L. E. Gordon, *J. Am. Pharm. Assoc. Sci. Ed.*, **46**, 124 (1957).
20. L. N. Christiansen, J. Deffner, E. M. Foster, and H. Sugiyama, *Appl. Microbiol.*, **16**, 133 (1968).
21. B. D. Church and H. Halvorson, *Nature*, **183**, 124 (1959).
22. R. E. Collier and N. M. Nakata, *Bacteriol. Proc.*, G55 (1958).
23. H R. Curran, *Bacteriol. Rev.*, **16**, 111 (1952).
24. R. Doi, H. Halvorson, and B. Church, *J. Bacteriol.*, 77, 43 (1959).
25. R. B. Edwards, L. J. Peterson, and D. G. Cummings, *Food Technol.*, 6, 284 (1954).
26. C. A. Friedman and B. S. Henry, *J. Bacteriol.*, **36**, 99 (1954).
27. H. Halvorson, *Spores II*, Burgess, Minneapolis, 1961.
28. W. A. Hardwick and J. W. Foster, *J. Bacteriol.*, **65**, 355 (1953).
29. W. Horwitz, *Official Methods of Analysis of the Association of Official Agriculture Chemists*, 10th ed., Association of Official Agriculture Chemists, Washington, D.C., 1965.
30. S. Jefferson, in *Massive Radiation Technique*, Newnes, London, 1964, pp. 61–96.
31. E. G. Klarmann, *Am. J. Pharm.*, **128**, 4 (1956).
32. W. Y. Koh, C. T. Morehouse, and V. L. Chandler, *Appl. Microbiol.*, **4**, 143 (1956).
33. C. A. Lawrence and A. L. Erlandson, Jr., *J. Am. Pharm. Assoc. Sci. Ed.*, **42**, 352 (1953).
34. A. G. Marr, in *The Bacteria*, (I. C. Gunsalus and R. Y. Stanier, eds.), Vol. 1, Academic Press, New York, 1960.
35. C. C. Moore and R. B. Hardwick, *Mfg. Chemist*, **27**, 305 (1956).
36. W. G. Murrell and W. Scott, *Nature*, **179**, (1957).

37. E. L. Oginsky and W. W. Umbreit, in *An Introduction to Bacterial Physiology*, 2nd ed., W. H. Freeman and Co., San Francisco, 1959.
38. L. F. Ortenzio, L. S. Stuart, and J. L. Friedl, *J. Assoc. Offic. Agri. Chemists*, **36**, 480 (1953).
39. R. C. Page and P. M. Borick, *Arch. Surg.*, **94**, 162 (1967).
40. R. E. Pepper, N. T. Buffa, and V. L. Chandler, *Appl. Microbiol.*, **4**. 149 (1956).
41. R. E. Pepper and V. L. Chandler, *Appl. Microbiol.*, **11**, 383 (1963).
42. C. S. Phillips, *Bacteriol. Rev.*, **16**, 135 (1952).
43. D. M. Portner, E. Mayo, and S. Kaye, *Bacteriol. Proc.*, 1954 p. 35.
44. J. F. Powell, *Biochem. J.*, 53, 210 (1953).
45. J. F. Powell and R. E. Strange, *Biochem. J.*, **63**, 661 (1956).
46. R. Quisno, I. W. Gibby, and M. J. Foter, *Am. J. Pharm.*, **118**, 320 (1946).
47. C. F. Robinow, in *The Bacteria* (I. C. Gunsalus and R. Y. Stanier, eds.), Vol. 1, Academic Press, New York, 1960.
48. K. F. A. Ross and E. Billing, *J. Gen. Microbiol.*, **16**, 418 (1957).
49. S. Rubbo and J. S. Gardner, in *A Review of Sterilization and Disinfection*, Lloyd-Luke, London, 1965, p. 224.
50. A. D. Russell, *Mfg. Chemist Aerosol News*, **36**, 38 (1965).
51. E. Shotton, in *Symposium on Recent Developments in the Sterilization of Surgical Materials,* The Pharmaceutical Press, London, 1961. pp. 1–6.
52. R. Slepecky and J. W. Foster, *J. Bacteriol.*, **78**, 117 (1959).
53. E. H. Spaulding, *Assoc. Operating Room Nurses J.*, 1, 36 (1963).
54. R. L. Stedman, *Am. J. Pharm.*, **128**, 84, 114 (1956).
55. H. Sugiyama, *J. Bacteriol.*, **62**, 81 (1951).
56. A. S. Sussmann and H. O. Halvorson, *Spores, Their Dormancy and Germination*, Harper & Row, New York, 1966.
57. W. Van Winkle, P. M. Borick, and M. G. Fogarty, *Proc. Intern. Conf. Sterilization of Medical Products, IAEA, Budapest, Hungary, 1967*, pp. 169–180.
58. V. Vintner, *Nature*, **189**, 589 (1961).
59. M. Willard and A. Alexander, *Appl. Microbiol.*, **12**, 229 (1964).
60. G. S. Wilson and A. A. Miles, *Topley and Wilson's Principles of Bacteriology and Immunology*, 5th ed., Vol. 1, Williams & Wilkins, Baltimore, 1957.
61. C. R. Woese, *J. Bacteriol.*, **75**, 5 (1958).

Author Citation Index

Subject Index